Clinical Reasoning and Decision-Making in Physical Therapy:

Facilitation, Assessment, and Implementation

Clinical Reasoning and Decision-Making in Physical Therapy:

Facilitation, Assessment, and Implementation

Edited by

GINA MARIA MUSOLINO, PT, DPT, MSED, EDD
Founding Program Director and Clinical Professor
Doctor of Physical Therapy Program
Department of Kinesiology & Community Health
College of Applied Health Sciences
The University of Illinois at Urbana—Champaign
Champaign, Illinois

GAIL M. JENSEN, PT, PHD, FAPTA, FNAP
Catherine Worthingham Fellow of the American Physical Therapy Association
Fellow of the National Academies of Practice
Dean, Graduate School and Vice Provost, Learning and Assessment
Professor of Physical Therapy and Faculty Associate
Center for Health Policy and Ethics
Creighton University
Omaha, Nebraska

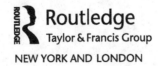

Routledge
Taylor & Francis Group

NEW YORK AND LONDON

Cover Artist: Lori Shields

First published in 2020 by SLACK Incorporated

Published in 2024 by Routledge
605 Third Avenue, New York, NY 10158

and by Routledge
4 Park Square, Milton Park, Abingdon, Oxon, OX14 4RN

Routledge is an imprint of the Taylor & Francis Group, an informa business

© 2020 Taylor & Francis Group

Library of Congress Control Number: 2019943696

ISBN:9781630914080(hbk)
ISBN:9781003523130(ebk)

DOI: 10.4324/9781003523130

Dedication

To our beloved families and friends, both professional and personal, thank you for providing tireless support for us to be able to dedicate ourselves to enriching the lives of others.

To our coauthors for persisting in the problem-solving process and making a difference through your undaunting explorations of clinical reasoning and decision-making and being brave enough to share your impressions, successes, and challenges to enhance movement and restore function.

To my coeditor, Gail M. Jensen, PT, PhD, FAPTA, FNAP, I am forever appreciative for your willingness to join the project and lend your insights in the midst of your many commitments to the profession.

To our patients and clients, we are grateful for the opportunities to collaborate with you to promote your strength, adaptability, and function. We appreciate you entrusting your care with physical therapists and your willingness to trust in yourselves, be courageous, and to believe in the possible to determine your maximum outcomes.

To our novice, former selves, may we always stay curious for the sake of our patients and clients. May we always strive to do better in service to society and be comfortable with not knowing. May we not get too hung up on fixed definitions of what any reality or life may or may not be … remaining open to the possibilities.

May we willingly forge pivotal conversations with our colleagues and those we mentor, being receptive to critically reflective feedback. May we be open to examining our curiosity, while having faith in the human spirit for the potentials that can be accomplished.

CONTENTS

ACKNOWLEDGMENTS

The initiation of a first edition of *Clinical Reasoning and Decision-Making in Physical Therapy: Facilitation, Assessment, and Implementation* is no small undertaking and was conceived as I began to study the learning outcomes of students in clinical education and noted the need to progress clinical reasoning (CR) for our doctoring profession. While serving as president of the American Physical Therapy Association Academy of Physical Therapy Education, we brought together a group of dedicated colleagues for a successful inaugural symposium focused on CR in physical therapy. The symposium was hosted by Creighton University, and many of the chapter contributors engaged for the summer with in-depth exploration of CR during 3 steamy days in Omaha, Nebraska. Our keynote speaker at that conference, Steven Durning, MD, PhD, internationally known expert in medical education research and CR, shared important insights into the teaching/learning and assessment of CR. He has continued to graciously and generously share his talent and time with our profession including a chapter in this text.

Prior to the CR symposium, well over 4 years ago, at a lunch meeting on a strikingly beautiful day in the desert mountains of Phoenix, Arizona, I shared with Tony Schiavo, Senior Acquisition Editor, the concept of the CR text. As always, he listened intently, encouraged an outline, floated the idea, and then we developed it into a full-fledged proposal. This is my second adventure in the publishing process with Tony and SLACK Incorporated and first endeavor for a first edition text. As we dedicated time and effort to bringing this text to fruition, I shared many other book concepts and potential authors for the continued progression of our profession. Tony was receptive to most and always interested in learning more. Tony keenly follows up on opportunities, has a strong sense of the profession, and remains highly professional and dedicated to the process, as a guide on the side with a strong moral compass. Tony was always prepared to chat when we encountered hurdles and offered viable solutions in addition to ensuring equity. Thank you, Tony, for providing the platform, following through, and being a stable support in the editorial process from start to finish! As a dedicated husband and father of 6 children, predominantly in teen-spirit mode, Tony's ability to multitask remains admirable!

Additionally, I have had the pleasure to share some delightful time with both Stephanie Arasim Portnoy, Senior Vice President, and Michelle Gatt, Vice President of Marketing. Both are lovely people that are at the pulse of the industry ensuring that health care publications are widely disseminated and timely distributed.

Sincerest appreciation goes to Allegra Tiver, Managing Editor, and Lori Shields, Cover Artist. Allegra and Lori amazingly took our written articulation of ideas and verbal concepts for the cover design and created a beautiful piece of art. The vibrant cover readily captures the often-changing, often-challenging, mosaic puzzle of CR and clinical problem-solving for human movement, while illustrating our collaborative works with our patients and clients for clinical decision-making.

Deepest gratitude is owed to Jennifer Cahill, Senior Project Editor, for doing the deep dive with attention to all the important details. Jenn remained patient with the process, ensured timely turn-arounds with a multiplicity of authors, and followed up precisely on any and all concerns. Jenn is an exceedingly steadfast professional who is a quick study of material and readily grasps intent, while providing manageable and effective solutions through the often-tedious copyedit process. Jenn never hesitated to ask a probing question or raise a point not considered. As a dedicated mother of teen twins, who are interested in the profession, we hope this text makes a difference in their preferred futures; it remains bright!

To our 39 coauthors, we are grateful for your dedicated contributions to this first edition. We hope that this work encourages continued pursuit of this line of inquiry and exploration, and we trust that others will come forward to join in for future works. To the initial 39, thank you for your time and efforts!

Our sincerest thanks to our esteemed colleague, Edelle (Edee) Field-Fote, PT, PhD, FAPTA, who took time from her dedicated research for spinal cord injury to read and review the first edition and provide meaningful insights in the Foreword. Dr. Field-Fote remains highly devoted to the profession. For more than 20 years, her studies have focused on the development of interventions to promote neuroplasticity and the use of adjuvant strategies to maximize the benefits of rehabilitation for improved function in persons with spinal cord injury. We are honored and blessed with her impressions.

Special thanks to the following individuals for your belief in the scholarship of teaching and learning for physical therapy: Nicholas Burd, PhD; Nicole Christensen, PT, PhD, MAppSc; Chad Cook, PT, PhD, MBA, FAPTA, FAAOMPT; Sonia J. Crandall, PhD, MS; Jeannette Elliott, PT; Thomas Elwood, DrPH; Cheryl Hanley-Maxwell, PhD; Sherril H. Hayes, PT, PhD; Joy Higgs, AM, PhD, MHPEd, BSc, PFHEA; Sara F. Maher, PT, DScPT, OMPT; Marilyn Moffatt, PT, PhD, FAPTA, CSCS, CEAAA; Michael Mueller, PT, PhD, FAPTA; Adam David Musolino, MA; Reneé Frances Musolino-Blattner, MSEd; Catherine Page, PT, MPH, PHD; William (Sandy) Quillen, PT, DPT, PhD, FACSM; Kathleen Rockefeller, PT, ScD; Mary Rogers, PT, PhD, FAPTA, FASB, FISB; Katherine Shepard, PT, PhD, FAPTA; Lee Shulman, PhD; Jacob Sosnoff, PhD; Alecia Thiele, PT, DPT, MSEd, ATC, LAT, DCE; Kenneth Wilund, PhD; and Amelia Mays Woods, PhD. Your leadership, influence, dedication, and friendship remain abundant and far-reaching—keep making a difference!

ABOUT THE EDITORS

Gina Maria Musolino, PT, DPT, MSEd, EdD, is Founding Program Director and Clinical Professor, Doctor of Physical Therapy Program with the Department of Kinesiology & Community Health, College of Applied Health Sciences, The University of Illinois at Urbana–Champaign, Champaign, Illinois. She received her BS in Physical Therapy from Washington University School of Medicine (WUMS PT) Program in Physical Therapy (St. Louis, Missouri); her MSEd from Southwest Baptist University (Bolivar, Missouri); her EdD with specialization in Curriculum Design, Development and Evaluation from Nova Southeastern University (NSU), Fischler College of Education (Ft. Lauderdale, Florida); and her post-professional Doctor of Physical Therapy (DPT) degree from Utica College (Utica, New York). Dr. Musolino has over 25 years as a physical therapy educator, director of clinical education, expert, and educational consultant.

Dr. Musolino was honored with the prestigious American Physical Therapy Association (APTA) Lucy Blair National Service Award (2012) for service of Exceptional Value to the Association. Dr. Musolino's published works focus on the scholarship of teaching and learning with focused explorations of professionalism, service learning, cultural competence, clinical reasoning, health policy leadership, and clinical education. Dr. Musolino has been awarded many grants and fellowships from numerous organizations in support of her research. She received the Beatrice F. Schulz Award for Outstanding Clinical Achievement, WUMS PT; the Southeast Region Division Clinical Practice Center of the Month and Outstanding Customer Service Awards as a clinical administrator with Rehability Corporation (Florida); the Research Excellence Award from the NSU, Fischler College for her dissertation works; the Award of Merit in Technology Delivered Instruction from the Utah System of Higher Education, Utah Electronic College Consortium (Salt Lake City, Utah) for her instructional design and development of online education courses; the Feitelberg Journal Founder's Award, APTA Academy of Physical Therapy Education (APTE), *Journal of Physical Therapy Education*, acknowledging excellence in publication by a first-time author for the research article "Enhancing Diversity Through Mentorship: The Nurturing Potential of Service Learning"; and the Alumnae Award (WUMS PT). She was also co-recipient of Outstanding Abstract with her colleagues by the APTA Annual Conference Program Committee for the abstract "Physical Therapist Tests and Measures for a Patient with Parkinson's Disease for Consultation With Referring Neurosurgeon."

Dr. Musolino has served on several voluntary boards in support of the health professions. She was elected for 12 years of Board leadership with the APTA APTE (formerly Education Section), two 4-year terms each as President, Vice-President, and Director-at-Large for Promotion. She led the voluntary APTA APTE Board of Directors (BOD) in transitioning to Academy status, collaborated with the Education Leadership Partnership as a founding member, with continuous component membership growth over 12 years. During her leadership, several new projects were initiated, a well-received clinical reasoning symposium, a successful mid-career faculty development workshop for educators, a robust social media presence, renewed website enhancements, expansions to 6 special interest groups, a major bylaw revision, increased funding opportunities for educational research, and translating the *Journal of Physical Therapy Education* from self-published to a full-fledged scholarly publication. Dr. Musolino served on the *Journal of Physical Therapy Education* member editorial BOD for 6 years and currently continues as peer reviewer.

Dr. Musolino is senior reviewer for the preeminent APTA *Physical Therapy Journal* (PTJ). Dr. Musolino previously served 2 BOD terms as Director of Scholarship for the APTA Health Policy and Administration Section—The Catalyst. Dr. Musolino has also served the APTA Florida Physical Therapy Association (FPTA) BOD as At-Large Director for 2 years and Chief Delegate for 4 years (2 elected terms) and elected delegate for 5 additional years. She was also previously Vice-Chair of the FPTA Southwest District. Dr. Musolino formerly chaired the APTA Academy of Neurologic Physical Therapy, Advocacy and Consumer Affairs Committee, for 6 years, serving as Federal Affairs Liaison to Congressional leaders and Key Contact for Florida Representatives. Dr. Musolino is an APTA Credentialed Clinical Instructor for both the APTA Level 1 and Level 2 Credentialed Clinical Instructor Programs, educating clinical instructors and health care professionals throughout the nation. Dr. Musolino also serves on the editorial board for the Association of Schools of Allied Health Professionals, *Journal of Allied Health*. Dr. Musolino is coauthor/author of chapters in *Clinical Education in Physical Therapy: The Evolution From Student to Clinical Instructor and Beyond* (2019) and *Finding Meaning in Civically Engaged Scholarship: Personal Journeys, Professional Experiences* (2009). Dr. Musolino is coeditor/author with esteemed colleague Carol M. Davis, PT, DPT, EdD, MS, FAPTA, of the bestseller *Patient Practitioner Interaction: An Experiential Manual for Developing the Art of Health Care, Sixth Edition* (2016), published by SLACK Incorporated.

Gail M. Jensen, PT, PhD, FAPTA, FNAP, is Dean, Graduate School and College of Professional Studies and Vice Provost for Learning and Assessment, Professor of Physical Therapy, and Faculty Associate for Center of Health Policy and Ethics at Creighton University in Omaha, Nebraska. She holds a BS in Education from the University of Minnesota, MA in physical therapy, and a PhD in educational evaluation both from Stanford University. Dr. Jensen served as principal investigator for the research on Physical Therapist Education for the Twenty First Century (PTE-21): Innovation and Excellence in Physical Therapist Academic and Clinical Education, that is the focus a 2019 SLACK Incorporated publication, *Educating Physical Therapists*. Dr. Jensen is a qualitative researcher well known for her scholarly publications related to expert practice, clinical reasoning, professional ethics, educational theory, and interprofessional education and practice. During her career she has held faculty appointments at Stanford University, Temple University, The University of Alabama at Birmingham, and Samuel Merritt University, and she was a part of the founding faculty of the first clinical doctoral program in physical therapy at Creighton University. She has coauthored/edited several books, including the Third Edition of *Handbook of Teaching for Physical Therapists*; *Leadership in Interprofessional Health Education and Practice*; *Realising Exemplary Practice-Based Education*; *Expertise in Physical Therapy Practice, Second Edition*; *Educating for Moral Action: A Sourcebook in Health and Rehabilitation Ethics*; and most recently, *Clinical Reasoning in the Health Professions, Fourth Edition*. Dr. Jensen is a Catherine Worthingham Fellow of the American Physical Therapy Association (APTA) and a fellow in the Physical Therapy Academy of the National Academies of Practice. In 2018, she received the Nicholas A. Cummings Award from the National Academies of Practice for extraordinary contributions to interprofessional health care. She is a recipient of the APTA's Rothstein Golden Pen Award and Lucy Blair Service Award, and she was the APTA's 2011 Mary McMillan Lecturer.

CONTRIBUTING AUTHORS

Heather Atkinson, PT, DPT, NCS (Chapter 10)
Board-Certified Clinical Specialist in Neurologic Physical Therapy
Center for Rehabilitation
The Children's Hospital of Philadelphia
Philadelphia, Pennsylvania

Andrew S. Bartlett, PT, PhD, MPA (Chapter 24)
Associate Professor in Physical Therapy
Nazareth College
Rochester, New York

Betsy J. Becker, PT, DPT, PhD (Chapters 26 and 27)
Associate Professor and Program Director
Division of Physical Therapy Education
College of Allied Health Professions
University of Nebraska Medical Center
Omaha, Nebraska

Lisa Black, PT, DPT (Chapters 15 and 16)
Associate Professor and Director of Clinical Education
Department of Physical Therapy
Creighton University
Omaha, Nebraska

Anita S. Campbell, PT, MPT, NCS, ATP (Chapter 22)
Board-Certified Clinical Specialist in Neurologic Physical Therapy
Assistant Teaching Professor
Department of Physical Therapy
School of Health Professions
University of Missouri
Columbia, Missouri

Nicole Christensen, PT, PhD, MAppSc (Chapters 4, 15, and 16)
Professor and Chair
Department of Physical Therapy
Samuel Merritt University
Oakland, California

N. Beth Collier, PT, DPT, OCS, FAAOMPT (Chapter 21)
Board-Certified Clinical Specialist in Orthopaedic Physical Therapy
Fellow of the American Academy of Orthopaedic Manual Physical Therapists
Clinical Assistant Professor
Department of Physical Therapy
Mercer University
Atlanta, Georgia

Chad E. Cook, PT, PhD, MBA, FAPTA, FAAOMPT (Chapter 13)
Catherine Worthingham Fellow of American Physical Therapy Association
Fellow of the American Academy of Orthopaedic Manual Physical Therapists
Program Director
Professor
Vice Chief of Research
Division of Physical Therapy
Duke University
Durham, North Carolina

Kyle Covington, PT, DPT, PhD (Chapters 6 and 13)
Associate Professor
Director of Assessment and Evaluation
Doctor of Physical Therapy Division
Duke University School of Medicine
Durham, North Carolina

Clare Delany, PhD, MHlth & MedLaw, MPhysio, BApp Sc (Physio) (Chapter 5)
Professor
Health Professions Education
Department of Medical Education
Melbourne Medical School
University of Melbourne
Children's Bioethics Centre
Royal Children's Hospital
Melbourne, Australia

Steven J. Durning, MD, PhD (Chapter 2)
Professor of Medicine and Pathology
Director of Graduate Programs in Health Professions Education
Uniformed Services University
Bethesda, Maryland

Ian Edwards, PhD, Grad Dip PT, BApp Sc (Physio) (Chapter 5)
South Australia

Wing Fu, PT, PhD, MA (Chapters 11 and 12)
Assistant Professor
Programs in Physical Therapy
Department of Rehabilitation and Regenerative Medicine
Columbia University
New York, New York

Jennifer Furze, PT, DPT, PCS (Chapter 16)
Board-Certified Clinical Specialist in Pediatric Physical Therapy
Associate Professor and Vice Chair
Pediatric Residency Program Coordinator
Department of Physical Therapy
Creighton University
Omaha, Nebraska

Margaret M. Gebhardt, PT, DPT, OCS, FAAOMPT (Chapter 21)
Board-Certified Clinical Specialist in Orthopaedic Physical Therapy
Fellow of the American Academy of Orthopaedic Manual Physical Therapists
Adjunct Clinical Instructor
Department of Physical Therapy
Mercer University
Physical Therapist
Fit Core Physical Therapist
Atlanta, Georgia
Dry Needling Instructor—Myopain Seminars

Sarah Gilliland, PT, DPT, PhD, CSCS (Chapters 8 and 9)
Certified Strength and Conditioning Coach
Associate Professor of Physical Therapy
West Coast University
Los Angeles, California

Gregory W. Hartley, PT, DPT, GCS, FNAP (Chapter 25)
Board-Certified Clinical Specialist in Geriatric Physical Therapy
Fellow of the National Academies of Practice
Assistant Professor of Clinical Physical Therapy
Department of Physical Therapy
University of Miami Miller School of Medicine
Coral Gables, Florida

Karen Huhn, PT, PhD (Chapters 17 and 18)
Associate Professor and Chair
School of Physical Therapy
Husson University
Bangor, Maine

A. Daniel Johnson, PhD (Chapter 24)
Teaching Professor
Department of Biology
Wake Forest University
Winston Salem, North Carolina

Daryl Lawson, PT, DSc (Chapter 23)
Associate Professor
Doctor of Physical Therapy Program
Department of Physical Therapy
College of Health and Human Services
Western Michigan University
Kalamazoo, Michigan

Alan Chong W. Lee, PT, PhD, DPT, CWS, GCS (Chapter 23)
Certified Wound Specialist
Board-Certified Clinical Specialist in Geriatric Physical Therapy
Professor
Mount Saint Mary's University, Los Angeles
Los Angeles, California

Theresa Najjar, PT, DPT, NCS, MS (Chapter 29)
Board-Certified Clinical Specialist in Neurologic Physical Therapy
Clinical Instructor
Kaiser Permanente Neurologic Physical Therapy Residency Program
Redwood City, California
Owner/CEO
Synaptic Physical Therapy, Inc
Sunnyvale, California

Peggy DeCelle Newman, PT, MHR (Chapters 19 and 20)
Academic Coordinator of Clinical Education
Professor
Physical Therapy Assistant Program
Division of Health Professions
Oklahoma City Community College
Oklahoma City, Oklahoma

Kim Nixon-Cave, PT, PhD, PCS, FAPTA (Chapter 10)
Board-Certified Clinical Specialist in Pediatric Physical Therapy
Catherine Worthingham Fellow of American Physical Therapy Association
Associate Professor and DPT Program Director
Program Director for Post-Professional Programs
College of Rehabilitation Sciences
Thomas Jefferson University
Philadelphia, Pennsylvania

Tricia R. Prokop, PT, EdD, MS, CSCS (Chapter 14)
Assistant Professor of Physical Therapy
Department of Rehabilitation Sciences
College of Education, Nursing and Health Professions
University of Hartford
West Hartford, Connecticut

Ken Randall, PT, PhD, MHR (Chapter 23)
Associate Dean and Professor
University of Oklahoma Schusterman Center
Tulsa, Oklahoma

Joseph Rencic, MD (Chapter 2)
Associate Professor of Medicine
Associate Program Director
Tufts Internal Medicine Residency Program
Tufts Medical Center
Tufts University School of Medicine
Boston, Massachusetts

Eric K. Robertson, PT, DPT (Chapter 26)
Associate Professor of Clinical Physical Therapy
Division of Biokinesiology and Physical Therapy
University of Southern California
Los Angeles, California

Trevor Russell, BPhty, PhD (Chapter 23)
Head of Physiotherapy (Acting)
Co-Director Centre for Research in Telerehabilitation
School of Health & Rehabilitation Sciences
The University of Queensland
Brisbane, Queensland, Australia

John Seiverd, PT, DPT (Chapter 25)
Chief of Physical Therapy
James A. Haley Veterans' Hospital
Tampa, Florida

Nancy Smith, PT, DPT, PhD, GCS (Chapter 24)
Board-Certified Clinical Specialist in Geriatric Physical Therapy
Associate Professor
Department of Physical Therapy
School of Health Sciences
Winston Salem State University
Winston Salem, North Carolina

Leslie F. Taylor, PT, PhD, MS (Chapter 21)
Professor and Associate Dean
Department of Physical Therapy
College of Health Professions
Mercer University
Atlanta, Georgia

Alecia Thiele, PT, DPT, MSEd, ATC, LAT, DCE (Chapter 28)
Associate Professor and Director of Clinical Education
Physical Therapy Department
Clarke University
Dubuque, Iowa

Yannick Tousignant-Laflamme, PT, PhD (Chapter 13)
Professor
School of Rehabilitation
Université de Sherbrooke
Sherbrooke, Québec, Canada

Susan Flannery Wainwright, PT, PhD (Chapters 7 and 16)
Professor and Chair
Department of Physical Therapy
Thomas Jefferson University
Philadelphia, Pennsylvania

Stephanie A. Weyrauch, PT, DPT, MSCI (Chapter 20)
Physical Therapy and Sports Medicine Centers
Orange, Connecticut

Brad W. Willis, PT, MPT, GCS (Chapter 22)
Board-Certified Clinical Specialist in Geriatric Physical Therapy
Assistant Teaching Professor
Department of Physical Therapy
School of Health Professions
University of Missouri
Columbia, Missouri

Steven L. Wolf, PT, PhD, FAPTA, FAHA, FASNR (Chapter 23)
Catherine Worthingham Fellow of American Physical Therapy Association
Fellow of the American Heart Association
Fellow of the American Society of Neurorehabilitation
Professor
Division of Physical Therapy Education
Department of Rehabilitation Medicine
Professor
Department of Medicine
Associate Professor
Department of Cell Biology
Emory University School of Medicine
Emory Rehabilitation Hospital
Professor of Health and Elder Care
Nell Hodgson Woodruff School of Nursing
Atlanta, Georgia
Senior Research Scientist and Associate Director for Training
Center for Visual and Neurocognitive Rehabilitation
Atlanta VA Health Care System
Decatur, Georgia

FOREWORD

Clinical reasoning (CR) taps into the essence of what makes physical therapy a unique profession. In this text, editors Drs. Musolino and Jensen have collaborated with an expert group of authors to decipher the CR process and provide the guidance needed to facilitate the development and assessment of these skills in learners at all levels. Both editors bring a long history of dedication to physical therapy education. Dr. Musolino has generously shared her expertise in education through her leadership of the Academy of Physical Therapy Education (APTE) of the American Physical Therapy Association (APTA), including 2 terms as president, vice president, and promotion director-at-large. While I had known Dr. Musolino for decades through her leadership roles in the APTA, it was because of her commitment to advancing physical therapist education that I came to truly know and admire her dedication to this cause.

Dr. Musolino has been a tireless ally in the effort to promote and support education research. Dr. Jensen is internationally respected for her contributions as a thought leader in physical therapist education, particularly related to the application of phenomenological approaches to ethics, gleaned from understanding the lived experiences of patients. Among her many accomplishments are leading the research team tasked with undertaking the study Excellence and Innovation in Physical Therapist Education, an initiative funded by the APTA, APTE, and several APTA components. For physical therapists of my generation who grew up reading her articles as part of our entry-level education, Dr. Jensen has always served as a beacon for patient-centered care, ethics, and morals in practice.

The CR process forms the essence of how we apply the knowledge and skills gained in our professional education programs, residency/fellowship training, and continuing education to the clinical problem presented by individuals with movement-related health conditions. In my role as editor-in-chief of the *Journal of Neurologic Physical Therapy*, one of my primary responsibilities is to devise the manuscript review criteria. I have advocated that a key review criteria for the evaluation of articles is how well the authors describe the theoretical rationale and the CR process for the selection of the interventions targeted in their studies. In this text, Drs. Musolino and Jensen and their colleagues break that CR process down into its constituent parts to provide the reader with the opportunity to closely examine cognitive and noncognitive theories and how they are integrated to form a framework for CR and decision-making.

Most people who are drawn to our profession come with an affinity for the sciences and the desire to work one-on-one with patients. The collaborative process of developing a treatment plan integrates our professional training and experiences with the patient's clinical presentation, goals, desires, and singular circumstances. In Chapter 1, the process of backward reasoning described by Musolino and Jensen bears a strong resemblance to the scientific method that has been ingrained in us since our earliest science classes. We ask a question, then we learn as much as we can about that question. We construct a hypothesis, test the hypothesis with an experiment, and analyze and interpret results. Based on these results, we draw conclusions and determine whether our hypothesis is true or false. If true, we can add this information to our knowledge base, and if false, then we reevaluate the hypothesis and begin again.

The clinical parallels to the scientific method are striking. As Nixon-Cave and Atkinson note in Chapter 10, the processes of clinical decision-making considers the whole patient and incorporates findings from evaluation at the level of body structure and function to activities through participation. We then construct a plan of intervention based on evidence of best practice to address the assessed impairments, limitations, and restrictions associated with the diagnosis. We collaborate with the patient to implement the intervention in the appropriate dose. Then we reevaluate the impairments, limitations, and restrictions to determine if the outcome was optimal. If yes, we conclude that the patient improved because the assessment, diagnosis, intervention, and dose were correct. Conversely, if the answer is no, and the patient did not improve, then we revisit the process. Perhaps the diagnosis missed the mark, the assessment did not capture the change, the selected intervention was not well suited to this patient, or the dose was insufficient. Through CR, we integrate our evaluation findings into a treatment and reevaluation plan.

A key element that differentiates the scientific method from CR and decision-making is that while the former is a one-way process, wherein the investigator works out the solution, clinical decision-making is enriched by the collaborative process that involves the patient. As Durning and Rencic note in Chapter 2, the development of a treatment plan to solve the movement problem is tailored to the patient's circumstances and preferences. The patient-centric process is strongly influenced by ethical considerations. As Delany and Edwards point out in Chapter 5, the expert clinician engages with the patient in a compassionate and nonjudgmental way, advocates for the needs of the patient, and works to improve his or her own skills to maintain the highest standards of practice. This theme of continually striving for the highest standards is echoed in Chapter 7, where, in her discussion of andragogy and transformative learning, Wainwright highlights the importance of critical reflection and dialogue with oneself and others to question assumptions and beliefs that influence clinical decisions.

Hartley and Seiverd expand on the concept of interprofessional collaboration in Chapter 25, noting that the clinical decision-making process is enriched by a learning environment that promotes transdisciplinary teamwork, wherein interactions with professional colleagues in other disciplines results in a whole that is greater than the sum of its parts. Relatedly, Gilliland in Chapter 8 describes the value of structuring the educational curriculum in a way that promotes integration across disciplines. Because the structure of the curriculum influences the way students organize their knowledge, reflective reasoning skills are best developed by thoughtful sequencing of courses and coordination across the curriculum. However, she adds the important caveat that even when all available information has been integrated, clinical decision-making will inherently have some element of uncertainty.

Returning to the theme of the parallels between the scientific method and the clinical decision-making process, evaluating the outcome of the process is an essential final step for both endeavors. In the scientific method, we assess whether the hypothesis was supported; in clinical decision-making, we assess whether the patient's movement improved. Likewise, with teaching clinical decision-making, evaluating the learning outcome is an essential step. In Chapter 10, Nixon-Cave and Atkinson describe the use of the Clinical Reasoning and Reflection Tool to probe the reflective process as a means to develop forward reasoning skills.

For times when CR skills require remediation, in Chapter 12, Wu describes a framework to discern the learner's remediation needs through a detailed interview to probe knowledge, communication, academic skills and support, as well as personal factors. In Chapter 25, Hartley and Seiverd also describe a systematic approach (FATE) to remediation that facilitates identification of the problem and the development of an action plan for remediation. In Chapter 28, Musolino and Thiele further describe how questioning strategies may be implemented with individualized, customized plans for clinical education and CR remediation.

Despite the striking parallels between the scientific method and clinical decision-making in physical therapist practice, there is one important difference. The APTA vision statement "Transforming society by optimizing movement to improve the human experience" hearkens to this difference. In the scientific method, it is incumbent upon the investigator to maintain a detached and dispassionate interest in the outcome of the process to maintain the necessary objectivity. However, it would be very rare to find a physical therapist who is dispassionate about the effects of his or her interventions on the patient's ability to move and function. Part of what draws people to become physical therapists is our knowledge that we have the skills to make a difference in our patients' lives by improving their experience of all that it means to be human by improving their ability to move and to interact with the world—and our passion for making this happen. In Chapter 1, Musolino and Jensen provide a model of the impacting components and varying influences for how clinical decision-making is realized in physical therapy, accounting for the human factors so important for the profession. So, while we look to science for the advanced technologies and scientific breakthroughs that define our modern society, we can feel invigorated as a profession with the awareness that we really do have the ability to transform society, and we do it one life at a time.

—Edelle [Edee] Field-Fote, PT, PhD, FAPTA
Catherine Worthingham Fellow of American Physical Therapy Association
Director, Spinal Cord Injury Research, Shepherd Center, Crawford Research Institute
Professor, Division of Physical Therapy, Emory University School of Medicine
Professor, School of Biological Sciences, Georgia Institute of Technology
Atlanta, Georgia
Editor-in-Chief, *Journal of Neurologic Physical Therapy*
Executive Editor, *Journal of Motor Behavior*

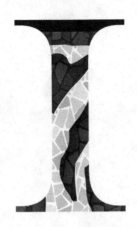

THEORETICAL FOUNDATIONS:
Guiding Practice for the Profession

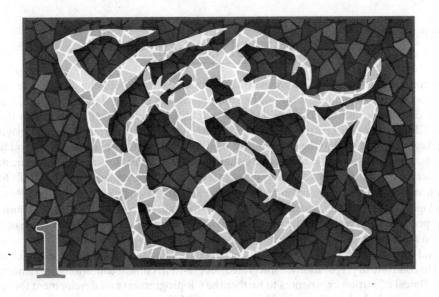

CLINICAL REASONING:
Why It Matters

*Gina Maria Musolino, PT, DPT, MSEd, EdD and
Gail M. Jensen, PT, PhD, FAPTA, FNAP*

On an important decision one rarely has 100% of the information needed for a good decision no matter how much one spends or how long one waits. And, if one waits too long, he has a different problem and must start all over. This is the terrible dilemma of the hesitant decision maker. —Robert K. Greenleaf, *The Servant As Leader*

OBJECTIVES

- Appreciate the challenges of creating a textbook to address clinical reasoning (CR), teaching, learning, and assessment within physical therapy.

- Conclude that CR is not well understood and remains a complex and iterative process with inherent linkages to learning, learning theories, and domains of learning (eg, affective, cognitive, psychomotor).

- Compare approaches for CR (eg, hypothetico-deductive, pattern recognition, forward thinking, systems thinking).

- Examine the interdependent relationship of CR, clinical problem-solving (CPS), and ongoing development of clinical knowledge.

- Appraise a conceptual figure that represents the many components of CR within the physical therapy profession.

- Support the reflective practitioner in proactively developing goals for CPS-CR, as he or she embarks on this journey of professional development for these foundational and essential elements of practice.

Musolino GM, Jensen GM, eds. *Clinical Reasoning and Decision-Making in Physical Therapy: Facilitation, Assessment, and Implementation* (pp 3-8).
© 2020 Taylor & Francis Group.

INTRODUCTION

CR is an important component for all health professions, yet many would comment that despite many years of research across disciplines, it is poorly understood.[1,2] CR cannot be seen merely as a generic skill or trait, but, rather, it is complex and tightly connected to the development of clinical knowledge as practitioners interact with patients in the context of care. The focus of our book is on CR and decision-making in physical therapy, yet more importantly, the underlying foundation for the book is about learning. Learning is central to the development of all aspects of CR from the teaching and facilitation of CR abilities in students, residents, and practitioners to the learning that is central to educators across academic and clinical settings as they understand more deeply the importance of the key concepts, learning theories, and practical tools for their work.

The purpose of this textbook is to provide a resource for health care professionals and especially within physical therapy. The text is designed for developing and practicing professionals to further their CR for best practice as both a foundational and essential element for professional practice for patients and clients. The content is best incorporated over the course of 2 to 3 semesters within entry-level programs, and serves as an excellent source for discussion and learning with academic, clinical development, residency and fellowship faculty, and residents and fellows-in-training to facilitate CR and in-depth conversations for learning over time. The text is especially helpful to complete in preparation for integrated, longer-term clinical education experiences, and revisiting during and following terminal clinical education experiences to further the CR progression and development for learners and facilitation by clinical instructors within clinical education and with residency and fellowship mentors.

Gruppen describes our challenge of creating a book that addresses the essential components when it comes to teaching, learning, and assessing CR:

> *Like the fable of the blind men and the elephant, each of whom, feeling a different part of the elephant, described it in very different ways, CR is a vast, complex construct that is described and used in different ways by different people.*[3(p4)]

We hope that this book will provide insights into the teaching, learning, assessment, research, and scholarship of CR for the physical therapy profession. The structure of the book has 3 sections, designed to assist our physical therapy colleagues across all settings, broaden their knowledge, and enhance their skills in the teaching and learning that is essential in the development of CR abilities.

- **Section I** focuses on the **theoretical foundations** that are important for understanding the breadth of CR as it applies to the practice of physical therapy, along with some key considerations from our interprofessional health colleagues.

- **Section II** has chapters addressing the **teaching, learning, and assessment strategies** that are essential for all learners, considering both qualitative and quantitative aspects of CR. Important CR tools are provided, along with examples to guide learners in the enhancement of CR.

- **Section III** includes chapters that provide the reader with **research, innovative projects, incorporating technology, including scholarly works and best practice exemplars across education and clinical settings,** with a special section devoted to the emerging area of **telehealth.**

CLINICAL REASONING: WHY IT MATTERS

Within physical therapy, CR is designated as a foundational element for practice and in need of progression along the learning continuum for a doctoring profession. CR has a long history and tradition of research across health professions, particularly extensive in medical education. CR is seen as central to the diagnostic and management decisions that physicians make, and to the development of expertise.[2,4] The study of CR is tightly linked to the diagnostic process, as the clinician must engage in problem-solving and categorization of clinical signs and symptoms to render a diagnosis and defined treatment. Much of the research and focus in medicine has been grounded in the cognitive science and the understanding of human cognition. This diagnostic process requires a dynamic interaction between knowledge and the ongoing creation of clinical knowledge and CR or critical thinking.[2,5,6] The CR research and theory development provides us with important background for understanding CR in physical therapy.

Much of the early work focused on the general problem-solving approaches to CR, as CPS skills were important for novices. The hypothetico-deductive reasoning or analytic process was generated from the medical problem-solving approach.[7,8] This hypothetico-deductive method has been incorporated into models that represent CR processes.

The process of collecting data or cues from the patient and generating hypotheses is considered a technique for transforming an unstructured problem (eg, a patient presenting with several complications) into a structured problem by generating a small possible set of solutions, often called *working hypotheses.* This structure is useful for novices, who need to develop a structured, analytical approach to sorting out patient cases, as they have scant experience from which to draw upon. The early work in reasoning labeled this process as *backward reasoning,* as the clinician worked backward from the working hypotheses. As research on experts continued, researchers found that in familiar or nonproblematic situations, experts did not typically display this analytical, hypothesis testing approach, but instead used rapid pattern recognition approaches. This process was called *forward reasoning,* which means clinicians see patterns, from cues gathered from patients in interviews or data collection, often recognizing prior patterns from experience. When experts are challenged by a complex case, they will then often engage in an analytical (backward) reasoning approach.[2,8,9]

Qualitative research in CR in female-dominated health professions[10-16] has been used to explore CR that occurs in everyday practice. This research has demonstrated how essential the understanding of the patient's perspective and context is in the act of clinical practice. For example, in physical therapy, Jensen and colleagues developed a grounded theory of expert practice in physical therapy.[15-17] In this model of expertise, CR is described as a collaborative process between the therapist and the patient. The patient, as a valued and trusted source of knowledge, was a non-negotiable element in the CR process, and collaboration with the patient was essential in the design and implementation of the intervention.

Ethnographic work by Edwards and colleagues[18,19] on expert physical therapists' CR strategies revealed an interplay of different reasoning strategies, in every task of clinical practice (eg, interactive reasoning, diagnostic reasoning, narrative reasoning, ethical reasoning, reasoning about teaching). Edwards made an important assertion for the physical therapy profession, as rather than contrasting the cognitively based, rationale models of reasoning and interactive models of reasoning, he proposed there was a dialectic model of CR that moves between the cognitive and decision-making processes required to diagnose and manage patients' physical disabilities, and the narrative or communicative reasoning and action are required to understand and engage patients and caregivers. A process of critical reflection is required with either CR process.

One way to understand this dialectic approach to CR is to frame the theories about CR into cognitive and noncognitive categories. Several chapters in the book will provide more in-depth discussion and application of these theories applied to education and practice. For example, cognitive theories include dual process theory for reasoning, which is simply described as slow or fast thinking. Fast thinking is nonanalytic reasoning and is much like pattern recognition or forward reasoning, also called Type I or System 1 thinking. Slow thinking or analytic reasoning is the hypothetico-deductive approach to reasoning or backward reasoning, also called Type II or System 2 thinking.[20,21]

Other cognitive theories are important in understanding the cognitive approach to CR that applies to cognition and knowledge, such as cognitive load (limits of our short-term working memory) and schema (mental structure for organizing knowledge).[2] While much of the emphasis and research in CR has focused on the analytical aspects and draws from well-known cognitive theories, for physical therapists, it is the noncognitive theories that are also important to consider in physical therapy practice, aptly described by Gilliland and Wainwright for physical therapists:

> *Patient cases are ambiguous by nature; thus, CR requires practitioners to develop a reasoning framework when not all the facts are known … approaches that therapists take to interacting with, examining, and assessing patients are shaped by the way the therapists frame the patients' problems.*[22(p500)]

To examine and frame patients' problems when not all the facts are known requires situation awareness, which is the ability and perception to see the elements in the environment—such as space, time, and patient factors—as critical components in framing the issues. We often call this *understanding the context of the situation.* This ability to see elements in a situation beyond one's own thinking and decision-making is particularly challenging for novice learners, who are generally rule governed and want structure, not ambiguity; they want black and white, not shades of grey. Social learning theories represent noncognitive theories that help us understand the reasoning that takes place through the dynamic interactions with patients, practitioners, and the environment.[2,23]

Now we return to our claim that learning is central to all our work in CR across academic and clinical settings. Understanding the central importance of being "adaptive" as it relates to both the adaptive learner and the development of adaptive expertise is critical to teaching and learning CR.[24] We know that expert clinicians have well-organized clinical knowledge structures, understand patients' needs and values, incorporate the social context, and can put all of this together in engaging their patients in collaborative CR toward successful assessment and treatment.[4,24] Expert clinicians can do this because of their use of higher-order processes or metacognitive thinking skills. These metacomponents are used to plan, monitor, and evaluate efforts for problem-solving, including progressive problem-solving. These metacognitive skills include problem recognition, definition, and representation; strategy formulation; resource allocation; monitoring; and evaluation of problem-solving.[25] Simply put, the learner's ability to self-assess, self-monitor, and reflect while thinking more deeply about that thinking is at the heart of metacognition.[26]

As educators, we are responsible for helping learners develop as adaptive learners who can engage in both self-assessment and self-directed learning, while recognizing errors and seeking greater understanding of one's abilities. Several chapters in this book provide ideas, structures, and teaching and learning strategies that help develop this important adaptive learner, foundational in the learning and teaching of CR.

CR is coupled directly with clinical decision-making (CDM) and CPS for patient and client management in health care, and we find these inextricably linked as foundational elements of physical therapy practice and key within the work of the physical therapist and physical therapist assistant team. CPS-CR-CDM must be considered at the highest levels of the cognitive learning taxonomy,[27-29] through creating plans of care, evaluating patient and client response to care, and analyzing the many aspects of patient/client information that is presented (eg, history, test and measures, response to care, social support, pharmacotherapeutics, imaging results, interprofessional care) for the best life course of care. As physical therapists and physical therapist assistants, we are also challenged on the higher levels of the learning taxonomies in the affective and psychomotor domains.[28,29]

Figure 1-1. CR in physical therapy.

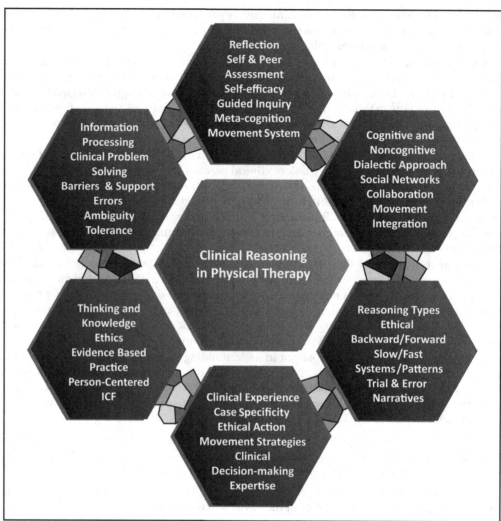

Within the affective domain,[26-28] physical therapy professionals go beyond the theory, internalizing the core values of the profession and incorporating the movement system concepts to resolve competing conflicts and collaborating with the patient/client and his or her families and caregivers. We work to understand the lived experience of our patients and incorporate the values and beliefs of the person-centered care, while working to evolve the health and wellness of the patient/client. This complex collaboration is accomplished through creative, self-actualizing change processes within the patient/client. The lifelong professional in physical therapy continues to challenge her or his own perspectives and beliefs and integrate past experiences with the current situation. As professionals, we must continue to engage in professional development activities that will facilitate highly skilled and innovative CPS-CR-CDM for contemporary practice.

Physical therapy health care providers often describe their own physical self as some of their best "tools." We are a hands-on profession and often incorporate not only our minds but also our bodies to effect a change within another's human movement system. Within the psychomotor realm, CR evolves to unconscious abilities to move and think on one's feet, with fluidity and the ability to compose, originate, vary, and adapt our movement. This leads to the embodiment of the more intuitive expert performance of movement, along with the protections for safer movement, for both the clinician and the patient/client. Facilitation of CPS-CR in an anticipatory manner with patient/client movement further allows physical therapy providers to proactively intervene to influence movement-in-action and guide purposeful and safer action in a participatory manner.

We posit that physical therapy CR may be inherently different, in some respects, than that of other health professions, yet has parallel processes, too. As you read this text, we trust you will have many moments of realization of how we reason similarly and yet differently. We hope you reflect on some of the thought-provoking queries sprinkled throughout the text to further challenge your learning, teaching, and clinical application for CPS-CR-CDM. A graphic representation of the many components of CR within physical therapy is provided for your considerations in Figure 1-1. Throughout the text, we will explore each of these CR components and examine how each part amalgamates with the whole, and the variability that occurs in our use of the CR components during clinical and educational encounters. Take a moment now to consider Figure 1-1 and how you incorporate the components for your CPS-CR-CDM.

As you are exposed or refamiliarized with the aspects of CR in physical therapy, you will also find that you begin to further synthesize and theorize about your own personal and professional CPS-CR-CDM development. You will find that you may sift through and begin to describe nuances in your CR, while at the same time discarding more novice ways of thinking. At times, you may also discover a "fit" with alternative approaches that you had not previously considered, as you uncover past experiences that align with the approaches being presented. We expect that at times you may be thinking more abstractly in a conceptual manner, while at other times you will be solidifying your viewpoints and CR practices. You may at times be cajoled to uncertainty, while at other times be comfortable with the complexities and ambiguities of CR in physical therapy, where conflicting approaches may present.

We hope that your repertoire will be expanded and your view of CR in physical therapy will be enhanced, called into question, expanded, and enlightened through the sometimes-differing viewpoints, unique scholarship, and varied experiences presented. As you examine and reexamine Figure 1-1, we believe you shall also find that it also represents the fluid nature where we may vacillate and shift within and among the components of CR based upon the nuances of the clinical problems in the real world of often-unpredictable practice.

Real-world problems in practice are messy indeterminate situations,[29] and physical therapy professionals must constantly think, reflect, and react in the art of practice with our hands, bodies, and minds to progress a patient safely through a plan of care and determine the best working clinical diagnosis relative to movement. While many problems are systematically organized and guided by algorithms and hypothetico-deductive approaches, some problems need to be seen from multiple perspectives by turning them upside-down and sidewise to see what is hidden for the true dissection of CPS-CR-CDM. It is this "professional artistry,"[29] as Schön describes, in which our skilful performance emerges to make all the difference. You will see throughout the text the incorporation of Schön's concepts of Reflective Practice[29] as a key component for CPS-CR-CDM. We believe that the more we think about CPS-CR-CDM, the more we realize there is more to learn and uncover. The mere act of thinking about thinking through our metacognitive processes and reflection-in-action will progress CR, yet how can we facilitate to bring about more exponential changes for the doctoring profession of physical therapy? We need to be more intentional with teaching, learning, practice, and application of CR-CDM throughout a career.

CR is an essential non-negotiable element for all health professionals. The health professional's ability to demonstrate professional competence, compassion, and accountability depends on a foundation of sound CR. The physical therapy profession's commitment to society is to define and promote the movement system as the foundation for optimizing movement for the patients we serve and the health of society. This concept demands intentional development of physical therapists' ability not only to think critically, but also to manage the uncertainty of practice. The CR process needs to bring together knowledge, experience, and understanding of people, the environment, and organizations along with a strong moral compass in making sound decisions and taking necessary actions.

While CR and the role of mentors have been a focus of the continued growth and development of residency programs in physical therapy, there is a critical need to have a broader, in-depth look at how educators across academic and clinical settings intentionally facilitate the development of CR skills across one's career. This book is designed to provide a comprehensive resource for the development of CR abilities across a career from professional education through residency education, as well as for directed, lifelong learning.

The text provides a wide-ranging and in-depth focus for development of CPS-CR-CDM patient/client management skills considering theory, assessment, facilitation frameworks, and technological applications, along with the continuum of development for physical therapy professionals. The aim and scope of the text are directed for physical therapy education, to enhance CPS-CR-CDM for developing professionals and post-professionals in both clinical and academic realms, and to develop clinical and academic faculty. The book addresses aspects of CR as a foundational patient management skill that has evolved considerably within the doctoring profession. The text uniquely offers both evidence-based approaches and pragmatic consultation from well-established and respected authors and clinicians, along with novel authors.

The authors have openly and painstakingly shared their direct practice experiences developing and implementing CPS-CR-CDM in practice applications for teaching students, residents, patients, and clinical and academic faculty in classrooms, clinics, and through simulation and telehealth. No other textbook addressing this element applies this breadth of practice applications of CR-CDM that are key for real-world practice and continuing competence as a health care professional within physical therapy.

As you begin your journey to enhance your CPS-CR-CDM abilities, after considering the chapter titles in Sections I through III of the text and contemplating Figure 1-1, please proactively consider 3 CR goals you hope to achieve for your professional development, and jot them down here to revisit later. You may wish to consider your goals in the realms of personal, professional, and future.

Goals for Clinical Reasoning

1. _____

2. _____

3. _____

Please note throughout the text you will be asked to reflect, and your active participation will assist in your learning along the way.

Most decisions are not binary, and there are usually better answers waiting to be found if you do the analysis and involve the right people. —Jamie Dimon, American businessman

REFERENCES

1. Loftus S. Rethinking clinical reasoning: time for a dialogical turn. *Med Educ.* 2012;46:1174-1178.
2. Trowbridge R, Recnic J, Durning S. *Teaching Clinical Reasoning.* Philadelphia, PA: American College of Physicians; 2015.
3. Gruppen LD. Clinical reasoning: defining it, teaching it, assessing it, studying it. *West J Emerg Med.* 2017;18(1):4-7.
4. Mylopoulos M. When I say … adaptive expertise. *Med Educ.* 2017;51:685-686.
5. Ericsson KA. Acquisition and maintenance of medical expertise: a perspective from the expert-performance approach with deliberate practice. *Acad Med.* 2015;90(11):1471-1486.
6. Schmidt H, Mamede S. How to improve the teaching of clinical reasoning: a narrative review and a proposal. *Med Educ.* 2015;49:961-973.
7. Elstein AS, Shulman LS, Sprafka SA. *Medical problem solving: an analysis of clinical reasoning.* Cambridge, MA: Harvard University Press; 1978.
8. Elstein AS, Shulman LS, Sprafka SA. Medical problem solving: a ten-year retrospective. *Eval Health Professions.* 1990;13:5-36.
9. Patel V, Kaufman D, Magder S. The acquisition of medical expertise in complex dynamic environments. In: Ericsson KA, ed. *The Road to Excellence.* Mahwah, NJ: Lawrence Erlbaum; 1996;12-165.
10. Benner P. *From Novice to Expert: Excellence and Power in Clinical Nursing Practice.* Menlo Park, CA: Addison-Wesley; 1982.
11. Benner P, Tanner CA, Chesla CA. *Expertise in Nursing Practice.* New York, NY: Springer; 1996.
12. Benner P, Hooper-Kyriakidis P, Stannard D. *Clinical Wisdom and Interventions in Critical Care.* Philadelphia, PA: WB Saunders; 1999.
13. Mattingly C, Flemming MH. *Clinical Reasoning.* Philadelphia, PA: FA Davis; 1994.
14. Fleming MH, Mattingly C. Action and narrative: two dynamics of clinical reasoning. In: Higgs J, Jones M, eds. *Clinical Reasoning in the Health Professions.* 2nd ed. Oxford, United Kingdom: Butterworth-Heinemann; 2000.
15. Jensen G, Gwyer J, Shepard K, Hack L. Expert practice in physical therapy. *Phys Ther.* 2000;80:28-52.
16. Jensen G, Gwyer J, Hack L, Shepard K. *Expertise in Physical Therapy Practice.* 2nd ed. St. Louis, MO: Saunders, Elsevier; 2007.
17. Jensen GM, Resnik L, Haddad A. Expertise and clinical reasoning. In: Higgs J, Jensen G, Loftus S, Christensen N, eds. *Clinical Reasoning in the Health Professions.* 4th ed. Edinburgh, United Kingdom: Elsevier; 2019.
18. Edwards I, Jones M, Carr J, Braunack-Mayer A, Jensen GM. Clinical reasoning strategies in physical therapy. *Phys Ther.* 2004;84(4):312-330.
19. Edwards I, Jones MA. Clinical reasoning and expert practice. In: Jensen GM, Gwyer JM, Hack LM, Shepard KF, eds. *Expertise in Physical Therapy Practice.* 2nd ed. Boston, MA: Elsevier; 2007:192-213.
20. Kahneman D. *Thinking, Fast and Slow.* London, UK: Allen Lane; 2011.
21. Marcum JA. An integrated model of clinical reasoning: dual-processing theory of cognition and metacognition. *J Eval Clin Pract.* 2012;18:954-961.
22. Gilliland S, Wainwright S. Patterns of clinical reasoning in physical therapist students. *Phys Ther.* 2017;97:499-511.
23. Halfer J, ed. *Extraordinary Learning in the Workplace.* New York, NY: Springer; 2011.
24. Cutrer WB, Miller B, Martin VP, et al. Fostering the development of master adaptive learners: a conceptual model to guide skill acquisition in medical education. *Acad Med.* 2017;92:70-75.
25. Higgs J, Jensen G, Loftus S, Christensen N, eds. *Clinical Reasoning in the Health Professions.* 4th ed. Edinburgh, United Kingdom: Elsevier; 2019.
26. Musolino GM. Fostering reflective practice: self-assessment abilities of physical therapy students and entry-level graduates. *J Allied Health.* 2006;35(1):30-42.
27. Bloom BS, Englehart MD, Furst EJ, Hill WH, Krathwohl DR. *The Taxonomy of Educational Objectives, Handbook I: The Cognitive Domain.* New York, NY: David McKay; 1956.
28. Krathwohl DR, Bloom B, Masia BB. *Taxonomy of Educational Objectives, The Classification of Educational Goals, Handbook II: Affective Domain.* New York, NY: David McKay; 1964.
29. Schön DA. *The Reflective Practitioner: How Professionals Think in Action.* New York, NY: Basic Books; 1983.

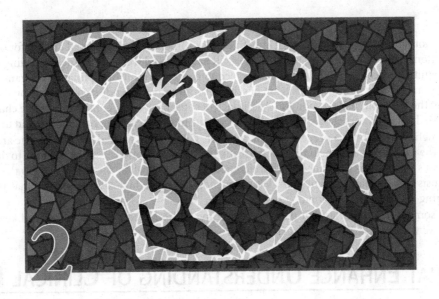

TEACHING CLINICAL REASONING:
"Lessons Learned" in Medical Education

Steven J. Durning, MD, PhD and Joseph Rencic, MD

OBJECTIVES

- Justify that clinical reasoning (CR) is both a process and an outcome, relevant for a variety of disciplines.
- Examine key aspects of CR in that it requires rich, content-specific and organized knowledge; more than one strategy; and flexibility with strategic approaches.
- Internalize that CR requires a prolonged and deliberate effort that is impacted by motivation and emotion.
- Conclude that CR is context specific, requiring lifelong and intentionally reflective learning.
- Appraise a conceptual figure of CR considering the dynamic and cyclical perspectives of self-regulated learning.

INTRODUCTION

Diagnostic errors are now reported as a leading cause of death.[1] The recent Institute of Medicine[2] report stresses that improved education and training in diagnosis must play a key role in reducing diagnostic error. Improvements in teaching CR can and should be made, but challenges abound. First, experience and practice are necessary for developing CR ability, yet experiences are often random, leading to gaps in clinicians' experiential knowledge of illnesses. In addition, expert clinicians do not necessarily teach CR effectively. Finally, assessment of CR has been termed the "Holy Grail"[3] because of the inability to measure it directly and the lack of a gold standard method. Without feasible and reliable methods with valid evidence for CR assessment, understanding the value of educational interventions becomes difficult.

Musolino GM, Jensen GM, eds. *Clinical Reasoning and Decision-Making in Physical Therapy: Facilitation, Assessment, and Implementation* (pp 9-21).
© 2020 Taylor & Francis Group.

Defining CR poses another challenge to teaching it effectively. For some, CR is an essential ability; for others, a core task; and for yet others, a foundational science.[4,5] Our understanding of CR has emerged from disciplines including expertise theory, educational psychology, cognitive psychology, neuroscience, and economics. This multidisciplinary amalgam of theories can lead to unclear or ill-defined boundaries for CR. Indeed, a team of scholars who recently conducted a definitional review of CR to better understand the scope of the term found 109 synonyms.[6] This lack of consensus likely contributes to the challenges of both teaching and assessing CR. Medical educators should clearly define CR within their teaching context to avoid unnecessary ambiguity.

For this chapter, we define CR as both a process and an outcome. CR is often divided into diagnostic and therapeutic reasoning; the former entails the steps up to and including establishing the diagnosis, and the latter pertains to developing a treatment plan that meets a patient's specific circumstances and preferences. CR begins when the patient enters the room, and ends with establishing the diagnosis and/or management plan. We have chosen a more inclusive definition that is consistent with this concept and the emerging literature on this topic.

We will begin with some salient theories that pertain to teaching CR followed by a brief review of key developments in the history of CR. Finally, we will discuss 5 "lessons learned" regarding teaching CR.

THEORIES THAT ENHANCE UNDERSTANDING OF CLINICAL REASONING

What theories are relevant to teaching CR? A number of theories are germane to this topic.[7] For example, dual process theory refers to the belief that we use 2 general processes to arrive at a diagnosis and/or management plan. The theory was popularized by the book *Thinking, Fast and Slow*.[8] Fast thinking in CR is known as Type 1, or nonanalytic, reasoning, and slow thinking is referred to as Type 2, or analytic reasoning. Nonanalytic reasoning is fast, subconscious, with low to no effort. On the other hand, analytic thinking is slow, conscious, and effortful. For example, you can immediately and easily identify a loved one among a group of 10 individuals. However, imagine having to write an essay on how a loved one walks, talks, and laughs. Interestingly, despite the ease with which people categorize things (eg, recognize a loved one), they often have limited introspection into how they do so (eg, the difficulty of describing how we recognize a loved one). For each of these 2 general cognitive processes, a number of strategies have been recognized.[9] Nonanalytic reasoning emerges from pattern recognition and heuristics, with useful rules of thumb such as "consider arthrocentesis in a patient who presents with acute monoarticular arthritis to rule out a septic joint." This knowledge is encoded in long-term working memory and rapidly accessible when triggered by an appropriate stimulus.[10] Strategies for analytic reasoning include evidence-based medicine, probabilistic reasoning, ruling out the worst-case scenario, and the key features approach. We discuss CR strategies in more detail during the lessons learned section.

Cognitive load theory relates to dual process theory. It pertains to our limited working memory capacity, which prevents us from processing more than a limited number of informational elements (classically 7 plus-or-minus 2).[11] Our minds overcome this information processing limitation by creating "chunks," which combine multiple pieces of related information into a larger conceptual category (eg, lateral shoulder pain, worst with movement or at night, with normal passive range of motion and a positive painful arc test, becomes rotator cuff syndrome). This only occupies one informational slot in working memory instead of four.[12]

Our brains constantly chunk information, which frees up our working memory space. The amount of information in a working memory "slot" appears limitless. Using the metaphor of the brain as a computer, one's working memory can be thought of as 7 Word documents. Each of these Word documents can contain a single word or sentence or represent a textbook. Thus, effective chunking of information enables one to pay greater attention to events in one's environment. Optimization of working memory through chunking helps to explain why expert chess players can play more than 10 games at once.

The health professions equivalent is the clinician who fills her or his working memory slots with highly chunked representations of relevant clinical information, leaving slots available for processing additional clinical findings and contextual factors. In contrast, the medical student may have single symptoms or findings in a given slot. Clinicians combine chunks about a given disease into schema, or illness scripts—mental representations of diseases that contain key information about diagnosis and treatment.[13] In terms of instruction, cognitive load theory emphasizes reducing extraneous load and needless noise within teaching that consumes mental effort (eg, having to flip a page to see a table to which the text refers) and leads to less efficient learning.[14]

Deliberate practice theory describes how a novice can become an expert performer. Deliberate practice involves the effortful practice of the component parts of an activity that at least initially is performed under the guidance of a coach or mentor.[15] Attainment of expert performance is believed to take 10 years or 10,000 hours of deliberate practice, not just time on task (eg, spending 2 hours in a clinic signing paperwork does not count as deliberate practice for CR). Deliberate practice has been extensively studied in sports, music, chess, and, more recently, medical education.[15,16] In other words, expert performance is an adaptation based upon accumulating knowledge and experience into chunks to free up working memory slots.

Situated cognition theory stresses the importance of contextual factors on CR. It posits that CR, or thinking in general, is a process that depends on the complex interactions between clinician, patient, and environmental factors.[17] These factors are interdependent, and they shape the outcome of the clinical encounter. For example, a clinician may easily diagnose cervical radiculopathy within a native English-speaking patient, but misdiagnose a non–English-speaking patient in a hectic, overbooked clinic. Context appears to powerfully impact a clinician's problem-solving and decision-making. Educators should account for situated cognition theory when considering how to maximize CR knowledge transfer into patient contexts.

Reflection Moment

What theory did you find most useful for your learning, teaching, and clinical practice of CR? How will you apply this theory to your teaching and clinical practice and patient care?

Next, we briefly describe some historical highlights in the development of CR, to provide context for understanding current opportunities and challenges in learning and teaching CR. This will be followed by a discussion of 5 lessons learned with an emphasis on teaching strategies for each lesson. Later, in Chapter 6, Covington provides an abridged literature review of CR.

HISTORICAL HIGHLIGHTS OF CLINICAL REASONING RESEARCH

Over the past several decades, researchers have explored CR in parallel with prevailing theories of the day. Here we outline the highlights of these experiments and the underlying theoretical perspectives that shaped their interpretation in each period. In the 1960s, medical education scholars hypothesized that CR expertise derived from superior general problem-solving skills. These problem-solving skills were believed to be both generalizable and teachable and, if acquired, would result in expert diagnostic performance. These predictions were incorrect. For example, studies using patient management problems[18,19] and other long-case formats indicated that an expert clinician (who presumably had these generalizable problem-solving skills) performed well on one case but did quite poorly on another. Indeed, the correlation of performance between such cases ranged from 0.1 to 0.3 (as a reference, the goal for a reliable test is at least 0.6 to 0.8).[20] Performance was discovered to be highly dependent on knowledge content within a given domain, rather than process,[21,22] thus establishing the concept of *content specificity*. A realization of this research era is that no gold standard process for CR in any given situation exists. This discovery led to the next era in CR theory.

Stimulated by the emergence of the computer and artificial intelligence, investigators adopted an information processing model for CR.[23] Information processing theory focused attention on knowledge organization (or how information is interconnected or chunked) in memory, rather than generalized problem-solving processes or algorithms.[20] Researchers explored forms of knowledge representation and organization,[24] such as illness scripts, to understand how the brain processed information. Like other professions, clinicians develop highly organized, associated chunks of information regarding diseases (ie, illness scripts) that they use in fast, or nonanalytic, thinking to recognize familiar patterns in a patient's presentation. Illness scripts were thought to derive from exemplars (ie, individual patients with the given disease) and prototypes (ie, a compilation of key features of a specific disease, based on experiences and reading into a general mental representation).[25,26]

Script theory provided insights into dual process theory by suggesting that clinicians use these idiosyncratic mental representations to make nonanalytic diagnostic and therapeutic decisions. Kahneman's research[8] demonstrated that the default pathway for reasoning is this nonanalytic pathway, with analytic reasoning recruited primarily for complicated or unfamiliar problems or situations where illness scripts are inadequately developed. He explored heuristics and biases extensively, illuminating their nonrationale and nonprobabilistic nature.[27] Indeed, a considerable body of research focused on describing and understanding heuristics and biases during this information processing era. Other researchers who explored the limitations of the brain's information processing capacity in this era developed cognitive load theory.[28] This theory has primarily focused on learning, but recently researchers have begun to recognize its relevance to CR performance.[29]

A significant historical breakthrough in CR research occurred with the discovery that content specificity (eg, clinician knowledge) provided an inadequate explanation for CR performance variation. Norman et al[30] demonstrated only moderate correlations in a clinician's performances on identical case presentations across 2 different occasions, suggesting that "context," the circumstances of a given occasion, rather than solely "content," influenced a physician's ability to apply knowledge to make accurate diagnoses. This research led to work that considers expertise as a state (limited to specific patient circumstances) rather than a trait (seen as a general or transferable "skill" within a profession).[21]

In other words, expertise as a state argues that CR performance is specific to the patient, other health professionals on the team, the environmental, and their emergent interactions (ie, the specific situation). Thus, *context specificity* captures the notion that something besides the clinical content of a case is influencing diagnoses and therapy. In seeking to explain context specificity and expand understanding of CR beyond the limits of information processing theory, researchers recognized that situated cognition theory may provide a valuable explanatory model. Situated cognition theory research shows that clinician factors account for only a small portion of the variance in predicting diagnostic success.[31] It stresses the importance of interactions between health care professionals, patients, and environments as fundamental in CR.[32] The implication of situated cognition theory is that both effective teaching and assessment of CR require a broad range of typical and atypical case presentations in patients of diverse backgrounds within a wide variety of clinical contexts.

FIVE LESSONS LEARNED

In this section, we outline 5 lessons learned in medicine, with an emphasis on teaching strategies. We also recommend that the reader considers reviewing other resources.[33,34]

Lesson 1: Clinical Reasoning Teaching Must Emphasize the Development of Rich, Content-Specific, Highly Organized Knowledge

Robust, well-organized knowledge is an essential element of effective CR.[20] Content knowledge and CR expert performance are difficult, if not impossible, to disentangle. For diagnosis, learners must acquire knowledge that allows them to discriminate one disease or health-related problem from another, because diagnostic reasoning is fundamentally a categorization exercise. Importantly, this knowledge must be rapidly, efficiently, and effectively recalled in clinical settings to enable optimal patient care. The ability to rapidly recall knowledge relates directly to knowledge organization, which refers to the interconnectedness of knowledge in memory.[10] Highly organized knowledge typically manifests as nonanalytic reasoning (fast thinking).

Insights into knowledge organization have emerged from other fields and analyzing clinicians' oral presentations, documentation, or thinking aloud. Steward et al's analysis[35] of physicians' and students' oral presentations discovered 4 general levels, or discourses, of knowledge organization.

1. At the lowest level is **dispersed knowledge**, in which a learner has difficulty demonstrating any meaningful knowledge about a given topic. These learners may benefit from test-enhanced learning strategies[36] that emphasize recall of learned information.

2. **Disorganized knowledge** is the descriptor for the next level. A learner with disorganized knowledge about a topic can often recite facts and figures about a problem or disease, but may struggle to independently define the nature of a patient's problem (ie, fail to see the forest for the trees) and apply that knowledge to a real patient encounter. These learners may benefit from exercises that require them to clearly define the patient's chief problem(s) or complaint(s), which may help them recall their own relevant knowledge or readily look up the necessary information.

3. The next level refers to **elaborated knowledge**, in which a learner demonstrates organized knowledge. Elaborated knowledge may manifest as semantic qualifiers and/or encapsulations. Semantic qualifiers are abstract, often binary terms that we use to describe a patient's complaint(s) as accurately and narrowly as possible.[37] The description of a patient who presents with a 4-hour history of a swollen, warm, and tender wrist with limited range of motion can be encapsulated by 4 semantic qualifiers for arthritis: acute, monoarticular, inflammatory, and arthritic. Learners use semantic qualifiers to translate a patient's story into a clearly defined clinical problem. Encapsulations often refer to chunking of multiple detailed biomedical findings into higher-order or higher-inference pathophysiological concepts, which subsume all of the relevant details (eg, a red, hot, swollen knee is recognized as an inflammatory arthritis).[12]

4. **Compiled knowledge** is the highest form of knowledge organization and is typically characterized by robust illness scripts. Illness scripts consist of idiosyncratic mental representations of the clinical findings, epidemiology, and pathophysiological considerations of diseases or health-related problems that a clinician has learned through reading and clinical experience.[13] Clinicians refine their illness scripts as they see additional patients or gain more "book" knowledge. Experienced clinicians typically employ illness scripts nonanalytically or unconsciously when they recognize the pattern of the clinical problem at hand, while novices likely often use analytic reasoning to consciously recall key elements of an illness script.

As another means of demonstrating the power of nonanalytic reasoning, one can read the excerpt below (as reading is typically a pattern recognition activity). This is what clinicians do with seeing patients: We sift through the signal, differentiating from the noise to effectively and efficiently arrive at a plan of care that is optimal for a patient's circumstances and preferences.

i cdnuolt blveiee taht I cluod aulaclty uesdnatnrd what I was rdanieg. The phaonmneal pweor of the hmuan mnid, aoccdrnig to a rscheearch at Cmabrigde Uinervtisy. It dseno't mtaetr in waht oerdr the ltteres in a word are, the olny iproamtnt tihng is taht the frsit and lsat ltteer be in the rghit pclae. The rset can be a taotl mses. Tihs is bcuseae the huamn mnid deos not raed ervey lteter by istlef, but the wrod as a wlohe. Azanmig huh? Yaeh and I awlyas tghuhot slpeling was ipmorantt!

TABLE 2-1

CLINICAL REASONING STEPS TO FOLLOW:
TEACHING STRATEGIES FOR ENHANCING KNOWLEDGE ORGANIZATION

OPTIMIZING COGNITIVE LOAD

1. Probe intermediate steps: syndrome, encapsulations, semantic qualifiers, problem lists
2. Create prototypical patient assignments
3. Change key features in the presentation
4. Construct compare and contrast assignments
5. Require self-explanation
6. Encourage visual diagnosis practice

EFFECTIVE CHUNKING

7. Use or create algorithms/flow charts/schemas or concept maps
8. Give the learner time to think (intentional pauses)
9. Discuss essential concepts multiple times and by multiple means
10. Consider near-peer teaching (particularly given a clinician's short introspection at times)
11. Provide worked examples (solved cases)
12. "Think aloud"
13. Start with common/classic (straightforward presentations) and gradually increase complexity
14. Limit feedback to no more than 1 to 3 areas for improvement

Adapted from Chamberland and Mamede,[45] Torre et al,[46] Mayer,[47] Ten Cate and Durning,[48] and Van Merriënboer and Sweller.[49]

Teaching strategies for this lesson (Table 2-1)[38-42] capitalize on probing the structure of a learner's illness scripts (a higher-order form of chunking strategies, Strategies 1 through 6) and optimizing cognitive load, which is important for effective chunking[43] strategies (Strategies 7 through 14). Probing intermediate steps, rather than asking only for the final diagnosis, allows insights into the learners' CR process. This process is similar to showing the long form of your math work or geometric proof to illustrate the problem-solving steps along the way.

Prototypical patient assignments refer to a teaching strategy in which the student provides the clinical findings for a typical presentation of a given disease either through a writing assignment or a role play. Changing key features of a presentation (eg, shoulder pain with intact passive range of motion becomes shoulder pain with loss of passive range of motion) also can improve categorization ability, because students recognize the importance of certain signs or symptoms in determining the diagnosis. This recall activity may strengthen learner illness scripts. Comparison and contrast assignments may further help learners to define and refine disease categories.[44]

Few clinicians know every symptom and sign for a given condition. Rather, they learn key features of diseases that help distinguish one from another. Multiple repetitions of comparison and contrast with a given clinical problem enhance learners' analytic and nonanalytic reasoning by strengthening illness scripts.[12] Given the haphazard nature and low number of repetitions available in clinical settings, these assignments can be provided through paper or online cases. Self-explanation, a process in which students explain the basis for their diagnostic and management decisions verbally or in clinical documentation, can enhance knowledge organization and categorization skills by requiring students to make connections between clinical findings and diseases that can lead to chunking.[45] Finally, algorithms can help learners develop methodical approaches for attacking specific clinical problems and, through the use of concept maps,[46] enable teachers to literally visualize a learner's knowledge organization.

With regard to optimizing cognitive load, allowing students time to process information is an important teaching technique. Because students have limited information chunks, they more typically use analytic reasoning, which requires more time. Teachers can allot the time either before the patient encounter by allowing the student to read about the patient's chief complaint to activate prior learning or review an algorithm or concept map about the patient's problem and/or after the encounter to allow the student to interpret and develop a self-explanation of the clinical findings.

Repetition of key concepts is essential to learning and should increase learners' ability to chunk information. In addition, learning often improves when both visual and aural sensory pathways are used.[47] CR should be taught with images and words when possible (eg, a picture of a patient with a dislocated shoulder supplements a verbal description of the typical symptoms). Visual diagnosis practice is a powerful teaching strategy that likely improves pattern recognition. Highlighting the importance of visual findings in clinical settings or in practice exercises can help students incorporate such strategies into their CR for learning.

Near-peer teaching (teacher and learner are close in training, such as a fourth-year medical student teaching a second-year medical student) may help learners improve their knowledge, because near-peers may explain their analytic reasoning processes better than experienced clinicians who may primarily use nonanalytic reasoning to make diagnoses.[48] Cognitive load theory demonstrates the benefits of enhanced learning when students see examples of solved clinical problems (worked examples).[49]

A practical way for a teacher to provide these examples is by "thinking aloud." The teacher who thinks aloud provides the learner with an approach to solving a clinical problem. A debrief after thinking aloud is important to allow the student to ask clarification questions and to allow the teacher to assess the learner's understanding. As they become more experienced with a health-related problem, learners can work through partially solved cases and then graduate to solving cases entirely on their own. Similarly, teaching students typical presentations of common diseases reduces cognitive load, but as students advance, providing atypical presentations of common diseases and typical presentations of uncommon diseases enables them to build their expertise for a given problem. Finally, excessive feedback can overwhelm a student, so teachers should emphasize 1 to 3 constructive points of feedback on CR points.[38]

Reflection Moment

What strategies in Lesson 1 did you find most valuable? How can you apply them to your teaching and learning? What challenges do you see in doing so?

Lesson 2: Clinical Reasoning Requires Multiple Strategies and Flexibility in Strategy Use

Clinicians use a range of analytic and nonanalytic CR strategies for problem-solving.[9] Examples of analytic strategies include using evidence-based medicine, thinking about one's thinking (metacognitive monitoring), ruling out the worst-case scenario for a condition, applying an algorithm or practice guideline, and employing a Bayesian approach whereby statistical principles are applied to specific patient circumstances.

Nonanalytic reasoning strategies include pattern recognition (the most common) and heuristics. Some strategies can fall into both categories. For example, heuristics, or useful rules of thumb, are sometimes subconscious and rapid (nonanalytic) and sometimes actively recalled and processed (analytic). Recent opinion views nonanalytic reasoning and analytic reasoning on a continuum, with clinicians toggling back and forth between the two or falling somewhere between the extremes in most clinical scenarios.[9,50] We recommend that the reader review the following cited references that provide additional detail regarding these strategies.[38,51-53] The teacher's goal should be to introduce students to these strategies for both nonanalytic and analytic reasoning and help them learn how and when to use them. With this knowledge, students can experiment to further develop their own practice style.

Discussion of reasoning strategies leads to the topic of cognitive diagnostic error. The reader is encouraged to review one of the several references on error and cognitive dispositions to respond.[54-56] The dominant discourse around cognitive error is that nonanalytic reasoning (eg, pattern recognition) leads to most diagnostic errors.[57] However, any strategy can lead to success or failure. To reduce diagnostic failure rates, some experts recommend universal use of cognitive forcing strategies (CFS),[58] in which clinicians force themselves to use an analytic reasoning doublecheck even when they are confident in their diagnosis. Consistent with Lesson 1, the literature currently supports knowledge-based analytic CFS (eg, structured reflection on the differential diagnosis specific to a given case) as likely the most effective in improving diagnostic accuracy rather than general debiasing CFS (eg, "Was I prone to any biases during my diagnostic process?").[59] Unfortunately, these data are limited to paper cases, and more research is required to determine optimal CFS for practicing clinicians. That being said, universal use of knowledge-based CFS, including use of structured reflection, can be recommended for learners, because evidence suggests that short-term diagnostic accuracy on paper cases improves, because such reflection likely serves as diagnostic reasoning practice that improves knowledge organization.[60] One practical approach for this recommendation is to require learners to demonstrate such reflection in clinical documentation, such as a structured reflection table (Table 2-2).[61] Following is an example applied to a clinical case scenario with application of Lesson 2 for your consideration, using multiple strategies while maintaining a flexible framework.

CLINICAL VIGNETTE

A 32-year-old, semiprofessional, right-handed baseball pitcher with no significant medical history presents with right shoulder pain. The pain is tingling in nature and radiates down his arm. It is not worsened by shoulder movement, but some neck positions make it worse. He denies weakness or numbness. On examination, his vital signs are normal. There is no tenderness in the shoulder or neck. He has full range of motion in his right shoulder. Compression of the head reproduces his symptoms, and distraction of his head reduces symptoms. Biceps reflex is 1+ in the right arm; the others are normal. Strength is 5/5 throughout. Sensation is intact to light touch, pinprick, and vibration sense.

TABLE 2-2
EXAMPLE OF A STRUCTURED DIAGNOSTIC REFLECTION EXERCISE

List 2 to 3 conditions on the differential diagnosis	1. Cervical radiculopathy	2. Rotator cuff syndrome	3. Superior labral anterior/posterior tear
List aspects of presentation that are concordant with diagnosis	• Shoulder pain • Paresthesia • Radiation • Symptoms changed by head and neck movements • Decreased biceps reflex	• Shoulder pain • Radiation down arm • Repetitive use (ie, pitcher) • Normal strength and sensation	• Shoulder pain • Repetitive use (ie, pitcher)
List aspects of presentation that are discordant with diagnosis	• Lack of neck pain	• Paresthesia • No pain with shoulder movement • Exacerbated by neck positions • Diminished biceps reflex	• Paresthesia • No pain with shoulder movement • Exacerbated by neck positions • Diminished biceps reflex
List aspects of presentation that are associated with diagnosis but are missing from presentation	• Worsened by cough or Valsalva	• Night pain	• Night pain • Decline in throwing velocity • Clicking

Adapted from Mamede et al.[61]

List clinical diagnoses in order of likelihood:

1. _____

2. _____

3. _____

The metaphor of a Major League Baseball player may be helpful for summing up this lesson learned. To be an effective professional pitcher, one throws faster pitches (nonanalytic reasoning) and slower pitches (analytic reasoning). Specific fast and slow pitches (eg, cutter, fastball or slider, and change-up or knuckle ball) represent specific nonanalytic and analytic reasoning strategies respectively. Throwing a strike (or arriving at the correct diagnosis and an optimal plan of care) will differ based on the situation. The same pitch is not thrown if the count is empty or full, if the first or eighth hitter is up, or if the bases are loaded or empty. The effective professional pitcher flexibly chooses which pitch to throw in what situation and we would argue that the expert performing clinician does the same thing—flexibly chooses which strategy (of many potential strategies) to use based on the specific situation.

In summary, teachers should encourage flexibility in strategy use and encourage structured reflection on clinical encounters. Teaching strategies for this lesson learned are displayed in Table 2-3.[41]

Reflection Moment

What strategies did you find most valuable from Lesson 2? How can you apply them to your teaching and learning? What challenges do you see in doing so?

TABLE 2-3

TEACHING STRATEGIES FOR INCREASING FLEXIBILITY IN CLINICAL REASONING

- Teach both processes (nonanalytic and analytic) and multiple strategies leveraging strengths as opposed to weaknesses.
- Think out loud to demonstrate your own reasoning strategies (pretend as if you have no frontal lobe, and state what comes to mind).
- Encourage use of knowledge-based cognitive forcing strategies for improving cognitive errors.

Adapted from Ledford and Nixon.[41]

Lesson 3: Clinical Reasoning Expert Performance Requires Prolonged and Deliberate Effort

The notion of prolonged effort is based on the theory of deliberate practice, which describes expert performance emerging over 10 years, or 10,000 hours of training in a specific field.[15] This practice should be designed, purposeful, and demanding. Early in training, learners do not know what such practice entails. Thus, the role of the teacher is best described as a coach. The teaching "coach" should provide clear goals and objectives, as well as practice exercises, that enable a learner to develop CR. Ideally, the coach has a longitudinal relationship with the learner to monitor CR ability over time and provide learner-specific feedback.

Reflection Moment

Do you view yourself as a teacher or coach? Does your role change with your peers and/or patients? If the former, would changing your viewpoint impact your teaching and learning? If so, how?

Coaches should understand key concepts related to CR and recognize that it is a complex learning task. For this type of learning, whole-task practice is essential to the development of CR, but it must be supplemented by part-task practice.[62] For example, one could teach individual sessions on history taking, physical examination, and the anatomy and pathophysiology of the shoulder (ie, part tasks), but without an integrative session on the approach to shoulder pain, students would likely struggle to master the "whole-task" ability to diagnose rotator cuff disease or glenohumeral arthritis. We would suggest that teachers should ensure that whole-task training exercises begin early, with a gradual increase as learners move closer to clinical practice (Figure 2-1).[62]

Reflection Moment

How would you design whole-task training for your more novice learners, given their limited knowledge base?

Once learners begin to understand what expert CR performance looks like through coaching and practice exercises, coaches should ensure that students "learn to learn" CR by encouraging them to apply self-regulated learning principles (Figure 2-2).[63] Self-regulated learning closely parallels deliberate practice. In self-regulated learning, students should set objectives for performing a task (eg, admit a patient with chest pain), choose strategies to help them achieve those objectives, monitor performance, and reflect on performance after task completion.[64] How will you employ your "before, during, and after" thinking in CR to alter your self-regulation?

Reflection Moment

Do you explicitly teach your learners (including your patients/clients) how to learn? How can you apply self-regulated learning theory to help your learners become better physical therapists/specialists, and/or more compliant as patients/clients, and/or more critical scholars?

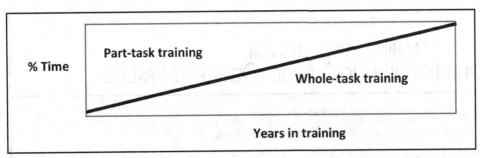

Figure 2-1. Emphasis on type of deliberate practice over training time.

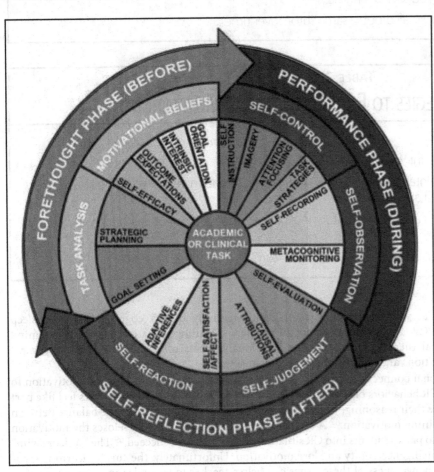

Figure 2-2. Self-regulated learning cycle. (Reprinted with permission from Artino AR Jr, Jones KD. AM last page: self-regulated learning—a dynamic, cyclical perspective. *Acad Med.* 2013;88[7]:1048, as adapted from Zimmerman BJ. Attaining self-regulation: a social cognitive perspective. In: Boekaerts M, Pintrich PR, Zeidner M, eds. *Handbook of Self-Regulation.* San Diego, CA: Academic Press; 2000.)

In some studies, successful application of self-regulated learning principles can account for as much as 90% of performance variation in noncomplex tasks.[65] Coaches can supplement learners' reflections-on-action with feedback, and learners should seek to calibrate their CR by following up on any patients' diagnoses and outcomes that are not obvious at the end of the clinical encounter. We will further discuss self-assessment concepts as applied for self-regulated learning for CR in Chapter 3.

In summary (Table 2-4), developing expert performance in CR requires deliberate practice. Teachers can help learners in these tasks by acting as coaches and teaching them how to learn.

Lesson 4: Clinical Reasoning Is Impacted by Motivation and Emotion

Traditionally, the teaching of CR focused only on cognitive processes, such as knowledge organization and reasoning strategies. However, this view of CR is incomplete. So how might motivation and emotion inform the teaching of CR?

Fields outside of medicine have stressed how "noncognitive" factors, such as motivation and emotion, are essential to CR performance (Table 2-5). Emotion and/or motivation influence our cognitive processes (ie, how we perceive, interpret, and act on information).[66] Working memory allocation is directed by motivation and emotion,[43] so these can improve working memory and, likely, deliberate practice capacity. Internal motivation emerges from a sense of purpose, autonomy, and mastery or self-efficacy, which can result in positive emotions.[67,68] Optimizing the learn-

---

TABLE 2-4
TEACHING STRATEGIES FOR PROMOTING EXPERT PERFORMANCE THROUGH DELIBERATE PRACTICE

- Act like a coach. Teach what activities to practice and in what situation.
- Teach students and patients/clients how to learn (self-regulated learning theory).
- Provide frequent, specific but limited feedback over time.
- Encourage longitudinal mentoring (eg, small groups, same tutors over time).

TABLE 2-5
TEACHING STRATEGIES TO ENHANCE INTERNAL MOTIVATION

- Optimize the learning environment.
  - Teach CR using engaging and relevant work activities.
  - Provide appropriate support to maintain learners' sense of self-efficacy and increase responsibility as learners progress in knowledge and ability.
- Capitalize on emotion with learning (tell a meaningful story [eg, patients, peers, former roles] and consider having learners teach each other).
- Consider how emotional and other situational clues may prompt learning and future performance.

---

ing environment to engender these feelings, as well as reducing factors that negatively impact cognitive load (eg, sleep deprivation and burnout), may help improve CR and its development in learners. Meaningful patient stories can remind learners of their purpose in choosing physical therapy. Debriefing the emotional aspects of positive or negative clinical encounters may help learners process their emotions and channel them in a positive way.

In addition, positive relationships and personal connections can also provide a strong source of purpose and motivation to learners because they will seek to emulate the CR behaviors of their supervisors. These relationships make learners feel like part of the team, and make them more likely to share their reasoning, which is essential to teaching CR. Finding the balance between supervision and autonomy is critical to maintaining motivation.[67] A learner who feels no autonomy often loses the motivation to learn. Regarding self-efficacy, teachers need to place students into CR situations where they can succeed.[69] The "sink or swim" approach can lead a learner to doubt her/his intelligence/ability and lose motivation. Unfortunately, the current learning environment is often less than optimal. However, an awareness of these issues can help a teacher to engender an environment that promotes internal motivation and positive emotions in learners.

Reflection Moment

What motivational and/or emotional strategies did you find most valuable? How can you apply the methods with your teaching and learning? What challenges do you see in doing so?

Lesson 5: Clinical Reasoning Is Context Specific

A more recent lesson in the medical education literature is emerging regarding context specificity (Table 2-6), which recognizes the need to teach and assess CR content and situations (or contexts) broadly.[70] The literature suggests that we should use the phrase "CR expert performance" as opposed to "CR expertise." In other words, expert performance is displayed in the specific situation (eg, clinic encounter) as opposed to being something inherent to the health professional. It is more a context-dependent state than a context-independent trait of a given health care professional. This final lesson impacts each of the previous 4 lessons, and educators should incorporate context specificity as each of the lessons are implemented. As educators develop both curricular and assessment strategies, as well as perform direct teaching, educators should account for situational factors,

---

TABLE 2-6
TEACHING STRATEGIES THAT ADDRESS CONTEXT SPECIFICITY

- Teach and assess CR with diverse cases across multiple diseases and health-related conditions in a broad array of patients and contexts.
- Stress to learners that expert performance is a dynamic state and requires lifelong learning rather than a static achievement.

---

such as the learner factors (eg, sleep deprivation), patient factors (eg, non-English speaker), environmental resources and influences, and the complex interactions among the learner, patient, and environment. For example, teaching differential diagnoses for rotator cuff syndromes should be done with cases involving each of the muscles with patients with different risk factors and in different settings. Such broad experiences have a greater chance of improving a learner's CR ability and also provide the teacher with a more accurate assessment of her or his performance.

Reflection Moment

How does knowledge of context specificity impact the manner and/or way that you teach and assess CR?

CONCLUSION

The recognition of diagnostic error as a leading cause of death has forced us to scrutinize how we teach CR. The theories and lessons from the literature described in this chapter provide valuable insights into potential strategies for teaching and learning CR. By employing these lessons, we have the potential to improve CR in our learners and reduce diagnostic and clinical decision errors. Perhaps the most valuable take-home point is to behave like a coach by demonstrating CR through "thinking aloud," providing "practice" and feedback to improve, and motivating learners through encouragement. While the physical therapy profession will have to continue to explore and uncover the unique elements of CR for physical therapists, we believe that the lessons learned from medical education have much to offer physical therapy in this journey. Now, just as a refresher, as you continue to embark on your own self-discovery of CR capabilities for practice, please keep in mind these five key lessons learned:

Five Clinical Reasoning Lessons Learned (Key Authors)

1. Requires rich, content-specific, and organized knowledge (Barrows, Fetlock, Schmidt, Bordage, Custers)
2. Requires a number of strategies and flexibility of strategy use (Schuwirth, Higgs, Ericsson)
3. Requires prolonged and deliberate effort (Durning, Ericsson)
4. Impacted by motivation and emotion (Artino, Kusurkar, Ten Cate)
5. Is context specific (state vs trait) (Eva, Norman)

REFERENCES

1. Makary MA, Daniel M. Medical error-the third leading cause of death in the US. *BMJ.* 2016;353:i2139.
2. Balogh EP, Miller BT, Ball JR. *Improving Diagnosis in Health Care.* Washington, DC: National Academies Press; 2016.
3. Schuwirth L. Is assessment of clinical reasoning still the holy grail? *Med Educ.* 2009;43(4):298-300.
4. Durning SJ, Artino Jr AR, Schuwirth L, van der Vleuten C. Clarifying assumptions to enhance our understanding and assessment of clinical reasoning. *Acad Med.* 2013;88(4):442-448.
5. Ilgen JS, Eva KW, Regehr G. What's in a label? Is diagnosis the start or the end of clinical reasoning? *J Gen Intern Med.* 2016;31(4):435-437.
6. Young ME, personal communication, September 2017.
7. Ratcliffe TA, Durning SJ. Theoretical concepts to consider in providing clinical reasoning instruction. In: Trowbridge RL, Rencic J, Durning SJ, eds. *Teaching Clinical Reasonig.* Philadelphia, PA: American College of Physicians; 2015.

8. Kahneman D. *Thinking, Fast and Slow.* New York, NY: Farrar, Strauss and Giroux; 2011.
9. Eva KW. What every teacher needs to know about clinical reasoning. *Med Educ.* 2005;39(1):98-106.
10. Ericsson KA, Charness N, Hoffman RR, Feltovich PJ. *Cambridge Handbook of Expertise and Expert Performance.* New York, NY: Cambridge University Press; 2006.
11. Miller GA. The magical number seven, plus or minus two: some limits on our capacity for processing information. *Psychol Rev.* 1956;63(2):81.
12. Schmidt HG, Rikers RM. How expertise develops in medicine: knowledge encapsulation and illness script formation. *Med Educ.* 2007;41:1133-1139.
13. Custers EJ. Thirty years of illness scripts: theoretical origins and practical applications. *Med Teach.* 2015;37(5):457-462.
14. van Merrienboer J, Sweller J. Cognitive load theory and complex learning: recent developments and future directions. *Educ Psychol Rev.* 2005;17:147-177.
15. Ericsson KA. Deliberate practice and the acquisition and maintenance of expert performance in medicine and related domains. *Acad Med.* 2004;79(10):S70-S81.
16. de Groot AD. *Thought and Choice in Chess.* 2nd ed. The Hague, Netherlands: Mouton Publishers; 1978.
17. Durning SJ, Artino AR. Situativity theory: a perspective on how participants and the environment can interact: AMEE guide no. 52. *Med Teach.* 2011;33(3):188-199.
18. McCarthy WH, Gonnella JS. The simulated patient management problem: a technique for evaluating and teaching clinical competence. *Med Educ.* 1967;1(5):348-352.
19. Rimoldi HJA. Rationale and applications of the test of diagnostic skills. *J Med Educ.* 1963;38:364-368.
20. Elstein AS, Shulman LS, Sprafka SA. Medical problem solving: an analysis of clinical reasoning. Cambridge, MA: Harvard University Press; 1978.
21. Eva KW. On the generality of specificity. *Med Educ.* 2003;37(7):587-588.
22. Eva KW, Neville AJ, Norman GR. Exploring the etiology of content specificity: factors influencing analogic transfer and problem solving. *Acad Med.* 1998;73(10):S1-S5.
23. Pauker SG, Gorry GA, Kassirer JP, Schwartz WB. Towards the simulation of clinical cognition: taking a present illness by computer. *Am J Med.* 1976;60(7):981-996.
24. Rosch E, Lloyd BB, eds. *Cognition and Categorization.* Hillsdale, NJ: Lawrence Erlbaum Associates; 1978.
25. Abbott V, Black JB, Smith EE. The representation of scripts in memory. *J Mem Lang.* 1985;24(2):179-199.
26. Charlin B, Boshuizen H, Custers EJ, Feltovich PJ. Scripts and clinical reasoning. *Med Educ.* 2007;41(12):1178-1184.
27. Tversky A, Kahneman D. Judgment under uncertainty: heuristics and biases. *Science.* 1974;184:1124-1131.
28. Sweller J, Van Merrienboer JJ, Paas FG. Cognitive architecture and instructional design. *Educ Psychol Rev.* 1998;10(3):251-296.
29. Durning SJ, Artino AR, Boulet JR, Dorrance K, van der Vleuten C, Schuwirth L. The impact of selected contextual factors on experts' clinical reasoning performance (does context impact clinical reasoning performance in experts?). *Adv Health Sci Educ Theory Pract.* 2012;17(1):65-79.
30. Norman GR, Tugwell P, Feightner JW, Muzzin LJ, Jacoby LL. Knowledge and clinical problem-solving. *Med Educ.* 1985;19(5):344-356.
31. Durning SJ, Artino AR, Schuwirth L, van der Vleuten C. Clarifying assumptions to enhance our understanding and assessment of clinical reasoning. *Acad Med.* 2013;88(4):442-448.
32. Durning SJ, Artino AR. Situativity theory: a perspective on how participants and the environment can interact: AMEE Guide no. 52. *Med Teach.* 2011;33(3):188-199.
33. Kassirer JP. Teaching clinical reasoning: case-based and coached. *Acad Med.* 2010;85(7):1118-1124.
34. Trowbridge RL, Rencic JJ, Durning SJ. *Teaching Clinical Reasoning.* Philadelphia, PA: ACP Press; 2015.
35. Steward D, Bordage G, Lemieux M. Semantic structures and diagnostic thinking of experts and novices. *Acad Med.* 1991;66(9):S70-S72.
36. Roediger III HL, Karpicke JD. Test-enhanced learning: taking memory tests improves long-term retention. *Psychol Science.* 2006;17(3):249-255.
37. Bordage G. Prototypes and semantic qualifiers: from past to present. *Med Educ.* 2007;41(12):1117-1121.
38. Bowen JL. Educational strategies to promote clinical diagnostic reasoning. *N Engl J Med.* 2006;355:2217-2225.
39. Bordage G. Elaborated knowledge: a key to successful diagnostic thinking. *Acad Med.* 1994;69(11):883-885.
40. Christensen N, Jones MA, Edwards I, Higgs J. Helping physiotherapy students learn clinical reasoning. In: Higgs J, Jones M, Loftus S, Christensen N, eds. *Clinical Reasoning in the Health Professions.* 3rd ed. Amsterdam, Netherlands: Butterworth-Heinemann Elsevier; 2008.
41. Ledford CH, Nixon LJ. General teaching techniques. In: Trowbridge RL, Rencic J, Durning SJ, eds. *Teaching Clinical Reasoning.* Philadelphia, PA: American College of Physicians; 2015.
42. Schmidt HG, Mamede S. How to improve the teaching of clinical reasoning: a narrative review and a proposal. *Med Educ.* 2015;49(10):961-973.
43. Shell DF, Brooks DW, Trainin G, et al. How the ULM fits. In: Shell DF, Brooks DW, Trainin G, et al, eds. *The Unified Learning Model: How Motivational, Cognitive, and Neurobiological Sciences Inform Best Teaching Practices.* Heidelberg, Germany: Springer; 2010:85-111.
44. Mamede S, van Gog T, Moura AS, et al. Reflection as a strategy to foster medical students' acquisition of diagnostic competence. *Med Educ.* 2012;46(5):464-472.
45. Chamberland M, Mamede S. Self-explanation, an instructional strategy to foster clinical reasoning in medical students. *Health Prof Educ.* 2015;1(1):24-33.
46. Torre DM, Durning SJ, Daley BJ. Twelve tips for teaching with concept maps in medical education. *Med Teach.* 2013;35(3):201-208.

47. Mayer RE. Applying the science of learning to medical education. *Med Educ.* 2010;44(6):543-549.
48. Ten Cate O, Durning S. Peer teaching in medical education: twelve reasons to move from theory to practice. *Med Teach.* 2007;29(6):591-599.
49. Van Merriënboer JJ, Sweller J. Cognitive load theory in health professional education: design principles and strategies. *Med Educ.* 2010;44(1):85-93.
50. Custers EJ. Medical education and cognitive continuum theory: an alternative perspective on medical problem solving and clinical reasoning. *Acad Med.* 2013;88(8):1074-1080.
51. Eva KW, Hatala RM, LeBlanc VR, Brooks LR. Teaching from the clinical reasoning literature: combined reasoning strategies help novice diagnosticians overcome misleading information. *Med Educ.* 2007;41(12):1152-1158.
52. Richardson WS. Integrating evidence into clinical diagnosis. In: Camacho PM, Gharib H, Sizemore GW, eds. *Evidence-Based Endocrinology.* 2nd ed. New York, NY: Lippincott Williams, & Wilkins; 2006.
53. Richardson WS. We should overcome the barriers to evidence-based clinical diagnosis! *J Clin Epidemiol.* 2007;60(3):217-227.
54. Graber ML. Educational strategies to reduce diagnostic error: can you teach this stuff? *Adv Health Sci Educ Theory Pract.* 2009;14(1):63-69.
55. Graber ML, Kissam S, Payne VL, et al. Cognitive interventions to reduce diagnostic error: a narrative review. *BMJ Qual Saf.* 2012;21(7):535-557.
56. Reilly JB. Educational approaches to common cognitive errors. In: Trowbridge RL, Rencic J, Durning SJ, eds. *Teaching Clinical Reasoning.* Philadelphia, PA: American College of Physicians; 2015.
57. Croskerry P. The importance of cognitive errors in diagnosis and strategies to minimize them. *Acad Med.* 2003;78(8):775-780.
58. Croskerry P. Cognitive forcing strategies in clinical decision making. *Ann Emerg Med.* 2003;41(1):110-120.
59. Norman GR, Monteiro SD, Sherbino J, Ilgen JS, Schmidt HG, Mamede S. The causes of errors in clinical reasoning: cognitive biases, knowledge deficits, and dual process thinking. *Acad Med.* 2017;92(1):23-30.
60. Mamede S, Schmidt HG. Reflection in medical diagnosis: a literature review. *Health Prof Educ.* 2017;3(1):15-25.
61. Mamede S, Van Gog T, Sampaio AM, et al. How can students' diagnostic competence benefit most from practice with clinical cases? The effects of structured reflection on future diagnosis of the same and novel diseases. *Acad Med.* 2014;89(1):121-127.
62. Van Merriënboer JJ, Clark RE, De Croock MB. Blueprints for complex learning: the 4C/ID-model. *Educ Technol Res Dev.* 2002;50(2):39-61.
63. Artino AR Jr, Jones KD. AM last page: self-regulated learning—a dynamic, cyclical perspective. *Acad Med.* 2013;88(7):1048.
64. Sandars J, Cleary TJ. Self-regulation theory: applications to medical education: AMEE Guide No. 58. *Med Teach.* 2011;33(11):875-886.
65. Kitsantas A, Zimmerman BJ. Comparing self-regulatory processes among novice, non-expert, and expert volleyball players: a microanalytic study. *J App Sport Psychol.* 2002;14(2):91-105.
66. McConnell MM, Eva KW. The role of emotion in the learning and transfer of clinical skills and knowledge. *Acad Med.* 2012;87(10):1316-1322.
67. Artino AR Jr, Holmboe ES, Durning SJ. Control-value theory: using achievement emotions to improve understanding of motivation, learning, and performance in medical education: AMEE Guide No. 64. *Med Teach.* 2012;34(3):e148-e160.
68. Pink DH. *Drive: The Surprising Truth About What Motivates Us.* New York, NY: Penguin; 2011.
69. Zimmerman BJ. Self-efficacy: an essential motive to learn. *Contemp Educ Psychol.* 2000;25(1):82-91.
70. Durning SJ, Artino AR. Situativity theory: a perspective on how participants and the environment can interact: AMEE guide no. 52. *Med Teach.* 2011;33(3):188-199.

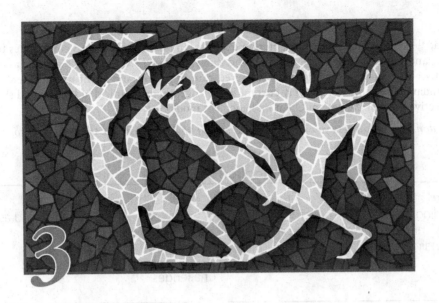

SELF-ASSESSMENT AND REFLECTIVE PRACTICE:
Evolutions for Clinical Reasoning

Gina Maria Musolino, PT, DPT, MSEd, EdD

OBJECTIVES

- Appreciate the theoretical underpinnings and relationship of self-assessment (SA), clinical reasoning (CR), and reflective practice (RP).
- Compare the process of CR models, self-regulated learning, and CR in physical therapy.
- Examine SA and CR concepts and examples.
- Appreciate the barriers and support for SA and CR for RP.
- Evaluate how habits of the mind and questioning strategies support SA, CR, and RP.
- Appraise potential CR bias errors.
- Synthesize newly acquired SA, CR, and RP learning with collaborative, person-centered care.

In this chapter, the focus is on SA as a building block and foundational skill for progression to Schön's[1-3] concept of RP. One must first look within to know thyself, to be self-aware. From self-awareness of one's skills, abilities, professionalism, and practice capacities comes the ability for RP. Drawing upon entry-level skills in SA and progressing through to becoming a "mature" reflective practitioner is emphasized for the professional in development. Discussion of the ability to self-assess one's application of CR with current knowledge, theory, and clinical judgment, and the patient's values and beliefs, are key discussion points within the CR cycles.[4] Considerations for critical reflection and considering the whole person, while recognizing limits for both the learner and profession, are emphasized. Classic theoretical foundations drawn upon and discussed include Schön,[1-3] Kolb,[5,6]

Musolino GM, Jensen GM, eds. *Clinical Reasoning and Decision-Making in Physical Therapy: Facilitation, Assessment, and Implementation* (pp 23-39).

Dewey,[7,8] and Bandura,[9-12] leading into the next chapter on expertise in practice. Chapter 3 emphasizes the need for the ability to self-assess, integrate, and reintegrate one's CR abilities, and know one's owns values and beliefs as a health care provider, to understand others' values and perspectives for person-centered care in patient and client management.[13,14] SA is definitively linked with CR as a fundamental construct to apply current knowledge, theory, clinical judgment and the patient's/client's values, beliefs, and perspectives within the patient/client management model.

It ain't what you don't know that gets you into trouble. It's what you know for sure that just ain't so. —Mark Twain

---

Reflection Moment

Reflect on this quote by Mark Twain for a moment, and then describe 2 assumptions and 2 challenges that you have regarding SA and CR. Discuss these with a peer or colleague. Keep these in mind as you continue your CR journey through the text, and especially this chapter, with respect to SA. Revisit at the end of the chapter to ascertain any changes or updates.

Assumptions   Challenges

1. _____   1. _____

2. _____   2. _____

SELF-ASSESSMENT FOR REFLECTIVE PRACTICE

Fundamentally, SA is the ability to assess one's own skills, to identify one's own educational needs, to evaluate one's own progress, and to determine one's performance.[15] SA requires one to not just be minimally qualified, but also to be seeking an "ever-more perfect understanding and performance of one's work."[16(p24)] To achieve the ability to be an RP,[1-3] one must be capable of honest SA as a stepping stone toward RP, with SA that is unencumbered by barriers.[14]

RP is rooted in the enlightenment theory and defined by Brookfield[17] as being able to "stand outside of ourselves and come to a clearer understanding of what we do and who we are by freeing ourselves of distorted ways of reasoning and acting. There are also elements that allow us to be in objective discoverable limbo."[17(p214)] Kirby and Teddlie[18] take RP a step further for the developing professional, indicating that one must have the ability to "integrate research with practice in response to the uncertainty and complexity that qualifies the practitioner for professional status."[18(p5)] This is vital in professions such as physical therapy, where theory is incomplete or where multiple, even conflicting, theories confront the practitioner.

According to Klevans et al,[19] the purpose of SA is to guide professionals to "better understand their learning needs so they can tailor their plans for professional development."[19(p17)] Using external profession-based criteria such as the American Physical Therapy Association (APTA) Clinical Performance Instrument (CPI), APTA Professionalism in Core Values Self-Assessment, and the Professional Behaviors for the 21st Century, provide learners a framework to begin to self-test against professional criteria to ascertain their learning needs. However, professional learners will initially be unconsciously incompetent in their SA abilities, as they have never before been professionals and do not have an appropriate barometer. Novice SA is generally over- or underestimated. Often revealing affective domain concerns, if it persists, it may likely be indicative of low self-esteem or inflated egos.

Self-esteem also relates back to self-regulation as a learner (see Figure 2-2) as a component of self-efficacy, which we use in the forethought phase of our clinical practice. Self-esteem is an important component of self-efficacy, for what motivates us to then perform again and again, then later reflect, in the regenerating cycle as a self-regulated learner. Hence, learners having challenges with self-esteem should seek assistance and guidance with their faculty, clinical faculty, student mental health services, and counseling as needed. Professionals in training should not hesitate to seek help for this fundamentally important aspect of their professional development. As many practicing professionals will also share with you, a little help goes a long way for a smart professional, and most of us need assistance in this area from time to time due to the many stressors of just being a day-to-day health care professional in today's complex health care systems.

Over time, with practice, those performing SA become more consciously competent and utilize their peers, faculty and clinical education faculty, mentors, and patients as collaborative partners, to guide their pathway toward RP. The constructive feedback from others calls for improvement of one's strengths, and identification and forthright feedback regarding one's areas for improvement. Learners must master SA relating to contemporary expectations of practice and meeting the needs and responsibilities of patients and clients.[13,14,20-23] Learners should thrive on feedback and seek the gift of feedback in relation to their own SA.

In Chapter 5, Delany and Edwards will expound on the ethical aspects of professional practice for us. Westberg and Jason[24] also note how the process of SA is inextricably linked to achieving the maximum benefit from professional education for stu-

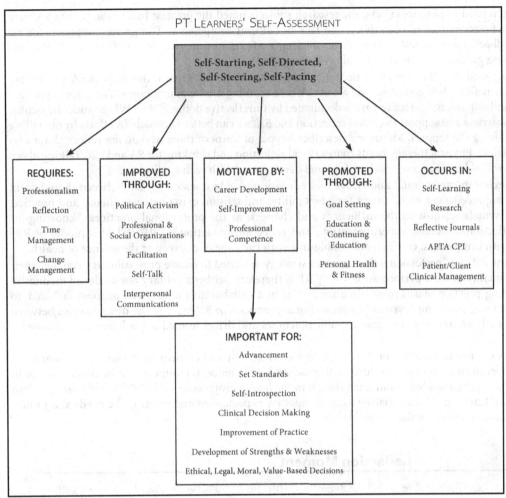

PT LEARNERS' SELF-ASSESSMENT

Self-Starting, Self-Directed,
Self-Steering, Self-Pacing

REQUIRES:
Professionalism
Reflection
Time
Management
Change
Management

IMPROVED THROUGH:
Political Activism
Professional &
Social Organizations
Facilitation
Self-Talk
Interpersonal
Communications

MOTIVATED BY:
Career Development
Self-Improvement
Professional
Competence

PROMOTED THROUGH:
Goal Setting
Education &
Continuing
Education
Personal Health
& Fitness

OCCURS IN:
Self-Learning
Research
Reflective Journals
APTA CPI
Patient/Client
Clinical Management

IMPORTANT FOR:
Advancement
Set Standards
Self-Introspection
Clinical Decision Making
Improvement of Practice
Development of Strengths & Weaknesses
Ethical, Legal, Moral, Value-Based Decisions

Figure 3-1. Musolino's conceptual model of SA. This figure represents the evolution of SA for developing physical therapist learners and the reciprocal determinism that occurs from the influence of the self, the environment, and one's own behaviors.[10,13-14] (Reprinted with permission from Musolino GM. Fostering reflective practice: self-assessment abilities of physical therapy students and entry-level graduates. *J Allied Health.* 2006;35[1]:30-42.)

dents to become safer and ethical providers of health care. Reflection and SA are fundamental to initiating appropriate self-directed learning and change. RP and SA must be cultivated and rewarded, and this takes some time in the already-hectic health professions. However, these collaborative efforts must be implemented to facilitate future professionals from:

> *Mindlessly repeating bad habits and failing to learn from their experiences ... Without the capabilities for SA the performance of professionals is at risk of stagnating, even deteriorating. Many of our health professions education, unfortunately, promote unreflective doing and mitigate against the kind of openness and trust needed for practicing and refining the skills of SA.*[24(pp278,281)]

Orest[25] first examined SA in physical therapist practice, and further refined the definition as "the clinicians' ability to assess their own skills, identify their own educational needs, and to evaluate one's progress, and be able to determine their own strengths and weaknesses of their own performance."[25(p51)] Four practicing physical therapist subjects participated in semistructured interviews, then Orest[25] identified 3 qualitative themes of SA: competence, patient outcome, and professional development as related to the clinicians' desires to improve their SA. Orest also found 4 prerequisites for SA in practicing physical therapists: self-starting, self-directed, self-paced, and self-steering. SA is no easy task, and novices may be caught up in mere survival in the fast-paced clinical environments. Therefore, it is important for all educators to find time, space, and places for SA, or the skill transference is likely not going to occur. The educator must promote active learning with students in professional development.[5-8] This is where the educator must effectively be the "guide on the side, not the sage on the stage."[26(pp30-35)]

Musolino[13,14] further explored SA capacities in both students and entry-level physical therapist graduates. She discovered core themes that emerged pertaining to specific aspects of SA, including requirements, areas for improvement, motivational and promotion factors, and activities that facilitate SA. Participants exhibited SA abilities, encountering obstacles and support, which are important to health care professionals, educators, and clinical faculty. Training needs were identified for physical therapist learners and for clinical and academic faculty.[13,14] These findings parallel with Schön's[1-3] concept of RP and Bandura's[9] Social Learning Theory. SA was improved and promoted through self-starting, self-steering, self-directed, and self-pacing activities (like Orest's[25] findings), with subjects' motivation for professional competence and self-improvement.[13,14] A resulting conceptual model of SA developed, illustrating the reciprocal determinism[9,10] that occurs in developing physical therapist professionals: the world and a person's behavior influence each other, or simply that one's environment causes behavior and behavior impacts the environment, likewise (Figure 3-1).

Musolino[13,14] discovered that, related to practice effects, the research subjects noted the greatest barriers for doing SA were time, complacency, negativity, self-esteem, lack of objectivity, and lack of cultural competence. The greatest supports for SA were taking the time, seeking feedback, being honest and objective, creating a safe environment for feedback, setting goals, supportive peers and faculty, and using guides for written and oral assessments.[13,14]

Westberg and Jason further expound that "Learners who do not value or who are not effective at the skills of SA and RP are unlikely to extract the maximum benefit of their education and are at risk for becoming unsafe practitioners. There are major barriers to learners being reflective and self-assessing. Health care is dominated by unreflective doing."[24(p27)] When students, faculty, and clinical faculty recognize the barriers and support to critical reflection and SA, we can better approach SA efforts by not falling prey to the barriers and by maximizing the support. Mezirow[27] describes 3 types of learners: those who do not reflect, those who reflect, and those who critically reflect. Physical therapy needs more critical reflection and thinking for SA and CR. Talking about how to do this and practicing SA will aid in your continued professional development with each application.

Schön[1,3] argued that a crisis exists in professional knowledge and education, due to a widening gap between thought and action. Today, there remains an unprecedented requirement for adaptability, and tension exists between theory and practice. Schön[2] contemplates how professionals readjust to the influences and changes, as the professional practices, "knowing-in-action, recognizing surprise, reflection-in-action, experimentation, and reflection-on-action."[2(pp119-140)] This model of RP[2] combines the art of health care with uniqueness, conflict, and ambiguity, with the zone of mastery or the science of health.

Osterman and Kottkamp define RP as a "professional development strategy designed to enable professionals to change their behavior, thereby improving the quality of their performance"[28(p66)] RP is therefore neither a solitary nor a relaxed meditative process. Rather, RP is a demanding practice that is most often successful in a collaborative mode. The purpose is 2-fold: to initiate a behavioral change and to realize an improvement in professional practice. An RP exposes the discrepancies between theory and practice, and creates a self-awareness of the unacceptable outcomes and drives toward a new behavioral change for development.

Much of what the future clinician needs to know for practice is not even known and consequently cannot necessarily be taught. Students do not begin to learn until asking questions of themselves.[5-8,23] Hence, the importance in education lies in being able to teach learners how to acquire knowledge and learn from it in the health professions.[13,14,17,20-23,26-29] Learners must master how to self-assess their own learning abilities relating to contemporary expectations and meeting the needs and professional responsibilities for the patients and society they serve.[13,14,20-23]

Reflection Moment

Let's stop for a moment and consider, as a result of your learning thus far in this chapter, whether as a teacher or learner or both, 2 ways in which you will change your SA in the classroom, in the clinic, on your own, and/or with your peers and colleagues. Make a commitment, jot down your ideas, and revisit.

1. _____

2. _____

In Figure 2-2, we examined the self-regulating aspects of learning and how we self-reflect, especially during and after clinical case encounters. As was shared by Durning and Rencic, through these encounters, we tend to rely more on self-control and self-observation while focusing our attention on tasks and thinking in metacognitive ways. Afterward, we rely more on self-reaction and self-judgment to guide us in our self-satisfaction, self-evaluation, and adaptations. Critical SA is made up of these components of self-judgment, self-evaluation, and adaptations. You should now be making these connections for why SA is important for RP and best expert performance in clinical practice.

Reflection Moment

Next, let's consider 1 or 2 of the statements below (eg, select statements A and D, or B and C, or any 2 statements you desire), and jot down a few impressions regarding your thoughts about the statement. Discuss your ideas about the statements with 2 to 3 of your peers or your faculty. Compare the concepts you elected to focus on with others' impressions.

Conceptual Statements

A. "An integral aspect of effective instruction planning is determining the questions to pose in class. Asking good questions is a sophisticated skill that needs practice and thoughtful planning."

B. "Effective instruction strives to take advantage of information obtained from all question types to improve learning."

C. "Both long-term and short-term instructional goals must influence the questions that are posed in class and their frequency."

D. "Both implicitly and explicitly, the content of a question is driven by a teacher's sense of what is important for learners to know and be able to do."

E. "Educators should include questions that are directed toward evaluating students' thinking. The educator's questions must give learners an opportunity to communicate their reasoning processes. These types of questions allow the educator to gather detailed data on how students think and what they learn from instruction."

Impressions

1. _____

2. _____

3. _____

These key concepts help to further elucidate that a shift in the classroom and clinical education needs to occur—we need to consider guiding questions to facilitate the learner's development for ourselves, our students, and our peers. Consider these simple guiding queries: "Can you consider another approach? Is there another way? What led you to go about it in that manner? What is your rationale for doing this test/intervention?" Instead of giving facts, we need to ask questions that lead to the facts, turning our teaching thoughts into guiding questions.

Peers should also work on this approach in their learning dyads and triads. We should be asking questions that require students to analyze, explain their thinking and reasoning, and reflect. We need to provide ample time for processing and thinking. It is not about rushing through multiple cases, but doing a case well and working toward efficiencies as a meaningful learning factor.

Try to use a variety of instructional strategies[5-8] to guide thinking and prepare for questioning. It does not always need to take a lot of time; you can take just 2 minutes to give feedback. Ask the learners verbally, or have them jot down or journal/blog, 2 things they are doing well, and 2 things they think they need to work on—then share your feedback. Get inside the metacognition of your learners. Fast feedback for SA is one way to get started. Then, as the students move along the learning continuum of SA from being consciously incompetent to becoming more consciously competent, build upon this fact and turn the question around. Ask them to name 2 things they would like to work on and 2 things they want to know more about, giving them credit for learning the fundamentals and advancing their learning responsibilities and SA.

Now it is time to reflect again. What are some guiding questions or responses from you as an educator that can encourage, facilitate, and promote SA? How can you facilitate the same in your patients for their progress? To get you started, in Table 3-1,[30-33] we have provided easy access ideas to encourage, promote, and facilitate SA for CR.[30-33] Some questions are more challenging than others; depending on the goal, you will want to match the level of question with where your learner or learning is on the learning curve, or challenge to the next level.

TABLE 3-1
ENCOURAGE, PROMOTE, AND FACILITATE SELF-ASSESSMENT FOR CLINICAL REASONING

Let's explore this …	How did you test out your theories?
Let's think this through …	What is still your muddiest point?
What happened? What were you thinking?	What were you feeling?
What did you learn?	Why did it happen?
How could you have approached it differently?	Describe what you think you do well.
Tell me about what you were thinking.	How does this compare to … ?
If it occurred again, what would you do differently?	How did the patient respond?
What did you do well? What would you like to improve upon?	How did you know what to do next?
Show me how you came to that decision.	How did it make you feel?
Walk me through your thinking about this.	How was your learning stimulated?
That is one option; let's explore some others.	What got in the way of your learning?
What are some possible outcomes of this approach?	Were you prepared?
Now let's consider all the possible options/solutions/outcomes.	What's next?
What impact did you have on the situation? Was that the intent?	Could it be different?
That is a good thought/answer/response/idea … let's expand on it.	What resources might you need?
Let's consider some alternatives.	Did you have a goal for the encounter?
Let's figure this out.	Would knowing results make a difference?
Tell me about what you have learned so far.	What biases impacted your encounter?
Great question—Where would you find the answer?	How did you tolerate the uncertainty?
Why don't you lead us through that process?	How will you prepare differently?
It's not just about the right answer; it's about the learning process.	What do you think about … ?
Good try; let's try again.	What do you think you need to do now?
Now that you've worked that out, let's try …	How does this compare to your expectation?
You're on the right track. Let's try something more challenging now.	Could it have been different?
Have you considered what would happen if … ?	How much do you trust the information?
What other causes might there be?	What makes you consider this vs that?
That is correct in this situation and for this person, but what if … ?	How might things change?
How do you know that is true? On what do you base your answer?	What else do you need to know?
What would you have done if it had not worked?	What might happen if you tried … ?
What will you do differently next time?	What would you do if the patient refused?

Adapted from Levett-Jones et al,[30] Rubenfeld and Scheffer,[31] Schell,[32] and Musolino and Mostrom.[33]

Reflection Moment

Consider the suggestions in Table 3-1. Note how you will implement these and which queries you believe to be most helpful.

As relayed by McManus,[34] SA provides learners the opportunity to care deeply about their own education, learn from and monitor their own learning, and collaborate and discuss with others to discover and construct new knowledge frameworks for new situations. Learners should be allowed to grapple with scenarios and cases as in real-world practice, and take time to self-assess their own learning through the process. In Chapter 4, Jensen and Christensen will reinforce these learner responsibilities and discuss how these responsibilities impact and inform one another. In Chapter 5, Delany and Edwards ask us to unpack the ethical aspects of CR within our roles in practice. Next we are going to explore ways in which we can continue to promote habits of the mind that will foster our SA abilities for CR.

As we have discovered, SA is comparing oneself with an ideal standard, and may be completed predictively, concurrently (in that moment), or summatively.[35] Concurrent (reflection-in-action) is believed to be a more accurate snapshot of SA than predic-

TABLE 3-2

PROMOTING HABITS OF THE MIND—REFLECTION MOMENT

HABIT	DESCRIPTION	EXAMPLE	YOUR SA REFLECTIONS
Confidence	Ensured of one's reasoning abilities.	My thinking was on track. I reconsidered and still thought I'd made the right decision. Clinical instructor knew my conclusion was well founded.	
Contextual Perspective	Considerate of the whole situation, including relationships, background, situation, and environment.	I took in the whole picture. I was mindful of the situation. I considered the possibilities. I considered the circumstances.	
Creativity	Intellectually inquisitive to generate, discover, or restructure ideas; able to imagine alternatives.	I let my imagination go. I thought "outside the box." I tried to be visionary.	
Intellectual Integrity	Seeking the truth through sincere, honest processes, even if the results are contrary to one's assumptions or beliefs.	Although it went against everything I believed, I needed to get to the truth. I questioned my biases and assumptions. I examined my thinking. I was not satisfied with my original conclusion.	
Intuition	Insightful patterns of knowing brought about by experience and pattern recognition.	I had a hunch. While I couldn't say why, I knew that from the last time this happened that ...	
Perseverance	Pursue learning and determined to overcome obstacles.	I was determined to find out. I would not accept that for an answer. I was persistent.	
Reflective	Contemplative of assumptions, thinking, and action for deeper understanding and self-evaluation.	I pondered my reactions. I considered what I had done and thought. I wondered what I could/should do differently next time. I considered how this would influence my practice.	

Adapted from Levett-Jones et al,[30] Rubenfeld and Scheffer,[31] and Scheffer and Rubenfeld.[36]

tive (reflection-for-action) or summative (reflection-on-action).[2] That is why your instructor may ask you probing queries in the midst of your learning and practice applications. You should do the same, but do not fall into the trap of paralysis by analysis.

Concurrent reflection, building upon Schön's RP model, is essentially reflection-in-action.[2] All 3 types of SA are relevant and important, but concurrent reflection is key to safer practice, and critical for learners to realize when they are beyond their abilities and seek assistance. As CR and clinical problem-solving (CPS) are foundational elements for physical therapy practice, the learner should keep reflection-in-action[2] at the forefront when working on the CR and CPS to ascertain progress and ensure safer practice. "Faking it to make it" is a huge barrier to honest SA and impedes good CR development. As a professional, your CR process depends mightily upon the veracity of your SA abilities, especially in terms of your personal disposition.[36]

Turning your attention to Table 3-2,[30,31,36] the first column provides the actual habit of the mind that we are trying to form, while the second column describes the habit, and the third column shares a learner's reflection on the habit. Please review each habit carefully, then continue your metacognitive development and self-monitoring by completing your own SA in the final column. You may wish to await a future opportunity for self-reflection based on a classroom or clinical case simulation, vignette, or real-world encounter. We encourage you to use the format regularly to promote your own SA for any learning opportunity. Practicing regular SA, promoting habits of the mind, will assist you in your progression toward RP; discussing it with a trusted peer, colleague, or clinical or academic faculty member will further progress your capacities for SA.

CLINICAL REASONING

CR is constantly occurring in clinical practice; indeed, once we are engaged in daily practice, we often are unaware that we are even doing CR. Do you consider yourself good at CR? What is your exposure to others doing CR? Exposure certainly helps for the translation of CR. However, can we do a better job of developing our capabilities for CR; how do we do it, and how do we know it is working?

For example, when we drive a car, we may be on autopilot until it is time to teach a 15-year-old with a permit. Then we quickly realize that the permit learner can steer, step on the brakes, and operate the controls in the car (especially the digital media), but is challenged putting all the pieces together, not only in a timely and responsive manner, but also in taking in the cues from the outside world that impact safety. They are not sure what to pay attention to, what to filter out and not be distracted by, or how the sensation of going from 5 mph to 60 mph and back down to 30 mph, for the first time as a driver, feels oddly like going in reverse.

Novice drivers can be very good with feed-forward actions, abilities, and thinking. They can start the car, know how to make it go faster, and know how to steer right vs left. However, the feedback loop is not inherent; they may not be considering the color of the stoplight, the fact that a pedestrian is still in the crosswalk, out of sync with the time allotted for crossing, and/or the presence of an oncoming car in the passing lane, still within 15 feet of the intersection.

You, on the other hand, as the experienced driver, who may also have benefited from the unfortunate experience of an accident, have much information, background, and exposure to draw upon. You can take in a variety of cues from the internal and external environment to anticipate safer and more defensive driving. In contrast, a novice is still working to put together all the different pre-motor and motor planning steps to arrive alive, and may be unable to process all the scanning cues from the environment. While driver simulation classes and/or virtual reality simulation help with this, it is not the same as a guided scenario with only so many forced choices and the pressure of being in the real world. Sometimes we must be allowed to make errors, or almost make errors, to learn. However, in many cases, safety is of the first concern—and others may need to step in to "take the wheel," as no patient, passenger, or pedestrian should be harmed for someone to learn.

For example, a student on clinical experience in acute care for the first week may be about to be tangled in two of the patient care lines in the simulation room. While we do not want the lines to accidently be "pulled out," we could allow the student to be caught up in the lines momentarily, rather than stop and pre-anticipate, then step in—if safety allows. A first-hand "entanglement" experience teaches volumes and offers ample opportunities for SA. Of course, if this is a live patient care situation, one may need to step in earlier to ensure safety and protect the patient from harm.

The same is true with CR—so many contextual pieces contribute to our abilities in this realm. Many clinicians in health care often make human and system errors that are due not to lack of knowledge and skills, but to the fact that we are not fully communicating and/or clinically reasoning. CR at its core is an activity rather than a cognitive structure or process.[37(p543)] CR is full of integration and re-integration of learning, skills, and abilities, promoted through SA for RP. Nursing has described CR as a logical process by which nurses and other clinicians collect cues, process the information, come to an understanding of a patient problem or situation, plan and implement interventions, evaluate outcomes, and reflect and learn from the process.[4,30] Yet, Levett-Jones[4,30] and her colleagues realize that this CR is not circular or even systematic; rather, it may be reactive, jump steps, and go forward and backward. For the novice, like the novice car driver, there are likely to be efforts to quickly move through a cycle using checklists, with abrupt stops and starts, jumping around, and some weaving (Figure 3-2). As you review the "big picture" of the CR cycle, you will begin to have some pattern recognitions with Figures 1-1 and 2-2. Now continue to consider how each figure is distinctive at the same time.

Often, much deep thought occurs to predict and match what to do as we struggle with SA within our own CR. Deep thought is often based on pattern recognition, past experiences, and learners' own internal systematic approaches. Novice professional learners often do not see the cognitive processes that occur, unless you are truly thinking aloud and sharing your reasoning along the way. Novices often miss the big picture or rely on their preferences rather than the patients' needs.[5-8] Dewey[7,8] often referred to these steps as the often indeterminate, forked-road scenarios where we must make a choice. Physical therapists' CR is clearly not a linear process, but tends to be more reciprocal, often times mosaic, and a constant reintegration (see Figure 1-1). Physical therapy is similar, in the patient/client management process, to the Levett-Jones CR model (see Figure 3-2). As physical therapists move through and shift backward and forward within the CR cycle, we are problem-solving with, for, and about our patients in a collaborative manner. As we move along in the text, we will continue to discuss each of the contributing elements for physical therapy CR.

Person-centered care drives us to work toward better CR abilities, and "thinking out loud" as educators and developing professionals helps to articulate and translate these abilities to others. This involves sharing your thoughts not only with the patient,

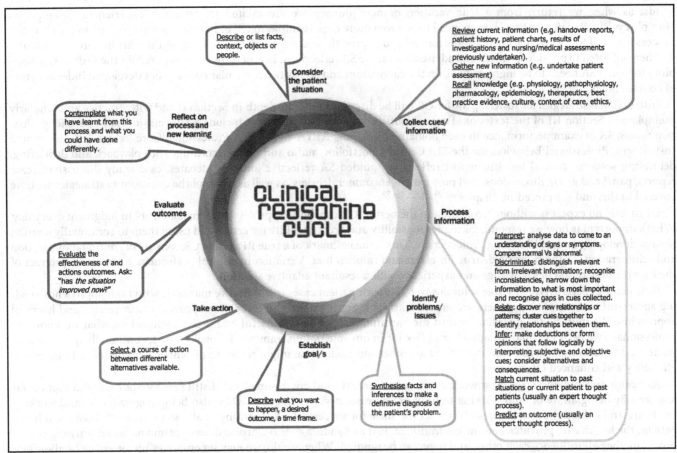

Figure 3-2. Levett-Jones clinical reasoning cycle. (Reprinted with permission from *Nurse Education Today*, 30, Levett-Jones T, Hoffman K, Dempsey J, et al. The "five rights" of clinical reasoning cycle: an educational model to enhance nursing students' ability to identify and manage clinically "at-risk" patients, 515-520, Copyright Elsevier 2010.)

but also with student learners. In Section II, author and educator Wing Fu will share an excellent case example of how this process was implemented to aid a learner to achieve the needed CR skills and capacities to successfully return to the clinical setting.

We often ask learners to stand back and look at the big picture, to help the student recognize the big pictures, patterns, relationships, and concepts, moving from whole to part, and then part to whole again. Students are more comfortable with the parts and the pieces, and are less likely to put them together to make sense of them. It is blurry to the students, and you need to help make it clearer by helping them zoom in and out on key areas of concern to discern the complexities. Letting others hear your SA and thought processes through CR will help.

Within the patient/client management model, what is the emerging big picture for the person-centered care, and where is the breakdown potentially occurring in the students' ability to SA and move toward CR? Consider in the descriptions with the CR model above: How do the cues and findings relate to the patients' story? How are the facts and information related to the potential outcomes? How do the cues impact your impressions? Predict—What is going to happen as a result of doing something? Doing nothing? Watching, waiting, vs intervening? Implementing minimally impacting interventions vs dramatic?

Physical therapist professionals make clinical diagnoses related to the movement system, considering impairments and functional limitations related to a person's disabilities and/or abilities. Goals are then established and related to the problems. Problems and goals should be prioritized and based again on your ability to CR, along with the patient's values, beliefs, and goals. This should be followed by reflection; professionals reflect regularly, and often all the time, so that it is challenging to turn off. Ask any true RP: we are not just CR when we are looking up evidence or chatting about a case. We reflect on our patients (or learners, for that matter) when exercising, swimming, in the shower, commuting, walking, and stopping at a traffic light. We are always working to problem-solve and reason to ensure we are providing the best care for our patients.

Examining the CR cycle when you are struggling, or your learning is struggling, helps break down where in the CR process there are blocks in the road, or detours in the thinking, or skills that may be lacking. While there are many ways to get from point A to point B, some are more efficient and effective, and some may take an inordinate amount of time, but a detour may be necessary. Turning the CR model descriptors into questions as you "talk aloud" with your case applications may also assist in moving CR along the learning continuum. It also gears students up to think about what is next and where they have come from—and remember what they have learned along the journey. Lots of opportunities exist for both feed-forward and feedback discussions for CR and SA processes within the cycle.

Just as when we return from a true vacation or new journey, we are excited to share our experiences. Kramp and Humphreys[38(p83)] maintain that learners need to be given more opportunities to tell of their experience in learning to meet the process needs of SA. These narratives allow for reshaping, growth, and reformulation of ideas in the learning process. Faculty are then obligated to provide feedback and advisement on the SA reflections. Learners must be prepared for the shift in responsibility for SA.[24] SA needs to be ingrained within the curriculum and across the curricular courses, not developed independently of course content.

Instructional strategies for fostering SA for CR will be discussed more in-depth in Section II and with practice and scholarly exemplars in Section III of the textbook. For now, suffice it to say that strategies include SA forms, journals, parallel evaluation forms, SA of exam performance in each domain of learning, APTA CPI, APTA Professional Core Values Self-Assessment Instrument, Professional Behaviors for the 21st Century, portfolios, audio and video recordings with playback and debriefing, debriefing sessions, critical incident report reflections, guided SA reflective journals, debates, case study discussions, case reports, panel and group discussions, and post-patient encounter debriefs, as well as many of the questioning strategies we have covered in this and the preceding chapter.[20,21,24,33,38-52]

Of course, no expert is without error. Even in the best of CR capabilities, professionals make errors in judgment every day. What's important is how we respond, taking responsibility and accountability for errors and using them to continually learn as always-developing and still-learning professionals. This is the hallmark of a true RP. While CR consists of continual integration and reintegration, so the same holds true for errors and implicit bias. Variation in clinical performance remains a product of the expert's integration of knowledge and experience with a resultant adaptive solution.[37]

How can 2 experts arrive at viable solutions, yet approach patient cases in alternative manners, with both approaches yielding successful outcomes? Often, there are many right ways. Yet there are also less safe, unproven, controversial, and harmful approaches. We must be the guardian against the harmful, discern what is useful and useless, and act on what we know. As professionals, we need to remain adaptable and flexible in our integration frameworks, avoid errors, continually question how we arrived at our solutions, and consider if there are other approaches that might serve our patients/clients better, with increased efficiency and enhanced effectiveness.

As health care providers, we must work in changing contexts and environments and still promote our CR and that of our learners. By being aware of (and working to limit or decrease) negative impacts, while also being cognizant of (and working to ensure and enhance) positive supports, we set the stage for successful CR. Durning et al[53] share that CR must include the patient, the health care provider, and the environment. Just as Bandura's[9-12] reciprocal determinism and social learning theory proclaim, they all influence each other, and none can be ignored. When we do, we may set ourselves up for errors or allow bias to become prejudice in our thinking or doing. As Epstein[54] implored, we must be mindful practitioners, and the process of SA helps to ensure we are continually mindful. Further, as Scott relays, everyone makes mistakes, but greater awareness of the causes will assist clinicians in avoiding errors as much as humanly possible.[55(p338)]

Now we ask that you turn your attention to Table 3-3.[30,55-58] As a developing RP, you will want to work to debias your thinking and actions by being aware of these CR bias errors. Realize, too, that if you are making a lot of errors in CR, you may need to manage your personal stress and any pressures or negativity that may impact your ability to be as objective as possible. Stress management is key for all health care professionals, and being able to SA when you need to get back in balance is also key to being a strong RP.[41] Thinking out loud through your CR process will assist you in your SA and peer assessment. Sharing your thinking with your clinical and faculty educators will also open a window to your CR and allow them a greater opportunity to facilitate your CR progress, working from the snapshot of where you are in your thinking and reasoning. Allow adequate time to receive constructive feedback on your CR. Remember to always keep your patient at the forefront of your CR and collaborate with them to discuss your impressions and plans to achieve the shared goals in health care.

TABLE 3-3	
CLINICAL REASONING ERRORS	
CR ERROR BIASES LIKELY TO RESULT IN FAULTY REASONING	**DESCRIPTION**
Anchoring bias	The tendency to lock onto salient features in the patient's presentation too early in the CR process, and failing to adjust this initial impression in the light of later information. Fixation on first impressions, selected signs, or simple results as predictors of a specific diagnosis. Compounded by confirmation bias.
Ascertainment bias	Thinking shaped by prior assumptions and preconceptions (eg, ageism, stigmatism, stereotyping).

continued

TABLE 3-3 (CONTINUED)
CLINICAL REASONING ERRORS

CR ERROR BIASES LIKELY TO RESULT IN FAULTY REASONING	DESCRIPTION
Availability bias	The tendency to suggest diagnoses, interventions, and plans that readily come to mind, due to ease of recalling a past similar case rather than on the basis of prevalence or probability.
Confirmation bias	The tendency to look for confirming evidence to support a diagnosis or treatment rather than look for disconfirming evidence to refute it, despite the latter often being more persuasive and definitive.
Commission bias	The tendency to do something (or seem to be doing something) even if the intended actions are not supported by robust evidence and may in fact do harm.
Diagnostic momentum	When repeated diagnostics, tests, or interventions are in vogue. Labels attached to patients tend to become stickier and stickier. What started as merely a possibility gathers increasing momentum until it becomes definite, and other possibilities are excluded or not even considered.
Extrapolation error	The tendency to generalize treatment experiences, clinical trials, clinical practice guidelines, or clinical decision-making rules to groups of patients in whom the treatment has not been properly evaluated or considered first as individuals.
Framing bias	Undue influence by the way the question or problem is framed (eg, if the clinical information suggests diagnosis, problem, or treatment "XYZ," there is a tendency to frame as "XYZ," and for benefits and risks to be perceived differently if expressed in relative vs absolute terms).
Fundamental attribution error	The tendency to be judgmental and blame patients for their illnesses (dispositional causes) rather than examine the circumstances (situational factors) that may have been responsible. Psychiatric patients, those from minority groups, and other marginalized groups tend to be at risk of this error.
Outcome bias	Naturally empathic inclination to favor a diagnosis that will result in a more favorable outcome for the patient, even if unsupported by evidence.
Overconfidence bias	A tendency to believe we know more than we do. Overconfidence reflects a tendency to act on incomplete information, intuition, or hunches. Too much faith is placed on opinion instead of carefully collected cues. This error may be augmented by anchoring.
Premature closure	The tendency to apply premature closure to the decision-making process, accept a diagnosis before it has been fully verified, and not consider alternatives or search for data that challenge the provisional diagnosis. This error accounts for a high proportion of missed diagnoses. The same can hold true for interventions.
Search satisfaction bias	The tendency to stop looking for additional abnormal findings once an initial probable diagnosis is identified, or to accept the current elected intervention and stop looking for evidence.
Unpacking principle	The failure to collect all the relevant cues in establishing a differential diagnosis; it may result in missing significant possibilities. The more specific a description of an illness that is received, the more likely the event is judged to exist. If an inadequate patient history is taken, unspecified possibilities may be discounted.
Zebra retreat	The inclination to hold back from making a rare diagnosis due to lack of confidence about reporting such an unusual condition, despite supporting evidence; reluctance to try a rare treatment intervention, due to lack of confidence, even though evidence supports it.

Adapted from Levett-Jones et al,[30] Scott,[55] Croskerry,[56] Bruno et al,[57] and Gaba and Howard.[58]

Time for Reflection...
Putting It Together: Application Practice and Analysis

Now, for the final activity in this chapter on SA, let's examine some examples of reflection provided in Table 3-4.

1. Select 2 of the reflections from Table 3-4 and review.
2. Discover what you can glean about the student's learning, and consider how you would guide the student if you were a faculty or peer.
3. Next, identify any Habits of the Mind (see Table 3-2) you see exhibited within the reflection.
4. Identify any errors in CR or bias (see Table 3-3) revealed in the reflection. If so, describe and discuss with a partner how you would guide the learning or what you might do next if you were the learner.

TABLE 3-4

EXAMPLES OF REFLECTION

EXAMPLE A

1. How are you continuing to challenge your own creativity with planning for your patients' care?
Each day is a brand-new day for me, and that is something I love at this center. I am never bored. In fact, I find new challenges each day. My biggest challenge is exercise progression for different body parts while considering patient age, comorbidities, prior level of function, and pain level. There is so much out there that I can use, but having a credible source is important. I love how (my clinical instructor [CI]) challenges me to find new exercises from reliable and credible sources. I like to be creative, and I can tell that I am growing in my craft because instead of my creating a "good exercise," I keep in mind function and how this new exercise can help the patient reach functional goals. I do find myself taking a lot of work home throughout the week, but it is helping me be more prepared for patients. I've learned thinking ahead helps save me time in clinic!

2. How are you ensuring your continued progression toward your post-midterm goals?
One goal was to start researching more articles that will help me in clinic with POC and finalize a topic for in-service. Both have helped me stay up-to-date on current research. I know that I won't be an expert or entry-level at the conclusion of week 10, but I feel confident that I will have a better understanding of tools that I can use to better assist patients. I know that I can do more reading on my own, but I am doing my best without burning myself out. I can truly admit that I will miss this clinic when I am done, because I have learned a lot about myself. One big accomplishment I am almost achieving is better pronunciation and clarity when communicating with patients. I have found that they take me a bit more seriously when I slow down and make each word clear to understand. The midterm goals have been a reference for me to improve and see what things I need to keep brushing up on. Each week I can tell more responsibility is given to me, but it is a great thing because I can tell my CI is trusting in me more.

3. How has your curiosity been stimulated to continue to learn?
Patients each week come in and leave me very curious about what all I can do to help! Most recently, a patient with bilateral shoulder pain and a hip replacement came in, and I thought I was not going to be able to treat her because I felt as if I was not ready. However, after having been thrown into the treatment session, I have learned that there is so much I can do because I know basic anatomy and standard protocols to ensure this patient is safe. After each visit with this patient, I am curious how I can challenge her more because she is such a "go-getter" and motivated patient. These are characteristics I love, but it challenges me to think out the box when trying to create appropriate interventions for her. I have become more stimulated to find good CKC that will help her become more ambulatory and less dependent on her assistive device. I have become so much closer with PubMed.

continued

Table 3-4 (continued)
EXAMPLES OF REFLECTION

4. Describe 2 ways in which you have exhibited professionalism in the clinic, and 2 ways in which you have witnessed your CI exhibit professionalism during CE1.

My 2 examples of professionalism:

1. Last week, I was under the weather, but I knew I could not slack off. I needed to leave earlier to get some rest. However, each morning I made sure to arrive early to finish notes and prepare for new and follow-up patients. I refused to let my sickness limit me from providing appropriate care to each patient and fulfilling my duties.

2. One patient was curious about a Baker's cyst and wanted to know if it would go away on its own. I was not familiar with this subject, so I kindly told her I was not sure and I would refer to my CI. My CI respected the fact that I responded in this way, but she recommended I tell the patient I would look it up for her during a break and be back with an answer.

My CI's 2 examples of professionalism:

1. Sometimes we have cancellations throughout the day. Instead of our taking an hour break, my CI would help a colleague by taking a patient off of his caseload. I like the fact that this branch of this center has such a family-oriented environment where they are always willing to help each other. Her colleague really appreciated the help, and he even thanked me for being willing to work with the patient as well.

2. Almost every clinic may have a morning that does not start off right. Last week, it happened to us: front desk staff were nowhere to be found. We had no printout of which patients were on whose schedule, so we had to wing it. My CI, who is also the office manager, started checking patients in and delegating tasks to me to help make things less stressful. She was a bit stressed out, but she did not allow patients to see it. I think she did a good job in helping get things under control until someone from the front desk showed up.

EXAMPLE B

1. How are you continuing to challenge your own creativity with planning for your patients' care?

I am coming up with my own ideas, using research, and using ideas from other physical therapists, instead of sticking with the same kinds of activities that my CI had in place before. I am still sticking with my patients' goals, but coming up with a different way to do a balance activity than just the balance beam, or figuring out a different way to mix up the plan of care to see if it works better or if we need to try again with something new. This is something that my CI and I have been working on to change up the routine.

2. How are you ensuring your continued progression toward achieving your post-midterm goals?

I am being completely on my own with my own caseload and only using my CI as a reference or to make sure I am on the right track with evaluations, plans of care, and changes to my patients' schedules. I have continued to be confident in my skills and report back to my CI on things that went well and things that I will continue to get better at, including baby handling skills, which have improved, but my CI told me that it took her even until she was out on her own to get better at those skills.

3. How has your curiosity been stimulated to continue to learn?

My curiosity has been stimulated to continue to learn by seeing the progress my patients have made, even the ones who have been there for years, so it makes me look more things up online and in research articles to see how we can keep improving to eventually discharge the patient. Every day is a new learning experience because our patient population is so dynamic, and one day a patient may present one way, and the next it is different. When I took the practice test for boards, I truly understood how this clinical has and will continue to help me learn more about pediatrics and prepare for boards.

4. Describe a concrete example of new learning that you have recently experienced.

We have a child with a complicated brain disorder that they are broad-terming "CP," but she will be more complicated than that. We are teaching her how to roll, and with my children who are hypotonic, I knew exactly how to approach this. As I was rolling the little girl with CP who is hypertonic on her right side, my CI asked me if the child was using more of her tone or actual musculature, and how to fix this issue and make her use more of her muscles than tone to achieve the skill. It clicked when my CI told me to flex her leg and hip up more to take out the tone, and have her use her abdominals and obliques more than her back muscles and hip flexor tone. It makes sense and is something I will never forget. So now we are working on not using tone but activating other muscles to meet gross motor milestones, which I thought was great.

continued

TABLE 3-4 (CONTINUED)

EXAMPLES OF REFLECTION

EXAMPLE C

1. How are you continuing to challenge your own creativity with planning for your patients' care?
To curtail any monotony with patient treatment, I constantly research treatment options. Obviously, I will do what has been shown to be effective, but sometimes patients cannot perform certain exercises, so I will research modifications or ask other therapists about alternatives that would still work.

2. How are you ensuring your continued progression toward achieving your post-midterm goals?
My CI and I do weekly progress forms, and we have been talking about what I need to work on in these last few weeks to achieve entry-level status.

3. How has your curiosity been stimulated to continue to learn?
I have been also following therapists who practice other types of therapies (eg, IASTM, dry-needling, vestibular), which has stimulated me to want to do certain continuing education studies post-graduation. Also, I have been doing research on certain treatment options that require certifications and continuing education.

4. Describe a concrete example of new learning that you have recently experienced.
I recently had a patient with TMJ issues, and we didn't get a ton of formal education on how to perform a good evaluation for that, so I had to do quite a bit of research prior to the initial evaluation. Although I am not TMJ-certified, I did get to assist with the evaluation and help come up with a diagnosis. This piqued my interest in TMJ treatment.

EXAMPLE D

1. How are you continuing to challenge your own creativity with planning for your patients' care?
As a side project, my CI has had me create a document for us both to have at the end of my clinical that contains creative ideas for functional skills. On my own time I research ideas via online sources, pediatric textbooks, PowerPoint presentations from class, and Peabody cards here at the clinic. This has allowed me to think outside the box and continue to improve upon efficiency during treatment sessions.

2. How are you ensuring your continued progression toward achieving your post-midterm goals?
We continue to set weekly goals, ensuring my independence in all aspects of my clinical rotation. In addition, continuous feedback after each session and at the end of the day keeps me on track.

3. How has your curiosity been stimulated to continue to learn?
Recently I had the pleasure of observing a PFFD evaluation and treatment session. I also had the chance to assist in treating the patient to better understand the diagnosis postoperatively and how to treat while distracting the patient from pain experienced postoperatively, secondary to the recent lengthening surgery. In addition, I had the opportunity to observe and assist in a burn evaluation.

4. Describe a concrete example of new learning that you have recently experienced.
During a co-treatment session with an occupational therapist, I had the opportunity to learn some neurodevelopment techniques for tone inhibition with a patient diagnosed with spastic CP. I have since incorporated it into my treatment session prior to working on functional skills to improve the quality of the patient's movement functionally. Since incorporating the techniques I learned, I have observed an improvement in the patient's bilateral foot posture in both static and dynamic standing positions.

EXAMPLE E

1. How are you continuing to challenge your own creativity with planning for your patients' care?
I feel that the SCI setting, and the neuro setting in general, can be a great place for creative treatment. I have attempted to create treatment plans for some of the higher-functioning patients by learning their interests and hobbies prior to their accidents. For example, I managed to create a home run derby for a patient who used to love baseball. I used hand grips, a dowel found in the clinic to use as a bat, and large foam softballs to hit outside. The activity worked on the patient's dynamic sitting balance and UE activity, as well as offering her the opportunity to participate in an activity she enjoys.

continued

TABLE 3-4 (CONTINUED)
EXAMPLES OF REFLECTION

2. How are you ensuring your continued progression toward achieving your post-midterm goals?

I am having conversations with my CI about areas in which I feel confident, and asking to continue to attempt things that I feel less confident about, such as wheelchair repairs and adjustments.

3. How has your curiosity been stimulated to continue to learn?

My curiosity has been stimulated by the notable differences between patients with the same diagnosis. I find it very interesting that 2 individuals of similar age with the same ASIA level injury can perform tasks so differently, but equally effectively. I enjoy talking about the differing strategies they use to perform tasks, then using the strategies to help advise patients when teaching them tasks such as bed mobility or wheelchair assembly/disassembly.

4. Describe a concrete example of new learning that you have recently experienced.

I recently had the opportunity to help trial a new type of FES LE cycle designed for SCI patients. It was a good experience to talk with the creators of the product and learn the science behind the machine. I was then able to attempt to use the device on all patients who were appropriate and compare the new device to the clinic's already-owned FES LE cycle.

EXAMPLE F

1. How are you continuing to challenge your own creativity with planning for your patients' care?

This has become a challenge with some patients within my patient caseload. Some of my patients have been to physical therapy for more than 100 visits due to the nature of their injury (SCI or TBI). Many will hit plateaus, which makes it difficult to determine if they have made all the progress that they can, or what other ways can we manipulate the POC to see if we can get continued results. Having the opportunity to follow a few different physical therapists in different settings, as well as being in a gym with at least 5 other physical therapists, gives me many opportunities to ask questions or observe other techniques. Also, by being in a neuro gym, I have many tools to use. I can change gait training over land to a BW support system over land to locomotor training.

2. How are you ensuring your continued progression toward achieving your post-midterm goals?

I have stopped misspelling words that I used to spell incorrectly with practice and identifying words that gave me difficulty. During evaluations, my CI has been able to just watch and not intervene. I have also improved on my efficiency of evaluations. I can continue to improve on being more efficient with time for more complex patients.

3. How has your curiosity been stimulated to continue to learn?

In the outpatient setting, I have had the opportunity to work with many different diagnoses. This has given me the chance to see how many diseases present and what impairments are associated with them. Seeing new diagnoses has kept me stimulated to continue to learn about each and every disease that I have come upon. I really enjoy the variety vs specializing in one area. Also, working with patients throughout their rehab has given me many opportunities to use different techniques and training methods. I have had the chance to work with different ambulation devices and ambulation types of training, learned about different wheelchairs, and worked on dependent lifts and slide board transfers.

4. Describe a concrete example of new learning that you have recently experienced.

Locomotor training. I worked with a physical therapist and her patient while they used a body weight support system over a treadmill. I had to control one of the patient's legs to help guide it through the proper motion. This showed me how taxing therapy can be, even on a therapist, for patients who are lower-level.

EXAMPLE G

1. How are you continuing to challenge your own creativity with planning for your patients' care?

I do chart reviews before my patient encounters to plan exercise progression. I discuss ideas with my CI to see whether she agrees or disagrees. In addition, I ask my CI to demonstrate skill sets or exercise ideas that she had learned from her previous CEUs. Recently, we discussed mobilization with movement and functional movement patterns. We will be going over these skills in the next 2½ weeks so I can acquire more ideas for my patient care. Also, I'm learning new exercises from observation and shadowing opportunities with other therapists in the clinic.

continued

TABLE 3-4 (CONTINUED)
EXAMPLES OF REFLECTION

2. How are you ensuring your continued progression toward achieving your post-midterm goals?

My CI and I continue to go over weekly student evaluations to make sure I'm on par with the requirement. I also seek feedback from other therapists when I'm shadowing them. I seek opportunities to be involved in the clinic, such as when I revised the scar tissue management handout. Currently, I'm revising the manual lymphatic drainage education handouts and creating a presentation to discuss physical therapy rehabilitation for post-breast reconstruction patients for the facilities' Health Plastic Surgeon Board. I am seeing 100% of my CI's caseloads. I am assisting the clinic in developing patient education materials and clinical projects to promote physical therapy services as well as interdisciplinary collaborations.

3. How has your curiosity been stimulated to continue to learn?

My clinical rotations provided exposure to acute inpatient care and pediatric and oncology rehabilitation. I have limited exposure to orthopedic caseloads, subacute inpatient care, and cardiopulmonary rehab. I asked my CI for opportunities to observe other physical therapists within this facility to observe and acquire more exposure. With these observation opportunities, I'm more encouraged to review certain materials and seek more resources to learn. Throughout this clinical rotation, I'm required to do a case presentation for every surgical procedure that I've observed. I would ask questions during surgery observation as well as additional research to learn more about the surgical procedures and potential complications from these operations.

4. Describe a concrete example of new learning that you have recently experienced.

On June 30, my CI had the day off, so I was working with an orthopedic therapist in the clinic. In our program, we have emphasized on "assess, treat, and reassess." The therapist whom I shadowed on Friday really emphasizes on this concept. He thoroughly explained that you must be able to make a point of how your services are benefiting these patients. He would "assess, treat, and reassess," then he would ask the patient how he or she feels. Objectively, we can measure and see the results of our treatments in improvement of a patient's deficits, either in range of motion, strength, or pain reduction. However, it is essential to know how the patient feels after our treatment. If the patient is feeling better, then he or she will be more compliant with physical therapy sessions as well as HEPs.

REFERENCES

1.   Schön DA. *The Reflective Practitioner: How Professionals Think in Action.* New York, NY: Basic Books; 1983.
2.   Schön DA. *Educating the Reflective Practitioner: Toward a New Design for Teaching and Learning in the Professions.* San Francisco, CA: Jossey-Bass; 1987.
3.   Schön DA: The theory of inquiry: Dewey's legacy to education. *Curriculum Inquiry.* 1992;22:119-140.
4.   Levett-Jones T, Hoffman K, Dempsey J, et al. The "five rights" of clinical reasoning: an educational model to enhance nursing students' ability to identify and manage clinically "at-risk" patients. *Nurse Educ Today.* 2010;30(6):515-520.
5.   Kolb D. *Experiential Learning: Experience as the Source of Learning and Development.* Upper Saddle River, NJ: Prentice Hall; 1984.
6.   Kolb DA. *Kolb Learning Style Inventory (LSI).* Version 4. Philadelphia, PA: Hay Group; 2007.
7.   Dewey J. *How We Think.* 1-13. London, United Kingdom: Heath; 1910:1859-1952.
8.   Dewey J. *How We Think: A Restatement of the Relation of Reflective Thinking to the Educative Process.* Boston, MA: DC Health & Co; 1933.
9.   Bandura A. *Social Learning Theory.* Englewood Cliffs, NJ: Prentice-Hall; 1977.
10. Bandura A. The self-system in reciprocal determinism. *Am Psychologist.* 1978;33:344-358.
11. Bandura A. *Self-Efficacy: The Exercise of Control.* New York, NY: WH Freeman; 1997.
12. Bandura A. Self-efficacy: toward a unifying theory of behavioral change. *Psychol Rev.* 1997;84:191-215.
13. Musolino GM. Readiness for reflective practice: peer and self-assessment. In: Davis CM, Musolino GM, eds. *Patient Practitioner Interaction: An Experiential Manual for Developing the Art of Healthcare.* 6th ed. Thorofare, NJ: SLACK Incorporated; 2016.
14. Musolino GM. Fostering reflective practice: self-assessment abilities of physical therapy students and entry-level graduates. *J Allied Health.* 2006;35(1):30-42.
15. Watts N. *Handbook of Clinical Teaching: Exercises and Guidelines for Health Professionals Who Teach Patients, Train Staff or Supervise Students.* New York, NY: Churchill Livingston; 1990.
16. Jonsen A. *The New Medicine and the Old Ethics.* Cambridge, MA: Harvard University Press; 1990:1-43.
17. Brookfield S. *Becoming a Critically Reflective Teacher.* San Francisco, CA: Jossey-Bass; 1995.

18. Kirby PC, Teddlie C. Development of the reflective teaching instrument. *J Research Dev Educ.* 1989;22(4):45-50.

19. Klevans DR, Smutz WD, Shuman SB, Bershad C. *Self-Assessment: Helping Professionals Discover What They Do Not Know. New Directions for Adult and Continuing Education.* San Francisco, CA: Jossey-Bass; 1992;55:17-27.

20. Barrows HS. *Practice-Based Learning: Problem-Based Learning Applied to Medical Education.* Springfield, IL: Southern Illinois University School of Medicine; 1994.

21. Barrows HS. *What Your Tutor May Never Tell You: A Medical Student's Guide to Problem-Based Learning.* Springfield, IL: Southern Illinois University School of Medicine; 1996.

22. Shepherd K. Jensen G. Attribute dimensions that distinguish master and novice physical therapy clinicians in orthopedic settings. *Phys Ther.* 1994;72:711-22.

23. West KM. The case against teaching. *J Medical Educ.* 1966;41:776-771.

24. Westberg J, Jason H. Fostering learners' reflection and self-assessment. *Family Med.* 1994;26:278-282.

25. Orest M. Clinicians' perceptions of self-assessment in clinical practice. *Phys Ther.* 1995;75:48-53.

26. King A. From sage on the stage to guide on the side. *College Teach.* 1994;41(1):30-35.

27. Mezirow J. *Transformative Dimensions of Adult Learning.* San Franscisco, CA: Jossey-Bass; 1991.

28. Osterman KF, Kottkamp RB. *Reflective Practice for Educators: Professional Development to Improve Student Learning.* 2nd ed. Thousand Oaks, CA: Corwin Press, Inc; 2004.

29. Musolino GM, van Duijn J, Noonan A, Eargle L, Gray D. Reasons identified for seeking the American Physical Therapy Association-Credentialed Clinical Instructor Program (CCIP) in Florida. *J Allied Health.* 2013;42(3):E51-E60.

30. Levett-Jones T, et al. *Clinical Reasoning: Instructor Resources.* University of Newcastle, Australia: School of Nursing and Midwifery, Faculty of Health; 2009.

31. Rubenfeld M, Scheffer B. *Critical Thinking Tactics for Nurses.* Boston, MA: Jones and Bartlett Publishing; 2006.

32. Schell K. Teaching tools: promoting student questioning. *Nurse Educ.* 1998;23:8-12.

33. Musolino GM, Mostrom E. Reflection and the scholarship of teaching, learning and assessment. *J Phys Ther Educ.* 2005;19(3):52-66.

34. McManus DA. The two paradigms of education and the peer review of teaching. *J Geoscience Educ.* 2001;49(6):423-434.

35. Schumacher DJ, Englander R, Carraccio C. Developing the master learner: applying learning theory to the learner, the teacher, and the learning environment. *Acad Med.* 2013;88(11):1635-1645.

36. Scheffer B, Rubenfeld M. A consensus statement on critical thinking in nursing. *J Nurs Educ.* 2000;39:352-359.

37. Woods NW, Mylopoulos M. On clinical reasoning research and applications: redefining expertise. *Med Educ.* 2015;49:542-544.

38. Kramp MK, Humphreys WL. *Narrative Self-Assessment and Reflective Learners and Teachers.* Knoxville, TN: Tennessee University. ERIC Document Reproduction Services; 1992.

39. Jensen G, Denton B. Teaching physical therapy students to reflect: a suggestion for clinical education. *J Phys Ther Educ.* 1991;5:33-38.

40. Klevans DR, Smutz WD, Shuman SB, Bershad C. *Self-Assessment: Helping Professionals Discover What They Do Not Know. New Directions for Adult and Continuing Education.* San Francisco, CA: Jossey-Bass. 1992;55:17-27.

41. Davis CM, Musolino GM, eds. *Patient Practitioner Interaction: An Experiential Manual for Developing the Art of Healthcare.* 6th ed. Thorofare, NJ: SLACK Incorporated; 2016.

42. Furgal KE, Norris E, Young SM, Wallman HW. Relative and absolute reliability of the professionalism in physical therapy core values self-assessment tool. *J Allied Health.* 2018;47:e45-e48.

43. Professionalism in physical therapy: core values. https://www.apta.org/uploadedFiles/APTAorg/About_Us/Policies/BOD/Judicial/ProfessionalisminPT.pdf. Accessed April 29, 2019.

44. Anderson D, Irwin K. Self-assessment of professionalism in physical therapy education. *Work.* 2013;44:275-281.

45. American Physical Therapy Association. *Physical Therapist Clinical Performance Instrument.* Alexandria, VA: America Physical Therapy Association; 2006.

46. American Physical Therapy Association. *Physical Therapist Assistant Clinical Performance Instrument.* Alexandria, VA: American Physical Therapy Association; 2006.

47. May WW, Morgan BJ, Lemke JC, et al. Model for ability-based assessment in physical therapy education. *J Phys Ther Educ.* 1995;9(1):3-6.

48. APTA credentialed clinical instructor program (CCIP) level 1 & level 2. http://www.apta.org/CCIP/. Accessed June 5, 2018.

49. Seif GA, Brown D, Annan-Coultas D. Video-recorded simulated patient interactions: can they help develop clinical and communication skills in today's learning environment. *J Allied Health.* 2013;42(2):e37-e44.

50. Peters JM. Strategies for reflective practice. *New Directions for Adult and Continuing Education.* 1991;51:89-96.

51. Smith FL, Barlow PB, Peters JM, Skolits GJ. Demystifying reflective practice: using the DATA model to enhance evaluators' professional activities. *Evaluation and Program Planning.* 2015;52:142-47.

52. McBee E, Ratcliffe T, Schuwirth L, et al. Context and clinical reasoning: understanding the medical student perspective. *Perspect Med Educ.* https://doi.org/10.1007/s40037-018-0417-x. Accessed April 29, 2019.

53. Durning SJ, Artino AR, Schwirth L, van der Vleuten C. Clarifying assumptions to enhance our understanding and assessment of clinical reasoning. *Acad Med.* 2013;88(4):432-438.

54. Epstein RM. Mindful practice. *JAMA.* 1999;282:833-839.

55. Scott IA. Errors in clinical reasoning: causes and remedial strategies. *BMJ.* 2009;338:1860.

56. Croskerry P. The importance of cognitive errors in diagnosis and strategies to minimize them. *Acad Med.* 2003;78(8):1-6.

57. Bruno MA, Walker EA, Abujudeh HH. Understanding and confronting our mistakes: the epidemiology of error in radiology and strategies for error reduction. *Radiographics.* 2015:35;1668-1676.

58. Gaba DM, Howard SK. Fatigue among clinicians and the safety of patients. *N Engl J Med.* 2002:347;1249-1255.

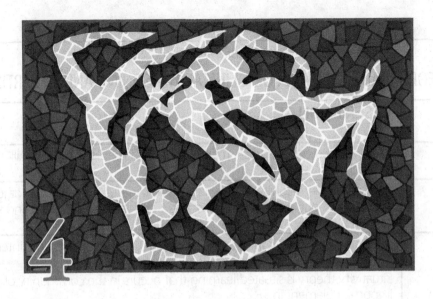

EXPERTISE IN CLINICAL REASONING:
Uncovering the Role of Context

Nicole Christensen, PT, PhD, MAppSc and
Gail M. Jensen, PT, PhD, FAPTA, FNAP

OBJECTIVES

- Describe the interdependence between clinical reasoning (CR) and the development of expertise.
- Discuss the influence of contextual factors on the characteristics and quality of CR among clinicians with differing levels of expertise.
- Propose teaching and learning strategies for the development of adaptive learners and adaptive expertise, to prepare clinicians to manage reasoning about contextual factors effectively in practice.
- Describe the link between adaptive learning and development of CR capability.

EXPERTISE AND CLINICAL REASONING

What are the connections between expertise and CR? Is CR the central concept or dimension of expertise, or is CR the Holy Grail? We know that expertise is not a static state or a list of attributes that one obtains through years of experience. Rather, expertise is a continuum of development and a dynamic process where reflection on that experience is central. Without learning mechanisms or reflection used to mediate improvement from CR experiences, there will be little acquisition of expertise.[1,2] If we consider expertise as an ongoing developmental process and way of being in practice, rather than an outcome or static state to be achieved, then we can begin to see the critical importance of learning in the context of professional development and expertise. The developmental pathway of expertise includes the building of various types of knowledge from foundational sciences to

Musolino GM, Jensen GM, eds. *Clinical Reasoning and Decision-Making in*
Physical Therapy: Facilitation, Assessment, and Implementation (pp 41-46).
© 2020 Taylor & Francis Group.

	TABLE 4-1
	THEORETICAL CONCEPTS FOR CLINICAL REASONING AND EXPERTISE
THEORETICAL CONCEPTS	**DESCRIPTION**
General problem-solving ability	Early work viewed expertise in CR as a "general problem-solving skill" that could be applied to any situation.[5]
Case specificity (knowledge organization)	Medical problem-solving work with physicians found that it was not just problem-solving skills, but also knowledge of the case that was organized and structured.[6]
Context specificity	Consideration of the context of the case, such as patient-provider interactions and the organization's factors, influence CR and the "diagnosis."[7] Situativity theory is situated learning that occurs in the community of practice as an important element in CR.[7]
Script theory (Organization/ chunking of knowledge)	Illness scripts are chunks that are part of the long-term memory as "scripts of how the patient will present," shaped by experience and refined as one practices over time.[8,9] Semantic qualifiers help clinicians sort and organize patient information (eg, acute or chronic).[10]
Dual processing theory **System 1** **System 2**	System 1—thinking fast is quick and subconscious or nonanalytic; an example strategy is pattern recognition (also called forward reasoning).[11,12] System 2—thinking slow and working analytically (also called backward reasoning) are key characteristics.[11,12]
Cognitive load theory	This theory describes limitations in short-term memory (which can hold 7 pieces of information); chunking uses long-term memory.[13,14]
Expert performance	Deliberate practice is a critical component for procedural performance; Ericsson[15] proposed that CR may benefit from deliberate practice.
Reflection	Reflection-in-action and reflection-on-action are 2 key concepts from Schön,[16] seen as essential for learners becoming professionals. Metacognition, or the act of thinking about your thinking, has also been seen as central to the reflective process.[17-19]
Adaptive expertise	This differentiates adaptive expertise from routine expertise.[1] Routine experts have mastery of knowledge in their domain and are efficient. Adaptive experts have mastery of knowledge in their domain and are efficient and innovative. This innovation occurs through reflective practice as one balances efficiency and innovation.[20]

clinical signs and symptoms, along with clinical skills. The complexity that comes with the interactions of thinking, reasoning, and building a knowledge base along with caring for patients can seem overwhelming, and goes well beyond the view of CR as a cognitive process.

Gruppen[3] would argue that thinking about CR only in terms of cognition leaves out critical dimensions of context, affect, and other organizational factors that are part of clinical practice. Young and colleagues[4] have recently observed that attempts to describe CR in the health professions are by nature influenced by the clinical context within which that practice is occurring. They propose that a potential explanation for the differences we see in individuals' understanding of CR is the presence of differing "boundary conditions"[4(p12)] within which reasoning occurs. Boundary conditions are those under which a given theory has explanatory power: the theory holds true for the specific situation or context within or for which it was developed. When recognizing that CR is a multifaceted construct with multiple coexisting understandings between individuals and across professions, the lack of consistency in its description may be a consequence of the broad range of factors beyond cognitive processing that are involved.

An overview of the multiple theoretical and conceptual perspectives of understanding CR and expertise demonstrates the complexity and heterogeneity of the related research, and a review summary is provided in Table 4-1.

CLINICAL REASONING AND CONTEXTUAL FACTORS

We know from research on expertise and CR in physical therapy that understanding contextual factors is a critical dimension of the CR process for physical therapists. Contextual factors include psycho-sociocultural aspects and personal aspects of the patient, in the context of their realms of participation in life, work, and society. These include factors such as language(s) spoken or not spoken, educational level and knowledge, literacy, financial status, social support systems, family roles and responsibilities, work situations, and relationship characteristics. In physical therapy, Jensen and colleagues developed a grounded theory of expert practice in physical therapy.[21,22] This model is a combination of multidimensional knowledge, CR skills, skilled movement, and virtue. CR skills were collaborative processes between therapists and patients or patients and their families. Expert therapists used the medical diagnosis as an additional piece of data, but not the focus of their interventions, as the patient's function and families' needs were central. Once the problems were identified and the context understood, the therapists engaged in collaborative problem-solving with the patient and family, teaching them about movement and function as the primary focus of the interventions.

Subsequent work by Resnik and Jensen[23] corroborated the presence of a patient-centred approach to care in collaborative CR and promotion of patient empowerment. At the foundation of the patient-centred approach, this research identified an ethic of caring and a respect for individuality, a passion for clinical care, and a desire to continually learn and improve. The primary goals of empowering patients, increasing self-efficacy beliefs, and involving patients in the care process are facilitated by patient-therapist collaborative problem-solving and enhanced through attentive listening, trust-building, and observation. Resnik and Jensen[23] reported that these efforts not only promoted patient empowerment and self-efficacy, but also resulted in greater continuity of services, more skilful care, more individualized plans of care, and, ultimately, better outcomes.

Edwards and colleagues[24] investigated expert physical therapists' CR strategies through in-depth ethnographic work and further described additional components of reasoning that were part of everyday practice (eg, interactive reasoning, diagnostic reasoning, procedural reasoning, narrative reasoning, ethical reasoning, reasoning about teaching, and predictive reasoning). They proposed a dialectic model of CR that moves between the cognitive and decision-making processes required to diagnose and manage patients' physical disabilities, and the narrative or communicative reasoning and action required to understand and engage patients and caregivers.[25] Therefore, this empirically derived model of expert CR and the variety of reasoning strategies included by expert reasoners was, in great part, characterized by ways in which experts were able to perceive, elicit, and construct a mutual understanding of the patient's particular contextual factors. Experts can integrate the understanding of contextual factors into their decision-making with patients along with their conclusions from the more traditional cognitive processing aspects of their reasoning.

Recent findings of educational research within medicine support that expert clinicians are more skillful in their abilities to consider and integrate management of contextual factors into their CR, and that overall the CR performance of all clinicians (experts and nonexperts) varies based on the specifics of the clinical context.[7,26] McBee and colleagues[26] found that when challenged with the presence of patient-related contextual factors, medical residents developed diagnostic uncertainty and resorted to gathering more, often irrelevant or unnecessary, information. Durning and colleagues[7] also identified that while both experts' and nonexperts' CR quality was influenced by the presence of contextual factors, and that when the clinicians studied recognized more than one contextual factor as relevant, clinicians across the board interpreted the situation as problematic and often frustrating. When reflecting on the clinical encounter, however, the more expert clinicians were much more aware of the presence of the contextual factors and their reactions to them than were the novices studied. The implications noted by these researchers collectively was that these findings indicate that a need for development of clinicians' abilities to cope with and effectively incorporate consideration of patients' contextual factors, and patients' perspectives, into their CR.[7,26]

For educators within physical therapy today, and for developing physical therapy clinicians, it has become clear that 2 important dimensions must be prioritized as a focus of CR education, considering what we know about CR, expertise, and context. One is the human or relationship side of practice, which is a central component of CR that continues to be addressed inadequately in much of professional entry-level CR education.[27] The second dimension is how central movement is to our interventions and our work as physical therapists. These 2 dimensions are interdependent, as most of our interventions require that the patient engage in movement. Human improvement and our outcomes, just like the work of many others such as teachers, psychologists, or other forms of therapists, depends on the human performance of the patient, client, or student.[28] How can we use what we know about what experts can do when reasoning with contextual factors to inform our educational strategies? How then do we facilitate the learning of CR such that clinicians can perform well in contextually rich, complex, and often-uncertain situations?

ADAPTIVE EXPERTISE:
FACILITATING LEARNING AND CLINICAL REASONING CAPABILITY

If we agree with the assertion that expertise is not a state of achievement, but, rather, a process of ongoing learning, and that CR is not simply a cognitive process and stand-alone concept, then the need to identify how we can best facilitate the development of adaptive learners becomes clear. Adaptive learners are described as able to thrive in changing environments by learning in, and for, practice and adapting as necessary.[29]

How do we facilitate the development of expert-like learners who can engage in progressive problem-solving characterized by a complexity and a variety of contextual factors, and are on a path toward the development of adaptive expertise? We know that adaptive expertise has the following attributes:

- An openness to reflecting on practice

- Metacognitive reasoning skills to recognize that a routine approach to the problem will not work

- Critical thinking to challenge current assumptions and beliefs

- The ability to reconstruct the problem space[29]

A central premise in these attributes is non-negotiable self-assessment skills (as described in Chapter 3) that require the learner to be open, engage in reflection or a metacognitive process in thinking about his or her thinking, challenge assumptions, and then reconstruct the problem space. Often our emphasis in the academic world is a focus on certainty and right answers, whereas everyday practice is one of uncertainty or the "swampy lowland of practice."[16] Our task then must be to facilitate a learning environment where learners are challenged to practice and adapt in the presence of progressively more complex contextual factors, as often as is necessary, to stimulate the building of continuous learning and self-improvement skills. Schumacher and colleagues[20] propose a visual that represents the integration of several of the learning concepts and theories that are factors in the development of the "master learner." Figure 4-1 is our adaptation of those factors.

One of the research areas within medical education is identification of the processes necessary for the development of the master adaptive learner.[1,20,29] These learners need to develop not just problem-solving skills but progressive, contextually rich problem-solving that includes efficiency as well as innovation to solve complex problems in new ways. Cutrer and colleagues[29] propose a 4-component model to guide a process of developing a master adaptive learner:

1. **Planning:** Identify a gap between what is and what should or could be, select an opportunity for learning, and search for resources for learning.

2. **Learning:** Engage in learning, critically appraise different sources for learning, and move beyond traditional learning strategies such as rereading or highlighting (mechanical learning processes) to more effective strategies such as spaced repetitions, elaboration, and concept integration.

3. **Assessing:** Try out what is learned and engage in informed self-assessment that uses external feedback.

4. **Adjusting:** Incorporate what is learned into daily routines, reexamine new learning, consider opportunities and barriers needed to adjust practice, and determine individual vs system implementation.

ADAPTIVE LEARNING AND CLINICAL REASONING CAPABILITY

Adaptive learners are characterized by engagement in continuous learning and self-improvement, achieved through active critical self-reflection and the motivation to change and grow to meet the challenges of new and unknown circumstances.[29] This concept of adaptive learners has been linked to another related educational concept: capability.[30] Capability[31] incorporates an explicit consideration of the types of meta-skills necessary for reasoning and experiential learning in practice characterized by uncertainty, introduced by an abundance of critically important contextual factors. Capability, in part, is characterized by a demonstrable and justifiable confidence, or self-efficacy, in the ability to make well-reasoned decisions collaboratively, in both known and unknown circumstances. Capability also includes a motivation to intentionally and continuously learn through reflection-on-practice.[32] The link to descriptions of adaptive learners here is clear. CR capability was described by Christensen and colleagues[33] as an extension of the model of capability, and is the confidence in the ability to effectively integrate key thinking and learning skills to make sense of and learn collaboratively from clinical experiences, in both known and unknown clinical contexts. The development of CR capability is thought to be facilitated when educators explicitly focus on building the thinking and learning skills observed in the CR of experts.[24] These include:

- **Reflective thinking:** Includes retrospection and thinking in action, or metacognitively[12,16,19]

- **Critical thinking:** Includes a focus on identification of blind spots, with correction of any erroneous assumptions or practice knowledge[34,35]

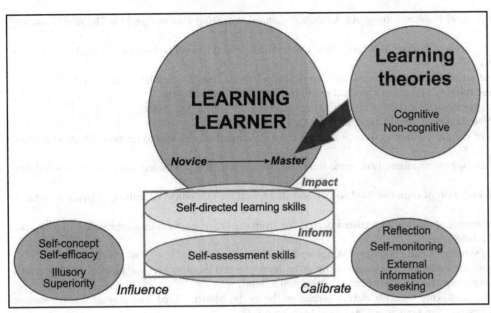

Figure 4-1. Factors in the development of adaptive learners. (Adapted from Schumacher DJ, Englander R, Carraccio C. Developing the master learner: applying learning theory to the learner, the teacher, and the learning environment. *Acad Med.* 2013;88[11]:1635-1645.)

- **Complexity thinking:** Recognition of dynamic interdependencies between all aspects of a situation and the ability to see a situation from multiple frames of reference[36,37]

- **Dialectical thinking:** A fluidity of reasoning between deductive, logical problem-solving strategies and inductive, narratively oriented communicative reasoning strategies[25]

Specifically, these skill sets for the facilitation of CR capability are linked to enhancing a learner's ability to develop practice knowledge (and eventually expertise) from learning from personal experiences in practice.[33]

CONCLUSION

The existing research about expertise, CR, and the role of context in CR performance all point to a critical need for educators to prepare clinicians as adaptive clinical learners, capable of CR in complex clinical situations characterized by a variety and combination of contextual factors. Learners also must be amenable to being adaptable for deeper learning with CR. Our challenge as educators and lifelong learning professionals, then, is two-fold:

1. **Develop educational strategies:** Advance explicit strategies informed by the existing research and educational theory.

2. **Education research:** Promote and support education research that investigates educational strategies to promote in our learners the capability to develop adaptive expertise.

Reflection Moment

Now consider and jot down your responses to the following points:

1. What educational strategies can be developed that are informed by research and educational theory?

2. What critical questions need to be addressed about how we develop learners with the capability to develop adaptive expertise?

REFERENCES

1. Mylopoulos M, Woods N. When I say … adaptive expertise. *Med Educ.* 2017;51:685-686.
2. Tsui ABM. *Understanding Expertise in Teaching.* Cambridge, MA: Cambridge University Press; 2003.
3. Gruppen LD. Clinical reasoning: defining it, teaching it, assessing it, studying it. *West J Emerg Med.* 2017;18(1):4-7.
4. Young M, Thomas A, Lubarsky S, et al. Drawing boundaries: the difficulty in defining clinical reasoning. *Acad Med.* 2018;93(7):990-995.
5. Newell A, Simon HA. *Human Problem Solving.* Englewood Cliffs, NJ: Prentice-Hall; 1972.

6. Elstein AS, Shulman L, Sprafka S. *Medical Problem Solving: An Analysis of Clinical Reasoning.* Cambridge, MA: Harvard University Press; 1978.

7. Durning S, Artino Jr AR, Pangaro L, van der Vleuten CP, Schuwirth L. Context and clinical reasoning: understanding the perspective of the expert's voice. *Med Educ.* 2011;45(9):927-938.

8. Custers EJFM. Thirty years of illness scripts: theoretical origins and practical applications. *Med Teach.* 2015;37(5):457-462.

9. Patel VL, Groen G. Knowledge-based solution strategies in medical reasoning. *Cogn Sci.* 1986;10:91-116.

10. Bordage G. Elaborated knowledge: a key to successful diagnostic thinking. *Acad Med.* 1994;69(11):883-885.

11. Kahneman D. *Thinking, Fast and Slow.* London, United Kingdom: Allen Lane; 2011.

12. Marcum JA. An integrated model of clinical reasoning: dual-processing theory of cognition and metacognition. *J Eval Clin Pract.* 2012;18:954-961.

13. Miller GA. The magical number seven, plus or minus two: some limits on our capacity for processing information. *Psychol Rev.* 1956;63:81-97.

14. Leppink J, van den Heuvel A. The evolution of cognitive load theory and its application to medical education. *Perspect Med Educ.* 2015;4(3):119-127.

15. Ericsson KA. Acquisition and maintenance of medical expertise: a perspective from the expert-performance approach with deliberate practice. *Acad Med.* 2015;90(11):1471-1486.

16. Schön DA. *Educating the Reflective Practitioner.* San Francisco, CA: Jossey-Bass; 1987.

17. Flavell JH. Metacognition and cognitivie monitoring: a new area of cognitive-developmental inquiry. *Am Psychol.* 1979;34(10):906-911.

18. Higgs J. Developing clinical reasoning competencies. *Physiotherapy.* 1992;78(8):575-581.

19. Mezirow J. Learning to think like an adult: core concepts of transformation theory. In: Mezirow J, ed. *Learning as Transformation: Critical Perspectives on a Theory in Progress.* San Francisco, CA: Jossey-Bass; 2000:3-33.

20. Schumacher DJ, Englander R, Carraccio C. Developing the master learner: applying learning theory to the learner, the teacher, and the learning environment. *Acad Med.* 2013;88(11):1635-1645.

21. Jensen GM, Gwyer J, Shepard KF, Hack LM. Expert practice in physical therapy. *Phys Ther.* 2000;80(1):28-52.

22. Jensen G, Gwyer J, Hack L, Shepard K. *Expertise in Physical Therapy Practice.* Philadelphia, PA: Saunders; 2007.

23. Resnik L, Jensen GM. Using clinical outcomes to explore the theory of expert practice in physical therapy. *Phys Ther.* 2003;83(12):1090-1106.

24. Edwards I, Jones M, Carr J, Braunack-Mayer A, Jensen GM. Clinical reasoning strategies in physical therapy. *Phys Ther.* 2004;84(4):312-330.

25. Edwards I, Jones MA. Clinical reasoning and expert practice. In: Jensen G, Gwyer J, Hack L, Shepard K, eds. *Expertise in Physical Therapy Practice.* Philadelphia, PA: Saunders; 2007:192-213.

26. McBee E, Ratcliffe T, Picho K, et al. Consequences of contextual factors on clinical reasoning in resident physicians. *Adv Health Sci Educ Theory Pract.* 2015;20(5):1225-1236.

27. Christensen N, Black L, Furze J, Huhn K, Vendrely A, Wainwright S. Clinical reasoning: survey of teaching methods, integration, and assessment in entry-level physical therapist academic education. *Phys Ther.* 2017;97(2):175-186.

28. Cohen DK. Professions of human improvement: predicaments of teaching. In: Nisan M, Schremer O, eds. *Educational Deliberations.* Jerusalem, Israel: Keter Publishers; 2005:278-294.

29. Cutrer WB, Miller B, Martin VP, et al. Fostering the development of master adaptive learners: a conceptual model to guide skill acquisition in medical education. *Acad Med.* 2017;92:70-75.

30. Christensen N, Jensen G. Developing clinical reasoning capability. In: Higgs J, Jensen G, Loftus S, Christensen N, eds. *Clinical Reasoning in the Health Professions.* 4th ed. Edinburgh, United Kingdom: Elsevier; 2019:427-434.

31. Stephenson J. The concept of capability and its importance in higher education. In: Stephenson J, Yorke M, eds. *Capability and Quality in Higher Education.* London, United Kingdom: Kogan Page; 1998:1-13.

32. Doncaster K, Lester S. Capability and its development: experiences from a work-based doctorate. *Studies in Higher Education.* 2002;27(1):91-101.

33. Christensen N, Jones M, Higgs J, Edwards I. Dimensions of clinical reasoning capability. In: Higgs J, Jones M, Loftus S, Christensen N, eds. *Clinical Reasoning in the Health Professions.* 3rd ed. Amsterdam, Netherlands: Butterworth-Heinemann Elsevier; 2008:101-110.

34. Brookfield SD. *Teaching Critical Thinking: Tools and Techniques to Help Students Question Their Assumptions.* San Francisco, CA: Jossey-Bass Wiley; 2012.

35. Paul R, Elder L. *The Miniature Guide to Critical Thinking: Concepts and Tools.* 4th ed. Berkeley, CA: The Foundation for Critical Thinking; 2006.

36. Plsek PE, Greenhalgh T. Complexity science: the challenge of complexity in health care. *Br Med J.* 2001;323:625-628.

37. Davis B, Sumara D. *Complexity and Education: Inquiries Into Learning, Teaching, and Research.* Mahwah, NJ: Lawrence Erlbaum Associates; 2006.

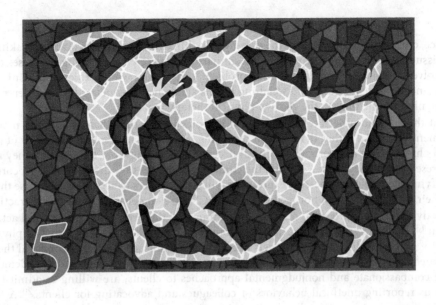

FROM ETHICAL REASONING TO ETHICAL ACTION

Clare Delany, PhD, MHlth & MedLaw, MPhysio, BApp Sc (Physio) and
Ian Edwards, PhD, Grad Dip PT, BApp Sc (Physio)

OBJECTIVES

- Identify and distill the core skills and thinking processes of clinical ethicists.
- Compare these skills with the core ethical thinking skills and reasoning processes apparent in physical therapy practice.
- Identify ways to merge the skills of a clinical ethicist and a practicing physical therapist.

INTRODUCTION

In health care practice, ethical reasoning refers to the step-by-step thinking processes involved in making and justifying decisions about an ethical issue or dilemma.[1,2] In recognition of the complexity of ethical dimensions of physical therapy practice, there is growing interest in examining processes of ethical reasoning. In this chapter, we identify and distill the reasoning skills of a clinical ethicist as an example of an expert practitioner in clinical ethics. Clinical ethicists identify and analyze ethical issues using formal codes of conduct and bioethical principles. A second role is more facilitative: to help others voice their concerns, and to help them identify ethically acceptable options in their own clinical context. We compare those skills to the ethical thinking and responses of physical therapists arising from their descriptions of ethical issues regularly encountered in diverse areas of practice. The comparison between the ethical deliberation skills and work of a clinical ethicist and those of a physical therapist point to the value (for physical therapy practice) of a subtle but important shift in focus: from ethical reasoning as a component of therapists' individual moral agency, to ethical reasoning as a process of working with others.

Musolino GM, Jensen GM, eds. *Clinical Reasoning and Decision-Making in Physical Therapy: Facilitation, Assessment, and Implementation* (pp 47-56).
© 2020 Taylor & Francis Group.

In health care practice, ethical reasoning refers to the step-by-step thinking processes involved in making and justifying decisions about an ethical issue or dilemma.[1,2] There are some similarities between the thinking processes of clinical and ethical reasoning.[1,3,4] Both involve gathering information about a problem, considering which ethical and clinical theories or guiding ethical and treatment principles[5] are relevant, and weighing harms and benefits associated with different responses.[4,6-8] Both clinical and ethical reasoning are intrinsic to the goals of physical therapy practice.

However, in physical therapy and other literature for health professionals, there has been much more research about the processes and development of clinical rather than ethical reasoning. For example, a substantial body of research has explored how expert practitioners hypothesize and formulate clinical decisions, including what information they regard as important,[1] the types of mental representations they create,[3,9,10] and the clinical experiences they draw upon.[3,11] A core assumption of these studies[3,12] is that identifying the thinking processes experts use will enable others to access and then use these clinical reasoning (CR) steps to develop their own reasoning and/or facilitate others' CR development and abilities for practice application.

In contrast to this body of research, processes of ethical reasoning and their relationship to ethical action have received less research-based attention.[13] There is a growing literature describing ethical challenges encountered by physical therapists in different clinical settings[14-17] and some discussion of models of ethical reasoning appropriate for physical therapy practice.[2,8,18,19] Some studies have explored the ethical dispositions of expert physical therapy practitioners and have demonstrated that experts habitually demonstrate compassionate and nonjudgmental approaches to clients, are willing to admit to mistakes, and take deliberate actions such as reporting unethical behaviors of colleagues and advocating for clients.[20] A further common and overriding characteristic of experts is a sustained commitment to continually improve and actively maintain high standards of practice.[21]

These same attributes are represented more broadly in the literature for health professionals, discussing the types of attitudes and sense of purpose and agency required to continue to learn and develop as excellent practitioners.[22-25] Expert practitioner characteristics in professionals are described as[25(p415)]:

- Deep engagement with the profession's public purposes, where intrinsic sense of meaning and satisfaction from professional work align with extrinsic and public-oriented purposes

- A strong professional identity

- Habits of salience whereby complex situations are understood or framed, at least in part, in moral terms

- Habitual patterns of behavioral responses to clients, authorities, and peers that are aligned with the profession's standards and ideals, not self-interest

- A capacity to contribute to the ethical quality of the profession with a sense of moral agency, moral imagination, and courage to create more constructive practices

However, there remains a gap in the literature about the moral dimensions of expert practice: to explore, from an empirical perspective, how practitioners move from perceiving an ethical issue or dilemma through **taking ethical action**. For the physical therapy profession, questions arising from this gap include:

- What types of moral problems do therapists perceive in their various practice contexts?

- What types of ethical reasoning strategies do physical therapists use to respond to and address these ethical issues?

- How can physical therapists be supported to develop the habits of salience to move from moral perception to moral action?

- What conditions might foster therapists to use their ethical reasoning to contribute to the ethical quality of the physical therapy profession (including to collaborate with physical therapist assistants) to address ethical dilemmas and ensure action when needed?

Exploring and unpacking expert CR has been a strong thread in the literature seeking to explicate CR processes leading to clinical decisions and actions. In this chapter we follow this same thread by unpacking the skills of a clinical ethics expert. Rather than focus on expert physical therapy practitioners who demonstrate ethically oriented attributes as an integrated aspect of their practice, we refer to literature about the role and practices of clinical ethicists to more distinctly illuminate the work of a practitioner who focuses only on clinical ethical issues.

Our goal is to identify and distill the core skills and thinking processes inherent in the clinical ethicist role. The identification of thinking skills associated with ethical reasoning, within ethics consultations, may be seen as conceptually and practically different to their integration and use within physical therapy ethical reasoning practice. However, our andragogical rationale for examining ethical reasoning processes used by a clinical ethicist is based on the idea that making "expert ethics" thinking skills and approaches more visible and concrete[12,26] will create a more visible path for physical therapists to access and then translate as habits of salience relevant to their own practice contexts.

TABLE 5-1	
ROLES OF A CLINICAL ETHICIST	
ETHICIST AS PROBLEM-SOLVER	**ETHICIST AS CRITICAL OUTSIDER AND INTERPRETER**
• Gather relevant information • Clarify concepts • Help parties voice concerns and define interests • Identify range and boundaries of ethically acceptable options • Provide an ethical justification for each option	• Exercise moral judgment • Advise and coach others in moral decision-making • Develop moral authority (respect from others about their views)

UNPACKING CLINICAL ETHICS EXPERTISE: THE ROLE AND SKILLS OF A CLINICAL ETHICIST

The American Society for Bioethics and Humanities[27] has identified core tasks of the clinical ethicist to:

- Identify and analyze the nature of ethical questions or value uncertainty
- Gather information to clarify ethical concepts
- Help people voice concerns and define interests
- Identify the range and boundaries of ethically acceptable options with justifications

These core tasks can be collapsed into 2 fundamental roles (Table 5-1). The first is a problem-solving role, because the goals are to identify and analyze the nature of an ethical question or value uncertainty. The second role is as a critical outsider, standing back from a problem and facilitating others to think and reason toward an ethical resolution.[28,29]

These 2 roles illustrated in Table 5-1 can be further classified as visible and less visible (or tacit) types of ethical reasoning. The more overt skills of clinical ethicists arise from their role as problem-solvers with expertise in moral theory (much like a physical therapist who has obvious clinical knowledge and expertise). The problem-solving role emphasizes ethical theory and guiding ethical principles as the underpinning knowledge framework. For the ethicist, this content-based knowledge is apparent when the ethicist draws from established bioethical principles (eg, respect for individual autonomy, beneficence, nonmaleficence, and justice),[5] or other ethical frameworks and analytic tools (eg, relational bioethics, virtue ethics), to shed light on and address complex moral problems. Ethical reasoning from this perspective focuses on logical and reasoned thinking steps.

The less visible skills of ethical reasoning arise from the role of an ethicist as an interpreter, facilitator, and critical outsider who uses questions to clarify moral positions and who aims to create a safe moral space within which differences can be "aired, understood, and resolved."[30(p2)] This also involves questioning directed toward generating common meanings—not for conformity with a particular clinical management plan, but to foster a level of understanding, tolerance, and respect about different clinical and ethical views.[31,32] These subtler skills require an ethicist to exercise moral judgment[33] and to have established the moral authority and respect necessary to be accepted to advise and coach colleagues in moral decision-making.[30,34] To establish this moral authority, the ethicist needs a commitment to building a type of communicative trust in which colleagues feel safe to contribute their own views. Casarett et al[30] refer to these skills as "moral augmentation" involving gathering data, facilitating discussion between people involved, and clarifying goals and perspectives. Verkerk and Lindemann[35] describe the same process and state more plainly that ethicists "construct, with those others, some good-seeming way to go on."[35(p301)] The same holds true in the coaching of CR.

The more tacit role of facilitating the building of a justified ethical resolution requires sensitivity to the world view of others—a commitment to establishing shared or common meanings and, where values differ, a capacity to sit with partial understanding of an issue or a person's perspective.[36] In this role, the clinical ethicist strives to understand a variety of moral positions that might be relevant by posing questions, suggesting strategies for thinking and framing problems, and helping participants see their own positions relative to others.[31] This type of ethical reasoning is a more relational process of working with people and acknowledging and integrating the perspectives and values they hold. This is in contrast to the analytic and deductive problem-solving role (see Column 1 in Table 5-1), where analysis and application of principles and values maybe abstracted from the specific context and circumstances.

Agich[37] uses the term *epistemic authority* to describe the combination of explicit knowledge required for ethical problem-solving and the tacit moral and relational authority needed to bring people together to discuss ethical issues. This type of authority generated by a clinical ethicist is based on authority in the field of ethics knowledge (which could be philosophical, ethical, or medically based) and an ability to use the relevant knowledge within consultations in ways that meet the needs of those who rely on such knowledge. Epistemic authority is therefore a type of authority that draws from and generates trust in others. People who rely on the advice of clinical ethicists trust that their advice and perspectives are authoritative, not only because they know about ethics in a formal sense, but also because they trust their integrity to think deeply and reflectively about an issue.

In physical therapy practice, most of the ethical frameworks and tools developed to help therapists think about ethical issues align closely with the problem-solving approach (see Column 1, Table 5-1) designed to support the therapist in individually recognizing and analyzing moral dimensions of a situation. For example, the active engagement model proposes a series of questions to help therapists recognize not only the ethical issues at stake in a clinical situation, but also the values and perspectives they (personally and professionally) bring to the encounter, and the views and values of their patients.[18] The ethical reasoning bridge demonstrates how therapists need to move between formal ethical knowledge (eg, codes of conduct and biomedical ethical principles) on one side of the bridge, and the knowledge and experiential perspectives of others regarding the same scenario on the other.[2] The phenomenological approach to ethical analysis[38] discusses how therapists should incorporate contextual elements, including richer notions of the lived experience of their patients, to assist in the their ethical reasoning.[39]

In this chapter, we examine how expert ethics roles might be used to illuminate and enhance the nexus between moral perceptions and moral actions of CR by physical therapists. To do this, we present findings from a qualitative study examining physical therapists' experiences of and responses to ethical challenges in their everyday practice. The data portray the ethical dimensions or landscape of different work contexts, and they provide examples of therapists' ethical reasoning and responses. These empirical data also allow us to distinguish between the ethical reasoning and deliberation strategies of clinical ethicists and those of physical therapy practitioners, with the end goal for each to inform the other.[40]

PHYSICAL THERAPY DATA: HOW ARE PHYSICAL THERAPISTS RESPONDING TO ETHICAL CHALLENGES?

The data presented in the following section derive from a project (Identifying Ethical Dimensions in Australian Physiotherapy Practice) funded by the Australian Physiotherapy Association (APA). Two key goals of the research were to:

1. Identify current ethical issues and dilemmas that physiotherapists encounter in their daily practice

2. Explore the responses (ethical reasoning) of physical therapists (how they perceive ethical issues and how they interpret and act) in relation to these ethical challenges

The project used interpretive qualitative research methodology[41] and involved focus group discussions with members of APA special interest groups (SIGs).[42] SIGs are voluntary groups of APA members who offer professional development and support in specific clinical areas of physiotherapy practice. Purposive sampling of committee members of these groups enabled the provision of rich information about ethical issues they encountered in their specific practice areas.[42] Data were collected (both face-to-face and via telephone) using group interviews. The interview questions were developed from the project objectives and with reference to questions used in previous research investigating the perspectives of health professionals about their ethical dimensions of their practice.[43,44]

The final project sample comprised 88 physiotherapists from 13 SIGs, 2 networks, and 1 committee. Most participants had been practicing as physiotherapists for at least 10 years, with the majority currently practicing in metropolitan regions (n = 81). Of the participants, 20 identified that they were currently practicing in a rural setting (either solely or in conjunction with metropolitan practice), and 8 reported previously practicing in a rural setting. Participants resided in all states and territories of Australia except the Northern Territory.

Data analysis drew from the interpretive narrative method.[45] This involved identifying each ethical concern raised by the focus group, within its wider context and circumstances of practice as narrated by the group participants. Table 5-2 lists the specific and central ethical concerns raised by each focus group. Further details about the narrative-based results have been published.[46]

The second method of data analysis was the thematic and constant comparative method.[47] This was used to compare the types of ethical issues raised across all groups, and to identify common ideas and patterns about the issues raised and therapists' responses. Five themes emerged from therapists' discussion of ethical dimensions of their practice and their responses and processes of deliberation:

1. Considering the working environment

2. Balancing diverse needs and expectations of patients and other stakeholders

3. Defining ethics

4. Striving to act ethically

5. Talking about ethics

TABLE 5-2
SPECIFIC ETHICAL ISSUES RAISED BY PARTICIPATING GROUPS

PARTICIPATING NATIONAL GROUP	SPECIFIC ETHICAL ISSUE
Acupuncture and Dry-Needling	Handling concerns about the impact of the physiotherapist's gender on the treatment encounter Dealing with conflicting views about (1) benefits and harms of acupuncture and (2) holistic and narrowly defined clinical treatment Managing risks associated with acupuncture and dry needling
Aquatic	Managing safety and risk in the aquatic physiotherapy practice context Negotiating available funding to meet patient needs Meeting diverse patient needs within the aquatic environment Managing emotional responses in the aquatic environment
Business	Balancing different drivers of clinical decision-making (funding, institutional guidelines, evidence-based practice) Managing conflicting financial relationships (funding models, product endorsement, other incentives) Integrating patient-centered and evidence-based practice Identifying and managing professional relationships with patients Keeping within professional boundaries when using social media for business purposes
Cancer, Palliative Care, and Lymphedema Network	Accessing rehabilitation in palliative care Managing inequitable health fund rebates Dealing with incidental findings of cancer and duty of care to patient Identifying philosophy and defining scope and role of palliative care physiotherapy Identifying risk and obtaining informed consent for treatment
Cardiorespiratory	Obtaining informed consent for treatment where patients may lack capacity Providing care that may be burdensome Handling pressure to discharge patients prematurely
Continence and Women's Health	Dealing with the sensitive nature of vaginal examination and treatment (patient expectations and physiotherapists' competencies) Balancing confidentiality and disclosure in the context of sexual abuse Balancing professional relationships and loyalties between patients and referring clinicians Defining scope of practice in women's health practice
Educators	Handling competing interests between student learning and patient care Making and justifying decisions about student clinical competence Understanding what to teach if little evidence exists for an area of practice
Emergency Department Network	Managing conflicts with doctors about treatment decisions Responding to policies that impact on quality of care in an emergency department Managing patient expectations to see a doctor Mitigating concerns about suboptimal care when using an interpreter Meeting performance targets without compromising patient care Responding to suspected domestic violence

continued

	TABLE 5-2 (CONTINUED) **SPECIFIC ETHICAL ISSUES RAISED BY PARTICIPATING GROUPS**
PARTICIPATING NATIONAL GROUP	**SPECIFIC ETHICAL ISSUE**
Gerontology	Defining and valuing physiotherapy-specific services in aged care facilities Responding to treatment restrictions based on financial pressures Assessing residents' competence for consent in aged care facilities Dealing with pressures to discharge residents prematurely Developing new models of physiotherapy in response to changing expectations and work opportunities in aged care sector
Indigenous Health Committee	Addressing inequitable access to physiotherapy for Aboriginal people and responding to discriminatory practice
Leadership and Management	Responding to reports of unprofessional practice Maintaining confidentiality and resolving conflict Identifying a need for more ethics training Managing conflict among multiple roles and responsibilities (eg, supporting and monitoring staff, primary and preventive practice)
Musculoskeletal	Managing competing duties to patients and referring clinicians (and coaches in sporting teams) Maintaining professional boundaries in different clinical contexts (eg, treating family members or students, meeting patients socially) Recognizing and avoiding overservicing
Neurology	Ensuring care is not compromised because of demands and restrictions imposed by funding models Managing differing or conflicting family and patient expectations Defining therapeutic relationships and boundaries of care in rehabilitation settings
Occupational Health	Maintaining professionalism in subcontractor working relationships Managing responsibilities to both employers and employees Sustaining personal and professional integrity in physiotherapy practice
Pediatric	Managing differing views about treatment when parents/family and health team disagree Managing trust in therapeutic relationship when mandatory reporting child abuse Responding to restrictions imposed by funding models and health policy decisions shaping practice Balancing confidentiality, privacy, and information needs of parents and adolescents Managing professional boundaries in partnership models of practice
Sports	Making clinical decisions when players disclose some but not all information Making clinical decisions when conflicting interests exist among players, coaches, and selectors Maintaining professional relationships when closely associated with a team

Themes 1 and 2 relate to the working environment and portray aspects of the ethical practice landscape for physical therapists at individual, organizational, and societal levels. Within the working environment (Theme 1), these included the influence of externally imposed constraints and affordances such as health insurance funding and governmental health policies restricting the scope of treatment. At the level of the patient and therapist encounter, many groups discussed ethical issues arising from increasing diversity of the individual patient's expectations of care (see Table 5-2).

The continence and women's health group raised a concern about how to best provide information and obtain informed consent for vaginal examination and exercise prescription. Participants acknowledged this treatment to be potentially sensitive for patients, and despite high levels of evidence for its effectiveness, they described how patients were sometimes surprised to find a physical therapist offering this treatment. These women's health specialist practitioners recognized it was ethically important to undertake assessment and treatment carefully to provide sufficient information to patients and to avoid misunderstandings. The aquatic group discussed the emotional reactions people sometimes had when they were immersed in water, and they described the challenge of emotionally supporting people while also ensuring therapeutic exercise goals were achieved within a session. The educators group discussed the challenge of meeting students' needs to see and practice their skills with patients while at the same time ensuring patients were safe.

Themes 3 (defining ethics), 4 (striving to act ethically), and 5 (talking about ethics) focus more closely on how physical therapists interpreted and responded to this landscape: how they defined ethics within their own practice, and the resources (including formal codes of conduct) they used to inform their ethical reflection and decision-making. For example, under theme 3, defining ethics, some participants defined ethics as a process of adhering to formal regulatory codes of conduct as their reference point for professional expectations and obligations.

> *... If you're a registered physio, then the code of ethics is part of your registration and that's part of what people understand they need. Their professional standing means embedding those codes of ethics into your practice. (Musculoskeletal SIG member)*

> *The Code of Conduct helps to draw the line about what should and shouldn't be done related to treatment and so it helps me draw lines. (Gerontology SIG member)*

Others spoke of "grey" areas in their practice, where they encountered complex relationships and differing values held by colleagues and/or with patients and third parties, which did not neatly align with the guidance and prescriptions of codes of conduct.

> *... It is very grey, and you can write a set of guidelines but when it comes to those actual patient scenarios ... [which] often have many shades of grey and where there's not always a right or wrong answer, I think that guidelines can be hard to interpret in those really challenging situations. (Neurology SIG member)*

Participants perceived codes and guidelines as having limited usefulness for ethical issues that required a dynamic and context-based response. Instead, participants described their ethical deliberation as being grounded in their particular context and relationships with patients and with colleagues and with health funders or through prior experience.

> *You also draw on your own experience, your expertise, your own views on it, your experience that you've had in the past with other patients or clients. (Acupuncture and Dry-Needling SIG member)*

Theme 4 (striving to act ethically) encapsulated discussions about striving to put the patient first and advocating for patients by helping them navigate complex health and health regulatory systems. However, it also highlighted feelings of discomfort and moral distress when therapists felt they were not able to adequately empower patients or did not have the authority to act in what they perceived to be patients' best interests.

A strong finding encompassed by Theme 5 (talking about ethics) was that practitioner groups who had forums for ethics discussions seemed to do a lot better in resolving ethical challenges than groups who had not developed processes for discussion forums. For example, participants highlighted that an important way of developing their understanding of ethical obligations was through talking through issues with more experienced colleagues and peers or through attending more formal ethics education.

> *Generally, one of the best coping mechanisms is not to feel like you are having to make that decision in isolation on your own. (Cardiorespiratory SIG member)*

> *... We've got a whole heap of legends in our field and they've been through a lot of things and so we'll often raise things with somebody who we know is very experienced. (Occupational Health SIG member)*

Mentoring early career physiotherapists was identified as an effective way of supporting development or "growing people up" (Indigenous Health Committee) in their ethical practice. The SIGs who had experience of regular discussion sessions either in formal continuing education sessions or more informally with their colleagues described less frustration and moral distress about the ethical issues they faced than those groups and individuals who faced ethical complexity without support. Therapists discussed how they valued ethics education at a professional development or post-graduate level. Suggestions for ongoing ethics education included lecture evenings, workshops, and webinars.

> *I certainly think it's [ethics education] something you need to do once you're out working. They probably could have tried to have some case studies or something at a university level where they tried to expose you to some of these kinds of issues. But I'm not sure it's something you can appreciate until you are at the bedside with an 85-year-old who's got multiple comorbidities and has got pneumonia and all those kinds of issues, but you get that emotional kind of interface as well. (Cardiorespiratory SIG member)*

FROM ETHICAL REASONING TO ETHICAL ACTION

At the beginning of this chapter, we posed 4 questions, and in this section, we will reexamine each one.

Question 1 asked, "What types of moral problems do therapists perceive in their various practice contexts?" The data affirm a complex ethical landscape, which has previously been noted by others.[14,16,48-54]

Question 2 considered, "What types of ethical reasoning strategies do physical therapists use to respond to and address these ethical issues?" The participant therapists were actively engaged in ethical reasoning processes, informed not only by normative principles and codes of conduct, but also according to their own analysis and ethical interpretation of their clinical experiences. However, the data also identified many grey areas of physical therapy practice—areas of ethical uncertainty where therapists were not sure of the scope and limits of their practice, or where they felt they were being constrained by others or by health funding policies that curtailed what they felt to be treatment in a patient's best interests. Although therapists recognized the benefit of seeking guidance from colleagues, this was framed in terms of seeking assistance to enable them to individually decide the most ethically appropriate response.

When these empirical data about ethical reasoning are compared with the roles and practices of a clinical ethicist, there is strong alignment with the first role of the clinical ethicist as a problem-solver—applying moral principles to specific contexts and individual patient circumstances. The second role of the clinical ethicist—to help others build an ethical resolution and to "construct with others, a good-seeming way to go"[35]—was less obvious in the data, although several groups discussed the importance and value of discussing and reflecting on ethical issues with colleagues and peers. Yet, it is this aspect of the ethicist's role that seems to be most relevant as a possible response to Question 3: "How can physical therapists be supported to develop the habits of salience to move from moral perception to moral action?"

A skilled ethicist gently and purposefully probes and encourages clinicians and patients to discuss their stories and articulate what matters to them. This communication strategy helps bring out different perspectives and ideas about a moral problem. It also situates ethical reasoning as a relational activity that involves working to establish common meanings through understanding, tolerance, and respect for the views and perspectives of colleagues, patients, and other stakeholders. This is a subtle but important shift in focus from ethical reasoning as a component of individual moral agency to ethical reasoning as a process of working with others to resolve ethical issues.

Cultivating this more facilitative and relational notion of ethical reasoning requires an environment of trust and safety, which encourages people to voice their perspectives, their ethical uncertainties, and their experiences. It is suggested that to become skilled at discussing ethical issues, "you have to do it, not sit back and watch someone else do it."[35(p300)]

There are 3 steps[35] to help clinicians do this moral reflection in their clinical practice, with reflection and dialogue focused on:

1. Seeing and discussing what is morally relevant in a given situation by seeking perspectives from a range of stakeholders in a specific clinical context

2. Knowing the particular point of view from which one sees it by explaining to others your own professional values and experience-informed perspective

3. Understanding that others involved in the situation may see it differently, and habitually discussing ethical concerns with colleagues to develop responses together

The benefits of workplace-based ethics discussions according to these steps are to encourage therapists to stand back from their personal assessment of an ethical situation and listen to other perspectives, find out different versions of the empirical details about a case, test out options, and become more aware of support available. All these activities are designed to enhance their self-awareness and confidence to move from ethical reasoning using an individual problem-solving process drawing from principles and moral theories to discussing ethics with others in their specific work context.

Verkerk and Lindemann[35(p291)] argue that if professionals are to practice their professions well, ethical reflection should not be left to a moral consultant, as "one might leave the care of the patient's heart to a cardiac consultant." The clinical ethics process of sharing ethical deliberation among all people within organizations involved in ethical challenges introduces the notion of shared accountability.[55] Ethical CR seen in this light draws on the collective wisdom of health teams, administrators, physical therapists, and others to ensure their ethical CR leads to ethical action. The research findings presented in this chapter demonstrate that therapists in many of the groups interviewed already recognize the value of dialogue with others and have used this method to explore and resolve ethical issues. These types of processes of collaborative and relational ethical reasoning are also relevant to address Question 4: "What conditions might foster therapists to use their ethical reasoning to contribute to the ethical quality of the physical therapy profession (including to collaborate with physical therapy assistants) to address ethical dilemmas and ensure action when needed?"

CONCLUSION

Chapter 5 has described the ethical reasoning strategies and professional dispositions of a clinical ethicist and compared them to physical therapists' experiences of ethical challenges and their ethical CR responses. Shulman[55] suggests that there is a great deal to learn from examining the signature characteristic forms of teaching and learning of different professions. We similarly conclude that there is a great deal to learn about ethical reasoning for physical therapists by examining the ethical reasoning strategies of an expert clinical ethicist. Based on the data presented, physical therapists' reasoning aligns closely with the ethical problem-solving work undertaken by a clinical ethicist. Therapists similarly draw from a range of sources (eg, formal codes of ethics, dialogue with peers and colleagues, their own experience and judgment) when making ethical decisions in their everyday practice. While physical therapists also recognized the need to seek and integrate the moral perspectives and understanding of others when addressing ethical challenges, their descriptions of moral engagement with others were (understandably) less developed than ethicists who actively facilitate moral resolution with others as a primary part of their role.

However, seeing ethical reasoning as clinical ethicists do—as a relational activity that seeks to establish common meanings through understanding, tolerance, and respect for the views of patients, colleagues, and other stakeholders—holds great promise for advancing the moral agency and expertise of physical therapists and for illuminating how to bridge the nexus between moral perception and analysis and moral action in the workplace. Reframing ethical analysis to encompass "sensitivity to the world view of others; a commitment to establishing shared or common meanings and, where there are differing values, a capacity to sit with partial understanding of an issue or a person's perspective"[36] builds on the current capacities of physical therapists. It has implications for ethics education development and progression of ethical CR and professional development programs to incorporate methods of moral deliberation with others as a component of professional ethics training and development. Importantly, it merges clinical ethics and clinical practice expertise.

Reflection Moment

Please consider how you will incorporate any of the 3 steps to enhance your moral compass with decision-making.

REFERENCES

1. Edwards I, Jones M, Carr J, Braunack-Mayer A, Jensen G. Clinical reasoning strategies in physical therapy. *Phys Ther.* 2004;84:312-330.
2. Edwards I, Delany C. Ethical reasoning. In: Higgs J, Jones M, Loftus S, Christensen N, eds. *Clinical Reasoning in the Health Professions.* 3rd ed. Amsterdam, Netherlands: Butterworth-Heinemann Elsevier; 2008:279-289.
3. Norman G. Research in clinical reasoning: past history and current trends. *Med Educ.* 2005;39(4):418-427.
4. Higgs J, Jones M, Loftus S, Christensen N, eds. *Clinical Reasoning in the Health Professions.* 3rd ed. Amsterdam, Netherlands: Butterworth-Heinemann Elsevier; 2008.
5. Beauchamp TL, Childress JF. *Principles of Biomedical Ethics.* Oxford, United Kingdom: Oxford University Press; 2001.
6. Rhodes R, Alfandre D. A systematic approach to clinical moral reasoning. *Clin Ethics.* 2007;2(2):66-70.
7. Jonsen AR, Siegler M, Winslade WJ. *Clinical Ethics: A Practical Approach to Ethical Decisions in Clinical Medicine.* 8th ed. New York, NY: McGraw Hill Professional; 2015.
8. Edwards I, Braunack-Mayer A, Jones M. Ethical reasoning as a clinical-reasoning strategy in physiotherapy. *Physiotherapy.* 2005;91(4):229-236.
9. Loftus S, Smith M. A history of clinical reasoning research. In: Higgs J, Jones M, Loftus S, Christensen N, eds. *Clinical Reasoning in the Health Professions.* 3rd ed. Amsterdam, Netherlands: Butterworth-Heinemann Elsevier; 2008:205-212.
10. Schmidt HG, Boshuizen HPA. On acquiring expertise in medicine. *Educ Psyc Rev.* 1993;5(3):205-221.
11. Ajjawi R, Higgs J. Learning to reason: a journey of professional socialisation. *Adv Health Sci Educ Theory Pract.* 2008;13(2):133-150.
12. Delany C, Golding C. Teaching clinical reasoning by making thinking visible: an action research project with allied health clinical educators. *BMC Med Educ.* 2014;14(1):20.
13. Irby DM, Cooke M, O'Brien BC. Calls for reform of medical education by the Carnegie Foundation for the Advancement of Teaching: 1910 and 2010. *Acad Med.* 2010;85(2):220-227.
14. Hudon A, Drolet M-J, Williams-Jones B. Ethical issues raised by private practice physiotherapy are more diverse than first meets the eye: recommendations from a literature review. *Physiother Can.* 2015;67(2):124-132.
15. Delany C, Gillam L, Spriggs M, Fry C. The unique nature of clinical ethics in allied health paediatrics and child health. *Camb Q Healthc Ethics.* 2010;19(4):471-480.
16. Praestegaard J, Gard G, Glasdam S. Practicing physiotherapy in Danish private practice: an ethical perspective. *Med Health Care Philos.* 2013;16(3):555-564.
17. Edwards I, Richardson B. Clinical reasoning and population health: decision making for an emerging paradigm of health care. *Physiother Theory Pract.* 2008;24(3):183-193.

18. Delany C, Edwards I, Jensen G, Skinner E. Closing the gap between ethics knowledge and practice through active engagement: an applied model of physical therapy ethics. *Phys Ther.* 2010;90:1068-1078.

19. Greenfield B, Jensen G, Delany C, Mostrom E, Knab M, Jampel A. Power and promise of narrative for advancing physical therapist education and practice. *Phys Ther Sport.* 2015;95(6):924-933.

20. Jensen GM, Gwyer J, Shepard KF. Expert practice in physical therapy. *Phys Ther.* 2000;80(1):28-43; discussion 44-52.

21. Jensen G, Delany C. Ethics and expert practice. In: Higgs J, Trede F, eds. *Professional Practice Discourse Marginalia.* Amsterdam, Netherlands: Sense Publishers; 2016:73-82.

22. Stichter M. Virtues, skills, and right action. *Ethical Theory Moral Pract.* 2011;14(1):73-86.

23. Benner PIE. Learning through experience and expression: skilful ethical comportment in nursing practice. In: Thomasma D, Kissell J, eds. *The Health Care Professional as Friend and Healer.* Washington, DC: Georgetown University Press; 2000:49-64.

24. Dreyfus H, Dreyfus S. The relationship of theory and practice in the acquisition of skill. In: Benner P, Tanner C, Chesla C, eds. *Expertise in Nursing Practice.* New York, NY: Springer; 1986.

25. Colby A, Sullivan W. Formation of professionalism and purpose: perspectives from the preparation for the professions program. *Univ St Thomas Law J.* 2008;5:404-426.

26. Ritchhart R, Church M, Morrison K. *Making Thinking Visible: How to Promote Engagement, Understanding, and Independence for All Learners.* Hoboken, NJ: John Wiley & Sons; 2011.

27. Tarzian AJ, Force ACCUT. Health care ethics consultation: an update on core competencies and emerging standards from the American Society for Bioethics and Humanities' Core Competencies Update Task Force. *Am J Bioeth.* 2013;13(2):3-13.

28. Dubler NN, Liebman CB. *Bioethics Mediation: A Guide to Shaping Shared Solutions.* Nashville, TN: Vanderbilt University Press; 2011.

29. Fox E, Myers S, Pearlman RA. Ethics consultation in United States hospitals: a national survey. *Am J Bioeth.* 2007;7(2):13-25.

30. Casarett DJ, Daskal F, Lantos J. The authority of the clinical ethicist. *The Hastings Center Report.* 1998;28(6):6-11.

31. Delany C, Hall G. "I just love these sessions:" Should physician satisfaction matter in clinical ethics consultations? *Clin Eth.* 2012;7:116-121.

32. Delany C. The role of clinical ethics consultations for physical therapy practice. *Phys Ther Rev.* 2012;17(3):176-183.

33. Priaulx N. The troubled identity of the bioethicist. *Health Care Anal.* 2013;21(1):6-19.

34. Archard D. Why moral philosophers are not and should not be moral experts. *Bioethics.* 2011;25(3):119-127.

35. Verkerk M, Lindemann H. Toward a naturalized clinical ethics. *Kennedy Inst Ethics J.* 2012;22(4):289-306.

36. Burbules N, Rice S. Dialogue across differences: continuing the conversation. *Harv Educ Rev.* 1991;61(4):393-417.

37. Agich G. Why should anyone listen to ethics consultants? *Philos Medicine.* 2002:117-137.

38. Greenfield B, Jensen GM. Beyond a code of ethics: phenomenological ethics for everyday practice. *Physiother Res Int.* 2010;15(2):88-95.

39. Bruce Greenfield P, Musolino GM. Technology in rehabilitation: ethical and curricular implications for physical therapist education. *J Phys Ther Educ.* 2012;26(2):81.

40. De Vries R. How can we help? From "sociology in" to "sociology of" bioethics. *J Law Med Ethics.* 2004;32(2):279-292.

41. Denzin NK, Lincoln YS. *The SAGE Handbook of Qualitative Research.* London, United Kingdom: SAGE Publications; 2005.

42. Krueger RA, Casey MA. *Focus Groups: A Practical Guide for Applied Research.* London, United Kingdom: SAGE Publications; 2014.

43. Finch E, Geddes EL, Larin H. Ethically-based clinical decision-making in physical therapy: process and issues. *Physiother Theory Pract.* 2005;21(3):147-162.

44. Sturman NJ, Parker M, van Driel ML. The informal curriculum—general practitioner perceptions of ethics in clinical practice. *Aus Fam Phys.* 2012;41(12):981-984.

45. Guillemin M, Gillam L. Telling moments. *Everyday Ethics in Health Care.* Melbourne, Australia: IP Communications; 2006.

46. Delany C, Edwards I, Fryer C. How physiotherapists perceive, interpret and respond to the ethical dimensions of practice: a qualitative study. *Physiother Theory Pract.* 2018;28:1-14.

47. Charmaz K. *Constructing Grounded Theory: A Practical Guide Through Qualitative Research.* London, United Kingdom: SAGE Publications; 2006.

48. Triezenberg HL. The identification of ethical issues in physical therapy practice. *Phys Ther.* 1996;76(10):1097-1107; discussion 1107-1098.

49. Carpenter C, Richardson B. Ethics knowledge in physical therapy: a narrative review of the literature since 2000. *Phys Ther Rev.* 2008;13(5):366-374.

50. American Physical Therapy Association. The code of ethics for the physical therapist. www.apta.org. Accessed October 31, 2018.

51. Hudon A, Laliberté M, Hunt M, et al. What place for ethics? An overview of ethics teaching in occupational therapy and physiotherapy programs in Canada. *Disabil Rehabil.* 2014;36(9):775-780.

52. Laliberte M, Hudon A. Do conflicts of interest create a new professional norm? Physical therapists and workers' compensation. *Am J Bioeth.* 2013;13(10):26-28.

53. Hunt MR, Carnevale FA. Exploring disability through the lens of moral experience. *Phys Ther Rev.* 2012;17(6):369-373.

54. Oyeyemi A. Ethics and contextual framework for professional behaviour and code of practice for physiotherapists in Nigeria. *J Nigeria Soc Physiother.* 2012;18(1-2):49-53.

55. Shulman L. Signature pedagogies in the professions. *Daedelus.* 2005;134:42-51.

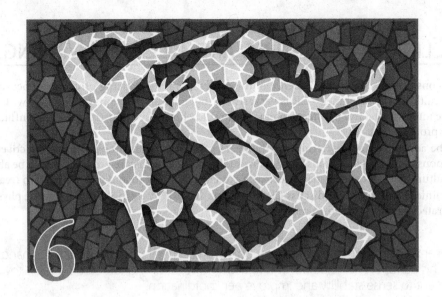

CLINICAL REASONING AND
DECISION-MAKING:
An Abridged Literature Review

Kyle Covington, PT, DPT, PhD

OBJECTIVES

- Examine an abridged review of the literature related to clinical reasoning and decision-making (CRDM).

- Compare predominant hallmark approaches for clinical reasoning (CR) within the health professions, considering both cognitive and interactive paradigms.

- Analyze how adaptive movement is used within physical therapy practice and education for CRDM.

- Critically examine a case study and how the origination of movement is a distinctive characteristic for CRDM within physical therapy.

This chapter provides a concise synthesis of the review of the literature-to-date reflective of CRDM. The review examines cognitive paradigms (ie, hypothetico-deductive, pattern, and intuitive) and interactive paradigms (ie, narrative reasoning and alternative forms). The chapter further examines the literature related to communicative and instrumental action in the paradigms and briefly describes the CR health discipline perspectives (ie, medicine, heuristics and context, occupational therapy, holistic tracks, and physical therapy collaborative CR). Discussion related to the importance of CR in relation to movement is provided, with a contemporary examination of a situational analysis in physical therapy. A proposed model within physical therapy of teaching and reasoning relationships for applications for human movement is introduced and explained.

Musolino GM, Jensen GM, eds. *Clinical Reasoning and Decision-Making in Physical Therapy: Facilitation, Assessment, and Implementation* (pp 57-70).
© 2020 Taylor & Francis Group.

Clinical Reasoning and Decision-Making

CRDM is a central consideration to the competence of the contemporary practicing professional because of the complexity of practice in today's health care environment. CR is pervasive throughout all decisions and actions within health professions practice. Therefore, one must understand its effects in practice to study how clinical instructors (CIs) influence students in their development as novice professionals.

Practitioners must be adept at quickly determining the needs of their patients, implementing effective plans for their care, and assessing their response to the interventions selected. In addition, the health care provider should be able to understand the social, personal, and cultural influences that may affect each patient's response to and participation in treatment.[1-6]

Consideration of a clinical scenario, as we discuss CR paradigms, helps provide insight into how the physical therapist's complex reasoning is integrated into his or her own movement.

Because of a recent stroke, an older woman struggles to coordinate her right arm and hand. Her physical therapist places his hands on her shoulder and forearm muscles, giving targeted pressure toward the hand, allowing the patient to sense stability and improve her coordination.

The woman's physical therapist has an infinite number of decisions to resolve during their interaction. What is the underlying pathology? Is the lack of motion solely caused by the stroke? Does she have other impairments from a previous injury? Exactly which muscles are affected, and why? Are they weak, absent of nerve input, injured in another way, tight, or painful? Is the lack of motion due to an injury at the joint? The therapist must consider all these questions as he begins to interact with the patient.

As treatment begins, the therapist starts to reason through other factors important to this patient. Does she have family, work, or community responsibilities, and how are those impacted by her injury? How is she impacted by the inability to perform these duties? How will these changes in her life affect her participation in rehabilitation?

Next, the therapist begins to interact with the patient by the use of his own movement. First, he feels the motion she has available in the joints of her arm as he moves the limb segments for her, with assistive and passive motions, considering quality and coordination of movement. Next, he palpates the joint and each muscle to assess its level of activity, continuity, and/or injury. He decides how, when, and where to place his hands to provide optimal data for his decisions, while at the same time considering the patient's needs, pain level, and personal preferences.

After a careful assessment, the physical therapist must begin to decide how to improve this woman's loss of movement in her arm. He decides where to place his hands, where to position his body, and in which directions to shift his weight to affect the change he desires in her arm. He carefully provides pressure in specific places, in chosen directions, and in a selected timing pattern to initiate activity in her arm. Simultaneously, his hands gather data about how her movement is affected, and he continues to adjust accordingly.

In an effort to describe this process, a juxtaposition of thinking, movement, response, rethinking, and reanalyzing occurs for CR in the health professions. CR is the sum of the thinking and decision-making processes associated with clinical practice; it is a critical skill in the health professions, central to the practice of professional autonomy, and it enables practitioners to take "wise" action, meaning taking the best judged action in a specific context.[7(p4)]

Arguably, the ability to employ CR is at the heart of all clinical practice.[7,8] It is precisely this position that makes CR such a complex concept. The assumption presented by Higgs and Jones[7] that CR is inextricably linked with every facet of practice implies that theoretical models of CR must encompass all decision-making and action taken by a practitioner. In addition, such theories should explain the time-consuming nature of the decision-making process of the novice clinician, compared to the seemingly automatic and rapid nature of the expert's clinical actions.[9-12]

Clinical Reasoning Paradigms

There has long been an emphasis on the acquisition and recall of knowledge, as well as the proper use of psychomotor skills, in the clinical care of patients.[13] The historical approach to scientific research, in which careful and methodical approaches to inquiry and discovery have been the norm, mirrors medicine's focus on CR.[14] Historically, some health professions, such as nursing, viewed their clinical decision-making (CDM) to include foci beyond a methodological search to answer a clinical question. They routinely sought options to include a broader interpretation of the impact of sociocultural and personal influences on the patient and practitioner in their clinical decisions.[15]

Though nursing long acknowledged the need for careful consideration of influences beyond the clinician in decision-making, until recently there remained a dominance of an analytic and positivist approach to studying and describing CR across all health professions. Now, many health care professions are more cognizant of the benefits involved in considering CR paradigms that include the patient's experiences.[14,16] As the body of knowledge about CR expanded, Higgs and Jones[7] proposed organizing the types of paradigms into 2 broad categories: those models that rely primarily on cognitive processes and those that are interactive by nature. Both paradigms have implications for understanding the learning relationship between CIs and their students.

COGNITIVE PARADIGMS

CR models developed primarily from the cognitive science literature.[17] These models represent a positivist paradigm, if the clinician can arrive at a decision that reflects an ideal truth. This truth is objective and measurable, and therefore can be generalized and used predictively.[1] The cognitive paradigms presented here are often collectively termed "diagnostic reasoning."[1(p314)] The theory development behind cognitive science, as applied to health professionals' reasoning, can be traced back to the mid-20th century as cognitive scientists began to study how people developed ideas, reasoned with conflicting information, and acted upon that information. In the early 1970s, these studies led to theories of problem-solving that described how a person, when confronted with a challenge, created a mental "problem space" that was influenced by context, available information, and experience.[18(pp148-149)]

A cognitive paradigm, or diagnostic reasoning, considers that the diagnostician places information into a mental classification system, grouping relative information together, and separating confounding information into its own class. Once clinicians consider these mental sets of information that arise from the patient's presentation, they compare these to known facts, witnessed events, and experiences to provide a prognosis, plan a treatment session, or begin to investigate more avenues of the patient's case.[19]

> When evaluating the woman after her stroke, the physical therapist needs to determine the exact causes for the lack of movement in her arm. Do tight muscles, inactive nerve input, pain, joint derangement, or a combination of all of these limit motion? Each possibility has a set of visible or testable signs and symptoms that the therapist must next seek to confirm or deny before proceeding in his treatment of the woman.

HYPOTHETICO-DEDUCTIVE REASONING

Elstein, Shulman, and Sprafka[20] proposed the hypothetico-deductive reasoning model as an explanation for the CR processes of physicians. This continues as a prominently used paradigm for analyzing, researching, and teaching CR in medicine.[1]

In hypothetico-deductive reasoning, the physician or other health professional delimits differential diagnoses based on the symptoms presented by the patient.[17] These diagnoses are derived from gathering information from the patient interview and examination. One question helps lead to another; one answer generates the next test.

> *To transform a problem from unstructured to structured by generating a small set of possible solutions [is] an efficient way to solve diagnostic problems.*[17(pp9-10)]

The hypothetico-deductive approach seeks to maximize cognitive efficiency by confirming or negating information presented with reliable measurement and testing.[1] The approach tends to be used by novice practitioners and experienced professionals encountering new or uniquely complex scenarios,[1] similar to the dynamic of student interns and experienced CIs. With more experience, questioning of the patient becomes more selective, and hypothesis generation happens more quickly and efficiently. The experienced clinician may not have more general hypotheses, as the novice might, but he or she can arrive at them with better efficiency, suggesting that the experienced clinician uses better "domain-specific knowledge," allowing the questioning of the patient and test selection to be better deduced to confirm or negate the hypotheses in question.[17(p10)]

The hypothetico-deductive reasoning method involves both inductive and deductive thought.[21] The clinician must move through a group of specific observations to generate hypotheses. This represents an inductive reasoning process. The practitioner, then, must also deductively test these generalizations on his or her specific case to confirm the hypothesis.

> *By this strategy, the induction problem is reduced to an issue of deduction, of the form "If the patient has X, then he must exhibit the following features."*[22]

As the physical therapist assists the woman attempting to raise her shoulder, he can feel that as she moves her arm to the side, a large indention appears in the surface of her skin, just as the muscles that cover this indention become inactive. He remembers this tactile feeling from many of his previous patients who had had a stroke, and he immediately knows the small rotator cuff muscles, which hold her arm to her shoulder blade, are extremely weak and incapable of stabilizing her joint as her more powerful shoulder muscles try to raise her arm.

Pattern Recognition

Pattern recognition is sometimes referred to as *nonanalytic reasoning*,[22] *forward reasoning*, or *illness scripts*.[1,22-24] In pattern recognition, "the clinician recognizes certain features of a case almost instantly, and this recognition leads to the use of other relevant information, including 'if-then' rules of production in the clinician's stored knowledge network."[1(p314)] The construction of cognitive representations of patient diagnoses demands experience; therefore, this method of reasoning tends to be used most by experienced clinicians.[23] Since the clinician can compare patient presentations to representations of previous experiences, this method of reasoning also tends to be faster.[22] When the experienced clinician has no recognizable pattern for comparing his or her current patient presentation, then the clinician may need to slow down and revert to hypothetico-deductive approaches to determining an answer to the clinical problem.[1] As demonstrated in the case vignette, the physical therapist's ability to use pattern recognition may be strongly influenced by the tactile information received from using his or her hands and body to work with patients. Using tactile information in CR pattern recognition, however, has not been extensively demonstrated in the literature, and it warrants investigation. Since pattern recognition relies on a significant experience base, this method is of little use to the novice clinician or student. Instead, it is a strategy that must develop with time and with more varied experiences in clinical practice. CIs, therefore, share their pattern recognitions to help guide novice learners.

One month ago, the experienced therapist was working with a patient whose lower leg would not move in a coordinated fashion after she had had a stroke. The therapist tried all the usual treatment methods. Knowing the patient had been an accomplished dancer throughout her life, he decided to play some of her favorite, upbeat music and encouraged her to tap her foot to the rhythm she heard. Ever so slightly, the otherwise inactive muscles began to twitch in synchrony to the beat. Now faced with a similar scenario with the woman's arm that lacks motion, he sits her in front of a piano, just like she does every Sunday morning at her church, and asks her to play. Though she doesn't have the strength to push the keys enough to make a sound, her fingers begin to flex.

Intuitive Reasoning

Some consider intuitive reasoning to be the same as pattern recognition. However, other researchers suggest this form of CDM relies on the practitioner using "instance scripts."[7] Instance scripts allow a clinician to compare a current patient presentation with a specific occurrence that he or she experienced previously with a patient. Whereas pattern recognition is formed by the compilation of many different similar cases, intuitive reasoning is derived from one specific instance. Similar to pattern recognition, however, it is only after previous unique cases are presented that the clinician is able to use intuitive processes in his or her reasoning. Once again, this is limited for the novice clinician, or even for the experienced clinician who has had little exposure to alternative scenarios or treatment approaches.

Interactive Paradigms

The cognitive paradigms each have limits. In addition, they all focus the locus of control to the clinician and do not consider the unique values and experiences of the patient. However, since the mid-1990s, researchers have paid greater attention to other forms of CR extending beyond the cognitive paradigms.[1]

In the late 20th century, as health information became readily available via technology to the lay public, consumers began to be more knowledgeable. In addition, sweeping governmental reform empowered the patient to play more of a role in the decision-making process for his or her health care. These factors combined to force change in the health professions. Where previously the practitioner was able to make clinical decisions based solely on his or her prior knowledge and experiences, now he or she needs to consider his or her patient's desires and integrate these into the plan of care.[25]

Many of these efforts in the health professions to integrate patients' values in CDM build out of an understanding of the benefits of reflection-in-action as a method for discovery and development of knowledge.[26] Reflection-in-action calls for the decision-maker to acknowledge that his or her choices and decisions have implications for the patient and, therefore, should attempt to incorporate the infinite, yet specific, variables that each individual patient presents. The interactive paradigm, therefore, shifts the clinician out of a positivist approach of knowledge generation and identification of truth, to an approach in which patients' values, social contexts, and experiences have merit and inform the clinician's diagnostic process. The interactive approach, sometimes referred to as interpretive, "...recognizes that truth or knowledge is related to meaning and the context in which it is produced and, therefore, concedes that in any given situation there may be multiple realities, truths, or perspectives."[1(p314)]

Through garbled speech, the woman begins to tell the physical therapist about her life. She tells him she is a wife, a mother, and a board member of a prominent company, all of which cause stress. She is active in her community, playing music weekly at her church and volunteering with a local women's club. Her favorite activity is spending time with her 3 grandchildren, and she especially loves to play catch with them in the park when the weather is nice. She becomes teary when she tells the physical therapist that in 6 weeks her youngest daughter will get married and wants her mother to play a prominent role in the ceremony and reception.

NARRATIVE REASONING

When patients tell their story or clinical history, many emphasize certain aspects, deemphasize others, and omit parts of the narrative altogether. Likewise, the practitioner engages in narrative reasoning when he or she enters into a process that seeks to understand the individual patient's experience.[27] The professional attempts to understand why his or her patients emphasize a portion of their symptomology in an effort to determine how this plays a role in the therapist's diagnosis and care. For example, the health care provider reasons narratively when he or she "want[s] to explain not whether someone has Parkinson's disease, but rather, why the patient's wife is so unwilling to have her husband be discharged home."[27(p999)]

By examining the patient's story and using narrative reasoning to attempt to understand it, better insight is gained into the patient's "experiences of disability or pain and his or her subsequent beliefs, feelings, and health behaviors."[1(pp314-315)] The cognitive paradigms presented earlier assume the practitioner unilaterally arrives at a decision based on the information presented. Conversely, narrative reasoning seeks to build consensus between the practitioner and the patient so that the health care professional realizes an understanding of the patient's experience to arrive at an optimal plan for the patient.[27]

ALTERNATIVE FORMS OF INTERACTIVE REASONING

Higgs and Jones[7(p9)] summarize several other forms of interactive reasoning that have been reported in the literature. These include multidisciplinary reasoning among a variety of health care providers simultaneously; conditional reasoning, which is used to gauge patient response to treatment and predict resultant outcomes; collaborative reasoning, which allows the practitioner and the patient to engage in shared decision-making; ethical reasoning, which includes how a clinician resolves political, moral, and economic dilemmas in the context of clinical patient care; and teaching as reasoning, in which the practitioner guides the patient through information with the intent to change his or her behavior. All these interactive reasoning strategies have many similarities with the hallmarks of narrative reasoning. Primarily, each interactive reasoning strategy assumes that there are multiple possible truths and that the patient's experiences and opinions have value in the diagnostic and treatment processes.

Communicative and Instrumental Action in the Paradigms

We must consider how these the cognitive and interactive paradigms work in concert. Edwards et al[1] associate these communicative and instrumental learnings and actions with the cognitive and interactive paradigms. According to the authors, knowledge—created from a positivist paradigm, including the diagnostic reasoning strategies of hypothetico-deduction and pattern recognition—generates instrumental learning and action. Conversely, knowledge generated out of an interpretive paradigm, such as narrative reasoning, leads to communicative learning and action.

DISCIPLINARY PERSPECTIVES ON CLINICAL REASONING

CR is also influenced by one's professional background and training. Professional roles and identity play a key part in how a health professional chooses to solve a problem.

[Practitioners'] interpretations of who they are and who they should be in their professional roles directly relate to how they frame situations or identify problems to be solved, and how they think through and act upon decisions they make. CR is a process that not only permeates each aspect of an individual clinician's practice, it is also a concept that crosses professional boundaries.[25(p39)]

		TABLE 6-1	
		CLINICAL REASONING ACROSS THE PROFESSIONS	
PROFESSION	HALLMARK APPROACH TO CR	DESCRIPTION	RELEVANT CITATIONS
Medicine	A multifaceted analytic approach	Physicians rely on a hypothetico-deductive reasoning and pattern recognition while incorporating specific aspects of their practice, the needs of the patient, and their past experiences during a specific patient encounter.	4, 8, 13, 29-36
Nursing	Heuristics and context	Nurses rely on building relationships with and empowering their patients to heal through reasoning strategies that consider the patient's past experiences, the current context of the patient's life and medical situation, and a reflective understanding of past clinical relationships with similar patients.	5, 15, 37-42
Occupational therapy	3 holistic tracts	Occupational therapists are concerned with teaming with the patient to find ways of adapting his or her environment to promote function through a balanced understanding of the patient's diagnosis, an understanding of the patient's unique needs, and an ability to alter needs to meet the changing environment.	11, 28, 43-47
Physical therapy	Collaboration in reasoning	Physical therapists use a metacognitive approach to reasoning, which relies on a collaborative relationship with the patient to understand the patient's functional goals and apply the patient's individual context with the therapist's own knowledge of treatment.	1, 3, 6, 26, 48-56

CR, therefore, is a pervasive topic that is reported throughout the health professions' literature, including medicine, nursing, occupational therapy, and physical therapy. Each discipline has historical research and theory perspectives that mirror the changing acceptance from a purely positivist paradigm to those that include aspects of interactive approaches.[1,16,23,28] We will now examine some of the key differences in how the professions of medicine, nursing, occupational therapy, and physical therapy employ aspects of the CR paradigms in contemporary practice (Table 6-1).

MEDICINE'S MULTIFACETED ANALYTIC APPROACH TO CLINICAL REASONING

In Flexner's 1910 report on the current state of medical education and his recommendations, the positivist influences on CR can clearly be seen.[29] Flexner encouraged programs to "train physicians to 'think like scientists' using scientific inquiry and research to solve clinical problems."[29(p221)] A century later, a follow-up report on the state of medical education still recognized a need to educate future physicians to embrace individualism in their clinical practice and to integrate clinical and social sciences as a way to combat a "fragmented understanding of patient experience."[29(p225)] The contemporary challenges in medical education outlined by Cooke et al[13] likely reflect the profession's continued primary reliance on cognitive, or diagnostic, paradigms for CDM.

In their review of CR models and educational implications in medicine, Schwartz and Elstein[30] summarize a 2-system model that recognizes that the clinician may use the benefits of the 2 approaches—pattern recognition and intuitive reasoning—to make quick decisions that are often accurate but remain susceptible to biases and the current emotional state of the clinician. The second employable system, however, is engaged in a slow analytic style using all available data, allowing for a flexible style of reasoning that may eventually lead to high cognitive load.[30] Advocates of the 2-system approach in medicine posit that it allows for the value of using multiple reasoning strategies in concert. However, this 2-system approach primarily relies on cognitive diagnostic paradigms for CDM.[30]

There is growing interest in the impact of cognitive load on the ability of learners to effectively prepare for the clinical learning experience and improve CDM.[31-35] These authors take a neurologic approach to understanding how memory works and considering how a student's brain manages different realms of incoming information and attempts to store pertinent information to be retrieved for later use. By decreasing extraneous information and carefully managing the key facts necessary to the learner at the moment, learning will be optimized and novices will more readily progress in their ability to integrate complex skills.[31]

Additionally, the medical profession has begun to recognize the multifaceted aspects of CR that occur in the practice of medicine.[4] Authors have acknowledged the importance of a nonlinear approach to understanding CR that accepts the influence of situativity theory as a way in which physicians incorporate aspects of the practice, the patient, their own experiences, and the encounter itself in their reasoning decisions.[36] Because of growing acceptance of the nonlinear nature of CDRM in medicine, authors are now calling for the medical profession to integrate training and assessment programs that combine multiple theoretical perspectives of CR that recognize its complexity.[8]

Heuristics and Context in the Clinical Reasoning of Nurses

CR in nursing has long embraced the profession's ideals of patient-centered care.[37] In nursing education, the rapidly changing role of the nurse in today's health care environment includes more responsibility as physicians function more as diagnosticians and prescribers, and "nurses, patients, and family members administer these treatment regimens."[15(p21)] This shift in responsibilities has led to an increased demand on the clinical judgment and decision-making required of today's practicing nurse.[15]

Recently, CR in nursing has been defined as a "complex task geared towards the identification and management of patients' health needs that requires a knowledgeable practitioner along with reliable information and a supportive environment."[38(p236)] In a qualitative study of critical care nurses asked to think aloud as they problem-solved a case study, researchers found that nurses form relationships between concepts and dichotomize between relevant and irrelevant data.[39] This process relied heavily on heuristic reasoning—thinking strategies acquired from similar patient case scenarios in the past. Other studies in nursing using a think aloud approach have found similar results.[40,41] Reviews of CR in nursing indicate that it is both intuitive and context-dependent. The nurse relies on past experiences and present information from his or her patient to make sound clinical judgments.[5,38] Because of this reliance on past experiences, nursing researchers studying early professionals have stressed the importance for early professionals to have supportive and nurturing environments to advance their CR skills.[42]

Three Holistic Tracks of Occupational Therapy Clinical Reasoning

As experts in assisting injured clients to participate in the activities required for daily living, occupational therapists approach patient care with a "holistic perspective, in which the focus is on adapting the environment to fit the person, and the person is an integral part of the therapy team."[43] As a profession, occupational therapy's historical roots in humanism are evident in contemporary approaches to clinical problem-solving.[44] CR in this profession integrates a 3-pronged reasoning approach inclusive of diagnostic reasoning, narrative reasoning, and pragmatic reasoning.[45] This form of reasoning acknowledges the contextual nature of the settings in which patient-client interactions occur and considers organizational constraints, values, resources, trends in practice, and reimbursement considerations as important players in the CR of the occupational therapist. Additionally, the use of evidence interweaves into the heuristic decision-making of the occupational therapist.[11,46,47] The occupational therapist has been described as having a 3-tracked mind consisting of the procedural track, concerned with the patient's diagnosis; the interactive track, focused on the patient as an individual; and the conditional track, which is provisional and holistic related to the patients' participation in their environment.[47]

Collaborative Clinical Reasoning in Physical Therapy

Physical therapists consider the patient's unique circumstances in the rehabilitation process, leading to a model of CR that is both "hypothesis-oriented and collaborative"[48] for sound CR. Physical therapists must use a wide range of scientific, procedural, and professional knowledge; employ cognitive processes in the form of data analysis, synthesis, and inquiry; and engage in metacognitive processes of self-awareness and reflection. This metacognitive process "allows clinicians to monitor their data collection, CR and clinical performance, also taking into account any knowledge limitations linking their broader societal and cultural beliefs and values that, along with propositional and craft knowledge, underpin their practice."[48(p236)]

Several authors have proposed models of CR in physical therapy that consider the plural nature of using a cognitive hypothesis-oriented approach simultaneously with collaborative and interpretive considerations of the patient's goals and personal circumstances.[1,3,49-51] The most contemporary models of CR in physical therapy include the World Health Organization's *International Classification of Functioning, Disability and Health* (ICF), which considers aspects of health and disability by focusing on the patient, his or her context, and factors that facilitate and inhibit his or her personal health condition.[52] Such patient-centered care models seem to have found a balance that reflects the dialectical nature of CR in physical therapy.[1,3,49]

The dialectical nature of CR in physical therapy requires a strong metacognitive reflective component.[1] Reflection-in-action is considered to be a significant contributory factor in professional development and progression toward expertise.[26] In the Jensen et al[53] study of expert physical therapists, it was found that collaboration is a vital component to optimal practice in physical therapy:

> *Collaboration between therapist and patient was central to the CR process. The patient as a valued and trusted source of knowledge was a critical focus in the assessment process ... Once the problem(s) are identified and the context understood, the therapist engages in collaborative problem solving with the patient and family and in educating them about movement and function ...*[53(pp37-38)]

Collaboration, context, and knowledge are demonstrated as key aspects of CR, which is inextricably linked with everything else. Though Jensen et al[53,54] noted it as a separate component of expertise, knowledge, virtues, and movement, all are influenced by reasoning, and in turn must influence the clinician's ability to reason. Building upon this idea, research focused on stating that simply considering physical therapists' CR as a combination of procedural and narrative is incomplete. Rather, physical therapists must deeply engage with the patient through a lived embodied approach for a comprehensive CR process.[6] When speaking of expert physical therapists, Jensen et al[54] state that, "the therapists welcomed challenges of tough patients and were comfortable with uncertainty and ambiguity—that is, not knowing the answer."[54(p161)] Experts who embraced ambiguity in their practice decision-making were further noted to use a metacognitive approach.[48,54,55]

MOVEMENT USE IN REASONING AND PRACTICE

In the scenario presented earlier of the physical therapist challenged by the treatment of a previously active businesswoman and grandmother, the physical therapist uses a collaborative and integrative approach to CR. As a physical therapist, he embodies the use of movement in practice in an effort to aid the movement and mobility of his patient, and therefore considers all aspects of her pathology, impairment, and life circumstances when making decisions about her care. If we could watch him treat, we would undoubtedly see demonstration of constant collaboration through his movements.

Most important, as his hands guided her shoulder, he noticed the dent in her skin. She may have winced in pain, and he gently returned her arm to her side. As she talked about her love of community and church involvement, he coupled his previous experiences with a dancer to try a new treatment strategy that used the current patient's interest in the piano. And as he reckoned with the prognosis, he assumed from his knowledge of the severity of her stroke that he would have to accelerate his expectations to achieve the patient's goal to fully participate in her daughter's wedding. These decisions are not just what he knows, but what he does. The treatments and movements he employs are not just facts and skills he possesses, but who he is as a physical therapist.

The ways in which physical therapists employ CRDM set us apart from other health professionals. Physical therapists draw on our training rooted in the basic, physical, behavioral, and clinical sciences to analytically determine the needs of our patients. We rely on the context of the patient's life to make decisions that will improve their function. We work in close connection, both physically and relationally, with our patients to understand their needs, address their pain, improve their movement, and provide functional restoration. Finally, our unique use of movement in practice clearly interplays with our CR. However, less is known about how these 2 aspects of patient management interweave.

A discussion of the role of movement and its influences on the development of CR in physical therapists would not be complete without consideration of the growing body of literature that seeks to describe how movement plays a role in learning. As movement permeates all aspects of human life and is central to the practice of physical therapy, commentary on how learning is influenced by movement pervades the literature in an infinite number of ways. The reciprocal influence of learning and movement is often described in the arts performance literature, sports enhancement and psychology, and physical education.

The dance performance literature addresses how movement through dance enhances cognitive skills, social awareness, and motor coordination of very young children as well as adults.[56-58] Likewise, the intricate movements associated with musical performance have been described in relation to how they are tied to learning and how injury affects that relationship.[59-62] Sports psychologists and physical education experts have historically described the intricate and crucial process learning played in performance of movement. Evidence demonstrates mental and physical practice strategies are key in the development of optimal movement.[63-66]

Much more familiar to the profession of physical therapy are the concepts of motor control and motor learning applied to patient care.[67] Motor control and motor learning theory are an integral part of physical therapist education and describe the complex interplay of the neurophysiologic processes involved in the production and sensation of movement, as well as psychology and its perspectives on how motor learning occurs and how skills are performed within the context of the environment. Physical therapists are the health care clinicians who must rectify problems of neurologic and anatomic pathology with treatment strategies that use movement in a variety of practice methodologies.[67] The study of motor control, motor learning, and athletic and artistic performance generally seeks to describe and understand how movement is performed, enhanced, or remembered. Though this information plays a key role in how a physical therapist learns to use movement in his or her practice, it is more crucial for the purposes of this chapter to examine how movement is experienced and integrated into one's existence as a professional.

An emerging body of literature now exists to describe the process by which adults experience and integrate movement into their existence.[2,68-70] This type of learning is "being labeled somatic or embodied learning—that is, learning through the body."[71(p190)] We may better understand the role of movement in physical therapy when we consider learning through the body, because "attending to these noncognitive dimensions of knowing can bring greater understanding to our lives; they enable us to make meaning of our everyday experiences."[71(p192)]

Many investigations have focused on the ability of physical therapists to examine and understand the movement, both normal and pathologic, of patients.[2,72,73] Studies have focused on how movement is involved in the teaching and learning process of the therapist–patient relationship. Skjaerven et al,[72,73] through a phenomenological approach, were able to better understand how an awareness of the therapist's own movement may promote better movement quality in his or her patients. "The ability to be mentally and physically attentive, here and now, was considered to be the basis for professional communication. The therapist's own movement awareness was considered a precondition for observing, understanding, and promoting movement quality,"[72(p1483)] and connecting this presence of mind to the learning process the patients go through. "A personal process of movement awareness learning for therapists that was similar to the process for patients provided basic support for clinical observation, reasoning, and action."[72(p1483)]

"Knowledge, especially knowledge used to solve life's ill-structured problems, may have to be constructed by the person, and this knowledge must be understood in the context in which it [is] generated."[71(p333)] Physical therapists face dilemmas in their decision-making every day in their clinical practice. The knowledge physical therapists must create to manage movement problems comes from within their professional context. It cannot always be gained from amassing facts from external sources. Instead, the physical therapist must use movement as his or her context for creating knowledge, through movement of his or her own body and of his or her patient's body. The concepts of movement of the physical therapist and in interaction with the patient, in combination with the importance of the expertise model[53,54] of physical therapy practice places on movement, indicate more attention should be paid to how physical therapists integrate movement in practice, as a way to enhance their knowledge and epistemological development on a pathway toward expert practice.

MOVEMENT USE AND REASONING IN PHYSICAL THERAPIST CLINICAL EDUCATION

Scant literature demonstrates how movement use is developed in physical therapists. Furthermore, little research has been published describing how movement use and CR are coupled. To date, one study has begun to examine how movement use is developed in physical therapist students by their CIs and how this influences how they embody movement use as an integrated component of their practice and decision-making.[74] The situational analysis examining how physical therapist CIs perceive and facilitate students' use of movement in practice revealed 3 important findings.

First, CIs must establish a learning environment supportive of students' unique needs as learners. By perceiving their individual needs, CIs are better able to facilitate their learning as the clinical education experience progresses. Second, CIs must be intentional when teaching students to use movement in clinical practice. Intentionality in teaching is best expressed when the instructor is able to express his or her tacit knowledge of movement usability for and with the patient encounter. And third, CIs play a vital role in establishing a foundation for students' trajectory of movement-related professional growth and development for practice. These findings are depicted graphically in Figure 6-1 as an upward trajectory of growth in a physical therapist student's progression toward an embodied use of movement in practice. As illustrated in Figure 6-1, the CI impacts this growth in 5 ways.

Five themes emerged from the study of movement use and reasoning in physical therapy clinical education: adapting and preparing, enhancing and connecting, and developing. Adapting and preparing help describe ways in which CIs perceived the needs of their students, as they established learning environments supportive of those unique needs. Enhancing and connecting signify methods for facilitating the students' development as they learn to use movement in their practice. Developing demonstrates the final way in which CIs help facilitate students' movement use as students begin to emerge with their own unique philosophy of movement use. The teaching and learning relationship among CIs, students, and patients influence these 5 themes, and each of these influences the other as the student progresses toward an embodied use of movement in practice.

CIs and students built a relationship of trust and communication that formed the foundation of the students' development and allowed them to perceive their students' needs. Once this foundation was in place, CIs adapted their teaching strategies to incorporate students' experiences. As students began to grapple with the complex and ambiguous nature of learning to use movement, they often displayed emotional responses to the stress, frustration, and feelings of being overwhelmed. CIs helped students by adapting to these emotional responses and guiding the students through understanding how to learn to use movement in clinical practice.

Figure 6-1. Through the learning relationship among the student, CI, and patient, the CI develops his or her student's use of movement in physical therapist practice. (Reprinted with permission from Covington K, Barcinas S. Situational analysis of physical therapist clinical instructors' facilitation of students' emerging embodiment of movement in practice. *Phys Ther.* 2017;97[6]:603-614.)

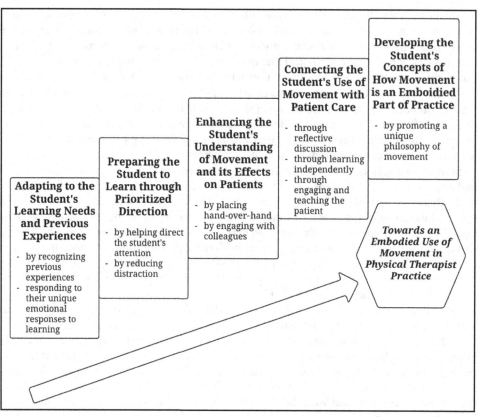

As CIs adapted to the needs of their students, they quickly began to prepare the students for the complexity of movement use required throughout the internship. First and foremost, CIs helped students understand how to use movement safely in the context of their patient caseloads. CIs also struggled to manage the cognitive loads the student faced initially, as the CIs sought to teach large amounts of information. CIs who were able to pace this load may have better promoted students to integrate movement use into practice later in the clinical education experience.

Once CIs were able to perceive their students' needs, they found ways to facilitate their development. CIs found a variety of teaching strategies useful to enhance student learning through the expression of their tacit knowledge of movement use. This frequently involved placing their own hands onto the students' hands or body to help them feel the desired movement as they simultaneously treated patients. Another commonly used intentional strategy was to allow students to spend time learning with other colleagues in the clinic. The opportunity to learn from therapists other than their primary CI enabled students to experience the tacit movement knowledge of other therapists and contrast that with the movements of the CI.

CIs helped students make connections between the movement of their bodies and their intended outcomes with patients. Through reflective conversations and pushing students to describe their own actions and CR, the CIs allowed the students to build a deeper understanding of why they used movement in practice. CIs allowed students to engage in self-discovery as they worked with patients free from constant input and realized the influence of their own hands, thereby deepening students' ability to make connections between their actions and their patients' outcomes. Also, CIs facilitated connections by engaging the patient in the process of teaching and learning, and encouraging their students to articulate their movement knowledge by teaching patients.

Finally, CIs were instrumental in allowing students the freedom to begin to develop their own unique movement philosophy and style of movement use with patients. By allowing their students the freedom to become a movement use professional, they helped initiate a trajectory of professional development that may lead to a fully embodied use of movement in expert physical therapist practice.

Though the themes have been presented in series and are depicted as such in Figure 6-1, there may be times when CIs moved between the themes as they worked with students. To conclude this chapter, let's examine a case study that demonstrates how a CI moves across these themes to help a student develop CR in conjunction with movement development.

Reflection Moment
Case Study: Clinical Reasoning of Movement Use

Claire is a third-year doctor of physical therapy (DPT) student on her second internship. She has been working with Graham, her CI, for 6 weeks in an inpatient rehabilitation facility. Graham, a neurologic certified specialist, is an experienced DPT with 20 years of practice experience, and for the past 15 years has worked primarily with neurologically impaired patients in the inpatient rehab environment. Graham has served as CI for 12 students, all of whom were on internships during their third year of their DPT programs.

Claire has been working diligently to understand the complex nature of caring for neurologically impaired patients in acute care. Most of the caseload she shares with Graham consists of patients who have had cerebrovascular accidents or other traumas resulting in intracranial bleeds. Over the past 5 weeks, her ability to do a thorough chart review has become very efficient and effective. Her awareness of safety concerns and precautions for patients with strokes takes only occasional reminders from Graham. While she has been working very hard to improve, Claire still finds it difficult to determine the patient's needs during gait training and to offer appropriate assistance to progress gait. Last week as Graham and Claire were revising her goals, Graham encouraged Claire to begin to think more about why she was making the choices she was in regard to her hand placement during gait training and to consider practicing at home in the evening with a roommate while describing out loud the reasoning for her hand placement and movements.

Today Graham has asked Claire to lead the treatment session for Mrs. Tucker, a 78-year-old lady who suffered a left middle cerebral artery infarct with hemiparesis and sensory loss of her right extremities. Claire, who has worked previously with Mrs. Tucker, accurately describes to Graham the patient's primary impairments limiting gait. After reviewing the chart from the weekend treatment sessions, Claire determines that the primary goal of today's treatment should focus on gait in the parallel bars to progress Mrs. Tucker to her stated goal of walking in her home from her bedroom to her sun porch.

Graham tells Claire to start the treatment without him, while he observes from the other side of the rehab gym. Claire first chats briefly with Mrs. Tucker and asks her how her weekend has been. She then asks Mrs. Tucker if she would like to work on walking today. Mrs. Tucker eagerly agrees, indicating her deep desire to be able to sit on her sun porch and watch the birds in her yard. Claire assists Mrs. Tucker in moving her wheelchair into the parallel bars and places a gait belt around the woman. Claire stands slightly to the side of Mrs. Tucker, tells her she is going to help her to stand, and places one hand on Mrs. Tucker's right thigh just above her knee and the other hand on Mrs. Tucker's lower back. On the count of "3," Mrs. Tucker stands with minimal assistance.

Graham comes over and indicates he will follow Claire and Mrs. Tucker with the wheelchair. Claire tells Mrs. Tucker to begin to walk whenever she is ready, and that she will help her as needed. Claire tightens her grip on the gait belt and places her other hand on Mrs. Tucker's right shoulder. Mrs. Tucker takes a step with her left leg, grips the parallel bar with her left hand, and attempts to swing her right leg. As she does, her trunk flexes slightly forward, her right knee hyperextends, and her right hip adducts. Claire uses her hand on Mrs. Tucker's shoulder to provide a manual cue to extend her trunk. She then verbally encourages Mrs. Tucker to swing her right leg. Once again, Mrs. Tucker tries, but, despite activating her hip flexors, cannot move her right leg forward.

From behind, Graham reaches over and places his hands on Claire's. He instructs Mrs. Tucker to stand up "very tall," and moves Claire's hand from Mrs. Tucker's shoulder to the woman's right hip abductors and gluteus medius. Using pressure directed toward the floor and medial, Graham's hand directs Claire to shift Mrs. Tucker's pelvis slightly toward her left foot. As Mrs. Tucker's pelvis begins to shift, Graham reduces the pressure from Claire's hand but whispers "keep going." As Claire continues to help Mrs. Tucker shift her weight toward her left foot, Mrs. Tucker slowly swings her right leg. After a few more steps, Mrs. Tucker sits down. Graham immediately asks Mrs. Tucker to provide Claire feedback on how it felt to be assisted during the gait training.

Following the treatment session, Graham and Claire discuss the experience. He asks Claire to describe what she was thinking as she started to help Mrs. Tucker walk. Claire describes her thought process, stating that she was concerned Mrs. Tucker's trunk flexion was preventing her from being able to get good activation of her hip flexors. Graham agrees with her reasoning but asks her to consider why, even with correction of the

continued

trunk, Mrs. Tucker was still unable to swing her right leg. Unable to answer, Graham asks Claire to consider what she felt when he placed his hand over hers and to comment on why the decision to cue the patient's movement at that time and direction in gait would help her to make a step.

Reflection Questions

What are notable differences between the CR processes of Claire and Graham?

What are ways that Claire collaborates with the patient, and how does this collaboration influence her CR?

What does Graham do to help Claire prepare for the gait training session with Mrs. Tucker? How does this preparation influence her CR?

During the gait training session, Graham decides to assist Claire with her movement use. What immediate influence do you think this has on Claire's CDM?

What strategies does Graham use to help Claire connect her movement decisions to the patient's care?

Which strategies do you believe are most influential in her progression of CR skills, and why?

REFERENCES

1. Edwards I, Jones M, Carr J, Braunack-Mayer A, Jensen GM. clinical reasoning strategies in physical therapy. *Phys Ther.* 2004;84(4):312-330; discussion 331-315.
2. Edwards I, Jones M, Hillier S. The interpretation of experience and its relationship to body movement: a clinical reasoning perspective. *Man Ther.* 2006;11(1):2-10.
3. Schenkman M, Deutsch JE, Gill-Body KM. An integrated framework for decision making in neurologic physical therapist practice. *Phys Ther.* 2006;86(12):1681-1702.
4. Durning SJ, Ratcliffe T, Artino AR Jr, et al. How is clinical reasoning developed, maintained, and objectively assessed? Views from expert internists and internal medicine interns. *J Contin Educ Health Prof.* 2013;33(4):215-223.
5. Menezes SS, Correa CG, Silva Rde C, Cruz Dde A. [Clinical reasoning in undergraduate nursing education: a scoping review]. *Rev Esc Enferm USP.* 2015;49(6):1037-1044.
6. Oberg GK, Normann B, Gallagher S. Embodied-enactive clinical reasoning in physical therapy. *Physiother Theory Pract.* 2015;31(4):244-252.
7. Higgs J, Jones M. Clinical decision making and multiple problem spaces. In: Higgs J, Jones M, Loftus S, Christensen N, eds. *Clinical Reasoning in the Health Professions.* 3rd ed. Amsterdam, Netherlands: Butterworth-Heinemann Elsevier; 2008.
8. Durning SJ, Artino AR Jr, Schuwirth L, van der Vleuten C. Clarifying assumptions to enhance our understanding and assessment of clinical reasoning. *Acad Med.* 2013;88(4):442-448.
9. Case K, Harrison K, Roskell C. Differences in the clinical reasoning process of expert and novice cardiorespiratory physiotherapists. *Physiotherapy.* 2000;86(1):14-21.
10. Doody C, McAteer M. Clinical reasoning of expert and novice physiotherapists in an outpatient orthopaedic setting. *Physiotherapy.* 2002;88(5):258-268.
11. Robertson D, Warrender F, Barnard S. The critical occupational therapy practitioner: how to define expertise? *Aust Occup Ther J.* 2015;62(1):68-71.
12. Woods NN, Mylopoulos M. How to improve the teaching of clinical reasoning: from processing to preparation. *Med Educ.* 2015;49(10):952-953.
13. Cooke M, Irby D, O'Brien B. *Educating Physicians: A Call for Reform of Medical School and Residency.* San Francisco, CA: Jossey-Bass; 2010.
14. Norman G. Research in clinical reasoning: past history and current trends. *Med Educ.* 2005;39(4):418-427.
15. Benner P, Sutphen M, Leonard V, Day L. *Educating Nurses: A Call for Radical Transformation.* Vol 15. Stanford, CA: Jossey-Bass; 2009.
16. Higgs J, Jones M, Loftus S, Christensen N. Amsterdam, Netherlands: Butterworth-Heinemann Elsevier; 2008.
17. Elstein AS, Shulman LS, Sprafka SA. Medical problem solving: a ten-year retrospective. *Eval Health Prof.* 1990;13(1):5-36.
18. Simon HA, Newell A. Human problem solving: the state of the theory in 1970. *Am Psychol.* 1971;26(2):145-159.
19. Charlin B, Tardif J, Boshuizen HP. Scripts and medical diagnostic knowledge: theory and applications for clinical reasoning instruction and research. *Acad Med.* 2000;75(2):182-190.
20. Elstein AS, Shulman LS, Sprafka SA. *Medical Problem Solving: An Analysis of Clinical Reasoning.* Cambridge, MA: Harvard University Press; 1978.
21. Ridderikhoff J. *Methods in Medicine: A Descriptive Study of Physicians' Behaviour.* Norwell, MA: Kluwer Academic Publishers; 1989.

22. Norman G, Young M, Brooks L. Non-analytical models of clinical reasoning: the role of experience. *Med Educ.* 2007;41(12):1140-1145.

23. Hack LM, Gwyer J. *Evidence Into Practice: Integrating Judgement, Values, and Research.* Philadelphia, PA: FA Davis; 2013.

24. Wheeler DJ, Cascino T, Sharpe BA, Connor DM. When the script doesn't fit: an exercise in clinical reasoning. *J Gen Intern Med.* 2017;32(7):836-840.

25. Christensen N, Jones M, Edwards I, Higgs J. Helping physiotherapy students develop clinical reasoning capability. In: Higgs J, Jones M, Loftus S, Christensen N, eds. *Clinical Reasoning in the Health Professions.* 3rd ed. Amsterdam, Netherlands: Butterworth-Heinemann Elsevier; 2008.

26. Schön DA. *Educating the Reflective Practitioner.* San Francisco, CA: Jossey-Bass; 1987.

27. Mattingly C. The narrative nature of clinical reasoning. *Am J Occup Ther.* 1991;45(11):998-1005.

28. Dutton R. *Clinical Reasoning in Physical Disabilities.* Baltimore, MD: Williams & Wilkins; 1995.

29. Irby DM, Cooke M, O'Brien BC. Calls for reform of medical education by the Carnegie Foundation for the Advancement of Teaching: 1910 and 2010. *Acad Med.* 2010;85(2):220-227.

30. Schwartz A, Elstein AS. Clinical reasoning in medicine. In: Higgs J, Jones M, Loftus S, Christensen N, eds. *Clinical Reasoning in the Health Professions.* 3rd ed. Amsterdam, Netherlands: Butterworth-Heinemann Elsevier; 2008.

31. Austin L. Scaffolding early clinical learning for students in communication sciences and disorders. *SIG 11 Perspectives on Administration and Supervision.* 2013;23(3):86-91.

32. Pociask FD, Morrison GR, Reid KR. Managing cognitive load while teaching human gait to novice health care science students. *J Phys Ther Educ.* 2013;27(1):58.

33. Morrison G, Goldfarb S, Lanken PN. Team training of medical students in the 21st century: would Flexner approve? *Acad Med.* 2010;85(2):254-259.

34. Schumacher DJ, Englander R, Carraccio C. Developing the master learner: applying learning theory to the learner, the teacher, and the learning environment. *Acad Med.* 2013;88(11):1635-1645.

35. White G. Mental load: helping clinical learners. *Clin Teach.* 2011;8(3):168-171.

36. Durning SJ, Artino AR. Situativity theory: a perspective on how participants and the environment can interact: AMEE Guide no. 52. *Med Teach.* 2011;33(3):188-199.

37. Benner P, Tanner C, Chesla CA. *Expertise in Nursing Practice: Caring, Clinical Judgment, and Ethics.* New York, NY: Springer Publishing Company; 1996.

38. Fonteyn ME, Ritter BJ. Clinical reasoning in nursing. In: Higgs J, Jones M, Loftus S, Christensen N, eds. *Clinical Reasoning in the Health Professions.* 3rd ed. Amsterdam, Netherlands: Butterworth-Heinemann Elsevier; 2008.

39. Fonteyn ME, Grobe SJ. *Expert nurses' clinical reasoning under uncertainty: representation, structure, and process.* Paper presented at: Proceedings of the Annual Symposium on Computer Application in Medical Care; 1993.

40. Lee J, Lee YJ, Bae J, Seo M. Registered nurses' clinical reasoning skills and reasoning process: a think-aloud study. *Nurse Educ Today.* 2016;46:75-80.

41. Johnsen HM, Slettebo A, Fossum M. Registered nurses' clinical reasoning in home healthcare clinical practice: a think-aloud study with protocol analysis. *Nurse Educ Today.* 2016;40:95-100.

42. Voldbjerg SL, Gronkjaer M, Wiechula R, Sorensen EE. Newly graduated nurses' use of knowledge sources in clinical decision-making: an ethnographic study. *J Clin Nurs.* 2017;26(9-10):1313-1327.

43. American Occupational Therapy Association. About occupational therapy. https://www.aota.org/About-Occupational-Therapy.aspx. Accessed June 17, 2017.

44. Chapparo C, Ranka J. Clinical reasoning in occupational therapy. In: Higgs J, Jones M, Loftus S, Christensen N, eds. *Clinical Reasoning in the Health Professions.* 3rd ed. Amsterdam, Netherlands: Butterworth-Heinemann Elsevier; 2008.

45. Schell BA, Cervero RM. Clinical reasoning in occupational therapy: an integrative review. *Am J Occup Ther.* 1993;47(7):605-610.

46. Cohn ES, Coster WJ, Kramer JM. Facilitated learning model to teach habits of evidence-based reasoning across an integrated master of science in occupational therapy curriculum. *Am J Occup Ther.* 2014;68(suppl 2):S73-S82.

47. Fleming M. The therapist with a three track mind. In: Mattingly C, Flemming M, eds. *Clinical Reasoning: Forms of Inquiry in a Therapeutic Practice.* Philadelphia, PA: FA Davis; 1994.

48. Jones M, Jensen GJ, Edwards I. Clinical reasoning in physiotherapy. In: Higgs J, Jones M, Loftus S, Christensen N, eds. *Clinical Reasoning in the Health Professions.* 3rd ed. Amsterdam, Netherlands: Butterworth-Heinemann Elsevier; 2008.

49. Atkinson HL, Nixon-Cave K. A tool for clinical reasoning and reflection using the *International Classification of Functioning, Disability and Health (ICF)* framework and patient management model. *Phys Ther.* 2011;91(3):416-430.

50. Embrey DG, Guthrie MR, White OR, Dietz J. Clinical decision making by experienced and inexperienced pediatric physical therapists for children with diplegic cerebral palsy. *Phys Ther.* 1996;76(1):20-33.

51. Gilliland S, Wainwright SF. Patterns of clinical reasoning in physical therapist students. *Phys Ther.* 2017;97(5):499-511.

52. World Health Organization. *International Classification of Functioning, Disability, and Health (ICF).* Geneva, Switzerland: World Health Organization; 2001.

53. Jensen GM, Gwyer J, Shepard KF. Expert practice in physical therapy. *Phys Ther.* 2000;80(1):28-43; discussion 44-52.

54. Jensen GM, Gwyer J, Hack LM, Shepard KF. *Expertise in Physical Therapy Practice.* Vol 2. St. Louis, MO: Saunders Elsevier; 2007.

55. McGlinchey MP, Davenport S. Exploring the decision-making process in the delivery of physiotherapy in a stroke unit. *Disabil Rehabil.* 2015;37(14):1277-1284.

56. Hanna JL. Learning through dance: why your schools should teach dance. *American School Board Journal.* 2000;187(6):47-48.

57. Keinänen M, Hetland L, Winner E. Teaching cognitive skill through dance: evidence for near but not far transfer. *J Aesthet Educ.* 2000;34(3/4):295-306.

58. Lorenzo-Lasa R, Ideishi RI, Ideishi SK. Facilitating preschool learning and movement through dance. *Early Child Educ J.* 2007;35(1):25-31.

59. Jankovic J, Ashoori A. Movement disorders in musicians. *Mov Disord.* 2008;23(14):1957-1965.

60. Palmer H. The music, movement, and learning connection. *Young Children.* 2001;56(5):13-17.

61. Pica R. *Experiences in Movement with Music, Activities, and Theory.* Albany, NY: Delmar Publishers; 1995.

62. Zatorre RJ, Chen JL, Penhune VB. When the brain plays music: auditory–motor interactions in music perception and production. *Nat Rev Neurosci.* 2007;8(7):547-558.

63. Blakemore CL. Movement is essential to learning. *J Phys Educ Recreat Dance.* 2003;74(9):22-25.

64. Rutherford OM, Jones DA. The role of learning and coordination in strength training. *Eur J Appl Physiol Occup Physiol.* 1986;55(1):100-105.

65. Singer RN. Strategies and metastrategies in learning and performing self-paced athletic skills. *The Sport Psychologist.* 1988;2(1):49-68.

66. Wulf G, Prinz W. Directing attention to movement effects enhances learning: a review. *Psychon Bull Rev.* 2001;8(4):648-660.

67. Schmidt RA, Lee T. *Motor Control and Learning: A Behavioral Emphasis.* Vol 5. Champaign, IL: Human Kinetics; 2011.

68. Amann T. *Creating space for somatic ways of knowing within transformative learning theory.* Paper presented at: Proceedings of the Fifth International Conference on Transformative Learning; 2003; Teacher's College, Columbia University; New York, NY.

69. Brockman J. *A somatic epistemology for education.* Paper presented at: The Educational Forum; 2001.

70. Horst TL. *The Body in Adult Education: Introducing a Somatic Learning Model.* Paper presented at: Proceedings of the 49th Annual Adult Education Research Conference; 2008.

71. Merriam SB, Caffarella RS, Baumgartner L. *Learning in Adulthood: A Comprehensive Guide.* Vol 3. San Francisco, CA: Jossey-Bass; 2007.

72. Skjaerven LH, Kristoffersen K, Gard G. How can movement quality be promoted in clinical practice? A phenomenological study of physical therapist experts. *Phys Ther.* 2010;90(10):1479-1492.

73. Skjaerven LH, Kristoffersen K, Gard G. An eye for movement quality: a phenomenological study of movement quality reflecting a group of physiotherapists' understanding of the phenomenon. *Physiother Theory Pract.* 2007;24(1):13-27.

74. Covington K, Barcinas S. Situational analysis of physical therapist clinical instructors' facilitation of students' emerging embodiment of movement in practice. *Phys Ther.* 2017;97(6):603-614.

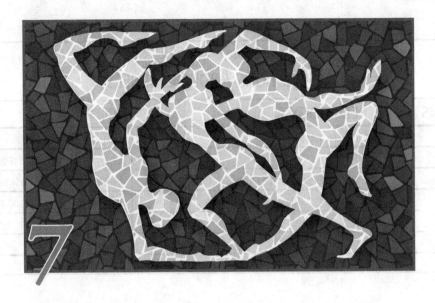

ANDRAGOGY:
Health Professions Clinical Reasoning Transitioning From Novice to Expert

Susan Flannery Wainwright, PT, PhD

OBJECTIVES

- Consider the relationship of andragogy for clinical reasoning (CR) and expertise.
- Explore CR assessment methods for adult learners.
- Discover the CR processes and the attributes used by novice and experienced practitioners within various health care professions.
- Examine how theories and models of CR relate to abilities and processes across the health professions.
- Discover the congruence of contemporary clinical practice with theoretical models.

INTRODUCTION

To conclude this first section of the text on the theoretical foundations, guiding practice for the professional, we now turn to Chapter 7, which includes further analysis of the literature of andragogy and observed CR in practice for the health professions. The role of CR in the development of expertise in practice, considering novice to experts, and including differences in CR abilities, is shared. Discussion of CR is presented within the context of the theoretical frameworks of CR in the profession of physical therapy.

Musolino GM, Jensen GM, eds. *Clinical Reasoning and Decision-Making in Physical Therapy: Facilitation, Assessment, and Implementation* (pp 71-88).
© 2020 Taylor & Francis Group.

TABLE 7-1			
ASSUMPTIONS ABOUT LEARNERS			
CONSIDERATIONS	**PEDAGOGY**	**ANDRAGOGY**
Self-concept	Dependency	Self-directiveness
Experience	Of little worth	Learners are a rich resource for learning
Readiness	Biological development social pressure	Developmental tasks of social roles
Time perspective	Postponed application	Immediacy of application
Learning orientation	Subject-centered	Problem-centered
Motivation	Extrinsic	Intrinsic
Adapted from Knowles.[1-3]			

Andragogy is defined as the art and science of any form of adult learning, including the methods and principles for adult education.[1] Knowles[2] has identified 4 principles of andragogy; learners:

- Are engaged in the planning and evaluation of their instruction

- Recognize that the opportunity to experience uncertainty and make errors as the foundation for learning activities

- Prefer to learn subjects that they can apply to work or personal life in meaningful ways

- Engage in learning that is problem-solving–oriented rather than content-oriented

Andragogy is characterized by assumptions about adult learners' attributes that enable them to engage as active learners. Adult learners have developed a sense of self-concept derived from their cumulative life and professional experiences. Self-concept places adult learners at a point along the developmental continuum where they are self-directed, motivated, and ready to learn and apply what they have learned.[1,3] The central premise that adult learning is learner-centric, initiated learning differentiates andragogy from pedagogy. Table 7-1 details the assumptions about the learners engaged in andragogy.[1-3]

Ingalls identified a 7-step process to apply the principles of andragogy and student learning to the classroom (Table 7-2).[4] What does this model and process of andragogy look like in physical therapy education? Imagine a doctor of physical therapy program faculty member entering a classroom with the goal of engaging with physical therapy students. The faculty member is likely to assume that the learners are motivated and self-directed to learn. It will be important for the faculty member to detail the nature and scope of what is to be learned, ideally engaging the students in how to proceed with learning activities and determine how to measure their success in learning. The instructor may query the students to ascertain their shared experiences and knowledge about the topic to be addressed. Throughout the learning activities, students will have the opportunity to apply their knowledge and experience to acquire new knowledge and skills that they can readily apply to practice.

The principles of andragogy span across all adult learners, not just those in structured academic settings, researchers, too, have applied the principles of andragogy to patient education.[5] Certainly, a patient who is motivated to improve and feel better is more likely to actively engage in therapy. An important component of clinical expertise in physical therapy is employing CR that is patient-centric and engages the patient. As physical therapists, we provide our patients with information and support, so that they have the capacity to become self-directed in their approach to their care. Each patient brings experience as a patient, as well as cumulative life experience, to a therapy interaction. When patients are self-directed and patient education is made relevant, patients can immediately apply what they are taught. Recognizing that our patients and family members and caregivers can engage as adult learners allows us to interact with them in a meaningful manner that may improve their ability to apply what they are taught for their daily lives.

For CR and expertise development to progress, reflection is required.[6,7] Andragogy and transformative learning (TL) originate from the common root of adult education. A premise of TL is that upon encountering a challenging question, issue, or belief, learners[8] will question their assumptions, test their justifications, and apply the resultant evidence to reach a decision.[8] TL occurs, in part, through critical reflection and dialogue with self and others to question assumptions and beliefs.[9] Through this critical reflection, the learner achieves new insight or understanding.

Assessment of our students' learning is both important and challenging to measure in an objective and meaningful manner. Application of both andragogy and TL gives credence to alternative assessment methods, such as peer assessment and self-assessment (SA), to describe or quantify CR within a learning context.[10] Engagement in the critical reflection and dialogue that are essential elements of TL is congruent with the use of SA and peer assessment, respectively.

Contextually rich experiential learning activities, such as service learning, and problem-based and case-based learning can all provide opportunity for explicit reflection and opportunity to explore roles as physical therapists.[11,12] Course design that

TABLE 7-2

SEVEN STEPS IN THE DEVELOPMENT, ORGANIZATION, AND ADMINISTRATION OF ANDRAGOGY

STEP			THE INSTRUCTOR'S ROLE FOR THE LEARNER IS TO …
Input	1	Setting a climate for learning	Establish a comfortable environment conducive to learning. Explain the purpose of the learning experience.
	2	Establishing a structure for mutual planning	Collaborate promoting interaction (rather than authoritative).
	3	Assessing needs, values, and interests	Query learners to determine needs and interests specific to achieving the learning outcomes.
Activity	4	Formulating objectives	Craft measurable, meaningful learning objectives.
	5	Designing learning activities	Create activities that move the learners from a problem-finding to a problem-solving mindset.
	6	Implementing learning activities	Engage with the learners to achieve the intended outcomes while making processes explicit.
Output	7	Evaluating results (reassessing needs, interests, values)	Assess learning through 3 lenses: knowledge, experience, and power: Learners demonstrate knowledge gained Through the learning experiences, learners share and communicate knowledge Learners are empowered to bring motivation to the learning activity

Reprinted from Ingalls JD. *A Trainer's Guide to Andragogy.* Rev. ed. Washington, DC: US Department of Health, Education, and Welfare; 1972.

incorporates some or all the 7 steps of andragogy can result in TL. For example, when a geriatrics course was intentionally redesigned to incorporate principles of adult learning, active learning, and reflection, pre- and post-assessment of student outcomes demonstrated increased student efficacy and confidence in their ability to effectively meet the needs of older adults.[13]

PROFESSIONAL FORMATION

The relevance and application of adult learning is congruent with a primary goal of professional preparation: "formation of a professional identity with a moral core of service and responsibility."[14] Three apprenticeships comprise professional education: the cognitive, the practical, and professional formation.[15] These apprenticeships are developmental in nature, requiring that learners be engaged and be capable of reflecting upon their experiences as they establish their professional identity. The educational experiences that are built around professional formation will lead students to develop habits of heart, head, and hands.[7] The beliefs, knowledge, and skills that derive from these 3 apprenticeships were evident in expert practice in physical therapy.[7] The learner's experiences shape the development of professional identity. An important context for students or novice clinicians is the community of practice in which they engage. Physical therapists entering practice are continuing their journey of professional formation beyond their formal professional education. The community of practice they enter shapes the development of their professional identity. The extent to which they actively engage in professional identity formation depends upon the extent that the culture of their practice setting values their professional development.[16] Novice physical therapists in their first year of practice who enter practice settings that foster professional identity formation report that their learning across the 3 apprenticeships occurs through work experience. Important elements of this work experience included the opportunity to practice and interact with coworkers, mentors, patients, and family and caregivers.

Culture and community of practice continue to strongly influence the development of identity formation as physical therapy practitioners enter their second year of practice. In clinical settings that facilitate and foster continued development, an expansion and deepening of beliefs, skills, and knowledge across the 3 apprenticeships is observed. Practitioners at this phase of professional practice express a growing confidence in themselves as professionals. This allows them to direct their learning beyond themselves to interact within the clinical environment.[17] A key ability that these practitioners possess is the ability to be self-reflective, taking time to engage in metacognitive activities.

APPRENTICESHIP APPROACHES

The Dreyfus model of skill acquisition addresses performance across these 3 apprenticeships. Learners progressing through the phases of novice ability to mastery of skills engage in contextually relevant and holistic thinking and analysis to reach a decision. Transition through the stages from novice to expert requires the learners to maintain a level of awareness to engage in ongoing SA.[18]

Steinberg's model suggests that the study of abilities (and the prerequisite building block skills) and achievements (consistent with expertise) can be effective measures of developing expertise in clinicians.[19] Certainly in physical therapist education, assessment of psychomotor performance of skills occurs across curricula. We do acknowledge that performance of clinical skills in isolation is not a measure of a student's CR abilities. Often educators who make clinical skills performance an explicit goal of the learning process may intend to create linkages for the learner to understand the importance of these skills in the decision reasoning process. We cannot assume that training in clinical skills will facilitate the novice learner in mastering strategies for CR consistent with the strategies used by experts. Caution should be taken when assessing skill acquisition, and by extension CR, when rubrics are not so detailed to objectify skill performance that they fail to measure the developmental nature of skill acquisition in a meaningful way.[20]

CLINICAL REASONING ASSESSMENT CONSIDERATIONS

The assessment of CR begins in the classroom. Let's discuss some of the more common methods used in today's practice of teaching, learning, and assessing CR.

Traditional pen-and-paper examinations can be innovative to assess CR. For example, in a written exam, using a key feature question with targeted follow-up questions allows the testing to focus on a difficult aspect on the diagnosis and management of a health issue. Through a review of the literature exploring the use of key factor questions in medical education, the internal consistency of key factor questions was reported as a range between 0.49 to 0.95. Internal consistency was higher when more cases were used. Content and construct validity of key factor questions was more likely evident when authored by educators with more experience, higher levels of education, board certification, and practice types. Like the instructional methods described earlier, key factor questions did not show any predictive validity regarding how a student would perform on a subsequent standardized patient experience.[21]

Scripts are a diagnostic concept using categorization to organize knowledge. The basic concept of scripts is that a diagnostician uses knowledge of pathologies to apply meaning to a new situation. New information is compared to the array of scripts that the practitioner has experienced and stored. Through the reasoning process, the practitioner can narrow down to just those scripts whose attributes fit the current patient. Signs and symptoms can be in many separate scripts (eg, fever or rash). These scripts are developed through experience. When medical students should begin forming scripts is a debated topic. But it is overwhelmingly agreed that it should occur well before clinical experiences.[22]

Mind maps are visual representations of information creating a graphic reconstruction of knowledge establishing relationships using a hierarchical process.[23] Mind-mapping supports a higher level of integration of material.[23] During a 4-month semester, physical therapy students were taught how to use mind mapping methods and received faculty feedback on their maps. Pre- and post-assessment using the Health Science Reasoning Test revealed scores increased by 1.7 points.[23] Mind-mapping, in this case, did not improve recall scores, yet notably improved CR.

Meaningful and relevant assessment has moved beyond these pen-and-paper measures to include think aloud[24] and reflective activities.[25,26] Think aloud activities have been used to explore how experienced pediatric nurses solve complex patient scenarios through CR.[24] Nurses were paired and recorded in a think aloud task involving a virtual patient in their area of pediatric practice. Content analysis of these dialogues identified the outcome of these think aloud activities. First, the nurses developed their hypotheses through pattern recognition in the clinical presentation and test results. Nurses used their extensive experience to reason deductively and with a holistic perspective. It is likely that these nurses' experience level provided insight into their thought processes that is likely not to be seen in more novice practitioners. Rather, novice practitioners are more likely to rely upon reflection-on-action activities about their CR.

Journaling is a common method used to afford students the opportunity to reflect on practice. Achievement of reflection includes assessment of the types and levels of reflection.[25,26] Review of physical therapy students' journals provided insight into the scope of their reflections while on a full-time clinical education experience. Topics that students reflected on included processes of making clinical decisions, complexity and richness of interactions with patients, effects of the practice environment on learning and patient care, acquisition of clinical and administrative skills, value of clinical experiences of validating and integrating previous learning, and acknowledgment and evaluation of learning methods.[26]

CLINICAL NARRATIVE

The use of narrative is central to human understandings, communication, and memory.[27] Narratives have a finite and longitudinal time sequence, presuppose a narrator and a listener with different viewpoints who collaborate to construct a story, are concerned with individual's feelings about the story, provide information beyond facts, and engross the listener. Narratives provide the ability for 2 individuals to develop an understanding that cannot be achieved in another way.[28]

In clinical practice, narratives are the ideal approach to obtain a patient history. All too often, unfortunately, patient interviews are fragmented and not interactive. Our current approaches to patient interaction that do not include narrative between practitioner and patient may lead acquisition of biomedical information at the expense of psychosocial context. Through narrative reasoning, clinicians are more likely to gain a complete and contextual patient history. Clinicians who use narrative to gain a more holistic understanding of the lived experiences of patients with diseases and to clarify the contextual nature of their physiological changes are more likely to develop an empathetic, patient-centered relationship.[29] The use of narrative in education of health professionals provides opportunity for reflection grounded in situated learning experiences.

The written narrative is a cognitive activity that provides opportunity for and develops the skills of reflection and reflexivity. These skills should be learned and practiced to develop critical reflection for expert practice.[30] Reflection is useful to probe a student's CR and metacognitive skills. Reflexivity focuses on how an individual's beliefs and values influence perspectives and behaviors.

Students have varying perception and skills about writing and reflection. Education and support are needed to allow students to develop the required skills.[31] Reflective abilities in the writings of medical students were found to be enhanced when provided instruction in effective reflection as compared to a comparison control group.[32] Explicit course work in developing skills in the use of reflective narrative in education has been demonstrated to change abilities and beliefs.[33]

In fact, final-year physiotherapy students reported enhanced skills of narrative reasoning upon completion of a narrative reasoning course. Reflective writing was implemented to promote students' application of the course content and skills gained on their clinical experiences. Emergent themes from focus groups revealed that students developed an understanding of patient experiences, of themselves, and clinical reflection skills.[34,35]

Traditional classroom assessment methods of CR such as key factor question,[21] script concordance test,[22] and mind-mapping[23] are limited in that they do not get to the theory of praxis. Psychomotor assessment evaluates the application of CR in the context of a patient encounter. The Objective Structured Clinical Examination (OSCE) is frequently used to assess student competence. In physical therapist education, OSCEs have been used to measure student competence.[36] More recent application of OSCE has explored if and how to effectively measure CR through OSCEs. Observed behaviors[37] and post-encounter reflective activities[38] have measured CR during OSCEs. Durning et al developed a post-encounter form that medical students completed after an OSCE. Grading of the students' post-encounter responses was compared to other components of the OSCE assessment and was found to be useful in evaluating CR.[38]

CLINICAL REASONING GRADING RUBRICS

Recently, several rubrics to assess CR have been developed and reported in the physical therapy literature. These rubrics focus on both practice-specific[39] as well as broad practice[40] assessment. The Think Aloud Standardized Patient Examination (TASPE)[39] assesses CR competency in novice physical therapy students during standardized musculoskeletal patient encounters. The assessment of the student's synthesis of data is used to inform think aloud sessions across the hypothetico-deductive reasoning process: hypothesis generation, hypothesis evaluation, and intervention. The TASPE assesses the student's performance consistent with Miller's Framework for Clinical Assessment (Figure 7-1).[41] Study of the tool with 26 physical therapy students, assessed by a pair of examiners, demonstrated interrater reliability among the examiners across TASPE items ranging from 0.63 to 0.98.[39] We will further exam utility of the TASPE by Fu in Section II of the text.

Grading rubrics quantify and evaluate CR through the assessment of observed clinical performance.[40,41] Furze et al have developed a grading rubric to assess CR in physical therapy students.[40] Constructs of the rubric pull heavily from the Dreyfus model of skill acquisition,[42] as well as the development of expertise in physical therapy.[43] This grading rubric assesses students across cognitive, psychomotor, and affective domains from low to high performance of knowledge, skills, and attitudes. The revised rubric has 2 purposes: to assess the CR skills of physical therapy students, and to evaluate readiness to progress to full-time clinical education. Initial pilot work using this assessment with entry-level physical therapy students revealed that more novice students demonstrated a beginner level of CR characterized by a student-centric focus and algorithmic thinking. As students were assessed across the curriculum, they progressed to an intermediate level of CR, ultimately achieving entry-level CR as they neared program completion. Exemplars of entry-level CR included dynamic patient interactions and a more adaptive approach to reasoning that fostered integration of context and patient interests into the clinical plan.[44] We will also further examine Furze's tool in Section II of the text.

Bridging Academic and Clinical Teaching and Assessment

Effective instructional strategies to develop CR require situational learning opportunities. This approach is consistent with the tenets of adult learning. Situated learning is the development of knowledge, skills, and behaviors within the context of engagement and learning in communities of practice.[45] Both the development and assessment of CR require meaningful and contextually relevant learning experiences.

Integrated clinical experience affords students the opportunity to transfer, apply, and reinforce what is learned in the classroom.[46] For adult learners in a professional program, these hands-on experiences create the opportunity for students to develop the knowledge, skills, and behaviors within the context of complexity and uncertainty of authentic practice settings. Integrated clinical experiences facilitate integration of assessment of CR across academic and clinical settings.[47,48] Students who have completed integrated clinical experiences have reported contributions to their academic success as well as preparation for full-time clinical education. When students are introduced to learning in clinical environments, there is an added dimension of collaboration and exploration of professional roles and responsibilities.[49] Interprofessional situated learning activities provide opportunity for students to learn about their role, as well as the roles of other members of the health care team, in addition to developing competency within their role.

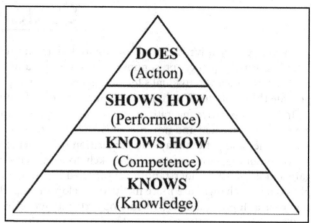

Figure 7-1. Framework for clinical assessment. (Reprinted with permission from Miller GE. The assessment of clinical skills/competence/performance. *Acad Med.* 1990;65[9]:S63-S67.)

Clinical Decision-Making

The development of clinical decision-making (CDM) abilities is an ongoing process that begins in entry-level physical therapy curricula and continues as physical therapists transition to their practice roles and pursue lifelong learning. CDM integrates the affective, cognitive, and psychomotor domains of learning. Spanning the learning domains are the constructs of SA, reflection, and experience.[50] It follows, then, that students and novice clinicians who have the opportunity to develop these skills will refine their CDM abilities. While CDM is the foundation for effective patient/client management, there is not always sufficient emphasis on the process and the development of decision-making abilities as an individual develops from a student to a novice, then on through to an experienced practitioner.[51] Professional disciplines have raised the issue of how individuals within the professions develop CR. Consider this scenario:

A physical therapist student on her final clinical experience was reporting in team rounds that a 19-year-old woman, status post-traumatic brain injury, continued to present with balance dysfunction. The attending physician asked the student to identify why she thought the patient had balance impairments. The student responded, "The patient's Functional Reach Test score indicated that the patient was at risk for falls." The physician then turned to the student's clinical instructor and repeated the question. The CI responded, "There are 2 primary issues. The patient has delayed perception of loss of balance. Also, due to the patient's strength impairment, she cannot generate sufficient amplitude or speed of force to maintain her center of mass within her base of support during dynamic activities. Combined with the range of motion impairment at the ankle and the sensory impairment throughout the left lower extremity, there are several issues to address to improve this patient's balance."

This exchange between team members, at a rehabilitation team meeting, illustrates the differences in CR between a novice and an experienced physical therapist. The student's response exemplifies how she reported data collected during examination, without the experience or clinical knowledge to put that data into a meaningful context for the physician's interpretations and the case for the patient's plan of care and discharge planning. Rephrasing the question, or posing follow-up questions, would likely not have facilitated a more accurate response. At this early stage of learning and experience, the novice is simply unable to construct a response reflecting a level of critical thinking and CR like the experienced clinician. The clinical instructor's response illustrates the experienced clinician's ability to integrate examination data into a contextually rich explanation of

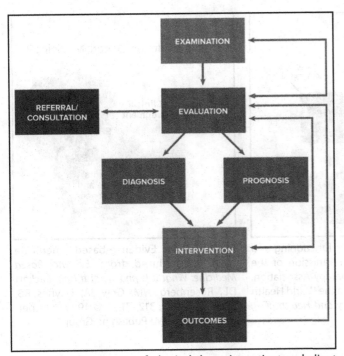

Figure 7-2. The process of physical therapist patient and client management. (Reprinted from http://guidetoptpractice.apta.org/, with permission of the American Physical Therapy Association. © 2018 American Physical Therapy Association. All rights reserved.)

the patient's clinical presentation that links impairment to functional assessment. These different responses illustrate that physical therapists progress through developmental stages of CDM as they grow from novice to more experienced practitioners.

Informed CDM and CR are the cornerstone of effective patient management. Whether a novice, experienced, or expert clinician, physical therapists strive to provide the best patient care and achieve the most meaningful outcomes for our patients. In physical therapist practice, the formal development of CR begins in entry-level curricula and continues through entry-level practice. Commonly, entry-level practice continues with formal education and mentorship in residency and/or fellowship programs, as well as places of employment.

Given the developmental nature of CR, refinement of CR is associated with evolving professional development. The current focus of studies describes the characteristics of the CR exemplified by novice and expert practitioners. How a practitioner approaches the CR process is shaped by educational experiences and practices that are unique to each professional. The approach that a practitioner uses to reason in a patient encounter is essentially consistent with the purpose of the intended outcome for that encounter. While CR lenses may differ, there are some similarities about how practitioners evolve their CR. The extent to which an individual achieves expertise within a given period of time appears to be shaped by both internal and external factors.[7,16-18,29,30,40-44]

Effective CR is guided by core documents within the profession. The APTA *Guide to Physical Therapist Practice* serves as a resource and establishes the standard for best practice across the spectrum of patient-client management.[52] The patient/client management model (Figure 7-2) of the CR framework is presented in the APTA *Guide*, serving as an additional road map for CR. The *International Classification of Functioning, Disability and Health* (ICF) model describes measures of health and disability at both the individual and population levels. The ICF (Figure 7-3) provides a framework for practitioners to contextualize the information they collect through communication with the patient and examination. Recent literature provides one example of how the ICF was applied to CR in stroke rehabilitation, resulting in effective communication across team members and structured service delivery within clarified team roles; these authors theorized that the results may contribute to enhanced CR.[53] In Section II, Chapter 10, Nixon-Cave and Atkinson will elaborate on a successful effort implementing a CR tool with the ICF to facilitate CR reflection for residents.

In addition to the documents that provide frameworks for effective CR, Sackett's model of evidence-based medicine (Figure 7-4) identifies inclusion standards for best practice. Evidence-based medicine is the confluence of application of the best available scientific literature, the patient values and preferences, and the clinical judgment of the practitioners.[54] This clinical judgment is grounded in the clinician's experience, knowledge, skills, and beliefs. The CR abilities of the practitioner inform this element of the evidence-based medicine triad. Certainly, there is great value in providing the best standard of care, while attempting to minimize unwarranted variation in the delivery of care.[55] The clinicians' abilities to appraise the literature and apply it accurately to an individual case scenario is essential,[56] again relying on effective clinical judgment. The impact that depth, breadth, and recency of practitioner experience has on CR is recognized in the clinical interactions and outcomes of our patients. In Section III, Chapter 26, Robertson and Becker will shine a contemporary lens on evidence-based practice in physical therapy.

PERSPECTIVE ON DEVELOPMENT OF EXPERTISE IN THE HEALTH PROFESSIONS

The development of expertise has been exemplified by characteristic reasoning abilities observed in practitioners across the professional development continuum. The research on CDM in medicine has focused on reasoning processes used by practitioners.[57-59] Studies in nursing have focused on quantifying the use of CDM[60-63]; within the profession of physical therapy, they have focused on clinicians' behavioral attributes.[64-72]

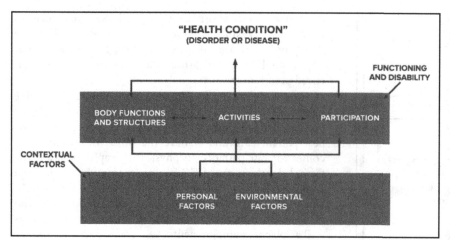

Figure 7-3. Interaction among the components of the ICF model of functioning and disability. (Reprinted from http://guidetoptpractice.apta.org/, with permission of the American Physical Therapy Association. © 2018 American Physical Therapy Association. All rights reserved. This APTA figure was adapted with permission from the World Health Organization, *Towards a Common Language for Functioning, Disability and Health [ICF]*, http://www.who.int/classifications/icf/icfbeginnersguide.pdf.)

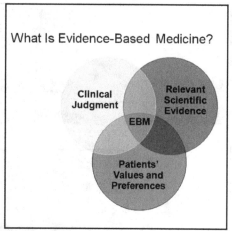

Figure 7-4. Evidence-based medicine triad. (Reproduced from *Evidence-Based Medicine: What It Is and What It Isn't*, Sackett DL, Rosenberg WM, Gray JA, Haynes RB, Richardson WS, 312, 71-72 © 1996 with permission from BMJ Publishing Group Ltd.)

Thus, to understand and describe expertise is to understand CR. The approach to the study of CR is framed in the theories and definitions of CR. One definition of CR expounds that it is simply "… reasoning that results in action."[73] Effective clinical practice assumes that several premises are met through this definition. The first is that thought, leading up to action, requires deliberation about appropriate course(s) of action, this deliberation occurs within a specific context, and there is an anticipated outcome. Second, the lens of this deliberation is framed by the practitioner's personal and professional experiences. Lastly, each practitioner's experiences provide a comparative reference framework against which an appropriate plan of action is determined.

In the broadest interpretation, these premises incorporate the scope of CR and the development of expertise. In medicine, these 3 premises elucidate the cognitive processes used to arrive at an appropriate medical diagnosis.[74] In physical therapy, the patient/client management model in the APTA guide outlines the process of deliberation that includes action to determine a physical therapy diagnosis, prognosis, and development of plan of care. Models such as these provide a means to evaluate and study professional formation across the continuum of experience and professional development.

CHARACTERISTICS OF EXPERT PRACTICE ACROSS THE PROFESSIONS

Development of Skills and Abilities

The nature of expert reasoning requires that these abilities be intertwined. Reflection is not only an activity in which experts engage; reflection is also an ability that is learned and honed with experience and intentional practice. Reflective practice (RP) is an ability consistently exemplified by expert practitioners.

Boud defines reflection in the context of learning. He states that reflection is "a generic term for those intellectual processes in which individuals engage to explore their experiences in order to lead to new understanding and appreciation."[75] Boyd and Fales emphasize the process of reflection, stating that: "Reflective learning is the process of internally examining and exploring an issue of concern, triggered by an experience, which creates and clarifies meaning in terms of self, and which results in a changed cultural perspective."[76] These 2 definitions explicitly link the process of reflection, with an outcome reflective of an altered or newly developed viewpoint that arises directly from experience. At the highest level of cognitive analysis, reflection is identified as the tool that can integrate theory and practice.[60] The metacognitive activity of reflection allows the learner (or practitioner) to link thoughts and ideas, to integrate new knowledge with existing knowledge, and to expand one's own CR and CDM framework. According to Goodman and Boud, 5 skills have been identified as necessary for effective reflection[75,77] (Table 7-3).

Expertise is an ongoing process, rather than explicit endpoint.[19] This suggests that the study of abilities and achievements (expertise) demonstrated in observation of practice may be effective measures of evolving expertise in clinicians.[19] Mindfulness is the process of thinking a practitioner uses to implement knowledge into clinical practice.[78] Epstein[78] suggests that mindfulness is necessary to develop the link between evidence-based and relationship-centered care. Practitioners demonstrate moral imagination when they assume an active role in thinking about and applying knowledge to clinical practice.[79] Experts do not achieve reflection; rather reflection is a central component in the always-present iterative, forward-thinking nature characterized in the expert CDM process.[78-83]

TABLE 7-3
GOODMAN AND BOUD'S MODEL OF SKILLS NEEDED FOR REFLECTION

SKILLS NEEDED FOR REFLECTION	
Self-awareness	The ability to assess how the situation has affected the person, and how the person has affected the situation.
Description	The ability to recognize and recall salient events.
Critical analysis	The ability to examine, identify, challenge assumptions, imagine, and explore alternatives.
Synthesis	The ability to integrate new knowledge with existing knowledge. The ability to use knowledge to solve problems and make predictions.
Evaluation	The ability to make judgments about the value of something.

Adapted from Boud et al.[75]

CLINICAL REASONING PROCESSES: THE NATURE OF CLINICAL DECISION-MAKING

There is a relatively extensive body of literature on CDM across the disciplines of medicine, nursing, and physical therapy. Many of the health professions have studied this construct across the spectrum of novice through experienced to expert clinicians, noting differences in the way that CDM has been studied. Let's examine a few perspectives from the health professions.

The study of CDM in the medical profession has evolved from the description of brief and superficial, unelaborated responses to systematic efforts to understand the problem-solver by gaining insight into his or her plans and intentions.[57] Early study within medicine approached the issue without a framework or preconceived hypotheses about physicians as problem-solvers. The lack of a conceptual framework is reflected in the unelaborated responses of the participating physicians. These unelaborated responses are characterized by superficial data that are not connected to themes. The response of the novice practitioner in the earlier physical therapist student case rounds vignette with the traumatic brain injury illustrates an unelaborated response. Elements of the unelaborated response include data, such as a Functional Reach score, that represent isolated bits of information. Novices' limited knowledge and experience limits their ability to understand the data within the context of the patient's functional limitation (ie, risk for falls). As the body of literature expanded and theories were developed, the research aims became more focused, and the research methods for acquiring the data were refined. In more recent studies, research methods have included interviews with thinking aloud processes that have provided systematic mapping of knowledge structures that guide the medical diagnosis process across the continuum from novice to intermediate to expert clinician.[57]

Contemporary views of CDM in medicine have focused on the transition from hypothetico-deductive reasoning processes used by novices to the forward-reasoning processes evidenced by expert clinicians.[57,84] Refer to Table 7-4,[3,9] which highlights the differences identified between novice and expert medical practitioners. The hypothetico-deductive reasoning processes allow novice clinicians to generate and test diagnostic hypotheses. These processes are prone to errors in problem-solving because novice clinicians have limited experience from which to develop and test their hypotheses. As the novice gains experience, the number of errors made is likely to decrease. At some critical point, novice practitioners gain sufficient experience and have success using their problem-solving strategies to transition from the hypothetico-deductive reasoning processes to more mature and efficient forward-reasoning processes.

The forward-reasoning processes employed by experienced physicians are characterized by a broad and structured knowledge base, the use of if/then prediction rules, the use of pattern recognition, and the development of a working diagnosis from the data.[57,84] The experienced physician's personal and professional experiences facilitate the development of an extensive knowledge base, and the ability to use this knowledge efficiently and accurately. An experienced physician's ability to shift to and from a forward-reasoning processes to and from a hypothetico-deductive reasoning processes is illustrative of the flexibility inherent in Schön's RP process.[80] The transition between reasoning processes is most likely to be observed when an experienced physician is confronted with a novel situation, for which an insufficient knowledge base exists.[85]

The study of CDM in the nursing profession has focused on the application of existing theory to nursing practice and education.[86-88] The clinical judgment of nurses is consistent with "engaged, practical reasoning first," and thought processes are grounded in experiences and responses of their patients as they cope with illness.[86] Expert nurses demonstrate CDM that is responsive to their patient's issues and concerns.[86] How nurses attend to salient factors about the patient's clinical presentation to inform CR is illustrated in a study of expert nurses.[87] The nurses' CR was examined while effectively administrating pain management, when caring for patients who were critically ill, nonverbal, and ventilator dependent.[87] Through direct observation of nurse-patient interactions, the nurses studied applied their biomedical knowledge to monitor each patient's physiologic status and response to interventions, inclusive of pharmacologic management and handling during care.[87] Attention to these

	TABLE 7-4	
COMPARISON OF NOVICE AND EXPERIENCED PHYSICIAN'S REASONING ABILITIES		
	NOVICE PHYSICIANS	**EXPERIENCED PHYSICIANS**
Method of reasoning	Hypothetico-deductive processes	Forward reasoning
Diagnostic hypothesis	Multiple hypotheses developed early in data collection phase	Data collection drives hypothesis generation
Atypical cases	Increased difficulty and increased errors with atypical cases	Less difficulty with atypical cases
Method of data collection	Less organized methods of data collection and errors of omission and commission	Selective in data collected
Recall	Inconsistent recall of data	Organized, bigger chunks; more "incidental recall" information
Relationship: Data collected to interpretation accuracy	Inconclusive data on correlation between thoroughness of data collected and the accuracy of data interpretation.	
Case specificity	Problem-solving expertise was highly variable and dependent upon mastery of a particular domain.	
Adapted from Knowles[3] and Taylor and Laros.[9]		

physiologic information sources allowed these expert nurses to anticipate patients' needs for pain management,[87] as many nurses presume great ownership and responsibility for what they often consider as "their" patients.

Comparison of similar critical care CDM was studied in novice and experienced nurses in making decisions to wean patients from mechanical ventilation. Novice nurses required a higher number of cues through patient interaction to achieve a level of certainty about their decisions.[88] The link between CDM and reflection has been identified as the means of integrating theory with clinical practice.[60,89] Specifically, reflection has been studied as the attribute that underlies effective CDM and patient management in a variety of clinical settings.[61-63,70,71,90-92]

Research within the profession of physical therapy has demonstrated an evolution in perspectives and methods with some of the earliest work exploring CR using the CR process described by Elstein et al[57] as a guiding framework. Payton[64] explored the CR processes employed by a convenience sample of 10 physical therapists who were identified as having some degree of expertise in some aspect of physical therapy. Audiotape of each participant performing an initial evaluation was used as an interview prompt in immediate subsequent interviews with these participants to determine "what exactly was going on in your mind as you worked with the patient."[64] These skilled physical therapists used CR processes primarily to develop problem lists. Overall, the CDM processes employed were more consistent with those previously documented in novice, rather than expert, physicians. Inconsistencies between the abilities of these expert physical therapists and those previously documented in expert physicians may be related to limitations in the use of a sample of convenience in selecting a cadre of expert clinicians, or the era of a more technically oriented profession.

Many later studies[66-72] used audiotaping and subject interviews as a means of understanding the behaviors and attributes of physical therapists. The premise for nomination and selection of expert clinicians was also refined in subsequent research, allowing more accurate description of expert practice. There may be evidence that CR abilities and processes, and subsequent expression of expertise, are not bounded by an individual's cognitive style. Cognitive style questionnaires were used as the means to measure the physical therapist's preferred way of thinking and organizing information. While it was hypothesized that those clinicians who worked in the intuitive mode would demonstrate better performance in history taking and physical assessment of patients, no difference was seen in the CDM between novice and experienced physical therapists[88]; rather differences were noted with respect to practice setting. Physical therapists in private practice responded less positively to a receptive data gathering style, characterized by sensitivity and attention to observed behaviors, as compared to those employed in hospital settings. Therapists in the private practice group also responded more positively to the systematic style and less positively to the intuitive style of information processing, as compared to therapists employed in rehabilitation centers. However, in the absence of any direct observation of clinicians in practice to determine if, and to what extent, their self-reported practices were employed, the authors' conclusions were limited to the participants' SA.[88]

Jensen and colleagues[66] used a qualitative methodology to study the CDM characteristics of novice and experienced physical therapists. The comparative differences between novice and experienced physical therapists are noted about the therapist–patient interaction in:

TABLE 7-5

KNOWLEDGE AND PERFORMANCE ATTRIBUTES THAT DISTINGUISH BETWEEN THE THERAPEUTIC INTERVENTIONS OF NOVICE AND MASTER CLINICIANS

ATTRIBUTE	NOVICE CLINICIAN	MASTER CLINICIAN
Confidence in predicting outcomes	Collect data and hope to find a clear direction; seek help from colleagues	Elaborate; comfortable schema for interpreting data and predicting outcomes
Ability to control environment	Interruptions not controlled	Interruptions controlled
Focuses verbal and nonverbal communication	Medley of approaches to gather data and maintain rapport	Intense patient-centered encounters
Evaluation and use of patient illness and disease data	Focus on finding the right data	Dynamic elicitation and use of data specific to the patient
Importance of teaching to hands-on care	Focus on patient rapport and hands-on skills	Reliance of teaching as an essential clinical skill

Adapted from Jensen et al.[66,67]

TABLE 7-6

TENETS UNDERLYING PATEL AND GROEN'S STUDY OF EXPERT CLINICAL DECISION-MAKING

FOUR TENETS OF EXPERT REASONING
1. Experts develop highly efficient ways of representing information in working memory.
2. Information in long-term memory is represented as a set of prediction rules.
3. Strong data collection methods grounded in heuristic strategies and tied to an extensive knowledge base are used.
4. Use of forward reasoning from the facts to the solution.

Adapted from Patel and Groen.[85]

- How the participants used their time with their patients
- The impact that the environment had
- The type of information collected and how it was applied
- The degree of responsive interaction
- The extent to which therapeutic and social interaction were integrated

The more experienced physical therapists were noted to spend more time in direct patient contact, engaging in social communication blended with education, explanation, and cueing. With the experienced participants, the flow of the treatment session was not affected by external environmental distractions and interruptions. The comparative results are summarized in Table 7-5. Notably, this was the first description of physical therapist attributes that was grounded in and guided by a conceptual framework. Subsequent study of expert and novice practice in physical therapy demonstrated that master clinicians were better able to control the treatment session through effective time management and attention to their patients, as compared to the novice clinicians; yet this was not necessarily attributable to years of experience.[67] The attributes consistent with greater expertise in clinical practice are detailed in Table 7-6, consistent with the work of Patel and Groen[85] in the discipline of medicine.

Embrey et al[68] identified 4 characteristics of CDM of expert physical therapists working with pediatric patients. Qualitative methods for data collection, including retrospective and concurrent think aloud procedures and semistructured interviews, were used to assess the nature of CDM by physical therapists working with a pediatric population. Embrey et al[68] identified attributes that the physical therapists used during the CDM process:

- The clinical application of domain-specific knowledge (movement scripts)
- The use of improvisation (practice without prior planning) as compared to formal decision analyses (procedural changes)

- Social responsiveness (psychosocial sensitivity)
- Ongoing SA as the key element within the CDM process (self-monitoring)

The experienced physical therapists in this study identified the use of self-monitoring twice as often as novice clinicians. Thus, in this revised framework, self-monitoring was portrayed as central to the CDM characteristics of improvisation, movement scripts, procedural changes, and psychosocial sensitivity. The frequent reporting of self-monitoring appeared to provide evidence of ongoing reflection (reflection-in-action) during patient management, providing insight into the link between CDM, in the context of the measurable attributes, and reflection.[68]

As Musolino discussed in Chapter 3, Orest[89] studied the importance of SA (including the prerequisites of self-starting, self-directed, self-paced, and self-steering behaviors) as related to continued clinical competence. SA was studied in a sample of 4 physical therapists.[89] Data collection methods included in-depth interviews in which questions were asked about the clinician's perceptions (emic perspective) regarding SA. Interviews with the subjects revealed that physical therapists felt clinical competence, patient outcome, and professional development were dependent upon accurate SA. While all subjects identified the need for SA, not all were confident that they used effective SA skills. All subjects felt that formal training in SA would allow them to use it more effectively and thus develop professionally into more effective and reflective practitioners. Orest's[89] study outcomes reinforce the central theme of the attribute of SA (self-monitoring) discussed by Embrey et al.[68] Orest's[89] study differs from the other studies previously described in that she selected and studied only the construct of SA as it related to CDM. While this study by Orest[89] contributes information about the CDM processes of physical therapists, the results only reflect the clinician's perceptions. Further study with multiple data sources is indicated to ascertain the link between SA and effective patient management.

The use of qualitative research methods reported in the physical therapy literature has provided an understanding of the attributes that an individual is likely to possess at the level of expert practice. The collective data provide guiding information about behaviors that are evident along the CDM continuum. Study of the phenomena from the emic perspective provides rich data that inform us about the attributes of novice and expert physical therapists.

THE PROCESS OF DEVELOPING CLINICAL REASONING CONSISTENT WITH EXPERTISE IN PRACTICE

What may or may not be as clearly understood is how expertise is developed. The traditional underlying assumption of the comparative study of CR in novices and experts is that different cognitive structures and mechanisms underlie organization of knowledge and CDM processes.[93] For example, functional magnetic resonance imaging has been used to study the neural basis of reasoning between internal medicine interns (novice) and board-certified staff internists (experts) while completing cognitive pen-and-paper assessments. Imaging results revealed both novices and experts share common neural processing networks while on task. The experts did demonstrate greater neural processing efficiency, particularly in regions such as the prefrontal cortex, during these cognitive, nonanalytical reasoning exercises.[94] Thus, imaging technology indicates that expertise is associated with efficiency of processes—with cognitive, nonanalytical reasoning—rather than differences in the processes, as traditionally thought. We should not constrain ourselves to assume that there is compulsory development of expertise with experience. In prior work exploring physical therapists' professionalism and core values, participants offered the following insight when describing experienced clinical peers: "I've worked with individuals who have 20 years' experience and those who have 1 year of experience 20 times."[95] So certainly factors are at play beyond our experience, with respect to years and/or duration of time vs experiences of exposures.

It is through clinical experience and practice that biomedical knowledge becomes encapsulated and eventually integrated into illness scripts. As Durning and Rencic discussed in Chapter 2, novice physicians (from medical students to entering residents) have neither sufficient biomedical knowledge nor experience to develop the illness scripts present in the CR framework of experienced physicians. Rather, novice physicians' approach to CDM is characterized by initial data collection that directs hypothesis generation in a hypothetico-deductive fashion, with errors often tied to nonanalytical reasoning.[96] Debate continues concerning the role of biomedical knowledge in clinical case processing.[97]

COMPARATIVE STUDY: NOVICE VS EXPERT

Not only are there differences in the volume of information[98] that novice and intermediate practitioners manage and apply, but there are also differences in how medical students (novices) as compared to physicians (experts) use this biomedical knowledge in clinical cases. When challenged with biomedical knowledge propositions, novice students demonstrated many inaccuracies in medical reasoning processes. These errors were not seen in expert reasoning processes. The proportion of biomedical propositions used in CDM decreased as expertise developed, with an intermediate effect seen in the mid-level physicians. The observed reduction in medical errors is theorized to be a product of RP seen in experts.[99] Further, expertise was evidenced using illness scripts to direct CDM. Shifting from using biomedical knowledge to using clinical knowledge seemed to be associated with the student's transition from preclinical to clinical education.[100]

A comparative, qualitative study of CR with 5 interns and 6 attending emergency department physicians across the novice to expert continuum characterized the cognitive differences between novice and expert emergency department physicians, as well as areas in which novices' skill and knowledge gaps are most pronounced. The novice physicians studied used linear thinking to identify a diagnosis quickly and were likely to discount and explain away data that was not consistent with their working diagnosis. In comparison, experienced physicians drew on expertise to recognize cues and patterns while demonstrating flexibility in reasoning to alter their initial diagnosis in response to data collected.[101]

More recent exploration of CR has included the concept of context specificity. Durning et al[102] studied expert internal medicine physicians, using the lens of situated cognition and cognitive load theories to explore the influence of selected contextual factors (eg, patient, encounter, and/or physician) on CR performance. Higher cognitive load measures were negatively correlated with effective CR. The presence of selected contextual factors that challenged cognitive load appeared to influence diagnostic reasoning more than therapeutic reasoning. Subsequently, contextual factors appeared to impact expert physician performance consistent with situated cognition and cognitive load theory predictions.[102]

Simulations have been used as well to explore the CR of physicians.[103] In one study, a low-intensity medical simulator exercise was used to assess the practitioner's ability to perform a preliminary study of the ability to recall and process patient information presented verbally. The physicians under study were divided into 3 groups based on time-dependent experience in critical care: novice (less than or equal to 8 weeks of critical care experience), intermediate (8 to 16 weeks of critical care experience), and expert (more than 16 weeks of critical care experience). The subjects were presented with 3 clinical cases. In the first case, the presentation contained 55 separate data points, and subject recall was analyzed. In the second and third cases, a patient report was given, and the subjects were asked by a "medical student" to outline and explain their treatment decisions. While the difference in experience between 8 weeks or less as compared to 16 weeks is limiting, as we traditionally think about the development of expertise, study findings indicate how these practitioners can manage, use, and apply biomedical knowledge to arrive at a medical diagnosis. There were no significant differences among the 3 groups regarding errors or total data points recalled. Differences were demonstrated in Cases 2 and 3 as intermediates and experts made significantly fewer errors, while employing forward-reasoning (hypothesis-based) process.[103] Noncognitive factors such as the nature of the knowledge domain, an individual's experience, and the acquisition of established group norms are likely to impact the development of expertise.[103]

Nurses often use CDM strategies to determine what clinical signs to attend to and how to organize the input, while novice nurses require more cues to arrive at the same decision-making.[104,105] In a study using a qualitative, descriptive design, researchers explored the influences that drive CDM among junior rheumatology nurses.[105] Findings of 4 distinct themes that influence CDM emerged, including professional development, patient-focused care, working in a specialty, and rheumatology nursing.[105] Development of experiential knowledge alongside access to specialized information and expert practitioners was also influential in informing decisions.[105]

Professional reasoning used by occupational therapists representing varied abilities along the spectrum of the Dreyfus model of skill acquisition, in the practice area of home modifications, was explored in a grounded theory study of occupational therapists.[106] Formal academic and learning through experience was found to provide the foundation for the reasoning systems and habits of practice described by these occupational therapy practitioners.[106] As participants gained expertise, they were able to shift their primary focus from systematic reasoning steps to focus on the comprehensive, client-centered, and contextual picture.[106] These observations of occupational therapists' CR are consistent with the hypothetico-deductive reasoning processes, observed in novice professionals with subsequent transition to forward-reasoning skills noted in more expert practitioners, as described in both the medical and physical therapy professions' literature.

The CDM of novice, intermediate, and expert therapists from various disciplines practicing in the pediatric rehabilitation setting was explored.[107,108] Expert and intermediate therapists differed from novices with respect to their content, self, and procedural knowledge. With increasing expertise, therapists transitioned to use a supportive, educational, holistic, functional, and strengths-based approach. These experts demonstrated heightened humility yet increased self-confidence in interacting with patients. Further, these experts described having an understanding about how to facilitate and support client change and adaptation by using principles of engagement, coherence, and manageability. Expert therapists used enabling and customizing strategies to ensure a successful therapeutic session, optimize the child's functioning, and ensure child and family adaptation and accommodation over the longer term.[107,108]

Literature exploring physical therapist practice in students through the first 2 years of clinical practice is providing description and insight into the professional formation of new professionals.[71,72,109,110] Study of the practice of student and novice physical therapists has focused on the CR process used during standardized patient encounters and patient interactions.

Study of novice physical therapists indicates that they use varied sources of information to inform and guide their CR. Like their novice physician counterparts, novice physical therapists employ hypothetico-deductive reasoning processes and are challenged when confronted with uncertainty.[109,110] When novice physical therapists use reflection, they are more likely to rely on reflection-on-action[80] rather than reflection-in-action[80] throughout a patient encounter.[70] Study of these novice clinicians, in practice for less than 18 months, demonstrated an intermediate effect and the impact of experience.[71,72]

Perspective and approaches to CR are shaped during entry-level education. Use of standardized patients in physical therapy education has provided insight into the development CR in physical therapy students.[110] Using observation and post-examination and post-intervention think aloud interviews, the nature of CR was explored in 8 second-year physical therapy students.[110]

All students demonstrated abilities and thought processes consistent with physical therapist CR models.[110] The most common reasoning strategy used was diagnostic reasoning, with 2 students attending to the patient's personal factors as well as the musculoskeletal impairments that were the focus of the remaining students.[110] The novice physical therapy students relied on a standardized approach/form to complete the examination, and all but one demonstrated use of hypothetico-deductive reasoning processes.[110] Specific findings in their reasoning about pain indicated that all students had a biomedical orientation to examining the patients' complaints of pain.[110] Only 2 of the students incorporated a behavioral approach to assessment of the pain, again incorporating patient personal factors into the interview and examination. The one student who did not have an organized approach to the patient encounter also did not demonstrate hypothetico-deductive reasoning processes like her peers. Rather, she employed a trial-and-error approach, collecting a variety of objective data.[110] She was unable to complete the examination or arrive at a diagnosis. Consistent with novice practice, these participants made errors in reasoning. Frequently (6 of the 8) participants did not generate an accurate hypothesis or diagnosis as they focused on one idea without exploring alternative hypotheses. Four of the 8 held on to an incorrect diagnosis despite disconfirming examination findings.[110]

The first year of practice is a period of ongoing development of clinical skills, knowledge, and behaviors. A study of novice therapists throughout their first year of practice demonstrated that the community of practice within these participants' practice was most influential on how these novices performed clinically. These participants learned through experience and social interaction afforded within their practice site, and learning was primarily directed toward self. The participants identified that evolving communication skills resulted in confidence. These novice physical therapists were engaged in professional identity formation and role transitions.[71]

Recognizing that there is no endpoint to professional development, study of the ongoing nature of development into the second year of practice has been examined. During that second year, formal and informal learning shifts from internal and self-focused to an outward view that leads to consolidation and elaboration of practice-based learning and skills. It is through the confidence gained with experience that these novice practitioners and their skills become more refined and they seek opportunities to engage in a clinical environment that fosters collaboration and opportunities for continued development in professional role formation.[72]

Development of expertise is driven by internal and external factors, as evidenced by the work of King et al,[107,108] who explored the development of expertise in 71 pediatric rehabilitation therapists. Participants were stratified by level of expertise as determined by a multifaceted assessment battery and their level of clinical experience.[108] Those who were identified as possessing expertise but less experience (less than 10 years) demonstrated the highest motivation, truth-seeking, and open-mindedness scores. The major differences between therapists who attain expertise quickly vs those who remain novices after many years of experience appear to be motivation and complexity of work experiences.[108]

Further study of the difference between experienced practitioners and those who demonstrate expertise explored attribute dimensions of practice.[111] Comparison of 6 therapists classified as expert and 6 therapists classified as average through retrospective analysis of an outcomes database revealed both differences and similarities about them as professionals.[111] All 12 therapists expressed a commitment to professional growth and an ethic of caring.[111] The physical therapists classified as expert were not distinguished by years of experience, but rather by academic and work experience, use of colleagues, use of reflection, view of their primary role, and pattern of delegation of care to support staff.[111] Therapists classified as expert had a patient-centered approach to care, characterized by collaborative CR and promotion of patient empowerment.[111]

The impact of length of clinical education experiences on CDM by cardiorespiratory physiotherapists has also been studied in the acute care hospital setting.[112] In this study, levels of experience were classified as having less experience (less than 2 years), intermediate experience (2.5 to 4 years), and more experience (more than 7 years). Level of experience influenced 4 dimensions of practice.[112] With increasing experience in cardiorespiratory physiotherapy CDM, these 4 dimensions were identified: an individual practice model, refined approaches to CDM, working in context, and social and emotional capability.[112] Underpinning these dimensions was evidence of reflection-on-practice, motivation to achieve best practice, critique of new knowledge, increasing confidence, and relationships with knowledgeable colleagues.[112]

It is clear that the development of CR is tied with expertise, and research across the professions has described the attributes, characteristics, and dimensions of expert practice, as well as the development of expertise. However, how to best facilitate the development of CR is still under investigation. Given that the work in physical therapy has identified the important role that collaboration has in professional identity formation, understanding teacher and learner perspectives on the development of CR provides insight. Durning et al[113] studied physicians' (internists faculty) and internal medicine interns' perspectives on how CR is developed, maintained, and objectively assessed. The interns were focused on knowledge acquisition activities and use of online resources to facilitate development of CR.[113] The faculty experts discussed the value of teaching for development and maintenance of CR. Both the faculty experts and intern participants both struggled with how to best measure CR, and direct observation was rarely mentioned as a strategy.[113]

Schmidt and Rikers[97] identified strategies that could contribute to the development of expertise for medical students, suggesting that it is important to teach the basic sciences in a clinical context, and to introduce patient problems early in the curriculum to facilitate CR.[97] In addition, time should be devoted to enabling reflection on patient problems with peers and expert doctors during experiential clerkships.[97] The recommended strategies could support the processes of encapsulation of information and illness script formation that is indicative of expert CR in physicians.[97]

Often the novelty, complexity, or uniqueness of a clinical scenario leads to uncertainty for novice practitioners.[114] Deliberate practice can be applied to contextual learning experiences. Review of the literature on applied deliberate practice—in both psychomotor tasks such as typing, and cognitive tasks such as proficiency in second language comprehension—reveals that deliberate practice is but one component of the developmental components of expertise.[114] Deliberate practice may provide meaningfulness to experience. Working memory was found to be more important when experiences or tasks were more complex or nonhabitual.[114]

CONCLUSION

CR is the cornerstone of effective patient management and optimal patient outcomes. The development and assessment of the habits of heart, hands, and head shape the how knowledge, skills, and attitudes and beliefs applied to CR manifest in patient–practitioner encounters. But the development of these habits does not occur serendipitously. The evolution of expertise in CR requires the intentional and explicit application of ongoing reflection for CDM in practice.

REFERENCES

1. Knowles MS. *The Modern Practice of Adult Education: From Pedagogy to Andragogy.* San Francisco, CA: Jossey-Bass Publishers; 1986.
2. Knowles MS. *Andragogy in Action.* San Francisco, CA: Jossey-Bass; 1984.
3. Knowles MS. *The Adult Learner: A Neglected Species.* 3rd ed. Houston, TX: Gulf Publishing; 1984.
4. Ingalls JD. *A Trainer's Guide to Andragogy.* Revised ed. Washington, DC: US Department of Health, Education, and Welfare; 1972.
5. Chesbro SB, Davis LA. Applying Knowles's model of andragogy to individualized osteoporosis education. *J Geriatr Phys Ther.* 2002;25(2):8-11.
6. Wainwright SF, Shepard KF, Harman LB, Stephens J. Novice and experienced physical therapist clinicians: a comparison of how reflection is used to inform the clinical decision-making process. *Phys Ther.* 2010;90(1):75-88.
7. Jensen GM, Gwyer J, Shepard KF, Hack LM. Expert practice in physical therapy. *Phys Ther.* 2000;80:28-43.
8. Mezirow J. Transformation theory in adult learning. In: MR Weldon, ed. In *Defense of the Lifeworld: Critical Perspectives of Adult Learning.* Albany, NY: SUNY; 1995.
9. Taylor EW, Laros A. Researching the practice of fostering transformative learning: lessons learned from the study of andragogy. *J Transform Educ.* 2014;12(2):131-147.
10. Beaman R. The unquiet … even loud, andragogy! Alternative assessments for adult learners. *Innov High Educ,* 1998;23(1):47-59.
11. Reynolds P. How service-learning experiences benefit physical therapist students' professional development: a grounded theory study. *J Phys Ther Educ.* 2005;19(1):41-54.
12. Kelly MJ. Beyond classroom borders: incorporating collaborative service learning for the adult student. *Adult Learning.* 2013;24(2):82-84.
13. Ruckert E, Plack MM, Maring J. A model for designing a geriatric physical therapy course grounded in educational principles and active learning strategies. *J Phys Ther Educ.* 2014;28(2):69-84.
14. Shulman LS. Foreword. In: O'Brien BC, Irby DM, Molly Cooke M, eds. *Educating Physicians: A Call for Reform of Medical School and Residency.* Stanford, CA: The Carnegie Foundation for the Advancement of Teaching; 2010.
15. Sullivan WM. In: Foster CR, Dahill LE, Golemon LA, Tolentino BW, eds. *Educating Clergy: Teaching Practices and Pastoral Imagination.* Stanford, CA: The Carnegie Foundation for the Advancement of Teaching; 2006.
16. Black LL, Jensen GM, Mostrom E, et al. The first year of practice: an investigation of the professional learning and development of promising novice physical therapists. *Phys Ther.* 2010;90:1758-1773.
17. Hayward LM, Black LL, Mostrom E, et al. The first two years of practice: a longitudinal perspective on the learning and professional development of promising novice physical therapists. *Phys Ther.* 2013;93:369-383.
18. Dreyfus HL, Dreyfus SL. The relationship of theory and practice in the acquisition of skill. In: Benner P, Tanner CA, Chelsea CA, eds. *Expertise in Nursing Practice.* New York, NY: Spring; 1986.
19. Steinberg R. Abilities are forms of developing expertise. *Educational Researcher.* 1998;27:11-19.
20. Carraccio CL, Benson BJ, Nixon LJ. From the educational bench to the clinical bedside: translating the Dreyfus developmental model to the learning of clinical skills. *Acad Med.* 2008;83(8):761-767.
21. Hrynchak P, Takahashi SG, Nayer M. Key feature questions for assessment of clinical reasoning: a literature review. *Med Educ.* 2014;48:870-883.
22. Charlin B, Roy L, Brailovsky C, Goulet F, Van der Vleuten C. The script concordance test: a tool to assess the reflective clinician. *Teach Learn Medicine.* 2000;12(4):189-195.
23. Zipp GP, Maher C, D'Antonio AV. Mind mapping: teaching and learning strategy for physical therapy curricula. *J Phys Ther Educ.* 2015;29(1):43-48.
24. Forsberg E, Ziegert K, Hult H, Fors U. Clinical reasoning in nursing, a think aloud study using virtual patients—a base for an innovative assessment. *Nurse Educ Today.* 2014;34:538-542.
25. Plack MM, Driscoll M, Blissett S, MeKenna R, Plack TP. A method for assessing reflective journal writing. *J Allied Health.* 2005;34(4):199-208.

26. Williams RM, Wilkins S. The use of reflective summary writing as a method of obtaining student feedback about entering physical therapy practice. *J Phys Ther Educ.* 1999;13(1):28-33.
27. Bolton G. *Reflective Practice—Writing and Professional Development.* 3rd ed. Los Angeles, CA: Sage Publishers; 2010:206.
28. Greenhalgh T, Hurwitz B. Narrative based medicine: why study narrative? *BMJ.* 1999;318:48-50.
29. Greenfield B. The role of narratives in the professional formation of students. In: Higgs J, Sheehan D, Currents JB, Letts W, Jensen GM, eds. *Realising Exemplary Practice-Based Education.* Rotterdam, Netherlands: Sense Publishers; 2013:163-170.
30. Greenfield BH, Jensen GM, Delany CM, et al. Power and promise of narrative for advancing physical therapist education and practice. *Phys Ther.* 2015;95:924-933.
31. Kurunsaari M, Tynjälä P, Piirainen A. Students' experiences of reflective writing as a tool for learning in physiotherapy education. In: van Steendam E, Tillema M, Rijlaarsdam G, van Den Bergh H, eds. *Writing for Professional Development.* Leiden, Netherlands: Brill; 2015:129-151.
32. Miller-Kuhlmann R, O'Sullivan PS, Aronson L. Essential steps in developing best practices to assess reflective skill: a comparison of two rubrics. *Med Teach.* 2016;38(1):75-81.
33. Cruz EB, Caeiro C, Pereira C. A narrative reasoning course to promote patient-centered practice in a physiotherapy undergraduate programme: a qualitative study of final year students. *Physiother Theory Pract.* 2014;30(4):254-260.
34. Caeiro C, Cruz EB, Pereira CM. Arts, literature and reflective writing as educational strategies to promote narrative reasoning capabilities among physiotherapy students. *Physiother Theory Pract.* 2014;30(8):572-580.
35. Greenfield B, Bridges P, Phillips T, et al. Reflective narratives by physical therapist students on their early clinical experiences: a deductive and inductive approach. *J Phys Ther Educ.* 2015;29(2):21-31.
36. Gorman SL, Lazaro R, Fairchild J, Kennedy B. Development and implementation of an objective structured clinical examination (OSCE) in neuromuscular physical therapy. *J Phys Ther Educ.* 2010;24(3):62-68.
37. Mitchell ML, Henderson A, Groves M, Dalton M, Nulty D. The objective structured clinical examination (OSCE): optimising its value in the undergraduate nursing curriculum. *Nurse Educ Today.* 2009;29(4):398-404.
38. Durning SJ, Artino A, Boulet J, et al. The feasibility, reliability, and validity of a post-encounter form for evaluating clinical reasoning. *Med Teach.* 2012;34(1):30-37.
39. Fu W. Development of an innovative tool to assess student physical therapists' clinical reasoning competency. *J Phys Ther Educ.* 2015;29(4):14-26.
40. Furze J, Gale J, Black L, Cochran TM, Jensen GM. Clinical reasoning: development of a grading rubric for student assessment. *J Phys Ther Educ.* 2015;29(3):34.
41. Miller GE. The assessment of clinical skills/competence/performance. *Acad Med.* 1990;65(9):S63-S67.
42. Dreyfus HL, Dreyfus SL. The relationship of theory and practice n the acquisition of skill. In: Benner P, Tanner CA, Chelsea CA, eds. *Expertise in Nursing Practice.* New York, NY: Spring; 1986:29-48.
43. Edwards I, Jones MA, Carr J, Brannack-Mayer A, Jensen GM. Clinical reasoning strategies in physical therapy. *Phys Ther.* 2004;84(4):312-335.
44. Furze J, Black L, Hoffman J, Barr JB, Cochran TM, Jensen GM. Exploration of student's clinical reasoning development in professional physical therapy education. *J Phys Ther Educ.* 2015;29(3):22-33.
45. Lave J, Wenger E. *Situated Learning: Legitimate Peripheral Participation.* Cambridge, MA: Cambridge University Press; 1991.
46. Hakim EW, Moffat M, Becker E, et al. Application of educational theory and evidence in support of an integrated model of clinical education. *J Phys Ther Educ.* 2014;28(suppl 1):13-21.
47. Weddle ML, Sellheim DO. Linking the classroom and the clinic: a model of integrated clinical education for first-year physical therapy students. *J Phys Ther Educ.* 2011;25(3):68-79.
48. Mai JA, Thiele A, O'Dell B, et al. Utilization of an integrated clinical experience in a physical therapist education program. *J Phys Ther Educ.* 2013;27(2):25-32.
49. Dubouliz CJ, Savard J, Burnett D, Guitard P. An interprofessional rehabilitation university clinic in primary health care: a collaborative learning model for physical therapist students in a clinical placement. *J Phys Ther Educ.* 2010;24(1):19-24.
50. Elstein AS. Shulman LS, Sprafka S. *Medical Problem Solving: An Analysis of Clinical Reasoning.* Cambridge, MA: Harvard Press; 1978.
51. Leighton R, Sheldon M. Model for teaching clinical decision making in physical therapy professional curriculum. *J Phys Ther Educ.* 1997;11:23-30.
52. American Physical Therapy Association. *Guide to Physical Therapist Practice.* 2nd ed. Alexandria, VA: American Physical Therapy Association; 2001.
53. Tempest S, McIntyre A. Using the ICF to clarify team roles and demonstrate clinical reasoning in stroke rehabilitation. *Disabil Rehabil.* 2006;28(10):663-667.
54. Sackett DL, Richardson WS, Rosenberg W, Haynes RB. *Evidence-Based Medicine: How to Practice and Teach EBM.* London, United Kingdom: Churchill Livingstone; 2002.
55. Mercuri M, Gafni A. Medical practice variations: what the literature tells us (or does not) about what are warranted and unwarranted variations. *J Eval Clin Pract.* 2011;17(4):671-677.
56. Sniderman AD, LaChapelle KJ, Rachon NA, Furberg CD. The necessity for clinical reasoning in the era of evidence-based medicine. *Mayo Clin Proc.* 2013;88(10):1108-1114.
57. Elstein AS, Shulman LS, Sprafka SA. Medical problem solving: a ten year retrospective. *Evaluation & the Health Professions.* 1990;13(1):5-36.
58. Schmidt HG, Norman GR, Boshuizen H. A cognitive perspective in medical expertise: theory and implications. *Acad Med.* 1990;65:611-621.

59. Elstein A. *Medical Problem Solving: An Analysis of Clinical Reasoning.* Cambridge, MA: Harvard University Press; 1978.

60. Atkins S, Murphy K. Reflection: a review of the literature. *J Adv Nurs.* 1993;18:1188-1192.

61. Pierson W. Reflection and nursing education. *J Adv Nurs.* 1998;27:165-170.

62. Burnard P. Nurse educators' perceptions of reflection and reflective practice: a report of a descriptive study. *J Adv Nurs.* 1995;21:1167-1174.

63. Saylor C. Reflection and professional education: art, science and competency. *Nurse Educ.* 1990;15:8-11.

64. Payton O. Clinical reasoning process in physical therapy. *Phys Ther.* 1985;65:924-928.

65. May B, Dennis J. Expert decision making in physical therapy—a survey of practitioners. *Phys Ther.* 1991;71:190-206.

66. Jensen G, Shepard KF, Hack L The novice versus the experienced clinician: insights into the work of the physical therapist. *Phys Ther.* 1990;70:314-323.

67. Jensen GM, Gwyer J, Hack L, Shepard KF. Attribute dimensions that distinguish master and novice physical therapy clinicians in orthopedic settings. *Phys Ther.* 1992;72:711-722.

68. Embrey D, Guthrie MR, White OR, Dietz J. Clinical decision making by experienced and inexperienced pediatric physical therapists for children with diplegic cerebral palsy. *Phys Ther.* 1996;76:20-33.

69. Wainwright SF, McGinnis PQ. Factors that Influence the clinical decision-making of rehabilitation professionals in long-term care settings. *J Allied Health.* 2009;38(3):143-151.

70. Wainwright SF, Shepard KF, Harman LB, Stephens J. Novice and experienced physical therapist clinicians: a comparison of how reflection is used to inform the clinical decision-making process. *Phys Ther.* 2010;90:75-88.

71. Black LL, Jensen GM, Mostrom E, et al. The first year of practice: an investigation of the professional learning and development of promising novice physical therapists. *Phys Ther.* 2010;90(12):1758-1773.

72. Hayward LM, Black LL, Mostrom E, et al. The first two years of practice: a longitudinal perspective on the learning and professional development of promising novice physical therapists. *Phys Ther.* 2013;93:369-383.

73. Mattingly C, Fleming M. *Clinical Reasoning—Forms of Inquiry in a Therapeutic Practice.* Philadelphia, PA: FA Davis; 1994.

74. Dowie J, Elstein A, eds. *Professional Judgment: A Reader in Clinical Decision Making.* New York, NY: Cambridge University Press; 1988.

75. Boud D, Keogh R, Walker D. *Reflection: Turning Experience Into Learning.* London, United Kingdom: Kegan Page; 1985.

76. Boyd E, Fales A. Reflective learning: key to learning from experience. *J Humanist Psychol.* 1983;23:99-117.

77. Foord-May L, May, W. Facilitating professionalism in physical therapy: theoretical foundations for the facilitation process. *J Phys Ther Educ.* 2007; 21(3):6-12.

78. Epstein R. Mindful practice. *JAMA.* 1999;282:833-839.

79. Coles R. The moral education of medical students. *Acad Med.* 1999;8(73):55-57.

80. Schön D. *Educating the Reflective Practitioner.* San Francisco, CA: Jossey-Bass Inc; 1987.

81. Crandall S. How expert clinicians teach what they know. *J Contin Educ Health Prof.* 1993;13:85-98.

82. Rikers RM, Loyens S, Schmidt HG. The role of encapsulated knowledge in clinical case representations of medical students and family doctors. *Med Educ.* 204;38:1035-1043.

83. Rikers RM, Schmidt HG, Boshuizen HP, et al. The robustness of medical expertise: clinical care processing by medical experts and subexperts. *Am J Psychol.* 2002;115:609-629.

84. Dowie J, Elstein A, eds. *Professional Judgment: A Reader in Clinical Decision Making.* New York, NY: Cambridge University Press; 1988.

85. Patel V, Groen G. Developmental accounts in the transition from medical student to doctor: some problems and suggestions. *Med Educ.* 1991;25:526-535.

86. Benner P, Tanner C, Chesla C. *Expertise in Nursing Practice: Caring, Clinical Judgment and Ethics.* New York, NY: Spring; 1996.

87. Gerber A, Thevoz AL, Ramelet RS. Expert clinical reasoning and pain assessment in mechanically ventilated patients: a descriptive study. *Aust Crit Care.* 2015;28(1):2-8.

88. May B, Dennis J. Expert decision making in physical therapy—a survey of practitioners. *Phys Ther.* 1991;71:190-206.

89. Orest M. Clinicians' perspectives of self-assessment in clinical practice. *Phys Ther.* 1995;75:824-829.

90. Hallett C. Learning through reflection in the community: the relevance of Schön's theories of coaching to nursing education. *Int J Nurs Stud.* 1997;34:103-110.

91. Powell J. The reflective practitioner in nursing. *J Adv Nurs.* 1989;14:824-832.

92. Kydonaki K, Huby G, Tocher J, Aitken LM. Understanding nurses' decision-making when managing weaning from mechanical ventilation: a study of novice and experienced critical care nurses in Scotland and Greece. *J Clin Nurs.* 2016;25:434-444.

93. Mylopoulos M, Woods NN. Having our cake and eating it too: seeking the best of both worlds in expertise research. *Med Educ.* 2009;43:406-413.

94. Durning SJ, Constanzo ME, Artino AR, et al. Neural basis on non-analytical reasoning expertise during clinical evaluation. *Brain Behav.* 2015;5(3):e00309.

95. McGinnis PQ, Guenther LA, Wainwright SF. Development and integration of professional core values among practicing clinicians. *Phys Ther.* 2016;96:1417-1429.

96. Norman G, Young M, Brooks L. Non-analytical models of clinical reasoning: the role of experience. *Med Educ.* 2007;41(12):1140-1145.

97. Schmidt HG, Rikers RM. How expertise develops in medicine: knowledge encapsulation and illness script formation. *Med Educ.* 2007;41(12):1133-1139.

98. Gobet F, Borg JL. The intermediate effect in clinical case recall is present in musculoskeletal physiotherapy. *Man Ther.* 2011;16(4):327-331.

99. Mamede S, Schmidt HG, Rikers R. Diagnostic errors and reflective practice in medicine. *J Eval Clin Pract.* 2007;13(1):138-145.

100. Boshuizan H, Schmidt H. On the role of biomedical knowledge in clinical reasoning by experts, intermediates and novices. *Cogn Sci.* 1992;16:153-184.
101. Schubert CC, Denmark TK, Crandall B, Grome A, Pappas J. Characterizing novice-expert differences in macrocognition: an exploratory study of cognitive work in the emergency department. *Ann Emerg Med.* 2013;61(1):96-109.
102. Durning SJ, Artino AR, Boulet JR, et al. The impact of selected contextual factors on experts' clinical reasoning performance (does context impact clinical reasoning performance in experts?). *Adv Health Sci Educ.* 2012;17(1):65-79.
103. Young JS, Smith RL, Guerlain S, Nolley B. How residents think and make medical decisions: implications for education and patient safety. *Am Surg.* 2007;73(6):548-553.
104. Kydonaki K, Huby G, Tocher J, Aitken LM. Understanding nurses' decision-making when managing weaning from mechanical ventilation: a study of novice and experienced critical care nurses in Scotland and Greece. *J Clin Nurs.* 2016;25:434-444.
105. Bryer DJ. Influences that drive clinical decision making among junior rheumatology nurses: a qualitative study. *Musculoskeletal Care.* 2006;4(4):223-232.
106. DuBroc W, Pickens ND. Becoming "at home" in home modifications: professional reasoning across the expertise continuum. *Occup Ther Health Care.* 2015;29(3):316-329.
107. King G, Currie M, Bartlett DJ, et al. The development of expertise in pediatric rehabilitation therapists: changes in approach, self-knowledge, and use of enabling and customizing strategies. *Dev Neurorehabil.* 2007;10(3):223-240.
108. King G, Currie M, Bartlett DJ, et al. The development of expertise in paediatric rehabilitation therapists: the roles of motivation, openness to experience, and types of caseload experience. *Aust Occup Ther J.* 2008;55(2):108-122.
109. Wainwright SF, Shepard KF, Harman LB, Stephens J. Factors that influence the clinical decision making of novice and experienced physical therapists. *Phys Ther.* 2011;91:87-101.
110. Gilliland S, Wainwright SF. Patterns of clinical reasoning in physical therapist students. *Phys Ther.* 2017;97:499-511.
111. Resnik L, Jensen GM. Using clinical outcomes to explore the theory of expert practice in physical therapy. *Phys Ther.* 2003;83(12):1090-1106.
112. Smith M, Higgs J, Ellis E. Effect of experience on clinical decision making by cardiorespiratory physiotherapists in acute care settings. *Physiother Theory Pract.* 2010;26(2):89-99.
113. Durning SJ, Ratcliffe T, Artino AR, et al. How is clinical reasoning developed, maintained, and objectively assessed? Views from expert internists and internal medicine interns. *J Contin Educ Health Prof.* 2013;33(4):215-223.
114. Kulamakan MK, Grierson LE, Norman GR. The roles of deliberate practice and innate ability in developing expertise: evidence and implications. *Med Educ.* 2013;47:979-989.

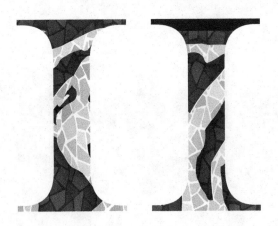

CLINICAL REASONING:
Teaching, Learning, and Assessment

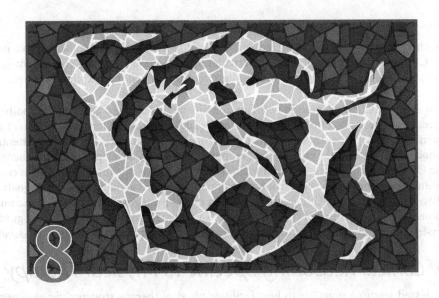

A CURRICULAR PERSPECTIVE ON
TEACHING CLINICAL REASONING IN
ENTRY-LEVEL EDUCATION

Sarah Gilliland, PT, DPT, PhD, CSCS

OBJECTIVES

- Describe the impact of integration of basic and clinical sciences within and across courses in an entry-level doctor of physical therapy program.
- Describe at least 3 ways that entry-level doctor of physical therapy programs can integrate clinical examples and experiences throughout the curriculum.
- Analyze the impact of implicit and explicit models of clinical reasoning (CR) and methods of assessment on students' developing understanding of CR.
- Integrate reflective learning activities across classroom and clinical learning to enhance students' development of CR.
- Evaluate how the 5 domains of curricular design can be enacted in traditional, systems-based, and problem-based curricular models.

INTRODUCTION

Entry-level physical therapist education must prepare students with the skills and dispositions required for effective physical therapists' specific CR. A curriculum for professional learning should be a continuous trajectory of growth, not disconnected pieces. Drawing on Dewey's proposition that a curriculum for professional learning should be a continuous trajectory of growth,

Musolino GM, Jensen GM, eds. *Clinical Reasoning and Decision-Making in Physical Therapy: Facilitation, Assessment, and Implementation* (pp 91-101).
© 2020 Taylor & Francis Group.

not disconnected pieces, this chapter draws on the literature in CR and professional development across professions to describe strategies for building a CR-focused curriculum. The 5 curricular strategies are described content integration, connection of theory to practice, consistent and explicit attention to CR, alignment of implicit and explicit messages, and an emphasis on reflective practice (RP).

Regardless of program design, content integration both horizontally (across courses) and longitudinally (throughout the program) is necessary for students' development of appropriate knowledge organization for CR. Consistent connections between didactic and clinical learning can improve students' transitions from classroom to clinic. Explicit attention to CR, including the use of a consistent model of CR across the curriculum, supports students in developing a comprehensive understanding of physical therapy-specific CR and provides a framework for application. Aligning the implicit messages communicated through curricular structure (timing and prioritization) and clinical examples with the curriculum's explicit goals supports students in developing a more cohesive understanding of CR. Finally, reflection must be integrated across the curriculum to inculcate habits of reflection for development of understanding of CR and ongoing learning. These principles provide a guiding but not prescriptive framework for entry-level program design and ongoing professional development to enhance the development of CR.

Importance of Clinical Reasoning Specific to Physical Therapy

Few studies have addressed teaching practices to best facilitate physical therapy students' development of CR skills. More studies have addressed the issue of diagnostic reasoning in medical students,[1-3] but 3 key differences in physical therapy practice suggest the need to examine teaching strategies specific to physical therapy CR.

First, the diagnostic process is only one aspect of the CR process for physical therapists.[4] The analysis of movement is central to experienced physical therapists' CR processes.[5] The current focus on the movement system shifts the attention of physical therapists' CR from the pathoanatomic to the pathokinesiological.[6] The focus on movement and understanding movement patterns, and their role in normal and pathological function, is central across physical therapy practice settings including pediatrics,[7] neurology,[8-10] and orthopedics.[11] Physical therapists must also consider contraindications and precautions to movement as they approach their examination and treatment with patients.[4]

Second, in addition to addressing issues of movement, physical therapists should address the consequences of the patient's disease process in addition to the pathology itself.[12] During the examination and assessment process, physical therapists also need to identify factors that contribute to the patient's problem,[4,13] as these factors often become the focal point for treatment.

Third, due to the ongoing and interactive nature of therapeutic work, concurrent with evaluating and developing strategies to address the patient's problems, the therapist ought to work collaboratively with the patient to determine ways to engage and motivate the patient in the treatment process.[9,14] Education for CR physical therapy should address these unique characteristics, in addition to the diagnostic process.

Clinical Reasoning as Analytical and Narrative

This chapter draws on Edwards et al's model[15] that characterizes CR as a complex interplay of deductive, inductive, and narrative reasoning processes. To engage in this type of complex reasoning, physical therapy students must develop appropriate knowledge organization; an understanding of collaborative, patient-centered reasoning; and the capacity to engage in reflection while working in uncertain contexts.

The importance of not only sufficient content knowledge but also appropriate knowledge organization has been described throughout the CR literature.[16-22] The organization and availability of the relevant content knowledge in their memory structure are primary determinants of clinicians' diagnostic reasoning.[16] Clinicians must have the appropriate content knowledge that is interlinked in clinically relevant patterns.[23-25] Practice-specific knowledge organization is evident in the movement scripts (a type of pattern recognition specific to the physical therapist's analysis of movement) engaged in by experienced physical therapists.[7,10] The type of knowledge organization needed for effective CR cannot be developed if content is taught as disconnected concepts.

Patient-centered collaborative reasoning is a hallmark of expert practice in physical therapy.[5] To engage in effective CR in physical therapy practice, physical therapists must have an orientation to reasoning that acknowledges the contributions all parties bring to the process.[26] Research with medical students has demonstrated that the students' conceptualizations of practice influence what they believe is valid to discuss with patients.[27] To engage in narrative reasoning, an integral component of CR, physical therapy students must develop an understanding of practice that values the patient-centered approach to care.

Finally, physical therapy students must develop the reflective abilities to engage in CR in uncertain contexts. Clinical decision-making always involves ambiguity and often involves value conflicts.[28] CR is a spiral process involving cognition, metacognition, and knowledge.[29] Regardless of how much research evidence is accumulated, clinicians will always ultimately have to make a decision, and that requires an element of uncertainty.[30] Overall, to engage in effective CR, students must integrate social and cognitive factors, while drawing on multiple knowledge sources including philosophy, personal, and propositional knowledge, to enhance their patient care.[31-33] Entry-level physical therapist curricula should facilitate students' development of knowledge organization, patient-centered reasoning, and reflective abilities such that they can engage in effective CR.

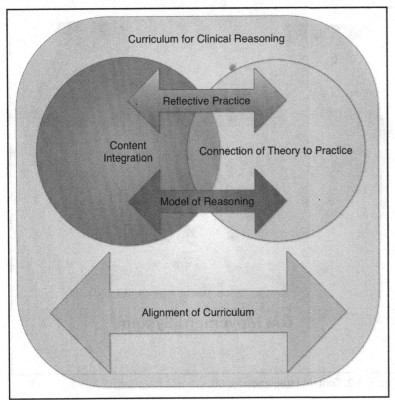

Figure 8-1. CR curricular model.

Need for Curricular Approach to Teaching Clinical Reasoning

Education for the development of CR should address the capacities required for effective reasoning.[34] As such, entry-level physical therapist education should address not only knowledge and efficient knowledge organization and integration, but also the integration of reflection and patient-centered practice. Further, these capacities should be developed with concurrent attention to students' orientations to practice, as a lack of alignment between elements may promote disconnections in students' development of reasoning abilities.

The current educational literature on CR addresses 3 broad categories of andragogical practices for teaching CR: cognitively directed teaching strategies including methods of content integration and the inclusion of case studies in classroom teaching[18,35,36]; explicit teaching of CR strategies in isolated CR courses[37,38] or clinical coursework and internships[39-42]; and the use of narrative and reflection in either classroom or clinical activities.[43-46] While each of these categories supports elements of the CR process, these teaching strategies in isolation leave disconnections between the classroom and clinic, and gaps in students' overall understanding of the reasoning process. A critical factor in the limitations of the current approaches to teaching CR stems from the clinical research approach. Most studies have designed and assessed the impacts of a single intervention. Further, many studies have been limited to an individual course in CR included late in the students' educational program.[47] The individual intervention level of these studies has also neglected to address the impact of curricular and program cultural factors on students' development of CR.[48] While these studies have contributed to our understanding of components of the learning process in the development of CR, we do not yet fully understand how they all work together for the most effective teaching of CR skills.

CR underlies all physical therapy practice, and thus, teaching of CR should be addressed at a programmatic level, not an individual classroom or clinical level. Individual courses in CR can support aspects of CR development, but classroom-to-clinic integration is needed for the most effective development.[34,49] Alone, each innovation described in the literature is insufficient to address the complex development of CR skills, but these studies provide insights that contribute to the development of a framework for addressing CR from a curricular perspective. A shift from the study of individual courses or interventions to informed program design and assessment is needed to fully address students' development of CR skills, because a curriculum for professional learning needs to encompass continuous growth, not disconnected pieces.[50]

A programmatic approach to teaching CR allows for the integration and consistency necessary for effective development of CR skills (Figure 8-1). Only when learning is coordinated across the curriculum can students consistently be exposed to the integrative ways of thinking that are necessary for effective clinical practice. The framework for curricular development described in this chapter draws on the existing research in teaching CR and models of professional learning across professions, and encompasses 5 dimensions that entry-level physical therapist educational programs should address in program design to promote students' development of CR capacities for patient-centered care. The dimensions include content integration, connection of theory to practice, consistent and explicit attention to CR, alignment of implicit and explicit messages, and an emphasis on RP (see Figure 8-1). This framework draws on content-specific concepts from the CR literature in medicine, nursing, and occupational and physical therapy, in conjunction with concepts of effective program design for professional development from the education literature. Drawing these bodies of literature together provides a physical therapist–specific framework for promoting entry-level and ongoing professional development.

Framework for Curricular Approach to Teaching Clinical Reasoning

Content Integration

The first dimension that programs must address is the integration of content areas (Figure 8-2). While a traditional approach to medical or physical therapy education addresses basic science, clinical science, and application separately, theories derived from the study of expert practice and cognitive science indicate that students will learn more effectively for practice if content teaching is integrated.[18,35,36] The type of integration needed for effective learning must happen at the programmatic level across courses, not within individual courses alone.

Expert clinicians consistently integrate knowledge from diverse sources to address the needs at hand.[31,51,52] Further, expert practice in physical therapy is characterized by consistent integration of analytical reasoning with strategic patient interactions. Interpersonal (narrative and collaborative) reasoning is not a separate process from ethical and deductive reasoning in clinical practice.[53] This practice suggests that training needs to be broad and interdisciplinary to promote the types of thinking expert therapists embody.[54]

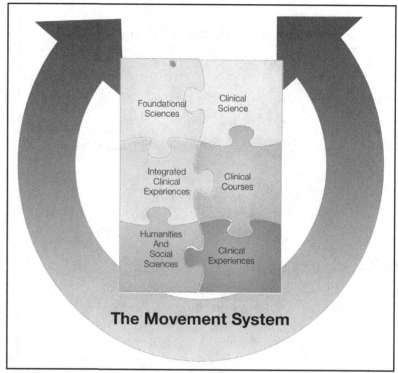

Figure 8-2. Content integration for CR.

To develop this cross-disciplinary thinking, students may benefit from programs in which initial basic science courses integrate clinical skills, professionalism, interpersonal skills, and practice-based learning.[18,36,55,56] The use of appropriate course sequencing can help promote the students' integration of ethical reasoning and technical practice, as the development of the capacity for moral agency develops alongside experience and skill development.[57,58] This type of integrated teaching not only promotes integration of content areas, but may also help students better organize their knowledge into systems/schema relevant to clinical practice that can promote better long-term retention and transfer.[24,56,59]

This type of cross-disciplinary integration, however, cannot happen at the level of individual courses. Integration of content areas requires informed decision-making about course sequencing and coordination across the curriculum.[57,60] This integration must extend to all areas of the curriculum, including clinical and reflective skills, in addition to content knowledge. Students tend to organize knowledge based on the structure of the curriculum,[41] and thus, when skills such as RP are taught in isolation, students do not incorporate them into their ongoing practice.[61]

Overall, this integrated teaching approach to program design may better assist students in developing big picture understanding (clinical gist) instead of learning disconnected facts.[62] Self-explanation during clinical cases (using unfamiliar cases) can guide students in integrating biomedical knowledge into clinical scripts.[63] Integration of content areas, including the basic sciences, social sciences, clinical skills, ethics, and RP, can support students in developing their content-specific reasoning capacities, understanding of the uncertainties in practice, and understanding of the types of patient interactions they will experience in practice. Content alone, however, is insufficient. Students must also have opportunities to develop an understanding of how their knowledge functions in clinical practice.

Connecting Theory to Practice

The second dimension that programs must address is the connection between classroom learning and clinical practice (Figure 8-3). Beyond classroom content integration, effectively incorporating clinical experiences helps students build contextual understanding and awareness of their role in the clinic. Studies have identified the disconnect between classroom learning and clinical experiences as a problem in physical therapy entry-level education.[46,64] Other researchers have suggested that cultural differences between the classroom and the clinic limit students' abilities to transfer their learning to clinical settings in which awareness of critical features of social and environmental context is critical for effective action.[64] Not only do students perceive this lack of coherence between their learning in the classroom and clinic,[65] but evidence also indicates that classroom performance (eg, grade point average, test scores) does not predict clinical performance,[66] nor does clinical performance predict

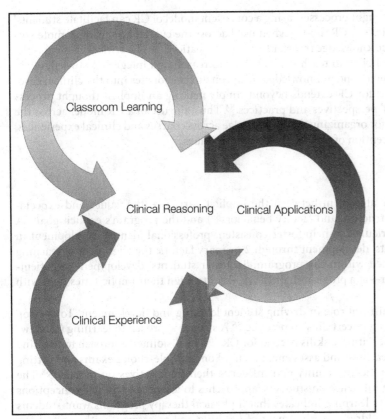

Figure 8-3. Connection from classroom to practice.

board exam performance.[67] While each setting offers its own affordances and constraints,[49,68,69] several factors, including the use of case studies and early incorporation of clinical experiences, that can be addressed at a programmatic level may contribute to bridging this gap.

Consistently bringing case studies into the classroom can help students in developing their understanding of the CR process and gaining specific examples to draw on in their own reasoning. Web-based patient simulation software may allow students to practice with many cases in an efficient manner. Further, software can allow instructors to analyze students' connections among exam findings, hypotheses, and intervention suggestions.[70] When students are provided with more details of the patient's life situation, they develop more detailed and individualized treatment plans and better situate their interventions in the social context.[71]

In another application of case study learning, students develop their own case studies and present them to the class for analysis of their deductive and interactive reasoning processes.[34,38,72] While each of these applications alone may support students in developing aspects of their reasoning abilities, the inclusion of innovative uses of case studies throughout the curriculum can support students' holistic approaches to CR.

While many studies have demonstrated the benefits of the use of case studies at a single point in the curriculum, including case studies throughout the curriculum may better promote students' capacities for integrating their content knowledge. A preliminary assessment of a longitudinal case study series across a physical therapy curriculum suggested that this type of case study may prompt the students to include greater consideration of psychosocial factors and integration of multiple knowledge sources in their patient care.[73,74] Bringing community patients into the classroom may further enhance the benefits of case study work, providing students, within the controlled environment of the classroom, with greater exposure to the types of interactive skills needed for clinical care.[75] The use of case studies and community patients within the classroom setting can provide students with a foundation of clinical skills; however, to effectively develop these skills, students must have opportunities to observe, learn, and practice within clinical settings.

Clinical experiences early in an entry-level program can help students develop appropriate contextual awareness, interactional skills, and knowledge organization for effective CR. These early clinical experiences, even experiences that include only observation, can help students in developing their conceptual models of physical therapy practice and reasoning.[76] The development of these conceptual models can influence students' later classroom learning, as students need a clear conceptual model of the entire task to understand a portion on which they may be focusing.[77] Clinical experiences included throughout the curriculum would enhance teachers' abilities to situate the task of CR and provide varied examples in practice,[78] better promoting students' understanding of the contextualized nature of CR.[4,79]

In addition to providing context, these early clinical experiences can enhance students' development of "illness scripts" and knowledge encapsulation.[17,18,80] Beyond supporting students' knowledge organization, clinical experiences can also help students understand the nature of clinical knowledge as a dynamic resource, not simply a collection of examples.[81] Finally, clinical experiences can support students in developing contextually appropriate interactional skills, an affordance not present in the classroom setting.[58] Clinical experiences must be coordinated with classroom coursework throughout the curriculum for students to most effectively reap these benefits. Strategic inclusion of clinical experiences supports students in further developing their content-specific reasoning skills, while building their interactive skills and gaining an understanding of the uncertainty inherent in clinical work.

Explicit and Consistent Attention to Clinical Reasoning

The third dimension that programs must address is the use of an explicit model for CR throughout the curriculum. Using an explicit model can help students develop an awareness of the thought processes clinicians typically enact at a subconscious level. Similar to the practices inherent in a cognitive apprenticeship,[78] the use of a framework for CR helps students and teachers identify the processes necessary for the abstract task of CR.

Beyond helping students understand the underlying thought processes, using a consistent model of CR can facilitate students' transfer of knowledge between courses and into the clinic.[82] A CR model, when used across the curriculum, can promote students' integration of varied content areas and may enhance knowledge transfer to clinical situations.[72] The critical element is the integration. A single class in reasoning processes is insufficient to teach students how to reason and integrate knowledge.[37,83] Effective courses in CR support students in integrating their content knowledge from concurrent courses into the clinical cases used in the reasoning course.[38] The influence of a model for CR extends beyond simply making an implicit thought process visible; the nature of that model also influences students' perspectives and practices.[84] Thus, the use of a CR model across the curriculum not only provides students with a framework for organizing their knowledge across courses and clinical experiences, but it also communicates an implicit message of the conception of practice the program values.

Implicit and Explicit Alignment

The fourth dimension programs must address is the alignment between the implicit curricula (the values and expectations communicated to students through the program structure and faculty behaviors[85]) and the program's explicit goals. A greater alignment between the implicit and explicit curricula can help foster consistent professional identity development in students.[86,87] The implicit curriculum influences students' development through 2 primary factors: the alignment of teaching and assessment, and the models of practice demonstrated within the program. To foster students' development of patient-centered orientations to practice, programs must consider—at a programmatic level—how to align their implicit messages with patient-centered practice.

The learning environment and assessment play a significant role in driving student learning and development. To develop effective CR abilities, students need capacities for managing uncertainty in practice.[86] A surface approach to learning (ie, viewing learning as an accumulation of facts) is not compatible with the skills needed for CR.[46] The disjointed approach to teaching and assessment currently employed in many programs (teaching and assessment focused on multiple-choice exams and getting the "right" answer) can limit students' development of reflective ability and influence their perspectives on practice.[88] The teaching and policies within a department exert a strong influence on students' approaches to learning and their conceptions of knowledge.[89,90] The research on students' approaches to learning indicates that if physical therapy programs want students to develop a deep approach to learning, then they must address the alignment of teaching and assessment with goals at the program level, as individual interventions or assignments seem ineffective at changing students' approaches to learning.[83,91-94]

One critical element for physical therapist education relates to content overload. In a profession in which students must develop a sufficient foundation of content knowledge, program directors need to consider how to effectively distribute coursework. Student perceptions of work overload influence their approaches to learning, primarily driving students toward a rote memorization approach to learning that is not compatible with effective CR.[90,92] Placing a higher focus on CR and communicating about reasoning may help reduce the implicit impact of emphasis on factual knowledge and technical skills, and can promote students' development of values consistent with patient-centered reasoning.[87] Physical therapy programs need to address assessment, learning environment, and workload from a programmatic perspective to best facilitate students' development of effective learning strategies for CR.

Not only do teaching practices and assessments influence students' conceptions of reasoning, but the models of practice to which they are exposed also shape their perspectives on CR. Students' development of CR skills is intertwined with their development of their understanding of the profession and their professional role.[95] Health sciences students enter their professional education with preexisting conceptions of their profession based on their experiences.[96,97] Professional development should support students' growth toward more expansive orientations to practice,[98,99] yet studies of medical students indicate that many do not change their conceptions of practice over the course of their education.[100] The development of students' conceptions of practice must be addressed at a programmatic level, as it is the aggregate influence of the faculty's implicit professional behaviors that determines what skills and values students develop.[101,102] The representations of practice (the examples of practice enacted within the educational program) influence what students learn to see from the disciplinary perspective.[103] Programs that emphasize students' technical skills and scientific knowledge over individual patient needs may sway students away from a patient-centered perspective.[104,105] Using an explicit model of practice may also help faculty offer representations of practice that better align with the overall mission.[102] Assessment at the program level can evaluate the influence of course ordering, emphasis, and organization on students' understanding of their professional roles to minimize implicit influences that counter the program mission.[104]

Overall, faculty must work together to expose students to models of practice consistent with the program's mission, and align their teaching and assessment to promote conceptions of knowledge and practice that support students in developing capacities for flexible patient-centered CR.

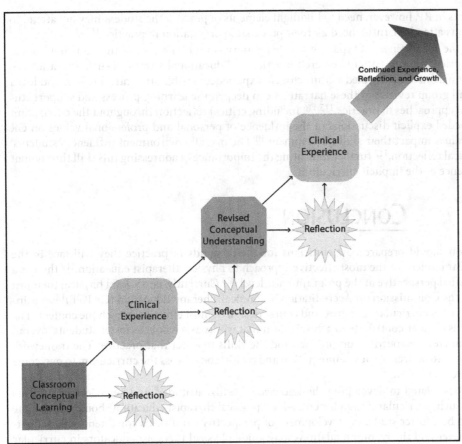

Figure 8-4. Cycles of reflection and growth.

Emphasis on Reflective Practice

The final dimension programs must address is the development of students' capacities for RP. While several researchers have developed frameworks and guidelines for RP in physical therapy,[43,44,93] teaching of RP is often limited to a single course, portfolio, or workshop.[61] An emphasis on RP not only helps students in developing skills of managing the uncertainty of clinical practice, but it can also help shape their perspectives on practice, deductive reasoning skills, and interactions with patients.

Reflection is a crucial skill in managing uncertainty in "real-world" clinical settings, but for students to effectively develop and integrate this practice, reflection must be addressed throughout the curriculum.[61] RP across classroom and clinical experiences can help students build the links they need between analytical reasoning and patient-centered care,[106] and transition their thinking to clinical applications.[40,52,107] Introducing students to a structured framework for reflection during their classroom work can provide them with support for reflection during clinical experiences.[43,44] Specifically integrating intentional reflection during students' clinical experiences through activities such as elaborating on their reasoning process with a mentor,[17] especially when students are supported in questioning their assumptions, can further help students move beyond simple repetition of previously learned concepts to develop their reasoning capacities.[44]

Reflection can also help students connect their classroom knowledge to the clinic. The practice of reflection during both classroom and clinical learning enables students to look back at their actions and better understand how their decisions and actions led to the outcomes they experienced.[108] Reflection must be integrated with classroom and experiential learning to provide students with opportunities to engage in activities, reflect on those activities, and compare their new experiences to their existing conceptual understanding (Figure 8-4).[109] Further, without the capacity for reflection, students will be limited in their ability to learn from experience, as it is not the experience itself that promotes learning but the process of thinking about the experience.[33,110] Reflection before, during, and after learning activities can better promote students' metacognition in reasoning.[72] Setting aside time during clinical experiences for reflection may help students better develop their experiential knowledge, the type of knowledge most depended on by clinicians.[46,64] The type of self-assessment that can be developed through reflection is crucial for ongoing professional learning, helping students develop the skills to identify their own strengths and limitations and engage in ongoing professional development.[43] Reflection may be the key to helping reduce the mismatch between classroom education and the type of knowledge needed for clinical practice.

Finally, reflection and analysis of practice can support positive shifts in students' orientations to practice. Interventions using video of participants' own practice and others' practice have enabled individuals in a variety of professions to become more reflective on their own practice, shift their perspectives on practice, and carry these new orientations into their actual practice.[111,112] Instructors guiding students in RP, however, need to highlight elements of practice the student may not attend to naturally, as the elements to which students attend are influenced by their preexisting orientation to practice.[113]

Further, guiding students to question the effectiveness of typically selected patterns of interaction and their attributions for success or failure may support shifts in orientation to patient-centered practice.[114] Educational strategies such as scaffolded, structured opportunities to write clinical narratives integrated within clinical experiences enable students to reflect and learn from individual patient experiences. Small group reviews of these narratives can deepen the learning process and support students in developing more patient-centered approaches to practice.[115,116] Including critical reflection throughout the curriculum can provide the opportunities for the needed explicit discussions of the influence of personal and professional values on CR to help students understand how these values impact their skill development.[10] The overall environment influences students' willingness and capacity to engage in critical reflection,[117] further indicating the importance of addressing this skill throughout the program while attending to the influence of the implicit curriculum.

CONCLUSION

Entry-level physical therapist education should prepare new clinicians for the demands of practice they will face in the future.[118] While there currently are no clear models for the most effective approach to physical therapist education,[119] there is a call to address education from a more unified perspective at the programmatic level.[120] Currently, entry-level physical therapist education programs have standards from the Commission on Accreditation in Physical Therapy Education (CAPTE)[121] outlining necessary content, but minimal guidance in curricular structure and course design to most effectively teach the content. The 5 domains (see Figure 8-1) described in this chapter contribute to a curriculum that works as a whole to foster students' overall professional growth, including patient-centered perspectives on practice and the skills to enact that practice. The framework described in this chapter can guide programs to address issues of integration and consistency across the curriculum to overcome the limitations of current teaching approaches for CR.

CAPTE[122] defines teaching as "activities related to developing the knowledge, skills, attitudes, and behaviors of students necessary for entry to the profession." As such, curricular design for entry-level physical therapist education should address the 5 dimensions described in this chapter to best foster students' development of perspectives and skills consistent with patient-centered care. The framework in this chapter and the recommendations may guide physical therapist educators in curricular design to provide students with the optimal experiences to enhance their development of patient-centered CR. This framework provides programs with greater direction for program design without prescriptive rigidity.

Reflection Moment

Reflect on how your program curriculum aligns with the 5 dimensional frameworks presented.

Where are the strengths? What could be strengthened?

How will you contribute to the enhancement potentials as an educator, student, peer, clinical instructor, or residency or fellowship leader?

REFERENCES

1. Coderre S, Jenkins D, McLaughlin K. Qualitative differences in knowledge structure are associated with diagnostic performance in medical students. *Adv Health Sci Educ Theory Pract.* 2009;14(5):677-684.
2. Norman G. Research in clinical reasoning: past history and current trends. *Med Educ.* 2005;39(4):418-427.
3. Patel VL, Groen GJ. Developmental accounts of the transition from medical student to doctor: some problems and suggestions. *Med Educ.* 1991;25(6):527-535.
4. Jones MA. CR in manual therapy. *Phys Ther.* 1992;72(12):875-884.
5. Jensen GM, Gwyer J, Shepard KF, Hack LM. Expert practice in physical therapy. *Phys Ther.* 2000;80(1):28-43; discussion 44-52.
6. Sahrmann SA. The human movement system: our professional identity. *Phys Ther.* 2014;94(7):1034-1042.
7. Embrey DG, Guthrie MR, White OR, Dietz J. CDM by experienced and inexperienced pediatric physical therapists for children with diplegic cerebral palsy. *Phys Ther.* 1996;76(1):20-33.
8. Riolo L. Skill differences in novice and expert clinicians in neurologic physical therapy. *Neurology Report.* 1996;20(1):60-63.
9. Wainwright SF, McGinnis PQ. Factors that influence the clinical decision-making of rehabilitation professionals in long-term care settings. *J Allied Health.* 2009;38(3):143-151.

10. McGinnis PQ, Hack LM, Nixon-Cave K, Michlovitz SL. Factors that influence the CDM of physical therapists in choosing a balance assessment approach. *Phys Ther.* 2009;89(3):233-247.

11. May S, Greasley A, Reeve S, Withers S. Expert therapists use specific CR processes in the assessment and management of patients with shoulder pain: a qualitative study. *Aust J Physiother.* 2008;54(4):261-266.

12. Jette AM. Diagnosis and classification by physical therapists: a special communication. *Phys Ther.* 1989;69(11):967-969.

13. Rothstein JM, Echternach JL, Riddle DL. The hypothesis-oriented algorithm for clinicians II (HOAC II): a guide for patient management. *Phys Ther.* 2003;83(5):455-470.

14. Mattingly C. What is clinical reasoning. *Am J Occup Ther.* 1991;45(11):979-986.

15. Edwards I, Jones M, Carr J, Braunack-Mayer A, Jensen GM. Clinical reasoning strategies in physical therapy. *Phys Ther.* 2004;84(4):312-330; discussion 331-315.

16. Bordage G, Grant J, Marsden P. Quantitative assessment of diagnostic ability. *Med Educ.* 1990;24(5):413-425.

17. Schmidt HG, Rikers RM. How expertise develops in medicine: knowledge encapsulation and illness script formation. *Med Educ.* 2007;41(12):1133-1139.

18. de Bruin AB, Schmidt HG, Rikers RM. The role of basic science knowledge and clinical knowledge in diagnostic reasoning: a structural equation modeling approach. *Acad Med.* 2005;80(8):765-773.

19. Rikers R, Schmidt HG, Moulaert V. Biomedical knowledge: encapsulated or two worlds apart? *Appl Cognit Psychol.* 2005;19:223-231.

20. Patel VL, Groen GJ, Frederiksen CH. Differences between medical students and doctors in memory for clinical cases. *Med Educ.* 1986;20(1):3-9.

21. Norman G. Reliability and construct validity of some cognitive measures of clinical reasoning. *Teach Learn Med.* 1989;1(4):194-199.

22. Norman G. Recall by expert medical practitioners and novices as a record of processing attention. *J Exp Psychol-Learn Mem.* 1989;15(6):1166-1174.

23. Schmidt HG, Norman G, Boshuizen HP. A cognitive perspective on medical expertise: theory and implication. *Acad Med.* 1990;65(10):611-621.

24. Mandin H, Jones A, Woloschuk W, Harasym P. Helping students learn to think like experts when solving clinical problems. *Acad Med.* 1997;72(3):173-179.

25. Furze J, Gale JR, Black L, Cochran TM, Jensen GM. Clinical reasoning: development of a grading rubric for student assessment. *J Phys Ther Educ.* 2015;29(3):34-45.

26. Edwards I, Jones M, Higgs J, Trede F, Jensen GM. What is collaborative reasoning? *Adv Physiother.* 2004;6:70-83.

27. Dall'alba G. Understanding medical practice: different outcomes of a pre-medical program. *Adv Health Sci Educ Theory Pract.* 2002;7(3):163-177.

28. Tanner CA. Thinking like a nurse: a research-based model of clinical judgment in nursing. *J Nurs Educ.* 2006;45(6):204-211.

29. Hendrick P, Bond C, Duncan E, Hale L. CR in musculoskeletal practice: students' conceptualizations. *Phys Ther.* 2009;89(5):430-442.

30. West AF, West RR. Clinical decision-making: coping with uncertainty. *Postgrad Med J.* 2002;78(920):319-321.

31. Rushton A, Lindsay G. Defining the construct of masters level clinical practice in manipulative physiotherapy. *Man Ther.* 2010;15(1):93-99.

32. Shepard KF, Hack LM, Gwyer J, Jensen GM. Describing expert practice in physical therapy. *Qual Health Res.* 1999;9(6):746-758.

33. Hayward LM, Black LL, Mostrom E, et al. The first two years of practice: a longitudinal perspective on the learning and professional development of promising novice physical therapists. *Phys Ther.* 2013;93(3):369-383.

34. Higgs J. Developing clinical reasoning competencies. *Physiotherapy.* 1992;78(8):575-581.

35. Beck AL, Bergman DA. Using structured medical information to improve students' problem-solving performance. *J Med Educ.* 1986;61(9 pt 1):749-756.

36. Eva KW. What every teacher needs to know about clinical reasoning. *Med Educ.* 2004;39:98-106.

37. Burnett CN, Pierson FM. Developing problem-solving skills in the classroom. *Phys Ther.* 1988;9:1381-1385.

38. Higgs J. Fostering the acquisition of clinical reasoning skills. *New Zealand J Physiother.* 1990;18:13.

39. Kelly SP. The exemplary clinical instructor: a qualitative case study. *J Phys Ther Educ.* 2007;21(1):63-69.

40. Crandall S. How expert clinical educators teach what they know. *J Contin Educ Health Prof.* 1993;13:85-98.

41. Bowen JL. Educational strategies to promote clinical diagnostic reasoning. *N Engl J Med.* 2006;355(21):2217-2225.

42. Goss JR. Teaching clinical reasoning to second-year medical students. *Acad Med.* 1996;71(4):349-352; discussion 348.

43. Donaghy ME, Morss K. An evaluation of a framework for facilitating and assessing physiotherapy students' reflection on practice. *Physiother Theory Pract.* 2007;23(2):83-94.

44. Donaghy ME, Morss K. Guided reflection: A framework to facilitate and assess RP within the discipline of physiotherapy. *Physiother Theory Pract.* 2000;16:3-14.

45. Brady DW, Corbie-Smith G, Branch WT. "What's important to you?" The use of narratives to promote self-reflection and to understand the experiences of medical residents. *Ann Intern Med.* 2002;137(3):220-223.

46. Jensen GM, Paschal KA. Habits of mind: student transition toward virtuous practice. *J Phys Ther Educ.* 2000;14(3):42-47.

47. Gay S, Bartlett M, McKinley R. Teaching clinical reasoning to medical students. *Clin Teach.* 2013;10(5):308-312.

48. Vidyarthi AR, Kamei R, Chan K, Goh SH, Lek N. Factors associated with medical student clinical reasoning and evidence based medicine practice. *Int J Med Educ.* 2015;6:142-148.

49. Terry W, Higgs J. Educational programmes to develop clinical reasoning skills. *Aust Physiother.* 1993;39(1):47-51.

50. Dewey J. The relation of theory to practice in education. In: Archambault RD, ed. *John Dewey on Education: Selected Writings.* Chicago, IL: University of Chicago Press; 1974.

51. Resnik L, Jensen GM. Using clinical outcomes to explore the theory of expert practice in physical therapy. *Phys Ther.* 2003;83(12):1090-1106.

52. Wainwright SF, Shepard KF, Harman LB, Stephens J. Novice and experienced physical therapist clinicians: a comparison of how reflection is used to inform the clinical decision-making process. *Phys Ther.* 2010;90(1):75-88.

53. Edwards I, Jones M, Hillier S. The interpretation of experience and its relationship to body movement: a CR perspective. *Man Ther.* 2006;11(1):2-10.

54. King G, Currie M, Bartlett DJ, et al. The development of expertise in pediatric rehabilitation therapists: changes in approach, self-knowledge, and use of enabling and customizing strategies. *Dev Neurorehabil.* 2007;10(3):223-240.

55. Gregory JK, Lachman N, Camp CL, Chen LP, Pawlina W. Restructuring a basic science course for core competencies: an example from anatomy teaching. *Med Teach.* 2009;31(9):855-861.

56. Norman G. Teaching basic science to optimize transfer. *Med Teach.* 2009;31(9):807-811.

57. Christensen N, Nordstrom T. Facilitating the teaching and learning of clinical reasoning. In: Jensen GM, Mostrom E, eds. *Handbook of Teaching and Learning for Physical Therapists.* 3rd ed. St. Louis, MO: Elsevier; 2013.

58. Benner P. Using the Dreyfus model of skill acquisition to describe and interpret skill acquisition and clinical judgment in nursing practice and education. *Bull Sci Technol Soc.* 2004;24(3):188-199.

59. Custers EJ. Long-term retention of basic science knowledge: a review study. *Adv Health Sci Educ Theory Pract.* 2010;15(1):109-128.

60. Weddle ML, Sellheim DO. An integrative curriculum model preparing physical therapists for vision 2020 practice. *J Phys Ther Educ.* 2009;23(1):12-21.

61. Delany C, Watkin D. A study of critical reflection in health professional education: "learning where others are coming from." *Adv Health Sci Educ Theory Pract.* 2009;14(3):411-429.

62. Lloyd FJ, Reyna VF. Clinical gist and medical education: connecting the dots. *JAMA.* 2009;302(12):1332-1333.

63. Chamberland M, Mamede S, St-Onge C, et al. Students' self-explanations while solving unfamiliar cases: the role of biomedical knowledge. *Med Educ.* 2013;47(11):1109-1116.

64. Richardson B. Professional development: professional knowledge and situated learning in the workplace. *Physiotherapy.* 1999;85(9):467-474.

65. Christensen N, Jones MA, Edwards I, Higgs J. Helping physiotherapy students develop clinical reasoning capability. In: Higgs J, Jones MA, Loftus S, Christensen N, eds. *Clinical Reasoning in the Health Professions.* 3rd ed. Amsterdam, Netherlands: Butterworth-Heinemann Elsevier; 2008:389-396.

66. Sisola SW. Moral reasoning as a predictor of clinical practice: the development of physical therapy students across the professional curriculum. *J Phys Ther Educ.* 2000;14(3):26-34.

67. Luedtke-Hoffmann K, Dillon L, Utsey C, Tomaka J. Is there a relationship between performance during physical therapist clinical education and scores on the National Physical Therapy Examination (NPTE)? *J Phys Ther Educ.* 2012;26(2):41-49.

68. Jensen GM, Shepard KF, Hack LM. The novice versus the experienced clinician: insights into the work of the physical therapist. *Phys Ther.* 1990;70(5):314-323.

69. Page CG, Ross IA. Instructional strategies utilized by physical therapist clinical instructors: an exploratory study. *J Phys Ther Educ.* 2004;18(1):43-49.

70. Huhn K, Deutsch JE. Development and assessment of a web-based patient simulation program. *J Phys Ther Educ.* 2011;25(1):5-10.

71. Neistadt ME, Wight J, Mulligan SE. Clinical reasoning case studies as teaching tools. *Am J Occup Ther.* 1998;52(2):125-132.

72. Higgs J. A programme for developing clinical reasoning skills. *Med Teach.* 1993;15(2/3):195.

73. Strunk V, Altenburger P, Bayliss AJ, Loghmani MT. It's all in the family: Making the case for instructional collaboration using the integrated longitudinal case-based learning model. Paper presented at: Combined Sections Meeting of the American Physical Therapy Association; February 2012; Chicago, IL.

74. Loghmani MT, Bayliss AJ, Strunk V, Altenburger P. An integrative, longitudinal case-based learning model as a curriculum strategy to enhance teaching and learning. *J Phys Ther Educ.* 2011;25(2):42-50.

75. Piper Kelly S, King HJ. The community patient resource group: a novel strategy for bringing the clinic to the classroom. *J Phys Ther Educ.* 2012;26(2):32-40.

76. Collins A, Brown JS, Newman SE. *Cognitive Apprenticeship: Teaching the Craft of Reading, Writing, and Mathematics.* Champaign, IL: Center for the Study of Reading; 1987.

77. Collins A. Cognitive apprenticeship. In: Sawyer RK, ed. *The Cambridge Handbook of Learning Science.* New York, NY: Cambridge University Press; 2006:47-60.

78. Collins A, Brown JS, Holum A. Cognitive apprenticeship: making thinking visible. *Am Educ.* 1991;15(3):6-11, 38-39.

79. Charlin B, Boshuizen HP, Custers EJ, Feltovich PJ. Scripts and clinical reasoning. *Med Educ.* 2007;41(12):1178-1184.

80. Norman G, Young M, Brooks L. Non-analytical models of clinical reasoning: the role of experience. *Med Educ.* 2007;41(12):1140-1145.

81. Mylopoulos M, Regehr G. Cognitive metaphors of expertise and knowledge: prospects and limitations for medical education. *Med Educ.* 2007;41(12):1159-1165.

82. Neistadt ME. Teaching strategies for the development of clinical reasoning. *Am J Occup Ther.* 1996;50(8):676-684.

83. Higgs J, Boud D. Self-directed learning as part of the mainstream of physiotherapy education. *Aust Physiother.* 1991;37(4):245-251.

84. Darrah J, Loomis J, Manns P, Norton B, May L. Role of conceptual models in a physical therapy curriculum: application of an integrated model of theory, research and clinical practice. *Physiother Theory Pract.* 2006;22:239-250.

85. Jensen GM, Paschal KA, Shepard KF. Curriculum design for physical therapy educational programs. In: Jensen GM, Mostrom E, eds. *Handbook of Teaching and Learning for Physical Therapists.* 3rd ed. St. Louis, MO: Elsevier; 2013:2-18.

86. Shepard KF, Jensen GM. Physical therapist curricula for the 1990s: educating the RP. *Phys Ther.* 1990;70(9):566-573.

87. Ajjawi R, Higgs J. Learning to communicate clinical reasoning. In: Higgs J, Jones MA, Loftus S, Christensen N, eds. *Clinical Reasoning in the Health Professions*. 3rd ed. Amsterdam, Netherlands: Butterworth-Heinemann Elsevier; 2008.

88. Coles R. The moral education of medical students. *Acad Med*. 1998;73(1):55-57.

89. Sheppard C, Gilbert J. Course design, teaching method and student epistemology. *High Educ*. 1991;22(3):229-249.

90. Newble DI, Entwistle NJ. Learning styles and approaches: implications for medical education. *Med Educ*. 1986;20(3):162-175.

91. Trigwell K, Prosser M. Improving the quality of student learning: the influence of learning context and student approaches to learning on learning outcomes. *Higher Education*. 1991;22(3):251-266.

92. Sadlo G, Richardson JTE. Approaches to studying and perceptions of the academic environment in students following problem-based and subject-based curricula. *Higher Education Research and Development*. 2003;22(3):253-274.

93. Mann K, Gordon J, MacLeod A. Reflection and reflective practice in health professions education: a systematic review. *Adv Health Sci Educ Theory Pract*. 2009;14:595-621.

94. Entwistle NJ. Approaches to learning and perceptions of the learning environment. *Higher Education*. 1991;22:201-204.

95. Ajjawi R, Higgs J. Learning to reason: a journey of professional socialisation. *Adv Health Sci Educ Theory Pract*. 2008;13(2):133-150.

96. Dall'alba G. Medical practice as characterised by beginning medical students. *Adv Health Sci Educ Theory Pract*. 1998;3(2):101-118.

97. Richardson B, Lindquist I, Engardt M, Aitman C. Professional socialization: students' expectations of being a physiotherapist. *Med Teach*. 2002;24(6):622-627.

98. Dall'Alba G, Sandberg J. Unveiling professional development: a critical review of stage models. *Rev Educ Res*. 2006;76(3):383-412.

99. Dall'Alba G, Sandberg J. Educating for competence in professional practice. *Instr Sci*. 1996;24:411-437.

100. Dall'Alba G. Understanding professional practice: investigations before and after an educational programme. *Stud High Educ*. 2004;29(6):679-692.

101. Threlkeld AJ, Jensen GM, Royeen CB. The clinical doctorate: a framework for analysis in physical therapist education. *Phys Ther*. 1999;79(6):567-581.

102. Santasier AM, Plack MM. Assessing professional behaviors using qualitative data anlaysis. *J Phys Ther Educ*. 2007;21(3):29-39.

103. Grossman PL, Compton C, Igra D, et al. Teaching practice: a cross-professional perspective. *Teach Coll Rec*. 2009;111(9):2055-2100.

104. Kieser JA, Dall'alba G, Livingstone V. Impact of curriculum on understanding of professional practice: a longitudinal study of students commencing dental education. *Adv Health Sci Educ Theory Pract*. 2009;14(3):303-314.

105. Shepard KF, Jensen GM, eds. *Handbook of Teaching for Physical Therapists*. 2nd ed. Philadelphia, PA: Butterworth-Heinemann; 2002.

106. Epstein RM. Mindful practice. *JAMA*. 1999;282(9):833-839.

107. Wainwright SF, Shepard KF, Harman LB, Stephens J. Factors that influence the clinical decision-making of novice and experienced physical therapists. *Phys Ther*. 2011;91(1):87-101.

108. Schön DA. *Educating the Reflective Practitioner*. San Francisco, CA: Jossey-Bass; 1987.

109. Simon MA, Tzur R. Explicating the role of mathematical tasks in conceptual learning: an elaboration of the hypothetical learning trajectory. *Math Think Learn*. 2004;6(2):91-104.

110. Shulman LS. The wisdom of practice: managing complexity in medicine and teaching. In: Shulman LS, Wilson SM, eds. *The Wisdom of Practice: Essays on Teaching, Learning, and Learning to Teach*. San Francisco, CA: Jossey-Bass; 2004:251-271.

111. Holmstrom I, Rosenqvist U. A change of the physicians' understanding of the encounter parallels competence development. *Patient Educ Couns*. 2001;42(3):271-278.

112. van Es EA, Sherin MG. The influence of video clubs on teachers' thinking and practice. *J Math Teach Educ*. 2010;13:155-176.

113. Larsson J, Holmstrom I, Lindberg E, Rosenqvist U. Trainee anaesthetists understand their work in different ways: implications for specialist education. *Br J Anaesth*. 2004;92(3):381-387.

114. Anderson RM, Funnell MM. Patient empowerment: reflections on the challenge of fostering the adoption of a new paradigm. *Patient Educ Couns*. 2005;57(2):153-157.

115. Greenfield BH, Jensen GM, Delany CM, et al. Power and promise of narrative for advancing physical therapist education and practice. *Phys Ther*. 2015;95(6):924-933.

116. Greenfield BH, Swisher LL. The role of narratives in professional formation for students. In: Higgs J, Sheehan D, Baldly Currens J, Letts W, Jensen GM, eds. *Realising Exemplary Practice-Based Education*. Rotterdam, Netherlands: Sense Publishers; 2013:163-170.

117. Poole G, Jones L, Whitfield M. Helping students reflect: lessons from cognitive psychology. *Adv Health Sci Educ Theory Pract*. 2013;18(4):817-824.

118. Wojciechowski M. The future of physical therapist education. *PT in Motion*. 2015;7(1):15-26.

119. Gwyer J, Hack LM. Editorial: in pursuit of best practice in physical therapy education. *J Phys Ther Educ*. 2015;29(1):3.

120. Graham CL. Pauline Cerasoli Lecture: Coming into focus: The need for a conceptual lens. Paper presented at: Combined Sections Meeting of the American Physical Therapy Association; 2015; Indianapolis, IN.

121. Commission on Accreditation in Physical Therapy Education. *Physical Therapy Standards and Required Elements*. Alexandria, VA: American Physical Therapy Association; 2016.

122. Commission on Accreditation in Physical Therapy Education. *Evaluative Criteria for Physical Therapy Programs*. Alexandria, VA: American Physical Therapy Association; 2014:viii.

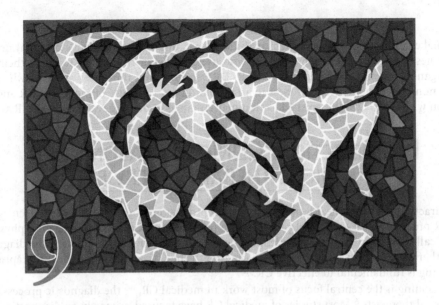

PATTERNS OF CLINICAL REASONING DEVELOPMENT IN ENTRY-LEVEL PHYSICAL THERAPIST STUDENTS

Sarah Gilliland, PT, DPT, PhD, CSCS

OBJECTIVES

- Analyze potential sources of variation in students' approaches to clinical reasoning (CR).
- Discuss the educational implications of 3 patterns of physical therapist students' reasoning errors.
- Describe the impact of structured models of CR on students' development of CR.
- Design a learning activity that provides opportunities for students to engage in a clinical activity, reflect on that experience, and revise the approach; this is also known as a reflective learning design.

Entry-level physical therapist students' development of CR is a nonhomogenous, nonlinear process of learning and development. Entry-level physical therapist education should support students in developing physical therapy–specific CR, including attending to movement, addressing contributing factors, and identifying patient-specific needs. Examination of the types of hypotheses and reasoning strategies students' use in the reasoning process can identify students' approaches to reasoning and shortcomings in developmental processing.

Over the course of the typical 3-year doctor of physical therapy (DPT) education program, students progress from a generalized process of identifying affected anatomical structures to a more specific physical therapist process of analyzing a patient's/client's movement and contributing factors affecting movement. At each stage in DPT students' education, students may take qualitatively different approaches to patient/client encounters. Some students maintain a focus on the biomechanical and technical aspects of the patient case throughout their education, while others consistently focus on the patient's specific contextual needs. Second- and third-year students make far fewer analytical reasoning errors than do first-year students, yet students at

Musolino GM, Jensen GM, eds. *Clinical Reasoning and Decision-Making in Physical Therapy: Facilitation, Assessment, and Implementation* (pp 103-110).

all stages may fail to make connections between their analytical reasoning and the patient's personal needs. During the first and second years of professional DPT education, students who use a model or framework to guide their reasoning processes demonstrate greater organization and purposefulness in CR. DPT second- and third-year students who incorporated greater reflection-in-action demonstrated more responsiveness to an unfolding case. The use of models of CR and purposeful integration of critical reflection within physical therapist education may enhance students' development of CR skills.

INTRODUCTION: CLINICAL REASONING IN PHYSICAL THERAPY OVERVIEW

CR shares many characteristics across health professions. Each profession, however, has unique factors that distinguish the profession's specific CR process. Studies of expert practice have provided frameworks for analyzing physical therapy–specific CR processes.[1,2] Specifically, 3 characteristics are evident in the CR of expert physical therapists: the diagnostic process is only one aspect of physical therapy CR; analysis of movement is central to the CR process of physical therapists; and collaborative, patient-centered reasoning is fundamental to effective CR.[1,2]

While diagnostic reasoning is the central focus of most work in medical CR,[3-5] the diagnostic process is only one aspect of the CR process for physical therapists.[6] Most studies of medical CR have focused primarily on diagnostic reasoning at the level of identifying the health condition (medical diagnosis).[7-12] In physical therapist practice, diagnostic reasoning must also identify the reason for the problem and the consequences of illness or disease process.[13-15] The analysis of movement is central to experienced physical therapists' CR processes.[16] This focus on movement, and understanding movement patterns and their role in normal and pathological function, is central across physical therapy practice settings.[17-21] In addition, physical therapists' analysis of movement must also address movement patterns that contribute to injury.[6,13] The literature on expert practice in physical therapy also indicates that effective physical therapists work collaboratively with their patients to determine ways to engage and motivate the patient in the treatment process.[19,22] This collaborative reasoning process includes gaining an understanding of the patient's context and perspective on the illness or injury.[15,23]

The literature on expert practice has shaped our understanding of CR in physical therapists; however, the literature indicates that expert practice is qualitatively different from novice practice.[24,25] Experience, socialization, interaction, and emerging confidence contribute to development in early professional practice.[26] Additional years of experience further develop the collaborative nature of practice and learning.[27] While entry-level physical therapist students are not expected to engage in CR with the same level of quality that expert physical therapists do, entry-level education should support students in developing ways of thinking that place them on a trajectory toward developing patient-centered, physical therapist–specific reasoning.

THE USE OF HYPOTHESES, REASONING STRATEGIES, AND REASONING ERRORS IN ANALYSES

The nature of the hypotheses and reasoning strategies physical therapists employ, and the reasoning errors they commit, provides insights into the organization and focus of DPT reasoning processes. The process of hypothesis formation and evaluation is central to CR.[28] A hypothesis is any diagnostic idea that may identify pathology, impairment, functional deficit, or causes of and factors influencing the patient's disability.[9,13,29] In physical therapist practice, hypotheses guide data collection during examination[14] and the development and implementation of interventions.[29] In clinical practice, a physical therapist's hypotheses should address factors related to the patient, the therapist, and the specific context.[30]

CR strategies have been defined as ways of "thinking and taking action within clinical practice."[1(p322)] Reasoning strategies specific to physical therapy have been identified in the literature.[1] These strategies further indicate the clinician's focus during the clinical encounter. Additionally, physical therapists demonstrate varying patterns of reasoning specifically about pain.[31] Broader reasoning patterns (including hypothetico-deductive and pattern recognition) have been well defined in medical literature and discussed in Section I of this textbook.[7,9] The hypotheses developed and CR strategies employed represent the clinician's knowledge structure and organization during the patient encounter.[32] The analysis of physical therapist students' hypotheses and reasoning strategies during a patient encounter provides insights into their progress toward physical therapist–specific CR.

Reasoning errors can indicate limitations in development of CR skills and can impact judgments about causal factors.[33] Extensive reliance on cognitive biases and heuristics can impact reasoning process and induce errors.[34,35] Finally, reasoning errors may be due to limitations in evaluation of data and inability to interpret clinical patterns.[36] The type and nature of reasoning errors students commit can provide educators with insights into students' needs for further growth. Specifically, errors can direct educators toward limitations in the student's knowledge access and organization, or limitations in the student's understanding of the scope and nature of the physical therapist's relations with patients.

CLINICAL REASONING DEVELOPMENT IN PHYSICAL THERAPY STUDENTS

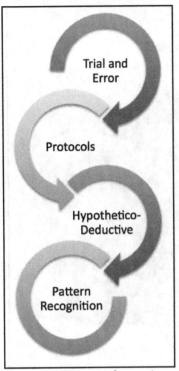

Figure 9-1. Patterns of reasoning.

Progress Toward Greater Specificity in Physical Therapy–Specific Reasoning

Physical therapist students demonstrate development toward the characteristics specific to physical therapist CR between their first and third years in entry-level DPT programs. Physical therapist students participating in a CR patient case during their first-year demonstrated hypothesis formation focused on identification of anatomical structures.[37] These first-year students also drew broad generalizations in their reasoning processes based on personal experience.[37] As a result of these generalizations, many students committed reasoning errors based on their inability to prioritize information or appropriately determine causal factors.

Students in their second and third years demonstrated greater specificity in reasoning and evidence of physical therapist–specific reasoning.[37] The second- and third-year students demonstrated well-established analysis of movement and consistent connection of movement to their reasoning strategies and hypothesis formation.[38,39] Second- and third-year students worked to analyze not only the patient's current health condition and movement patterns but also contributing biomechanical factors and target treatment plans toward these factors.[37,38] Finally, the second- and third-year students demonstrated use of established patterns of reasoning (hypothetico-deductive and pattern recognition), while first-year students demonstrated trial and error and a process of ruling ideas in or out (Figure 9-1). Students at all stages of their education used aspects of protocols to help guide their reasoning processes (see Figure 9-1).[37-39] First-, second-, and third-year students also used the patient's pain reports to guide their reasoning, but varied in specificity and interpretation of the information.[37-39] As described in the following section, some students used the pain reports with a purely biomedical interpretation, while others took a biopsychosocial perspective on the patient's pain descriptions.

Qualitatively Different Approaches to Clinical Reasoning

While the emergence of physical therapist–specific CR was evident in the second- and third-year students, at all levels, qualitatively different patterns were evident in the students' reasoning processes (Figure 9-2).[38-40] Students at each level varied in the amount of attention they gave to the patient's personal needs.[38,39] Many students focused exclusively on the biomechanical nature of the patient's health condition and paid little attention to the patient's personal goals, values, or life situations that impacted his or her level of participation. Other students, however, focused primarily on the patient's level of participation and identified areas to educate the patient for self-management. These different approaches suggest that some students are working from a primarily biomedical model, while others have embraced a biopsychosocial model.[41,42]

The DPT students' qualitative differences in CR were also apparent in their interpretation of examination data. Students in their second and third years collected similar examination data (eg, patient pain reports, observations of posture and movement), yet they provided different interpretations of their findings. For example, some students used the patient's pain reports (at rest and during activity) from a biomedical perspective as indicators of tissue damage and severity.[38] Other students (at the same educational level) used this pain information as an indicator of the patient's perspective and behavioral response to the injury.[38] Each student was consistent in his or her approach, and those who took a behavioral interpretation of the patient's pain responses integrated greater patient education and behavioral change strategies into their intervention plans.[38]

The students whose CR focused primarily on biomechanical factors created interventions worked on addressing impairment level issues, such as strength and range of motion and pain management.[38,39] A few students demonstrated a middle ground approach wherein they focused their assessment primarily on the patient's biomechanical needs, yet also acknowledged the impact of the patient's psychological state and need for emotional support.[38] The spectrum of approaches to CR (from strictly biomedical to biopsychosocial) was evident not only at each educational level but also across 2 entry-level DPT programs.

Reasoning Errors

The number and nature of the reasoning errors students committed during their first year compared to later in the program indicate progress in analytical reasoning, yet limitations in narrative reasoning (Figure 9-3). Second- and third-year students made fewer analytical errors, yet they continued to demonstrate errors related to addressing unique, personal-level patient issues[38,39] The students' analytical errors fell into 3 primary categories: jumping to conclusions (premature closure[35]), perseveration, and disregard. You may recall that each of these error types was also introduced with other potential errors in CR in Section I, Chapter 3, Table 3-3.

Students' analytical reasoning errors frequently stemmed from a limited understanding of the interrelations of their knowledge. Students who committed the error of jumping to conclusions (premature closure[35]) took one piece of information that was necessary but not sufficient to draw a certain conclusion, and jumped to that evaluation without considering the other findings necessary for drawing that conclusion.[37,39] These patterns suggest limitations in the students' understanding of how they must triangulate from multiple findings to assess their patient. This pattern was evident in the first- and second-year students.

Another error that indicated students' limited understanding of necessary and sufficient conditions for drawing a conclusion was perseveration. Students who committed this error took an examination finding that was necessary but not sufficient to rule in a particular hypothesis, and then continued to rationalize the stated hypothesis as other information was collected, even when later examination findings ran counter to the stated hypothesis.[37] The pattern of perseveration was evident primarily in first-year students.

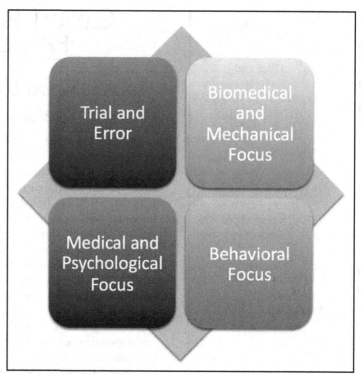

Figure 9-2. Qualitative differences.

The final analytical reasoning error evident in the students reasoning processes was disregard. The first-year students who demonstrated disregard selected to ignore an examination finding because they were unsure of the implications of the finding and chose to move on in their examination process because of uncertainty regarding how to integrate the finding into their reasoning process.[37] These errors suggest the students' inability to determine if an examination finding is a critical finding or not. The inability to prioritize findings often resulted in excessive focus on and distraction by cues that were not critical to the assessment of the patient.[37]

These analytical errors parallel medical students' noted errors, including jumping to conclusions (premature closure[35]), lack of prioritization, and trial-and-error data collection.[43] The difficulties the students demonstrated in organizing and prioritizing the information they collected have also been noted in novice classroom teachers.[44] The similarities in reasoning errors across professions suggest commonalities in the development process in professions that require complex real-time data collection, analysis, and decision-making.[45]

Students at all stages of their education demonstrated reasoning errors that indicate limited development of narrative reasoning and the process of integrating the patient's perspective into their CR. The error that consistently persisted into the second- and third-year students' work was a lack of attention to connections between the patient's personal situations (eg, values and personal interests for participation) and the CR process.[39] The error of limited connections was evident in the lack of connection between any personal information collected about the patient and the impact of the patient's condition on his or her day-to-day life. This error was evident in students at all stages (first- to third-year) of their education as well as across 2 DPT programs.[37-39]

Structured models of CR or examination procedure guidelines may support students in their development of CR. At each stage in their education, students who were able to use a protocol or model provided from class were better able to connect reasoning and data collection.[37] While overreliance on protocols may limit the flexibility within the CR process, models or routines may provide the structure necessary for students to initiate the reasoning process.[46] The value of external supports or structures was specifically evident in the CR work of the first-year students. First-year students who were able to recall an examination template provided in their coursework to support their preliminary reasoning processes used more sophisticated strategies (ie, less trial and error) during their patient examination. Students at all stages of their education indicated relying on their memory of examination templates they had used in courses or clinical experiences (CE). The second- and third-year students, however, demonstrated greater ability to diverge from the template procedures than did the first-year students. Black et al[26] noted a similar progression away from external examination guidelines in their study of physical therapist clinicians during their first year of practice.

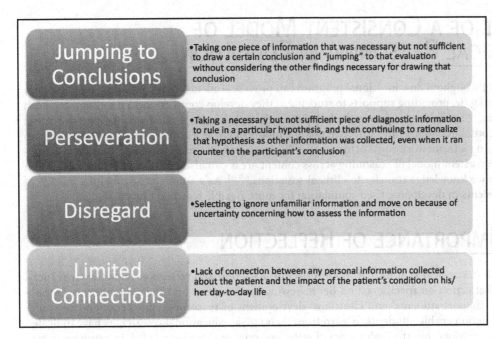

Figure 9-3. Reasoning errors.

Jumping to Conclusions
• Taking one piece of information that was necessary but not sufficient to draw a certain conclusion and "jumping" to that evaluation without considering the other findings necessary for drawing that conclusion

Perseveration
• Taking a necessary but not sufficient piece of diagnostic information to rule in a particular hypothesis, and then continuing to rationalize that hypothesis as other information was collected, even when it ran counter to the participant's conclusion

Disregard
• Selecting to ignore unfamiliar information and move on because of uncertainty concerning how to assess the information

Limited Connections
• Lack of connection between any personal information collected about the patient and the impact of the patient's condition on his/her day-to-day life

Use of Reflection

The second-year students' CR processes were analyzed for evidence of reflective practice, specifically reflection-in-action (an ongoing metacognitive awareness) and reflection-on-action (looking back and analyzing prior actions).[47,48] All participants demonstrated elements of reflection-on-action as they reviewed and commented on specific actions they had taken after the patient encounter.[38] Reflection-in-action has been less commonly noted in novice clinicians and students.[48,49] The students who exhibited greater use of reflection demonstrated greater flexibility in their progress through the case and were able to adapt their tests and measures to the unfolding situation.[47,48] The students who demonstrated reflection-in-action demonstrated a greater ability to adapt their examination and evaluation process to the unfolding findings,[38] suggesting greater development toward the type of practice evident in experienced clinicians.[25]

SIGNIFICANCE AND IMPLICATIONS FOR EDUCATION

This chapter has described the patterns of CR demonstrated by entry-level DPT students across 2 different programs and stages of their education. The DPT students in the second and third years of their education demonstrated characteristics of CR specific to physical therapist practice. At each stage, however, students demonstrated qualitatively different approaches to the patient. The following section describes the implications of these qualitative differences and proposes the importance of the use of models of CR and guidance for reflection in entry-level physical therapist education to support students' development of CR.

DIFFERENT MODELS OF PRACTICE

The qualitative differences in the students' approaches to CR suggest they are working from different models of practice.[50] Specifically, some students focused primarily on biomechanical and pathoanatomical factors indicative of a biomedical perspective on practice.[41,42] Other students prioritized patient education and focused on factors that impacted the patient's level of participation, suggesting they were working from a biopsychosocial model.[41,42] Physical therapist students have also demonstrated qualitatively different understandings of the purpose of physical therapist practice.[51] Research in dental education indicates that course ordering, methods of assessment, and models of practice all communicate values to the students and can influence their understandings of practice.[52] Educational program factors that support students in developing a biopsychosocial view alongside the skills to act on that model may enhance students' development of patient-centered CR.

For example, the integration of reflective activities within a community of practice can support students in developing a patient-centered view of practice and the skills to engage in patient-centered care.[53] Opportunities to develop conversational routines compatible with patient-centered reasoning may further support students in developing the types of verbal interactions they need to effectively engage patients in their care.[54-56] The nature of models of CR demonstrated within an educational program can influence students' perspectives and practices.[57] The use of a patient-centered CR model (such as the Edwards and Jones model[2]) that integrates narrative reasoning can provide students with a scaffolding that guides their development toward patient-centered reasoning.

USE OF A CONSISTENT MODEL OF CLINICAL REASONING IN EDUCATION

The use of a consistent model of CR throughout an educational program can provide students with scaffolding for their early development of CR. The use of scaffolding (ie, providing supports to students as they develop complex understandings) has been well established in the learning sciences.[58] Scaffolding supports the learner in accomplishing tasks that would otherwise be out of reach at that student's level of conceptual development.[59] Effective use of a model of CR as a scaffold to student learning can guide the students not only in developing a framework to structure their CR processes but also in learning from their experiences with reasoning.[59] The use of a consistent model of reasoning across content areas can also promote students' integration of varied content areas and may enhance knowledge transfer to clinical situations.[60,61] As a source of scaffolding, models of reasoning and protocols can guide students in developing their foundation for more flexible reasoning processes.

IMPORTANCE OF REFLECTION

At all stages of education, reflection is a critical skill for CR. Both reflection-in-action and reflection-on-action are crucial for the development of effective CR. Reflection on specific action (ie, reviewing one's actions and the consequences of those actions after a patient encounter) can support students' and clinicians' development of reasoning and metacognitive strategies.[62,63] Engagement in reflection-on-action enables students to learn from their CE, as educational researchers have indicated that students do not learn from experience alone, but through the act of reflecting on those experiences.[64] The intuitive flow of CR in experienced clinicians depends on their application of knowledge through moment-to-moment decisions that are often not directly expressed.[47] Ongoing reflection on experience can support students in the development of illness and incidence scripts for pattern recognition in reasoning.[65,66] While students must engage in reflection-on-action as they develop their CR abilities, they must also have guidance in reflection-in-action, such that they can question and revise their reasoning processes and change course, if needed.[47] Clinical instructors can play a key role in students' development of CR by allowing students appropriate amounts of freedom in their CE to try out their reasoning processes and receive coaching instead of direct instruction.[67] We will examine this more closely in CE in Section III, Chapter 28, practice exemplars.

DPT students demonstrate a trajectory of learning and development in their engagement in CR. Learning trajectories are broad, nonlinear pathways of progressively more sophisticated ways of thinking.[68] Learning trajectories are inextricably intertwined with the curricular tasks that promote students' learning.[69] Students' individual characteristics, such as their superficial or deep orientation to learning, also impact their learning trajectories within a given curriculum.[70] The varied stages of the students' engagement in CR point to the impacts of both their personal factors and curricular opportunities (such as CE) for development of CR. Critical components of these learning trajectories are students' opportunities to engage in activities, reflect on those activities, and compare their new experiences to their existing conceptual understanding.[71] The cyclical nature of reasoning, reflection, and goal modification in the revised model of CR highlights this crucial aspect of learning for professional practice.

CONCLUSION

The development of CR in DPT students entails interactions of students' personal background, prior experiences, and curricular factors. Students in the second and third years of their entry-level DPT education demonstrate characteristics of physical therapist–specific CR. At all stages of their education, however, students demonstrate qualitative differences in their approach to the patient encounter, suggestive of different models of practice.

Entry-level DPT physical therapist education should prepare new clinicians for the demands of practice they will face.[72] To best prepare physical therapist students, entry-level programs should work to integrate models of CR and practices in reflection to support students' development of physical therapist–specific patient-centered CR.

Reflection Moment

Consider the specific CR errors (see Figure 9-3) discussed in this chapter, and discuss how you will address each to avoid in your learning, teaching, and practice.

Discuss how you have learned from your CR errors or near errors, or those of others.

What models or frameworks do you find helpful for your CR?

REFERENCES

1. Edwards I, Jones M, Carr J, Braunack-Mayer A, Jensen GM. Clinical reasoning strategies in physical therapy. *Phys Ther.* 2004;84(4):312-330; discussion 331-315.
2. Edwards I, Jones M. Clinical reasoning and expert practice. In: Jensen GM, Gwyer J, Hack LM, Shepard KF, eds. *Expertise in Physical Therapy Practice.* 2nd ed. Boston, MA: Elsevier; 2007:192-213.
3. Barrows HS, Feltovich PJ. The clinical reasoning process. *Med Educ.* 1987;21(2):86-91.
4. Bowen JL. Educational strategies to promote clinical diagnostic reasoning. *N Engl J Med.* 2006;355(21):2217-2225.
5. Elstein AS. Thinking about diagnostic thinking: a 30-year perspective. *Adv Health Sci Educ.* 2009;14(1 suppl):7-18.
6. Jones MA. Clinical reasoning in manual therapy. *Phys Ther.* 1992;72(12):875-884.
7. Elstein AS, Shulman LS, Sprafka SA. *Medical Problem Solving: An Analysis of Clinical Reasoning.* Cambridge, MA: Harvard University Press; 1978.
8. Bordage G, Grant J, Marsden P. Quantitative assessment of diagnostic ability. *Med Educ.* 1990;24(5):413-425.
9. Patel VL, Groen GJ. Knowledge based solution strategies in medical reasoning. *Cogn Sci.* 1986;10:91-116.
10. Norman G. Research in clinical reasoning: past history and current trends. *Med Educ.* 2005;39(4):418-427.
11. Coderre S, Jenkins D, McLaughlin K. Qualitative differences in knowledge structure are associated with diagnostic performance in medical students. *Adv Health Sci Educ Theory Pract.* 2009;14(5):677-684.
12. Patel VL, Groen GJ. Developmental accounts of the transition from medical student to doctor: some problems and suggestions. *Med Educ.* 1991;25(6):527-535.
13. Rothstein JM, Echternach JL, Riddle DL. The hypothesis-oriented algorithm for clinicians II (HOAC II): a guide for patient management. *Phys Ther.* 2003;83(5):455-470.
14. Jette AM. Diagnosis and classification by physical therapists: a special communication. *Phys Ther.* 1989;69(11):967-969.
15. Christensen N, Black L, Jensen GM. Physiotherapy clinical placements and learning to reason. In: Higgs J, Sheehan D, Baldry Currens J, Letts W, Jensen GM, eds. *Realising Exemplary Practice-Based Education.* Rotterdam, Netherlands: Sense Publishers; 2013:135-142.
16. Jensen GM, Gwyer J, Shepard KF, Hack LM. Expert practice in physical therapy. *Phys Ther.* 2000;80(1):28-43; discussion 44-52.
17. Embrey DG, Guthrie MR, White OR, Dietz J. Clinical decision making by experienced and inexperienced pediatric physical therapists for children with diplegic cerebral palsy. *Phys Ther.* 1996;76(1):20-33.
18. Riolo L. Skill differences in novice and expert clinicians in neurologic physical therapy. *Neurology Report.* 1996;20(1):60-63.
19. Wainwright SF, McGinnis PQ. Factors that influence the clinical decision-making of rehabilitation professionals in long-term care settings. *J Allied Health.* 2009;38(3):143-151.
20. McGinnis PQ, Hack LM, Nixon-Cave K, Michlovitz SL. Factors that influence the clinical decision making of physical therapists in choosing a balance assessment approach. *Phys Ther.* 2009;89(3):233-247.
21. May S, Greasley A, Reeve S, Withers S. Expert therapists use specific clinical reasoning processes in the assessment and management of patients with shoulder pain: a qualitative study. *Aust J Physiother.* 2008;54(4):261-266.
22. Mattingly C. What is clinical reasoning. *Am J Occup Ther.* 1991;45(11):979-986.
23. Jensen GM. Learning what matters most. 2011 McMillan Lecture. *Phys Ther.* 2011;91(11):1674-1689.
24. Jensen GM, Shepard KF, Hack LM. The novice versus the experienced clinician: insights into the work of the physical therapist. *Phys Ther.* 1990;70(5):314-323.
25. Jensen GM, Shepard KF, Gwyer J, Hack LM. Attribute dimensions that distinguish master and novice physical therapy clinicians in orthopedic settings. *Phys Ther.* 1992;72(10):711-722.
26. Black LL, Jensen GM, Mostrom E, et al. The first year of practice: an investigation of the professional learning and development of promising novice physical therapists. *Phys Ther.* 2010;90(12):1758-1773.
27. Hayward LM, Black LL, Mostrom E, et al. The first two years of practice: a longitudinal perspective on the learning and professional development of promising novice physical therapists. *Phys Ther.* 2013;93(3):369-383.
28. Holdar U, Wallin L, Heiwe S. Why do we do as we do? Factors influencing clinical reasoning and decision-making among physiotherapists in an acute setting. *Physiother Res Int.* 2013;18(4):220-229.
29. Rothstein JM, Echternach JL. Hypothesis-oriented algorithm for clinicians. A method for evaluation and treatment planning. *Phys Ther.* 1986;66(9):1388-1394.
30. Yeung E, Woods N, Dubrowski A, Hodges B, Carnahan H. Establishing assessment criteria for clinical reasoning in orthopedic manual physical therapy: a consensus-building study. *J Man Manip Ther.* 2015;23(1):27-36.
31. Smart K, Doody C. The clinical reasoning of pain by experienced musculoskeletal physiotherapists. *Man Ther.* 2007;12(1):40-49.
32. Jones MA, Jensen GM, Edwards I. Clinical reasoning in physiotherapy. In: Higgs J, Jones MA, Loftus S, Christensen N, eds. *Clinical Reasoning in the Health Professions.* 3rd ed. Amsterdam, Netherlands: Butterworth-Heinemann Elsevier; 2008:245-256.
33. Fernbach PM, Darlow A, Sloman SA. Neglect of alternative causes in predictive but not diagnostic reasoning. *Psycho Sci.* 2010;21(3):329-336.
34. Wilcox G, Schroeder M. What comes before report writing? Attending to CR and thinking errors in school psychology. *J Psychoeduc Assess.* 2015;33(7):652-661.
35. Croskerry P. The importance of cognitive errors in diagnosis and strategies to minimize them. *Acad Med.* 2003;78(8):775-780.
36. Doody C, McAteer M. Clinical reasoning of expert and novice physiotherapists in an outpatient orthopaedic setting. *Physiotherapy.* 2002;88(5):258-268.
37. Gilliland SJ. Clinical reasoning in first- and third-year physical therapist students. *J Phys Ther Educ.* 2014;28(3):64-80.

38. Gilliland SJ. Believing, thinking, and doing: Physical therapist students' CR and conceptualizations of practice [Dissertation]. Irvine, CA: School of Education, University of California, Irvine; 2015.

39. Gilliland SJ. Physical therapist students' development of diagnostic reasoning: a longitudinal study. *J Phys Ther Educ.* 2017;31(1):31-48.

40. Furze J, Black L, Hoffman J, Barr J, Cochran TM, Jensen GM. Exploration of students' clinical reasoning development in professional physical therapy education. *J Phys Ther Educ.* 2015;29(3):22-33.

41. Daykin AR, Richardson B. Physiotherapists' pain beliefs and their influence on the management of patients with chronic low back pain. *Spine (Phila Pa 1976).* 2004;29(7):783-795.

42. Stenmar L, Nordholm LA. Swedish physical therapists' beliefs on what makes therapy work. *Phys Ther.* 1994;74(11):1034-1039.

43. Audetat MC, Laurin S, Sanche G, et al. Clinical reasoning difficulties: a taxonomy for clinical teachers. *Med Teach.* 2013;35(3):e984-e989.

44. Livingston C, Borko H. Expert-novice differences in teaching: a cognitive analysis and implications for teacher education. *J Teach Educ.* 1989;40:36-42.

45. Rowan B. Comparing teachers' work with work in other occupations: notes on the professional status of teaching. *Educ Researcher.* 1994;23(6):4-21.

46. Delany C, Golding C. Teaching clinical reasoning by making thinking visible: an action research project with allied health clinical educators. *BMC Med Educ.* 2014;14:20.

47. Schön DA. *The Reflective Practitioner: How Professionals Think in Action.* New York, NY: Basic Books, Inc; 1983.

48. Wainwright SF, Shepard KF, Harman LB, Stephens J. Novice and experienced physical therapist clinicians: a comparison of how reflection is used to inform the clinical decision-making process. *Phys Ther.* 2010;90(1):75-88.

49. Burbach B, Barnason S, Thompson SA. Using "think aloud" to capture clinical reasoning during patient simulation. *Int J Nurs Educ Scholarsh.* 2015;12(1):1-7.

50. Dall'alba G. Understanding medical practice: different outcomes of a pre-medical program. *Adv Health Sci Educ Theory Pract.* 2002;7(3):163-177.

51. Gilliland SJ, Wainwright SF. Physical therapist students' conceptualizations of practice. *J Phys Ther Educ.* In press.

52. Kieser JA, Dall'alba G, Livingstone V. Impact of curriculum on understanding of professional practice: a longitudinal study of students commencing dental education. *Adv Health Sci Educ Theory Pract.* 2009;14(3):303-314.

53. Hayward LM, Li L. Promoting and assessing cultural competence, professional identity, and advocacy in doctor of physical therapy (DPT) degree students within a community of practice. *J Phys Ther Educ.* 2014;28(1):23-36.

54. Ball DL, Forzani FM. The work of teaching and the challenge of teacher education. *J Teach Educ.* 2009;60:497-511.

55. Lampert M, Beasley H, Ghousseini H, Kazemi E, Franke M. Using designed instructional activities to enable novices to manage ambitious mathematics teaching. In: Stein MK, Kucan L, eds. *Instructional Explanations in the Disciplines.* New York, NY: Springer; 2010:129-141.

56. Holmstrom I, Rosenqvist U. A change of the physicians' understanding of the encounter parallels competence development. *Patient Educ Couns.* 2001;42(3):271-278.

57. Darrah J, Loomis J, Manns P, Norton B, May L. Role of conceptual models in a physical therapy curriculum: application of an integrated model of theory, research and clinical practice. *Physiother Theory Pract.* 2006;22:239-250.

58. Collins A. Cognitive apprenticeship. In: Sawyer RK, ed. *The Cambridge Handbook of Learning Science.* New York, NY: Cambridge University Press; 2006:47-60.

59. Reiser BT. Scaffolding complex learning: the mechanisms of structuring and problematizing student work. *J Learn Sci.* 2004;13(3):273-304.

60. Higgs J. A programme for developing clinical reasoning skills. *Med Teach.* 1993;15(2/3):195.

61. Neistadt ME. Teaching strategies for the development of clinical reasoning. *Am J Occup Ther.* 1996;50(8):676-684.

62. Kuiper R. Self-regulated learning during a clinical preceptorship: the reflections of senior baccalaureate nursing students. *Nurs Educ Perspect.* 2005;26(6):351-356.

63. Jensen GM, Paschal KA. Habits of mind: student transition toward virtuous practice. *J Phys Ther Educ.* 2000;14(3):42-47.

64. Shulman LS. The wisdom of practice: managing complexity in medicine and teaching. In: Shulman LS, Wilson SM, eds. *The Wisdom of Practice: Essays on Teaching, Learning, and Learning to Teach.* San Francisco, CA: Jossey-Bass; 2004:251-271.

65. Schmidt HG, Norman G, Boshuizen HP. A cognitive perspective on medical expertise: theory and implication. *Acad Med.* 1990;65(10):611-621.

66. Mandin H, Jones A, Woloschuk W, Harasym P. Helping students learn to think like experts when solving clinical problems. *Acad Med.* 1997;72(3):173-179.

67. Schön DA. *Educating the Reflective Practitioner.* San Francisco, CA: Jossey-Bass; 1987.

68. Clements DH, Sarama J. *Learning and Teaching Early Math: The Learning Trajectories Approach.* New York, NY: Routledge; 2009.

69. Empson SB. On the idea of learning trajectories: promises and pitfalls. *The Mathematics Enthusiast.* 2011;8(3):Article 6.

70. Spiers JA, Williams B, Gibson B, et al. Graduate nurses' learning trajectories and experiences of problem based learning: a focused ethnography study. *Int J Nurs Stud.* 2014;51(11):1462-1471.

71. Simon MA, Tzur R. Explicating the role of mathematical tasks in conceptual learning: an elaboration of the hypothetical learning trajectory. *Mathematical Thinking and Learning.* 2004;6(2):91-104.

72. Wojciechowski M. The future of physical therapist education. *PT in Motion.* 2015;7(1):15-26.

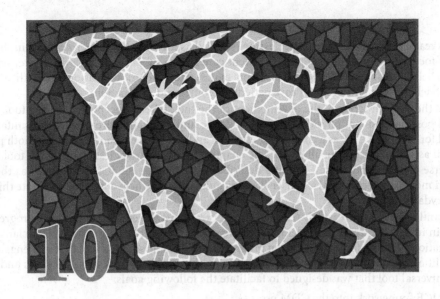

10

THE CLINICAL REASONING AND REFLECTION TOOL:
Clinical Application for Clinical Decision-Making

Kim Nixon-Cave, PT, PhD, PCS, FAPTA and Heather Atkinson, PT, DPT, NCS

OBJECTIVES

- Analyze the development and implementation of the Clinical Reasoning and Reflection Tool (CRT).
- Interpret the CRT for clinical reasoning (CR) and reflection in the clinical decision-making (CDM) process.
- Integrate the *International Classification of Functioning, Disability and Health* (ICF) framework into the CDM process at various levels of clinical practice.
- Apply the CRT for clinical reflection for clinicians of all abilities and levels of clinical experience to advance CR.
- Describe how the CRT facilitates critical inquiry and professional development among mentors and mentees.

INTRODUCTION

CDM and the ability for physical therapists to use CR skills to provide high-value care and services to patients are essential aspects of professional development and the practice of physical therapy. As the physical therapy profession continues to evolve in autonomous practice along with recent changes in health care, physical therapists must provide high value and efficient quality care. As the profession embraces the new American Physical Therapy Association (APTA) vision of "Transforming society by optimizing movement to improve the human experience," more emphasis is being placed on the development of advanced CDM and CR skills.

Musolino GM, Jensen GM, eds. *Clinical Reasoning and Decision-Making in
Physical Therapy: Facilitation, Assessment, and Implementation* (pp 111-132).

Over the last several years, the physical therapy profession—as well as most health care professions in the United States—has adopted a more patient-focused framework to approach patient care and to support CDM. This chapter will describe the CRT, which was developed to help clinicians, students, and residents make effective clinical decisions using the ICF and patient/client management (PCM) model as a foundation to improve patient outcomes and satisfaction.

This chapter reviews the CRT, in terms of the development of the tool, CDM concepts within the tool, and ways the tool is being used in pre- and post-professional physical therapy academic and clinical environments to facilitate clinical decisions. Strategies are presented for using the CRT as a conduit for effective and practical decision-making in both pre- and post-professional education, as well as with clinicians of all levels. The chapter discusses strategies for using the tool from a shared CDM perspective with a diverse patient population. Examples describe how to merge the ICF framework, as the foundation for the CRT, into existing CDM models, as a universal and user-friendly guide that may help clinicians integrate this new way of critical thinking (CT) into everyday practice.

Although reflection and mentorship are widely regarded as important instruments to facilitate the progression of CR and may further help clinicians in integrating the ICF model into practice, little structure exists to assist clinicians with these essential needs. As more organizations develop formal mentoring programs, the need arises for a tool that will engage mentors, protégés, and clinicians of all abilities in thoughtful reflection and discussion that will help to develop CR skills and realize the vision of APTA. The CRT is a universal tool that was designed to facilitate the following goals:

- To integrate the ICF framework into the CDM process
- To provide a worksheet for clinical reflection for clinicians of all abilities
- To propose discussion points for mentors or colleagues to facilitate critical inquiry and professional development
- To help clinicians identify important clinical questions that could add to the body of evidence
- To facilitate the provision of high-quality patient care

BACKGROUND

As physical therapy evolves as a profession and strives to meet the needs of a changing health care landscape, excellence in CDM skills is paramount for success. CDM is a key foundation to the APTA vision statement ("Transforming society by optimizing movement to improve the human experience") and relates directly to the guiding principles of identity, quality, collaboration, value, innovation, and consumer-centricity.[1] Greater emphasis is placed on quality, value, and patient outcomes, and it is critical to educate both students and post-professionals in ongoing and lifelong advancement of CR and reflective practice (RP).

Strategies to Advance Clinical Reasoning

Multiple avenues exist for physical therapists to advance their CR skills and improve their RP. One effective method is to participate in a credentialed residency or fellowship program, which provides structured mentoring as well as a deliberate focus on CR advancement to achieve measurable goals and objectives.[2] The CRT was developed to support CR in a residency program, but has been found useful in many practice settings.

The Reflective Practitioner

RP is a cornerstone for professional development. Although clinical reflection methods and associated CR strategies have been widely studied, little existed in the way of a user-friendly guide to probe reflection and reasoning for patient situations, and this ultimately drove the need for the development of the CRT. In real-world clinical environments, clinicians move among reflection and reasoning styles in nonlinear and dynamic ways.[3,4] As novice clinicians enrich their repertoire from reflection-on-action and hypothetico-deductive reasoning to reflection-in-action and forward reasoning, it is important to engage in deliberate reflection, facilitated by a skilled mentor if possible, to minimize error and develop expertise.[5]

Tools and Models to Advance Clinical Reasoning and Reflection

A variety of models and algorithms have been published to organize and guide CR into optimal CDM.[4] These models may be used in pre-professional education, in residencies and fellowships, or by practicing physical therapists looking to improve personal CR or reason through a challenging problem. While planning for the development of a residency program in a large academic health care setting, it became clear that it would be helpful to integrate some of the most often used CR models into the curriculum for the residency as well as the practice setting, and to supplement that with deliberate thought-provoking questions designed to advance the resident's CR and reflection skills.

DEVELOPMENT

CDM applies the cognitive thoughts, or evaluation, about a patient after completing a systematic process of examination that results in action. It incorporates CT and clinical problem-solving (CPS) to make effective decisions about patient management that considers the patient's individual circumstances and environment.[6] The CRT was developed to facilitate the CDM, CR, and reflective skills—initially of physical therapist residents, and subsequently of doctor of physical therapy (DPT) students and physical therapist clinicians—to make effective and appropriate decisions for patients/clients.[7] The foundation of the tool was based on established CDM models, such as the Hypothesis-Oriented Algorithm for Clinicians (HOAC), and classification schemes, such as the PCM model in the effort to improve patient outcomes and satisfaction. The tool is a concept map showing the relationships between the ICF classification system and the APTA *Guide to Physical Therapist Practice* PCM model, and incorporates the reflective model of clinical practice. The tool also serves as a graphical conduit for organizing and representing CDM and CR based on clinical knowledge and clinical reflection.

The main goal in developing the CRT was to facilitate CDM by applying a cognitive thought process incorporating CT and CPS while considering the patient's individual environment and circumstances. The tool includes and facilitates the ability to reason through complex multifaceted clinical decisions, which often require nonlinear goal-directed CR, while incorporating CT and CPS. Both CDM and CR require that the thought process include the influence of the patient factors, clinical and nonclinical, and the environment. Clinical factors that must be considered are the ones that clinicians typically consider, such as the patient's health condition, clinician's knowledge and skill, and practice setting. Nonclinical factors include the patient's cultural beliefs, values and traditions, religious beliefs, socioeconomic status, health behavior, and family and caregivers. The CRT attempts to address the contextual dependent nature of CDM, which directly impacts the CR of the therapist. The CRT considers the nature of the clinical decision, attributes, the decision-maker, and environment of where the decision takes place.[8]

PURPOSE

The CRT (Figure 10-1) is designed to advance the CR and CDM skills of clinicians of all abilities by synthesizing CDM models into a user-friendly guide intended to probe RP and collaborative discourse. Key features include:

- The CRT moves the clinician from a basic CDM and systematic reasoning approach, such as the HOAC deductive approach, to a more advanced CR approach of inductive reasoning, such as forward reasoning, equating more to the advanced reasoning strategy employed by progressive clinicians and experts.

- The CRT promotes the use of evidence-based practice in terms of critical inquiry and emphasizes the use of evidence and theory to support CDM and CR.

- The CRT facilitates reflection-in-practice with the use of reflective questions and points as a core component. The reflective component of the tool can be used as a personal reflection tool or in mentoring and supervising situations.

COMPONENTS

The components of CRT (see Figure 10-1) include the PCM model from the APTA *Guide to Physical Therapist Practice*, which allows for an ongoing, iterative process for physical therapist CDM and reasoning while managing a patient/client.[9] The CRT allows for collaborative and reflective reasoning and seeks to integrate the ICF framework into the PCM model while incorporating the hypothesis-driven basis of CDM models. The tool was designed to develop forward reasoning and reflective decision-making for pre- and post-professionals, specifically in residency programs. The tool is applicable to other health care practitioners. Its design aims to probe reflection and discussion for both the novice and master clinician, and may be used as a mentoring tool for specific patient cases. The CRT incorporates Schön's model of RP and seeks to develop the skill of reflection—including reflection-for-action, reflection-in-action, and reflection-on-action—in physical therapists at all levels.[7,10]

In the PCM model, clinicians are offered an overall concept map for practice in any setting or with any population. Using the PCM model enables the individual to develop knowledge and reasoning skills while considering all patient factors that may impact the plan of care. The 6 essential components of the *Guide to Physical Therapist Practice* PCM—examination, evaluation, diagnosis, prognosis, intervention, and outcomes—are the foundation of the CRT, and all assist in the CDM and CR about the care of patients/clients.[9]

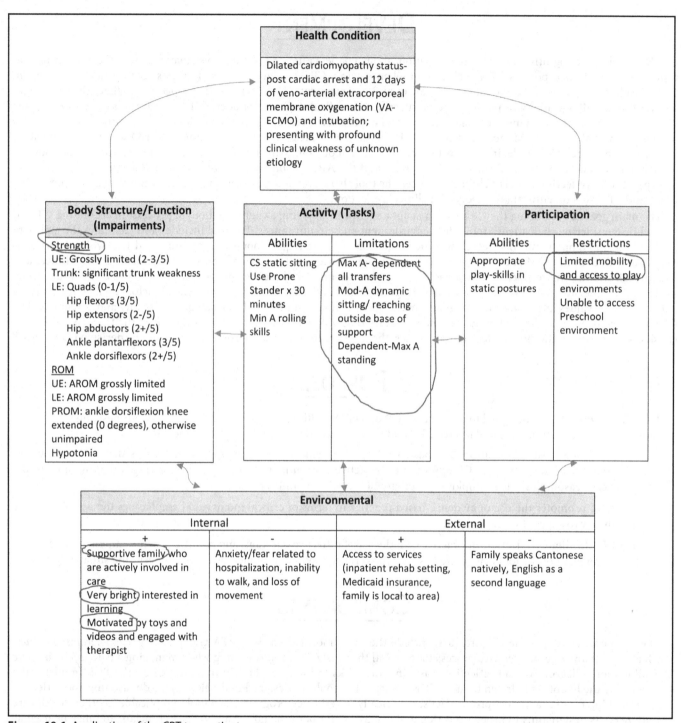

Figure 10-1. Application of the CRT to a patient case.

CRT Reflection Points:
Initial Data Gathering/Interview

History and present function:

4 year old boy with a history of dilated cardiomyopathy presented with hypoglycemia. He arrived at the emergency department with fatigue and decreased appetite and was admitted in severe heart failure. He had a cardiac arrest requiring multiple rounds of chest compressions and epinephrine to return to normal sinus rhythm. He was canulated for veno-arterial extracorporeal membrane oxygenation (VA-ECMO) and intubated x 12 days. He was extubated, decanulated and then weaned off inotropic support. He developed hypoactive delirium and a head CT showed cerebral atrophy which did not correlate with clinical presentation of profound weakness. Medical diagnostic work-up is ongoing; etiology unclear but presumed to be due to metabolic disorder. He was admitted to inpatient rehab for comprehensive therapies and further testing was decided to be postponed due to his significant UE and LE weakness with limited active movement and need for rehab.

Reflection Points:

➢ **Assess how the patient's medical diagnosis affects your interview.** Unfortunately, patient's Mom did not attend the initial evaluation due to his increased behaviors when she is present. History was obtained through chart review

➢ **What is the value of the data you gathered?** Understanding that future diagnostic tests will be completed but have not occurred yet may provide a challenge for PT treatment. It is unclear what his diagnosis and prognosis are at this time and if his strength is likely to return.

➢ **Have you verified the patient's goals and what resources are available?** Patient talked about playing with different toys and was engaged in activities. His family live locally which may allow possible day-hospital and/or outpatient therapy to be feasible for the family. He lives in a two story house with bedroom and bathroom on second floor with mother, father, and 2 siblings. At this time, he is small and able to be carried, however in the future the family may need to consider housing modifications.

➢ **What is your assessment of the patient's/caregiver's knowledge and understanding of their diagnosis and need for PT?** It is unclear how much patient's Mom understands about his diagnosis and his potential for return of strength and functional motor skills. This may need to be addressed at team planning meetings in the future to set realistic expectations while leaving room for hope with his unknown medical diagnosis and prognosis at this time. Patient did say "I can't stand" and "I can't walk" which indicates that he has some level of understanding about his current functional ability.

Generation of Initial Hypothesis

a. Body structures/functions: See ICF model above
b. Impairments
c. Activity limitations
d. Participation restrictions

Reflection Points:

➢ **Can you construct a hypothesis based on the information gathered?** Because he does not have a medical diagnosis, his prognosis for strength return is unclear. Based on his current impairments, he will require a wheelchair for ambulation and a stander for weight bearing. If his strength returns during inpatient rehab, he may need orthotics and/or an assistive device to improve his safety and independence.

➢ **What do you anticipate could be an outcome for this patient?** I anticipate that he will have some strength gains, however it is unclear if he will be able to functionally ambulate. He may require bracing to provide LE support, however the weight of the bracing may also be a limiting factor in his functional independence. He may need a wheelchair, and training to be able to propel it with assistance for steep inclines and curbs. He may have other equipment needs, such as a stander or gait trainer to encourage weight bearing and strengthening in a supported way.

➢ **What is your approach/planned sequence/strategy for the examination?** Initially I want to observe his movements, passive and active ROM in gravity eliminated and against gravity positions. I want to observe his seated posture, seated balance statically and dynamically, monitor his vital signs and any signs of fatigue. I want to see what he looks like with assisted weight-bearing, and observe him in prone, supine, and side-lying, ring-sitting and short-sitting positions. I would like to do an outcome measure, but I need more information about his current abilities before choosing the most appropriate measure to assess his functional skills.

Figure 10-1 continued. Application of the CRT to a patient case.

Examination

---

a. Tests and measures

Reflection Points:

➢ **Appraising the tests and measures you selected for your examination, how and why did you select them?** I completed AROM, PROM, strength testing, observation in functional positions (prone, supine, side-lying, supported standing, ring sit, short sit), bed mobility, seated balance, standing balance. The Weefim is used for all patients admitted to inpatient rehab. At the time of the initial examination, I did not complete an outcome measure, however as I continued to re-assess the patient, I chose to complete the Expanded Hammersmith Functional Motor Scale for SMA (HFMSE) and Gross Motor Function Measure (GMFM). These measures were chosen because both evaluate the patient in a variety of functional positions and had potential to capture his current skill level and his progress over time. Other standardized assessments that would have been appropriate based on his age, were not chosen because he would be unable to complete a majority of the tasks (PDMS-2) and therefore the test would not be a good measure of his functional skills.

➢ **Can the identified tests and measures help you determine a change in status? Are they able to detect a minimum clinically important difference?** There are no identified minimum clinically important differences for the HFMSE or for his specific diagnosis on the GMFM. However, both assessments include functional skills and positions, therefore any changes on either measure would be indicative of improved function.

➢ **How does your selection of tests and measures relate to the patient's goals?** His Mom would like him to be back to his baseline of level of activity which includes walking, jumping, playing with friends. At his baseline, he has age-appropriate gross motor skills as per his Mom's report. The outcome measures that I selected will be able to track his changes over time (GMFM and HFMSE) however they will not assess higher level gross motor skills (jumping, running) or higher level balance activities. As he progresses, we can complete additional outcome measures (PDMS-2, Bayley) that assess age-appropriate gross motor skills.

Evaluation

Diagnosis: Decreased strength of core and LE, Limited ROM, impaired static and dynamic balance, impaired tone, impaired posture, decreased endurance

Prognosis: Fair, unclear of potential for strength and mobility recovery

Reflection Points:

➢ **What factors might support or interfere with the patient's prognosis?** The possible underlying metabolic disease may interfere with his ability to gain strength. He also may have an underlying myopathy or neuropathy that could be interfering with his potential for strengthening and therefore weight bearing and ambulation. He does have significant cardiac impairments including cardiomyopathy with an ejection fraction of 48% which leads to earlier fatigue and decreased endurance. His motivation to move, his intelligence, and his playfulness are all positive factors that will influence his participation in therapies.

➢ **What is your rationale for prognosis, and what are the positive and negative prognostic indicators?** His prognosis is guarded, I feel there is potential to make strength gains and improve function, however it is unclear if he will plateau at a certain point. Positive prognostic indicators include his participation in therapies, if he is able to increase endurance, if he can tolerate using his stander in the evenings to increase standing tolerance and achieve weight-bearing through LE, maintaining full ankle ROM and increasing strength throughout his UE, trunk, and LE. Negative prognostic indicators would be any significant decrease in function or movement, behaviors, LE or neuropathic pain.

➢ **How might any cultural factors influence your care of the patient?** He is Asian, Mom and Dad speak Cantonese as primary language and English as a second language. They decline interpreters, however, sometimes it seems that Mom may have trouble understanding the rehab team.

➢ **What are your considerations for behavior, motivation, and readiness?** At his initial evaluation, he was very willing to play and did not exhibit any avoidance behaviors. However, during the course of his therapies, when he becomes frustrated or perceives an activity to be challenging, he will become tearful, say "I'm scared", or swat at therapist. Behaviors strategies such as "first, then" or using a picture schedule helped with these behaviors, but it is most effective to distract him with toys and games.

➢ **How can you determine capacity for progress towards goals?** This is a challenge due to the unknown underlying diagnosis. At this time, there is no evidence or testing that says that he can't get better or back to his baseline, and therefore his long-term goals support a full return to age-appropriate functional skills. However, with the significant strength deficits at his initial evaluation, it is reasonable that it may take a long time to achieve those skills. The challenge is to be both optimistic and realistic with his potential for recovery, which is more challenging because of the potential for an unknown underlying diagnosis.

Figure 10-1 continued. Application of the CRT to a patient case.

Plan of Care

a. Identify short and long-term goals

b. Identify outcome measures
   1. Gross Motor Function Measure (GMFM)
   2. Expanded Hammersmith Functional Motor Scale (HFMSE)
   3. WeeFim

c. PT prescription (frequency/intensity of service, include key elements)
   1. 7x/week, 90-120 minutes of therapy per day

Reflection Points:

➢ **How did you determine the PT prescription or plan of care?** Based on his current level of function and the role of inpatient rehab to make daily progress, I chose to provide therapy services 7 days per week for 90-120 minutes on weekdays and 45 minutes on weekends as per the department procedures. The intensity will vary depending on the activity and his level of fatigue. He will also receive OT 90 minutes per day and ST initially 3 times per week then decreased to 2 times per week for 60 minutes.

➢ **How do the patient's personal and environmental factors affect the PT plan of care?** His age and high level of fatigue affects his plan of care. While he would benefit from two 60-minute therapy sessions per day, some days he is tired and a 30 minute afternoon session is preferred. He also naps in the afternoon and falls asleep around 2:00 which limits flexibility in his schedule.

Interventions

a. Describe how you are using evidence to guide your practice
   1. While there is in general limited pediatric intervention research, I am using evidence to support aquatic therapy, FES bike, motor learning strategies, and outcome measures

b. Identify overall approach/strategy
   1. Overall goal is to improve functional mobility which includes participating in strengthening (therapeutic exercise/activities and aquatic therapy) along with participating in gait training with different equipment to optimize his access to environment with the least restrictive assistive device. I try to include standing every day through an evening stander program as well as during therapy to maintain adequate ankle ROM and for the strengthening benefits.

c. Describe and prioritize specific procedural interventions
   1. Strength training
   2. Endurance training
   3. ROM
   4. Gait training
   5. Aquatic therapy
   6. Functional mobility training
   7. Transfer training
   8. Parent Education
   9. DME

d. Describe your plan for progression
   1. My plan is to progress weight bearing activities from static standing to dynamic standing and then to ambulation outside of an assistive device along with strengthening in both open and closed chain positions, progressing through increased ROM and decreasing the level of assistance. The plan for progression of interventions depends on his progress in rehab.

Reflection Points:

➢ **Discuss your overall PT approach or strategies? How will you modify principles for this patient? Are there specific aspects about this particular patient to keep in mind? How does your approach relate to theory and current evidence?** I am focusing on strengthening of LE and core/trunk musculature along with balance, postural control, standing tolerance, and ambulation using equipment/assistive devices as necessary. I am trying to combine part and whole task practice to achieve functional skills such as bed mobility and transfers.

➢ **How might you need to modify your interventions for this particular patient and caregiver?** Because of his cardiac history and limited endurance, I need to monitor strengthening and endurance activities to challenge him enough to achieve the goal of the exercise, but avoid over-exertion that leads to significant fatigue or cardiac stress. I also modify interventions to try to find activities that are most effective and efficient. He seemed to benefit most from aquatic therapy and therefore a large amount of therapeutic time was devoted to aquatics. However, that was balanced by weight-bearing activities on land along with therapeutic exercises on a mat table. The balance of different interventions is changing each week based on his needs and also his behaviors and interests.

➢ **What are the communication needs with other team members?** Communication with the medical team about his LE strength is important because the medical team is considering further diagnostic testing. In addition, I communicate regular with occupational therapy, speech therapy, child life services, and his family. We are able to meet as a team once per week to discuss his plan of care and his potential discharge date and anticipated discharge needs.

Figure 10-1 continued. Application of the CRT to a patient case.

Reexamination

a.   When and how often

Reflection Points:

➤ **Evaluate the effectiveness of your interventions. Do you need to modify anything?** _Gait training:_ Initially, I attempted gait training in the parallel bars with KI and solid temporary aquaplast AFO's, however he was unable to hold onto the bars to stabilize his trunk and was dependent for the trial. I modified the activity to use a rifton pacer gait trainer, using the forearm prompts, trunk prompt and hard seat. He required mod-max A to move the gait trainer forward and would tolerate it for 10-15 minute intervals before becoming frustrated. I also tried the Kidwalk which allows him to use his UE to push the large wheels and take steps with his LE, and he enjoyed ambulation with this device, however his step-pattern was less functional with short step-length and slight seated position on saddle. As he improved with tolerance to gait training in the Kidwalk, I transitioned back to the gait trainer for a more functional gait pattern. I also tried gait training with the body-weight supported treadmill, and he was able to take steps, however the quality of the movement was better in the gait trainer. _Therapeutic exercise:_ During the first 2 weeks of treatment, I was focused primarily on ways to encourage standing and weight bearing and I did not focus enough of therapeutic exercises such as assisted hip bridges, hip abduction/adduction in gravity eliminated positions. I modified my plan of care to include more therapeutic exercises as he began gaining LE strength. _NMES and FES Bike:_ His quad strength continued to be 0-1/5 after 2 weeks of PT and I wanted to see if he was able to a achieve a muscle contraction with the assistance of NMES. Over 3 sessions the intensity of the stim was increased, while he was in a side-lying gravity minimized position and completed 10 minutes of active-assisted knee flexion and extension with NMES. He tolerated the NMES, however there was no strong muscle contraction most likely due to the intensity of the e-stim. On the FES bike, he was able to tolerate the e-stim along with passive pedaling, and when encouraged to use his muscles to pedal the bike, he was able to achieve several revolutions at low power. Due to his age and limited tolerance of the stim, he did not achieve a strong muscle contraction and therefore the FES bike did not seem to be the best use of his time in therapy. _Aquatic Therapy_: When he was approved by the medical team, I initiated aquatic therapy for 60 minutes. He enjoyed playing in the pool and had significantly increased LE movement including palpable quad contraction with knee extension. He was also able to ambulate in the pool with ankle cuff weights and holding onto a flotation barbell with minimal assistance at his trunk. He was initially very fatigued from playing in the pool and therefore tolerated less land therapy, however his endurance improved over a 2-week period and he was able to tolerate 1 hour of land and 1 hour of aquatic therapy most days.

➤ **Is there anything that you overlooked, misinterpreted, overvalued, undervalued, and what might you do differently? Will this address any potential errors you have made?** I initially undervalued mat exercises in favor of focusing on standing and gait-training. However, because of his significant strength deficits, the mat exercises were necessary to work on strengthening in gravity minimized positions.

➤ **How do the characteristics of the patient's progress affect your goals, prognosis, and anticipated outcome?** Although his progress is slow, he is continuing to make steady gains in strength and mobility. However, it is unclear if there will be a time when his strength gains plateau, potentially due to an underlying myopathy or neuropathy that has not been diagnosed. I modified his goals at his re-evaluation due to his limited progress. While his initial goals were appropriate, they were not sensitive enough to show his daily progress.

Outcomes

a.   Discharge plan (include follow-up, equipment, school/work/community re-entry, etc.)

Reflection Points:

➤ **Was PT effective, and what outcome measures did you use to assess the outcome? Why or why not?**

➤ **What barriers (physical, personal, environmental) if any, are there to discharge?** There are physical and environmental barriers to discharge. It is anticipated that he will need a wheelchair for community level ambulation, and his family lives in a 2 story home with stairs to enter. While he is small at this time and can be carried, he will continue to grow and Mom may be unable to carry him in the future. Similarly, at this time he has adequate trunk control to sit in a vehicle with a standard seatbelt, however for community outings, his family will need to bring a wheelchair and complete a car transfer. His Mom and Dad both speak English as a second language (Cantonese is their primary language) and therefore there may be a language barrier when planning his discharge (although family declines interpreter whenever offered). He will benefit from continued services both through the IU and outpatient. The family lives locally, which may make the transition to outpatient more smooth. He also has expressed that he loves being in rehab and playing here, and does not want to go home, which may be challenging for the family during the transition process.

Figure 10-1 continued. Application of the CRT to a patient case.

Examination

The examination component focuses on the history and review of the systems to enable the physical therapist to gather information about the patient. From a CR perspective, forward reasoning, or pattern recognition, can be used to identify salient subjective information, which expert practitioners use to recognize patterns and formulate hypotheses.[5,7,11,12] In a qualitative research report examining CDM for balance assessment, McGinnis and colleagues suggest that a nonlinear thought process is involved in selecting specific tests and measures.[3] The authors describe 3 stages of CR for balance assessment CDM, including initial impressions and movement observation, data gathering, and diagnosis and treatment planning.[3] The therapists involved in the study frequently looked ahead to their possible diagnoses and treatment plans when selecting tests and measures during the examination, indicating a nonlinear thought process.[3]

Clinicians may also use backward reasoning, or hypothesis-guided inquiry, which facilitates the process of systematically negating or supporting generated hypotheses,[3,7,12] and is a key ingredient in differential diagnoses. The CRT also incorporates concepts relating to the HOAC II, which provides clinicians and students with a framework for science-based clinical practice.[13] It focuses on the remediation of functional deficits and how changes in impairments relate to these deficits.[13]

Evaluation

At the evaluation stage, the clinician synthesizes the subjective and objective information, and considers all the clinical and nonclinical factors that may help identify impairments, limitations, and restrictions. The CRT uses the ICF classification model to illustrate and classify the patient's problems and to generate a diagnosis or diagnoses, prognosis, and plan of care. During this component, the clinician prioritizes patient problems and links them to the ICF framework, which is essential in determining whether and how physical therapy may benefit the patient. This process is challenging for novice clinicians and difficult to teach. By writing thoughts down on paper in a flow chart or conceptual map, therapists can organize information, identify priority problems that are keeping the patient from reaching his or her goals, and start to highlight which problem areas should be the focus for the intervention plan.[7,12,13]

Intervention

Prioritization and progression of procedural interventions are an integral component of a systematic CR process.[7,9,12] CDM skills are a key ingredient to competent appraisal of the available evidence and subsequently selection of the most appropriate treatment. This complex, multifaceted ability includes the asking of a specific and clinically relevant question, an accurate and effective search of the available literature, the interpretation of the strength and relevance of the findings, and ultimately the translation of the evaluation of the literature into practice and specific clinical situations. While scientific evidence is emphasized in guiding decisions, clinicians must also make decisions when receiving advice from colleagues, being guided by mentors, or relying on experience.

Outcomes

Positive outcomes depend upon integrating collaboration with the patient into the CR process.[7,14-17] Physical therapist expertise may be less related to years of experience, and instead more closely linked with health-related quality of life outcomes and patient satisfaction.[14-16] Features of expert physical therapist practice include collaborative goal-making and reasoning and advocating for patient empowerment through active participation and education.[16] Furthermore, although outcome measurement is widely regarded as a critical piece of professional practice, many clinicians self-report falling short of this goal and may require more focused education and mentorship to integrate this essential component into routine care.[17] The CRT seeks to probe clinicians to collaborate with patients through all stages of care, and to select and administer the most appropriate outcome measures to help judge patient progress and effectiveness of care.

Clearly, physical therapists must use a variety of CDM strategies throughout the elements of physical therapist practice. By considering reasoning strategies used in various aspects of care and the PCM model, the CRT aims to help clinicians think broadly, collaboratively, and in nonlinear ways to reach a higher proficiency in CR.

The ICF is an integral part of the foundation of the tool. The ICF is a classification of health and health-related domains, which helps describe the individual's health condition or changes in body function and structure. The ICF also describes an individual's level of capabilities in his or her environment, as well as his or her level of performance in usual environments.[18] It is an effective framework for physical therapists to better understand each person's experience with his or her disablement, and assists in prioritizing treatment selection. The explicit acknowledgment of personal and environmental factors aids in addressing potential barriers. The ICF model integrates well with other models of practice such as evidence-based practice, the rehabilitation cycle, and Edwards and colleagues' CR model.[4,18]

Another foundational component of the CRT is the HOAC II, which is a CDM diagnostic process using procedural reasoning to generate hypotheses or clinical impressions about the patient's problems.[13] This approach focuses on process and typically is used by less experienced clinicians or with complex patient situations. It also has been found to assist novices or students in focusing on patient-centered outcomes and identifying impairments, functional limitations or deficits, and environmental constraints to determine the cause or source of the issues. The HOAC II uses an iterative process of testing the hypotheses, collecting further data, choosing an intervention plan, and evaluating the outcomes while moving from generalization toward specific conclusions.[13]

The research done by Jensen et al on novice vs expert CDM and practice behaviors helps inform some of the underpinning philosophy of the CRT.[14,19] The researchers found clear differences in dimensions for experienced clinicians vs novice or new clinicians. Dimensions identified focused on treatment time, information gathering, the therapeutic environment, and therapeutic and nontherapeutic interactions.[19] In subsequent work, the similarities and differences that focused on the inexperienced decision-maker vs the experienced decision-maker focused on the clinician's experiences, sources of information gathered, and, most important, reflective skills in making clinical decisions.[20] The evidence from these research articles assisted in the development of the CRT to help design a tool that allowed for reflection, as well as CR and CDM skills, especially for new clinicians, but also for clinicians at all levels.

Lastly, Schön's model of RP is a central theme of the CRT.[7,10] It provides the basis for facilitating the development of clinicians in regard to fostering the ability for continued learning and problem-solving throughout their career. Schön's theories about reflection in clinical practice focused on "active engagement in intellectual processes, exploration of problems or experiences, and a subsequent changed perspective or new insights."[10,20] The CRT incorporates Schön's RP model to facilitate reflection through questioning and mentoring strategies focused on the elements of the RP model, incorporating "knowing-in-action, surprise, reflection-in-action, experimentation, and reflection-on-action."[10] The concept of reflection in CDM was further developed by more recent work on reflection-for-action.[20] All these key strategies for reflection were reviewed and considered during the development of the CRT with the goal of helping users become RPs.

IMPLEMENTATION

The CRT was piloted in the pediatric residency program of a large academic health care network. The post-professional DPT-licensed resident spends 4 months each in acute care, inpatient rehabilitation, and outpatient, with a mentor in each rotation. The mentors collaborate to provide continuity and to advance the resident's CR skills as he or she transitions from setting to setting. The CRT is used throughout the experience to move the resident along the continuum from entry-level clinician to advanced practitioner, and to support the goals of both the resident and the program, which include mastery in CDM for pediatric practice and preparing to sit for the pediatric specialty practice exam from the APTA American Board of Physical Therapy Specialties.[21,22] The tool is used to probe reflection, stimulate clinical questions, and facilitate discussion between resident and mentor to advance CR skills.

Residents and mentors may choose to use specific sections or reflective questions in the CRT to facilitate CPS or to serve as a springboard for discussion. The tool may be used in part or in its entirety, depending on the individual need of the resident and scenario being discussed. Sections to highlight with the mentee may vary depending on the patient case, the clinical setting, or where the resident is from a CT point of view.

Selecting Sections Based on Patient Case

Figure 10-1 provides the CRT, and Figure 10-2 provides a detailed example applying some of the sections and reflective points of the CRT and how it can be used for dialogue around a specific patient. In this case, the resident was challenged by a complex patient with new neurologic dysfunction of unknown etiology, resulting in significant weakness and impaired mobility. Unclear pathology and medical prognosis created uncertainty with the physical therapist prognosis and plan of care. By using relevant sections of the CRT with her mentor, the resident could identify primary problem areas to work on and review and predict prognostic indicators that would help drive her plan of care. Pertinent questions on the CRT helped guide her strategy to prioritize and progress intervention and prompted her to select sensitive tests to measure the patient's response to treatment so she could reassess and modify her plan accordingly.

Selecting Sections Based on Practice Setting

Different sections of the CRT may have more relevance for certain practice settings or for where the patient is on the continuum of care. For example, the outcomes section can probe questions for discharge planning. Alternatively, the evaluation and intervention sections may have significance for a resident struggling with treatment planning in an inpatient rehabilitation setting. See Table 10-1 for a mentor's perspective.

RESIDENCY AND POST-RESIDENCY CLINICAL REASONING AND REFLECTION WITH THE CRT

During residency

"The CRT was helpful when organizing my thoughts about a complex patient with significant rehab needs. It is initially overwhelming because of the volume of questions, but it was helpful that my Mentor and I looked through together to highlight some of the questions we thought would best relate to my patient. The next time I used the CRT I was able to make those decisions more independently based on the patient case and the goals of using the tool.

For my patient, I wanted to organize my thoughts related to the patient history due to his complex medical history and unclear medical diagnosis. I also wanted to organize my thoughts and intervention plans to get the most out of my patient's rehab sessions. It was helpful identify the interventions that I had been using and then think about additional interventions that I hadn't tried. It was also helpful to think about the time spent with each intervention, and how I was modifying the interventions.

I gained the most from the evaluation, intervention, and reexamination sections. We also talked in our mentor meeting about thinking more deeply about the order of the interventions and not just the progression of each individual intervention".

Three years post-residency

"My main take-home points regarding the CRT have to do with the idea of cultivating meta-cognition. With an awareness about how you came to the hypotheses or decisions you made, one can better understand where the pitfalls, biases, etc may lie. Similarly, thinking aloud (either as a mentee or mentor) allows for in the moment reflection and learning, as well as the opportunity for informed discussion following a patient interaction. I always think to the research on creating good teachers, and all of that research shows that teachers get better by being observed and getting immediate feedback. Large parts of me strongly disliked being watched for a year during the residency and having to talk out my clinical reasoning, but I am certain that I am better for having done it. Now, as a clinical instructor, I think frequently about how to coax out my student's thought process, as well as when my own thought process can become a teaching moment. The CRT serves as tool to initiate dialogue surrounding these clinical decisions".

Six years post residency

"In my current roles as a clinical instructor for DPT students, mentor in a residency program, and as a clinical trainer for our new employee developmental competency training program, I refer to this document and tool frequently. The reflection points are helpful to use either individually or as a unit and help drive many clinical reasoning conversations I have with trainees, and I continue to use them for my own clinical reasoning! On occasion I have also shared the pages of reflection points with my trainees and have had them choose several to comment on while writing a reflective journal entry.

I reference the ICF frequently during my own practice and use it often with the students, residents, and new employees I work with. I particularly like the ICF model provided in the appendices because it clearly highlights the activity limitations AND abilities, the participation restrictions AND abilities and the barriers AND facilitators for the internal and external environmental factors. I often feel that we, as clinicians, are not as strengths-based in our clinical practice as we should be, and I love that this chart calls us to that mission. I also appreciate the fact that the environmental factors box is more sizeable than is often found in other ICF charts. I feel that the environmental factors often are down-played in importance when they frequently ARE the prognosis".

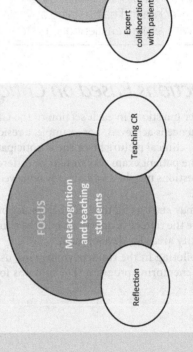
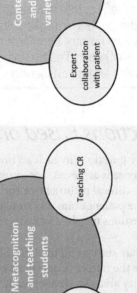

FOCUS
Contextual factors and teaching a variety of learners

Expert collaboration with patient

Philosophy of practice

FOCUS
Metacognition and teaching students

Reflection

Teaching CR

FOCUS
Clinical problem-solving

Clinical skill development

Integrating cognitive, psychomotor, affective

Proficient

Expert

Figure 10-2. Residency and post-residency CR and reflection with the CRT.

TABLE 10-1
A MENTOR'S PERSPECTIVE
USING RELEVANT SECTIONS OF THE CLINICAL REASONING AND REFLECTION TOOL Sections to focus on for CR development may depend on where the mentee is in terms of CDM abilities or even practice setting. For example, a resident in a pediatric inpatient rehabilitation setting was working with a 12-year-old patient with right hemiparesis due to stroke. The patient was being seen for 90 minutes per day, and he was able to ambulate with supervision, with gait deviations consistent with right-sided weakness (ie, toes first for initial contact, steppage pattern during swing, and knee hyperextension in late stance). The resident developed a treatment plan that focused on high-level balance activities but lacked exercises designed to develop strength and control of the hemiparetic side. By using the CRT and categorizing and prioritizing the patient's impairments, limitations, and abilities using the ICF, and by reflecting on the intervention questions with her mentor, the resident was able to reflect that her treatment plan was inadequately addressing one of the primary problem areas influencing the patient's mobility: right lower extremity strength. She adjusted her treatment plan to include focal strengthening and motor control of the right anterior tibialis, quadriceps, and hip extensors, and integrated those changes to over ground gait training as well. The patient began to progress faster and was able to ambulate greater distances with a more efficient gait pattern, which related directly to his goals for rehab.

Selecting Sections Based on Critical Thinking

In addition, deeper questions in each section of the CRT can allow the mentor and mentee to explore even richer CT once basic clinical competence is achieved. For example, a resident in the beginning of the experience may use the initial hypothesis section to explore the clinical picture he or she is anticipating based on medical history or chart review alone, and then discuss with a mentor how the patient exam was similar or different to what was expected. For a resident further along on the learning continuum, these questions may be more quickly reviewed, but then a deeper discussion of the why may occur, such as how bias may enter into CDM.

Finally, mentees may start using the CRT before-action and after-action with the guidance of their mentors, but ultimately the goal is to integrate the reflective questions into the clinician's repertoire in-action.[10] Through practice and exploration, users of the CRT can identify areas for development.[7]

After successful piloting in the residency program, use of the CRT was expanded to the neonatal fellowship program and the new professional mentoring program. The tool was found to be useful and versatile for various types of users, patient situations, and settings.[7]

USE

The CRT was initially published as a case report with the purpose of disseminating a tool that would support physical therapists' professional development to address CDM and reflection through mentorship.[7] The CRT was designed to be used in the post-professional arena as a clinical reflection tool to assist clinicians through mentoring, with the essential needs of making clinical decisions. From 2014 to 2015, we conducted a survey on how, where, with whom, and for what purpose the tool was being used. Since publication of the case report, the tool has been used in various ways (including publications, practice settings, and academic and clinical environments) and in various formats. The survey found that the CRT has received unexpected and surprising success. The survey uncovered that the tool is used by physical therapists with various levels of experience including faculty (academic and clinical), clinical leadership, and mentors. The CRT is used in all areas of physical therapy practice settings, from pediatrics to geriatrics, inpatient and outpatient, and at all levels of acuity and chronicity. The tool has been used with preprofessional students, residents, fellows, new professionals, those in remediation, and experienced clinicians. Surprisingly, the tool has also been used by occupational therapists, speech therapists, and recreational therapists.

The CRT is primarily used in residency and fellowship programs as well as DPT programs. Examples of use of the tool in entry-level and transitional DPT programs include integration into the curriculum via specific CDM courses and clinical experiences to facilitate reflection and patient-centered CDM. Residency and fellowship programs have embraced the tool both formally and informally. The American Board of Physical Therapy Residency and Fellowship Education highlighted the CRT in the *Mentoring Resource Manual,*[22] and the CRT has also been featured in their online training course "Successful Mentorship for Residency and Fellowship Education."[23] It is used in training mentors to structure and facilitate mentoring sessions, as well as in part of the practical live patient examination process and documentation. In the clinical post-professional arena, the tool is used to develop and mentor new and experienced professionals through in-services, journal clubs, and activities focused on evidence-based practice. Lastly, the tool has also been used for research projects both nationally and internationally to examine and investigate CR of clinicians and the use of the APTA guide and ICF for PCM.

As with any tool or model, users identified positive aspects as well as challenges. The most commonly identified positive aspects of using the CRT are that it offers the following benefits:

- Helps students/clinicians organize data and identify key areas to address during interventions with patients
- Includes environmental and personal factors that impact patient care
- Promotes objective CR
- Challenges students to think
- Promotes a more holistic approach to care
- Focuses on reflection, helps newer clinicians see the big picture
- Improves description of thought process with improved organization
- Encourages better dialogue and improved succinct communication
- Facilitates a transdisciplinary approach to patient management
- Improves documentation
- Encourages an organized stepwise format along with the ICF table
- Increases RP at all levels of clinicians
- Facilitates professional development, moving the physical therapist and/or student along the continuum of development
- Improves CDM and CR skills
- Increases focus on patient-centered care

Challenges identified with the CRT primarily focused on the length of the tool and the time to complete it. Some users indicated that the form was awkward, and they felt the need to answer all questions in each section. Most of the challenges appear to be related to lack of understanding on how to use the tool and its intent and adaptability for specific learning needs.

JOURNEY FROM NOVICE TO EXPERT

Understanding the process of CR and CDM has been the subject of much research and discussion over the past 30 years in the health professions. CR has been defined as "an inferential process used by practitioners to collect and evaluate data and to make judgments about the diagnosis and management of patient problems."[24(p101)] CR includes not only the application of cognitive and psychomotor skills based on theory and evidence, but also the ability to reflect and modify care to maximize patient response.[25] Integrating the application of knowledge and skill with the intuitive ability to modify care based on patient response to maximize outcome is a core attribute that separates experts from novices.[12,14,19,25]

Several investigators have sought to better understand the development of professional expertise to better teach CDM to student and novice clinicians. The CRT seeks to move clinicians along the continuum of professional development by highlighting these important hallmarks of expert practice.[14] A case sample of convenience reveals some beginning understanding of how the use of the CRT may evolve during the course of professional development (see Figure 10-2).

In this figure, a resident reviews how she uses the tool for organizing and prioritizing her thoughts, demonstrating a focus on CPS and skill development. Her CR elucidated by the CRT represents proficiency in practice and analytical decision-making. A clinician 3 years post-residency reports a deeper reflection, cultivating metacognition, and using the CRT to probe CR in her students. By teaching CR in a deliberate way, she is continuing to advance her CDM skills and consolidate her own mastery of practice. Finally, a clinician 6 years post-residency discusses using the CRT for a spectrum of different learners, adeptly using the tool for various stages of CR. She also emphasizes her use of contextual factors and collaboration with families in driving CDM and has developed a philosophy of practice, all of which represent the hallmarks of expert practice.[14] While more remains to be explored, these insights may shape use and adaptation of the CRT.

EVOLUTION: AN UPDATE AND THE FUTURE OF THE TOOL

The CRT has been in use for more than 7 years, and this experience has allowed the developers to revise and update the tool. The revised and updated version of the CRT is under development with the goal of including current health care concepts and strategies that focus on patient-centered care and increased reflection by clinicians. These concepts include shared decision-making and cultural competence that were identified from the results of the survey, as well as anecdotal findings from use of the tool.

In addressing CR and CDM, it is important to recognize that decisions are contextually dependent. Many contextual factors must be considered that can directly or indirectly influence the clinical decision and reasoning strategies. In general, when looking at contextual aspects of clinical decisions and reasoning, the factors that must be considered include the nature of the decision or task, the attributes of the decision-maker, the skill and knowledge of the decision-maker, and the context in which the decision takes place.[26]

There are 2 main categories when considering the contextual factors that influence clinical decisions: clinical and nonclinical influences.[8] Clinical influences include information such as patient's health condition, clinician's knowledge and skill, clinician's use of evidence-based strategies, practice setting, patient's age and race, and patient's adherence. The types of clinical decisions these influences would address include the following[8]:

- What are the patient's main impairments?
- What are the patient's abilities and limitations?
- Does the patient need treatment, and why?
- What are the expected outcomes of intervention?
- What outcome measures would be most appropriate?
- What interventions, if any, are needed?
- What is the appropriate dosing for the patient?
- How many sessions are needed to address the problem?

The nonclinical influences on clinical decisions include both patient and clinician factors, both of which can have a direct and indirect influence on clinical decisions.[8] The patient factors include the following:

- Cultural beliefs, values, and traditions
- Religious beliefs
- Communication style and language
- Age, race, ethnicity, and gender
- Socioeconomic status
- Health behavior
- Health literacy
- Adherence
- Attitudes and behavior
- Goals and preferences
- Family and caregivers
- Patient's trust of the health care system

The clinician factors include:

- Personal characteristics such as age, race, ethnicity, gender, and faith
- Cultural beliefs, values, and traditions
- Interpersonal skills
- Communication style and language
- Clinician's use of evidence (evidence-based practice)
- Professional interaction

- Practice setting
  - Type of practice
  - Time constraints
  - Workload
  - Available resources
  - Management policies

By integrating more explicit guidance for reflection on these contextual factors and influences into the updated CRT, mentors and mentees can have deeper discussions around striving for cultural competence in CDM at different points of care.

CONCLUSION

It is important to consider all influences when making clinical decisions and reasoning to best serve the patient. The CRT allows for the physical therapist to use CDM models, the guide, and ICF to improve outcomes for patients while delivering effective health care services.[7,10] The usability and versatile features of the CRT have been embraced by educators, mentors, students, mentees, and practicing physical therapists. Its focus on CR and reflection traverses practice setting, and the depth of questions allow it to be helpful regardless of years of experience.

However, as the health care landscape continues to change, so does the profession and the drive for clinical excellence. A revised and updated version of the CRT is under development, and it will integrate concepts in shared decision-making and cultural competence, and formulate them into reflective questions to improve practice. Finally, further exploration into how the CRT is used by clinicians of varying levels of expertise may provide insight into how the tool can evolve for individual users and perhaps provide a window into the inner workings of CR along the journey from novice to expert practitioner. The CRT supports the ongoing development of CR, cultural competence, and family-centered care by providing a guide for RP that ultimately may lead to improved patient outcomes.

Reflection Moment

Describe how CRT is an effective tool for teaching CDM and CR skills in physical therapy.

Discuss ways in which the CRT can be used with various levels of physical therapists from students to expert clinicians.

Explain how the CRT facilitates reflection in CR, moving the clinician along the continuum of professional development from basic deductive reasoning to higher CR strategies of inductive reasoning.

Discuss how the CRT facilitates shared decision-making and addresses diversity of values, beliefs, and needs of different patient populations.

Consider whether you believe that the CRT is a nimble and flexible clinical tool that can be modified as the practice of physical therapy and health care demands change.

REFERENCES

1. American Physical Therapy Association. Vision statement. http://www.apta.org/vision. Accessed August 15, 2016.
2. American Physical Therapy Association. Professional development: residencies and fellowships. http://www.apta.org/AM/Template.cfm?Section=Residency&CONTENTID=30116&TEMPLATE=/CM/ContentDisplay.cfm. Accessed April 19, 2009.
3. McGinnis PQ, Hack LM, Nixon-Cave K, Michlovitz SL. Factors that influence clinical decision-making of physical therapists in choosing a balance assessment approach. *Phys Ther.* 2009;89:233-247.
4. Edwards I, Jones M, Carr J, Braunack-Mayer, Jensen G. Clinical reasoning strategies in physical therapy. *Phys Ther.* 2004;84:312-330.
5. Shepard KF, Jensen GM. Techniques for teaching and evaluating students in academic settings. In: Shepard KF, Jensen GM, eds. *Handbook of Teaching for Physical Therapists.* 2nd ed. Waltham, MA: Butterworth-Heinmann; 2002:71-132.
6. Leighton D, Sheldon M. Model for teaching clinical decision-making in a physical therapy professional curriculum. *J Phys Ther Educ.* 1997;11(2):23-30.
7. Atkinson HL, Nixon-Cave K. A tool for clinical reasoning and reflection using the *International Classification of Functioning, Disability and Health (ICF)* framework and PCM. *Phys Ther.* 2011;92(3).

8. American Physical Therapy Association. Clinical decision-making in diverse patient populations. E-learning course. https://iweb.apta.org/purchase/ProductDetail.aspx?Product_code=LMS-822. Accessed May 1, 2019.

9. American Physical Therapy Association. Guide to physical therapist practice. http://www.apta.org/guide. Accessed August 20, 2016.

10. Schön DA. *The Reflective Practitioner*. New York, NY: Basic Books, 1983.

11. Eva KW. What every teacher needs to know about clinical reasoning. *Med Educ.* 2004;39:98-106.

12. Tichenor CJ, Davidson JM. Post professional clinical residency education. In: Shepard KF, Jensen GM, eds. *Handbook of Teaching for Physical Therapists*. 2nd ed. Waltham, MA: Butterworth-Heinemann; 2002:473-502.

13. Riddle DL, Rothstein JM, Echternach JL. Application of the HOAC II: an episode of care for a patient with low back pain. *Phys Ther.* 2003;83:471-485.

14. Jensen GM, Gwyer J, Shepard K, Hack LM. Expert practice in physical therapy. *Phys Ther.* 2000;80:28-43.

15. Resnik L, Hart DL. Using clinical outcomes to identify expert physical therapists. *Phys Ther.* 2003;83:990-1002.

16. Resnik L, Jensen GM. Using clinical outcomes to explore the theory of expert practice in physical therapy. *Phys Ther.* 2003;83:1090-1106.

17. Jette DU, Halbert J, Iverson C, Miceli E, Shah P. Use of standardized outcome measures in physical therapist practice: perceptions and applications. *Phys Ther.* 2009;89:125-135.

18. World Health Organization. International classification of functioning, disability and health (ICF). http://www.who.int/classifications/icf/appareas/en/index.html. Accessed March 6, 2009.

19. Jensen GM, Shepard KF, Gwyer J, Hack LM. Attribute dimensions that distinguish master and novice physical therapy clinicians in orthopedic settings. *Phys Ther.* 1992;72:711-722.

20. Wainwright S, Shepard K, Harmon L, Stephens J. Novice and experienced physical therapist clinicians: a comparison of how reflection is used to inform the clinical decision-making process. *Phys Ther.* 2010;90:75-88.

21. American Board of Physical Therapy Specialties. http://www.abpts.org/home.aspx. Accessed November 9, 2017.

22. American Board of Physical Therapy Residency and Fellowship Education. Mentoring resource manual. http://www.abptrfe.org/uploadedFiles/ABPTRFEorg/For_Programs/ABPTRFEMentoringResourceManual.pdf. Accessed April 23, 2018.

23. American Physical Therapy Association. Successful mentorship for residency and fellowship education. E-learning course. http://learningcenter.apta.org/student/MyCourse.aspx?id=e659bff6-1199-4287-a9c8-6a5a1ce9ceb0&programid=dcca7f06-4cd9-4530-b9d3-4ef7d2717b5d. Accessed April 23, 2018.

24. Lee JE, Ryan-Wenger N. The "Think Aloud" seminar for teaching clinical reasoning: a case study of a child with pharyngitis. *J Pediatr Health Care.* 1997;11:101-110.

25. Palisano RJ, Campbell SK, Harris SR. Evidence-based decision-making in pediatric physical therapy. In: Campbell SK, Palisano RJ, Orlin MN, eds. *Physical Therapy for Children*. 3rd ed. St. Louis, MO: Saunders Elsevier; 2006:3-32.

26. Smith M, Higgs J, Ellis E. Physiotherapy decision-making in acute cardiorespiratory care is influenced by factors related to the physiotherapist and the nature and context of the decision: a qualitative study. *Aust J Physiother.* 2007;53:261-267.

APPENDIX
CLINICAL REASONING AND REFLECTION TOOL

Clinical Reasoning and Reflection

Appendix.
The Physical Therapy Clinical Reasoning and Reflection Tool (PT-CRT)[a]

I. Initial Data Gathering/Interview

a. History and present function

REFLECTION POINTS:

➢ Assess how the patient's medical diagnosis affects your interview.

➢ How might your personal biases/assumptions affect your interview?

➢ Assessing the information you gathered, what do you see as a pattern or connection between the symptoms?

➢ What is the value of the data you gathered?

➢ What are some of the judgments you can draw from the data? Are there alternative solutions?

➢ What is your assessment of the patient's/caregiver's knowledge and understanding of their diagnosis and need for PT?

➢ Have you verified the patient's goals and what resources are available?

➢ Based on the information gathered, are you able to assess a need for a referral to another health care professional?

II. Generation of Initial Hypothesis

a. Body structures/functions

b. Impairments

c. Activity limitations

d. Participation restrictions

REFLECTION POINTS:

➢ Can you construct a hypothesis based on the information gathered?

➢ What is that based on (biases, experiences)?

➢ How did you arrive at the hypothesis? How can you explain your rationale?

➢ What about this patient and the information you have gathered might support your hypothesis?

➢ What do you anticipate could be an outcome for this patient (prognosis)?

➢ Based on your hypothesis, how might your strategy for the examination be influenced?

➢ What is your approach/planned sequence/strategy for the examination?

➢ How might the environmental factors affect your examination?

➢ How might other diagnostic information affect your examination?

(Continued)

Clinical Reasoning and Reflection

Appendix.
Continued

III. Examination

    a. Tests and Measures

RELECTION POINTS:

➤ Appraising the tests and measures you selected for your examination, how and why did you select them?

➤ Reflecting on these tests, how might they support/negate your hypothesis?

➤ Can the identified tests and measures help you determine a change in status? Are they able to detect a minimum clinically important difference?

➤ How did you organize the examination? What might you do differently?

➤ Describe considerations for the psychometric properties of tests and measures used.

➤ Discuss other systems not tested that may be affecting the patient's problem.

➤ Compare your examination findings for this patient with another patient with a similar medical diagnosis.

➤ How does your selection of tests and measures relate to the patient's goals?

(Continued)

Clinical Reasoning and Reflection

Appendix.
Continued

IV. Evaluation

HEALTH CONDITION

BODY STRUCTURES/FUNCTION (IMPAIRMENTS)

ACTIVITY (TASKS)	
Abilities	Limitations

PARTICIPATION	
Abilities	Restrictions

ENVIRONMENTAL			
Internal		External	
+	−	+	−

(Continued)

Clinical Reasoning and Reflection

Appendix.
Continued

IV. Evaluation (continued)

a. Diagnosis

b. Prognosis

REFLECTION POINTS:

➢ How did you determine your diagnosis? What about this patient suggested your diagnosis?

➢ How did your examination findings support or negate your initial hypothesis?

➢ What is your appraisal of the most important issues to work on?

➢ How do these relate to the patient's goals and identified issues?

➢ What factors might support or interfere with the patient's prognosis?

➢ How might other factors such as bodily functions and environmental and societal factors affect the patient?

➢ What is your rationale for the prognosis, and what are the positive and negative prognostic indicators?

➢ How will you go about developing a therapeutic relationship?

➢ How might any cultural factors influence your care of the patient?

➢ What are your considerations for behavior, motivation, and readiness?

➢ How can you determine capacity for progress toward goals?

V. Plan of Care

a. Identify short-term and long-term goals

b. Identify outcome measures

c. PT prescription (frequency/intensity of service, include key elements)

REFLECTION POINTS:

➢ How have you incorporated the patient's and family's goals?

➢ How do the goals reflect your examination and evaluation (ICF framework)?

➢ How did you determine the PT prescription or plan of care (frequency, intensity, anticipated length of service)?

➢ How do key elements of the PT plan of care relate back to primary diagnosis?

➢ How do the patient's personal and environmental factors affect the PT plan of care?

(Continued)

Clinical Reasoning and Reflection

Appendix.
Continued

VI. Interventions

a. Describe how you are using evidence to guide your practice

b. Identify overall approach/strategy

c. Describe and prioritize specific procedural interventions

d. Describe your plan for progression

REFLECTION POINTS:

➢ Discuss your overall PT approach or strategies (eg, motor learning, strengthening).

- How will you modify principles for this patient?
- Are there specific aspects about this particular patient to keep in mind?
- How does your approach relate to theory and current evidence?

➢ As you designed your intervention plan, how did you select specific strategies?

➢ What is your rationale for those intervention strategies?

➢ How do the interventions relate to the primary problem areas identified using the ICF?

➢ How might you need to modify your interventions for this particular patient and caregiver? What are your criteria for doing so?

➢ What are the coordination of care aspects?

➢ What are the communication needs with other team members?

➢ What are the documentation aspects?

➢ How will you ensure safety?

➢ Patient/caregiver education:

- What are your overall strategies for teaching?
- Describe learning styles/barriers and any possible accommodations for the patient and caregiver.
- How can you ensure understanding and buy-in?
- What communication strategies (verbal and nonverbal) will be most successful?

(Continued)

Clinical Reasoning and Reflection

Appendix.
Continued

VII. Reexamination

a. When and how often

> **REFLECTION POINTS:**
>
> ➢ Evaluate the effectiveness of your interventions. Do you need to modify anything?
>
> ➢ What have you learned about the patient/caregiver that you did not know before?
>
> ➢ Using the ICF, how does this patient's progress toward goals compare with that of other patients with a similar diagnosis?
>
> ➢ Is there anything that you overlooked, misinterpreted, overvalued, or undervalued, and what might you do differently? Will this address any potential errors you have made?
>
> ➢ How has your interaction with the patient/caregiver changed?
>
> ➢ How has your therapeutic relationship changed?
>
> ➢ How might any new factors affect the patient outcome?
>
> ➢ How do the characteristics of the patient's progress affect your goals, prognosis, and anticipated outcome?
>
> ➢ How can you determine the patient's views (satisfaction/frustration) about his or her progress toward goals? How might that affect your plan of care?
>
> ➢ How has PT affected the patient's life?

VIII. Outcomes

a. Discharge plan (include follow-up, equipment, school/work/community re-entry, etc)

> **REFLECTION POINTS:**
>
> ➢ Was PT effective, and what outcome measures did you use to assess the outcome? Was there a minimum clinically important difference?
>
> ➢ Why or why not?
>
> ➢ What criteria did you or will you use to determine whether the patient has met his or her goals?
>
> ➢ How do you determine the patient is ready to return to home/community/work/school/sports?
>
> ➢ What barriers (physical, personal, environmental), if any, are there to discharge?
>
> ➢ What are the anticipated life-span needs, and what are they based on?
>
> ➢ What might the role of PT be in the future?
>
> ➢ What are the patient's/caregiver's views of future PT needs?
>
> ➢ How can you and the patient/caregiver partner together for a lifetime plan for wellness?

IX. Mentor Feedback:

Strengths:

Opportunities for development:

a PT=physical therapy, ICF=*International Classification of Functioning, Disability and Health.*

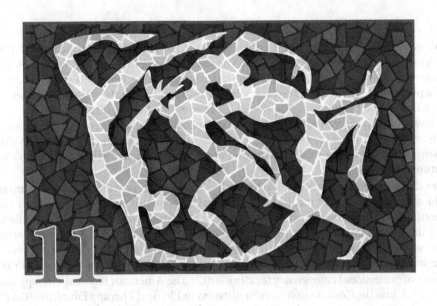

Using a Comprehensive Framework to Assess Clinical Reasoning

Wing Fu, PT, PhD, MA

Objectives

Upon completing this chapter, you will be able to:

- Describe the clinical reasoning (CR) assessment framework and its 4 levels.

- Identify assessment tools for the 4 levels of the CR assessment framework.

- Explain how to use the CR assessment framework and its assessment findings for your andragogical reflection and evaluation.

- Explain how to use the CR assessment framework and its assessment findings for student remediation.

- Consider how to use the CR assessment framework and its assessment findings for a programmatic or curricular review.

Introduction

CR is a critical attribute that student physical therapists must develop to become autonomous practitioners in the current health care environment.[1] Physical therapist education programs are obligated to ensure CR as an educational outcome[2,3] by adopting and implementing appropriate instructional methods and assessment strategies. CR is a complex and multidimensional construct[4]; therefore, CR assessment requires a carefully combined set of instruments for a comprehensive review of CR skills and abilities. Assessment frameworks have been recognized as a means to provide a structured conceptual map,[5] which directs the overall evaluation of educational outcomes and the specific choices of assessment instruments.

Musolino GM, Jensen GM, eds. *Clinical Reasoning and Decision-Making in Physical Therapy: Facilitation, Assessment, and Implementation* (pp 133-142).
© 2020 Taylor & Francis Group.

In this chapter, a hierarchical CR assessment framework is delineated to guide the assessment of DPT student physical therapists' CR in both a systematic and comprehensive manner. The CR assessment framework was developed primarily based on Miller's pyramid[6] (a hierarchical structure established for clinical assessment; see Figure 7-1) and was customized to address the assessment of CR for the purpose of physical therapist entry-level education. The author provides rationales for adopting the CR assessment framework, followed by a thorough description of the framework architecture. The CR assessment framework allows users to assess CR at 4 levels, employing various assessment instruments. The instruments applicable to each of the 4 levels are described to further illustrate the utility of the CR assessment framework. The chapter concludes with a discussion of the applications of the CR assessment framework in student education and remediation, as well as programmatic or curricular review, with suggestions for future developments.

Assessment is "the bridge between teaching and learning."[7(p15)] The bridge provides educators a means of discovering and measuring students' educational outcomes. In medical education, assessment also protects the public by identifying incompetent practitioners.[8] The identification through assessment is supported by 2 studies, which demonstrated a significant correlation between performance at the student phase and the post-graduation phase. Papadakis et al[9] revealed a strong association among practicing physicians between unprofessional behavior in medical school and disciplinary action by medical boards. Carr et al[10] found that academic performance of medical students predicted their workplace performance as junior doctors.

CR is a vital component of professional competency for clinicians.[11] The American Physical Therapy Association (APTA) recognizes the importance of CR, and the Commission on Accreditation in Physical Therapy Education (CAPTE) Standards specify CR as an educational outcome for graduates of physical therapist education programs.[2,3] To protect the public, it is imperative to assess CR among student physical therapists and to identify any incompetent or struggling individuals. The assessment of student physical therapists' CR has been gaining more national attention, with the Clinical Reasoning Curricula and Assessment Consortium created within the recently formed APTA American Council of Academic Physical Therapy.[12] One of the goals of the consortium is to develop best-practice standards for CR curricula and assessment.

The revised APTA Physical Therapist Clinical Performance Instrument (CPI) (version 2006)[13] includes CR as a performance criterion and a red flag item, a foundational element of practice, in assessing student physical therapists' performance during clinical education experiences.[14] Assessing CR is unquestionably crucial, but the assessment task is not easy. CR is a complex and multifaceted phenomenon.[4] The inherent complexity and intricacy make it challenging to measure CR by a single assessment. CR requires multiple assessment tools to reveal and reflect the phenomenon comprehensively. This is in line with the recommendation of the Middle States Commission on Higher Education: "to triangulate around important learning goals, assessing them through various means, and through tests of various formats."[15(p39)]

The multiple assessment tools also need to be selected and combined in a careful and thoughtful manner by following a framework that guides the evaluation of the educational outcome. While assessment tools have been developed to assess student physical therapists' CR,[13,16,17] scant attention has been paid to establish a pertinent assessment framework. Based on Miller's pyramid,[6] the author specifically developed a CR assessment framework that is applicable to the entry-level physical therapist education.

ASSESSMENT FRAMEWORKS

To begin, let's examine the definition of an assessment framework. Pearce et al provided this detailed description:

> *Assessment frameworks provide a structured conceptual map of the learning outcomes of a programme of study. Where curriculum frameworks detail what is to be taught, assessment frameworks detail what is to be assessed as evidence of learning described by the requisite curriculum content. Built into an assessment framework are assessment concepts (and their definitions), along with theoretical assumptions that allow others to relate to the framework and potentially adapt it to other domains of assessment. Further an assessment framework details how an assessment is to be operationalized. It combines theory and practice, and explains both the "what" and the "how."*[5(p110)]

Based on this description, an assessment framework is essentially a conceptual structure that provides theoretical and practical guidance for the assessment of relevant educational outcomes.

In addition to describing assessment frameworks, Pearce et al[5] offered rationales to support the use of assessment frameworks in medical education. Drawing upon Pearce's justifications, the author developed the following rationales to advocate for using a framework in the assessment of CR. A CR assessment framework can convey the CR constructs to be measured and provide a clear illustration of the relationships among the constructs. The articulation and illustration serve as a conceptual map to operationalize the assessment tasks, produce robust assessment tools more easily, and improve the validity and reliability of the assessment. If a common CR assessment framework were developed and adopted across institutions, both educators and learners could increase the consistency of CR assessment and generate comparable assessment data, not only within but also across institutions. In a survey study,[18] 46% of responding accredited physical therapist education programs reported that the assessment of CR within or between programs was not consistent. The finding validates the need to adopt a common CR assessment framework across education programs.

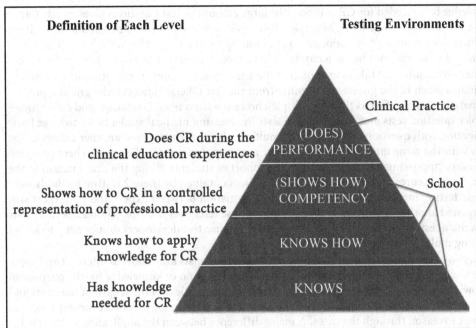

Definition of Each Level

Testing Environments

Clinical Practice

(DOES) PERFORMANCE

Does CR during the clinical education experiences

(SHOWS HOW) COMPETENCY — School

Shows how to CR in a controlled representation of professional practice

KNOWS HOW

Knows how to apply knowledge for CR

KNOWS

Has knowledge needed for CR

Figure 11-1. The CR assessment framework.[6,19] (Reprinted with permission from Fu W. Development of an innovative tool to assess student physical therapists' clinical reasoning competency. *J Phys Ther Ed.* 2015;29:14-26, as adapted from Miller GE. The assessment of clinical skills/competence/performance. *Acad Med.* 1990;65[9]:S63-S67.)

THE CLINICAL REASONING ASSESSMENT FRAMEWORK

Miller[6] proposed a pyramidal framework for assessing medical students, which was introduced in Chapter 7 of this text (see Figure 7-1). The framework is divided into 4 hierarchical levels. Moving from the base of the prism or pyramidal structure, "knows" represents medical students' knowledge base or factual information. The next level up is "knows how," which assesses whether medical students know how to apply the knowledge that they have accumulated.

The upper 2 levels are "shows how" and "does." Miller[6] defined these upper 2 levels as "how medical students perform when faced with a patient" (usually assessed via clinical teachers' observations) and "what medical students do in clinical practice after they graduate" (workplace-based assessments). Rethans et al[19] redefined the upper 2 levels and labeled them as competency and performance, respectively, with competency referred to as what an individual is capable of doing in a controlled representation of professional practice, and performance equivalent to what an individual does in the actual professional practice.

The pyramidal structure is also identified as moving along a continuum from novice to expert. The pyramid puts the novice at the base, progresses through the middle levels with demonstrations of learning, and then places the individual as more expert in the performance phase, as the learner incorporates knowledge, skills, and attitudes moving into integration of performance for practice.

The author developed a CR assessment framework based on Miller's pyramid[6] and the modified definitions of its upper 2 levels from Rethans et al.[19] The CR assessment framework, as illustrated in Figure 11-1, has 4 hierarchical levels: knows, knows how, competency, and performance, from the bottom up. The derived CR assessment framework is designed to guide the assessment of student physical therapists' CR in entry-level education.

The knows, knows how, and competency levels are tested in the academic or simulation settings during the didactic component of the education programs. The performance level is assessed during the clinical education experiences, which are in real-world situations.

The CR assessment framework allows users to assess student physical therapists' CR at 4 different levels, in an ongoing fashion, employing various assessment tools. Limited CR assessment tools have been developed for physical therapist education. Assessment tools developed for learners in other health professions, particularly medicine and nursing, are also applicable to the framework. The current understanding suggests that CR cannot be measured independent of pertinent content knowledge.[20] Therefore, even within a single level of the assessment framework, multiple assessment tools are needed to measure CR in relation to specific knowledge sets of individual clinical domains. Clinical domains can be either clinical specialties or settings. Moreover, before we select an assessment tool at a certain level, we need to investigate the CR construct that the tool is designed to measure, to ensure the construct fits the assessment need.

As with Miller's pyramid, the knowledge level represents whether student physical therapists have the basic factual knowledge required as a basis for CR. Any assessment tools testing students' ability to recall the knowledge base are applicable. Examples include multiple-choice question tests,[21] free-response tests,[22] and oral examinations that focus on verbal regurgitation of the related building blocks of knowledge. Automated machines can grade multiple-choice question tests easily and quickly.[23] This allows the test developers to include a large amount of test questions without worrying about the time involved in the grading process. Since the knowledge base needed for CR is broad, the large amount of test questions gives an advantage to using multiple-choice question tests for the knowledge level. Multiple-choice question tests can also be used to test a large number of students without much human intervention.[24] A major critique of multiple-choice question tests is that test takers can guess the answers.[25] Therefore, the test score may not be an accurate reflection of individual test takers' knowledge base.

Free-response tests and oral examinations require test takers to construct the answers and express them either in a written or verbal format. The construction eliminates much of the guesswork coming from the test takers. However, the grading process for free-response tests and oral examinations is not as fast as that of multiple-choice question tests. Damjanov and colleagues[22] compared the abilities of multiple-choice question tests and free-response tests in assessing medical students' knowledge base. One cohort of students took an examination with questions written in the multiple-choice format, while another cohort in the subsequent year took the examination with the same questions written in the free-response format. The researchers provided a reference list of potential uncued answers (approximately 200 words) to the cohort of students taking the examination in the free-response format. Both the students' mean scores and the discrimination indices obtained by these 2 testing methods were comparable. However, the free-response testing method provided a better discrimination between expert and nonexpert students. Damjanov and colleagues[22] suggested another advantage of using free-response tests over multiple-choice question tests at the knowledge level: It is easier to write questions in the free-response format because test developers do not need to spend time on creating distractors, as in writing multiple-choice questions.

The application of knowledge (knows how) level assesses whether student physical therapists know how to interpret and apply the knowledge for CR. The knowledge level demands assessment tools that test the application of knowledge for the purpose of CR, instead of testing the recall of knowledge. All the tools at this level are case based, regardless of the length of the cases and the test format. Typical test formats are paper based and computerized. The clinical cases provide a context for test takers to apply their knowledge when they attempt to reason through the cases. A major difference between the application of knowledge (knows how) level and the competency level is that the former level does not require test takers to work with a standardized patient (a patient actor) in a controlled representation of professional practice, while the latter level does. Multiple-choice question tests[24] and free-response tests are appropriate as long as the questions are constructed to assess the taxonomically higher-order, cognitive processing and application of knowledge. Multiple-choice question tests based on rich case descriptions are widely used,[26] but they are criticized for the low face validity, as well as the educational concern and implication of limiting test takers' response to one correct or one best answer per question.[27] Compared to grading multiple-choice question tests, grading free-response tests at the knows how level is not only more time consuming, but also less objective. Even with training, it is challenging to remove the subjectivity from the objective examination of student-constructed responses.

Using panels may assist in grading objectivity and produce multiple responses, but the approach is even more time and labor intensive. Free-response tests do have a huge advantage over multiple-choice question tests when testing CR at the application of knowledge (knows how) level. Incorrect answers to the free-response tests can be used to identify test takers' misconceptions and misunderstandings of the relevant materials. Asking test takers to clarify their thinking on misjudgments remains a rich learning opportunity that is often left to chance. Debriefing with student learners provides an opportunity to investigate the CR process and where the learners are led astray or why they may have stayed the course to arrive at the best response, even in errant reasoning.

Well-structured research designs or method models for the assessment of CR at the application of knowledge level have yet to be described in the physical therapist education arena. In Section III of this text, we will explore additional innovative and novel works in this area. Examples of applicable existing assessment tools are script concordance tests (SCTs),[28] key features tests,[29,30] virtual patients,[31] patient management problems,[32,33] and CR problems.[34] They are created primarily for education in health care professions other than physical therapy. Only the first 3 examples are discussed in this chapter based on contemporary usage.

SCTs ask test takers to respond to a series of items following each brief case scenario in the context of ambiguity by making use of the related organized knowledge (script).[28] Each series of items is composed of a lead-in that provides a hypothesis (diagnostic or management), followed by a new piece of information. The test takers need to evaluate the impact of the new information on the likelihood of the hypothesis. The test measures the degree of concordance by comparing the responses of the test takers with those of expert clinicians. SCTs are typically claimed to measure CR in uncertain situations.[28] When applying the test to the CR assessment framework, it should be classified to the knows how level, owing to the associated application of knowledge. In a literature review of validity evidence, Lubarsky et al[35] reported that SCTs have a strong validity in both areas of content and internal structure. With regard to test construction and implementation, Dory and colleagues[26] conducted a systematic review and concluded that 25 ill-defined cases, with approximately 4 items per case reflecting clinical practice in the selected domain, are required to obtain reliable scores. In addition, the recommended size of the panel of expert clinicians is noted as 10 to 20. Kelly et al[36] compared an SCT to a multiple-choice examination on a core internal medicine clerkship. Both tests covered the same content areas in 20 questions. The medical students' SCT performance correlated with their clinical performance, while the students' multiple-choice examination performance did not have such correlation.

Dawson et al[37] applied an SCT to evaluate CR in nursing students and found it to be standardized, reliable, and easy to administer. Although Dawson et al[37] claimed that SCT has been used in training programs including physical therapy, they did not include any supporting evidence. To the author's knowledge, no research has been published on using SCT to examine student physical therapists' CR, despite the strengths of the test. The author wonders if the necessary resources (eg, test construction skills and panel size) are barriers for its implementation in physical therapist education. While the Federation of State Boards of Physical Therapy provides courses in item writing and test construction, it has been limited thus far to the multiple-choice format. Multi-institutional collaboration may be necessary to overcome the barriers and should be considered.

Another application of knowledge or mid-level assessment tool is the key features test. The Medical Council of Canada commissioned a 6-year research and development project to create the test, which measures CR.[38] The test was developed to replace the patient management problems format in the qualifying examination for medicine. A key feature is "a critical step in the resolution of a clinical problem."[29(p194)] Each clinical case scenario is briefly stated and followed by questions that focus only on the key features. The response format and the answer key are flexible. The test may ask the test takers to write their response or select the response from a list of options. The answer key for each question can vary from one to more responses. The short length of the case scenarios allows a broader sampling of clinical problems. The broader sampling can, in turn, enhance the reliability of the test scores.[39] The key features test is estimated to require 40 questions and slightly above 4 hours of examination time to achieve a reliability coefficient of 0.8.[38] Hrynchak et al[40] conducted a literature review and reported that the test has moderate to high face and content validity, good construct validity, and the ability to successfully predict future physician performance. As with the SCT, the author was not able to locate any published studies demonstrating the application of key features tests with student physical therapists.

Monnier et al[41] investigated the relationship between either SCTs or key features tests and global performance measures with 129 obstetrics-gynecology clerkship students. The SCT correlated positively with the in-training CR score extracted from supervisors' evaluation reports. Surprisingly, the key features test was only associated with the preclinical evaluation score, which was deemed to link more with factual knowledge.

The remaining application of knowledge assessment tool on which we will focus is called virtual patients. Virtual patients, when developed and implemented for the purpose of assessment, are defined as "computer-based simulations of patient management, incorporating narrative and media, designed to examine candidate skills in patient management."[31(p759)] Gesundheit et al[42] studied medical students' acceptance toward using virtual patients to assess their clinical skills and reasoning. The preclinical (second-year) students rated virtual patients higher than standardized patients for both patient portrayal and the quality of being appropriately challenged." The students found virtual patients more realistic because the associated simulation allowed the introduction of abnormal findings. Cook and Triola[43] published a literature review on the use of virtual patients in 2009 and found that only 5 studies reported the generation of an assessment outcome representing CR of health professions students.

VirtualPT Clinician is a virtual patient software designed specifically for student physical therapists.[44] After a student works through a patient case online, the software can provide a quantitative assessment of the student's performance by rendering a few scores, including the CR score.[45] However, no validity and reliability data for VirtualPT Clinician are available. Researchers proposed potential benefits[46] of using computerized simulations for the development of student physical therapists' CR. Some of the benefits apply to the assessment of CR and include the following: simulations make the assessment easily accessible regardless of location and time, predetermined criteria can provide immediate and individualized feedback after students complete the associated assessment, and simulations eliminate cost and logistic issues as well as safety problems typically associated with incorporating real or standardized patients in student assessment.[46] Nonetheless, the production cost of virtual patients is high in terms of time and money.[47] We will take a closer look at the use of instructional technologies in Section III.

Next up on the CR assessment framework (see Figure 11-1) is the competency level, which demonstrates whether student physical therapists are able to show how to do CR in a controlled representation of professional practice, such as in a simulated clinical environment. Standardized patients are individuals who have been trained to portray specific clinical cases in a standardized way.[48,49] They have been used in examinations to provide simulated clinical encounters,[6] which is a requirement for testing competency.[19] The author developed and examined an innovative assessment tool for the competency level.[16] This Think Aloud Standardized Patient Examination (TASPE) tool incorporates the think aloud method into a standardized patient examination to assess student physical therapists' CR competency.[6] The CR construct to be measured was defined as "the ability to think and make clinical decisions following a hypothetico-deductive reasoning model (novice approach) with the application of propositional knowledge."[16(p15)] The think aloud method asks individuals to verbalize their thinking underpinning a standardized patient encounter.[50] The think aloud method has been recognized as useful in understanding internal cognitive processes,[51] like the mostly invisible CR.[52]

When taking the TASPE, each student is required to examine a standardized patient and verbalize the cognitive processes for diagnostic and treatment decisions, with the performance scored by an onsite examiner. The examination was found to have a modest interrater reliability at the level of the think aloud item scores, and a high interrater reliability at the level of the total think aloud score in 3 of the 4 pairs of onsite and independent examiners. The ordinal alpha was 0.93, which demonstrated internal consistency of the examination. The students and onsite examiners appeared to support the usefulness of the examination. The TASPE was used to assess the CR competency of student physical therapists in the musculoskeletal domain. The transferability to other clinical domains has not been tested. Another limitation of the assessment tool originates from case specificity, which has been a concern among developers of case-based examinations in health professions education.[53] The implication of case specificity is that "a successful reasoning strategy in one situation may not apply in a second case, because the practitioner may not know enough about the area of the patient's problem."[54(p125)] To address the concern of case specificity, the author advocates combining and integrating assessment results from various levels of the assessment framework for a fuller understanding of an individual's CR. The use of the TASPE is further discussed with an application in an upcoming chapter.

The Objective Structured Clinical Examination (OSCE) may also serve as an assessment tool for the competency level, provided it has an explicit component of CR assessment. The examination includes a mixed circuit of short assessment stations that allow uniform testing of test takers for a wide range of clinical skills.[55] The examination typically makes use of standardized patients to allow clinical history, examination, and counseling sessions in the stations.[55] Park and colleagues[56] demonstrated that the OSCE score did not reflect medical students' CR abilities. The researchers further stated that the "OSCE (especially with a checklist scoring system) could not differentiate students who asked appropriate history questions with appropriate CR from others who asked history questions with insufficient CR."[56(p65)] The author argued that due to the invisibility of CR,[52] OSCE must include a written or verbal channel for the test takers to express their internal cognitive processes. The channel minimizes or even eliminates any needs to infer the examiners' thinking on the test takers based on the observed clinical performance.

The triple jump examination, which includes a case-based oral, written, and practical examination introduced by McMaster University in physiotherapy education, is another in-depth assessment method. It mimics real-world practice while going more in-depth with time and assessing all 3 learning domains to ensure understanding of the learners' CR processes. The triple jump is used frequently within problem-based learning programs and has been implemented in nearly all the health professions. The triple jump is usually somewhat time intensive, yet ensures higher-level learning assessment in all domains.

As we continue to move up the CR assessment framework (see Figure 11-1), we finally get to its top level. This performance level illustrates how student physical therapists perform or do CR during clinical education experiences in real-world situations. The assessment is done using direct observation by clinical instructors (CIs) and self-assessment by the student learners. The APTA PT CPI[13] is the standardized and widely used instrument assessing student physical therapists' clinical performance in the United States. CR is 1 of the 18 performance criteria and is a red flag foundational element of practice.

According to Christensen et al,[18] it lacks the detail and specificity for various aspects of CR. The APTA PT CPI provides a single rating of a student's CR based upon sample behaviors and a criterion-referenced rating scale with distinct measures of a student's performance considering the performance criteria of quality, consistency, efficiency, and effectiveness of performance, along with the amount of supervision required and caseload considerations. Additionally, each APTA PT CPI performance criteria rating requires both the rich narrative comments provided for further insight by the CI, along with the students' self-assessment. The APTA PT CPI instrument demonstrated construct validity and good internal consistency; its rater reliability was not examined.[14] Both students and instructors complete proficiency training, with competency of 85% or higher, to use and implement the standardized APTA PT CPI.[14] We will look further at the APTA PT CPI with several student and CI examples in Chapter 29.

Applications of the Clinical Reasoning Assessment Framework

The CR assessment framework can provide comprehensive assessments of CR at multiple points within a physical therapist education curriculum, as shown in Figure 11-2. The selection of these points depends on the assessment needs of the physical therapist education program. For instance, if the program is interested in finding out if its students are ready for the next clinical education experience, the program may want to undertake a comprehensive assessment of its students' CR prior to the experience by following the assessment framework to test and combine assessment results of the available levels. Other examples of time points are at the end of an academic year and at the time of graduation.

We can test and combine assessment results from different levels of the framework, as long as all test components are based on the same blueprint in terms of content knowledge and CR construct. For each didactic course series of the same clinical domain, the author recommends testing students at the bottom 3 levels: the knows, knows how, and competency levels. To make the testing more pragmatic, course instructors may consider reviewing and revising their current tests. For example, if multiple-choice or free-response examinations have been the primary testing instrument in the course series, instructors may want to evaluate the examination questions and make sure that they test students' knowledge base (the knows level) as well as ability to apply the accumulated knowledge (the knows how level). Ultimately, developing and adopting either SCTs or key features tests for assessing student physical therapists' CR at the knows how level is more ideal considering the validity and reliability of the 2 testing methods. Practical examinations are common in didactic course series of clinical domains. If a practical examination has been in place, course instructors may want to convert it to a TASPE, triple jump, or OSCE with an explicit component of CR assessment to test their students' CR at the competency level. Testing students at the bottom 3 levels within didactic course series of clinical domains may provide the course instructors better insights on the effectiveness of their andragogical approaches in facilitating CR. For example, if students do well at the knows level but do fairly or poorly at the knows how and competency levels, the instructors may need to reflect upon their andragogical approaches and consider adopting those that facilitate the development of CR at the higher levels.

Assessing students at the bottom 3 levels may also help the course instructors identify students who struggle with CR and the exact levels of any CR deficiency. The assessment findings may be useful in designing and delivering a "just-in-time" (timely and preferably before the students struggle with any other higher-level CR tests) and "just-for-you" (customized to the students' levels of CR deficiency) remediation to those in need. For students who struggle with CR for more than one level, it seems logical to put more focus on the lowest level of deficiency before or while addressing any higher levels during the remediation. When the remediation effort fails, the 3 systematic levels of assessment of CR may serve as a justified gatekeeper in preventing unprepared or underprepared students to manage patients safely in the real world, even with supervision.

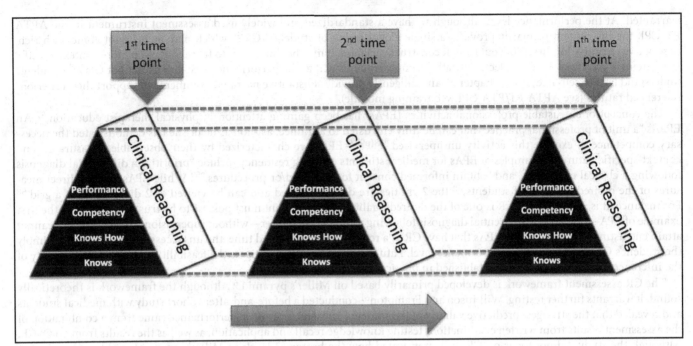

Figure 11-2. The progression of a physical therapist education curriculum.

To apply the CR assessment framework as described above, course instructors may need training and resources to revise and convert their current tests as well as to develop any new ones. It is not uncommon to have more than one instructor teaching a didactic course series of the same clinical domain. In that case, it is imperative for the instructors to collaborate with each other to develop a blueprint for the assessment of CR in the series despite the potential challenges of finding time to meet and building consensus.

Once students' CR has been evaluated at the bottom 3 levels of the CR assessment framework within individual didactic course series of the same clinical domains, education programs can obtain a more complete picture of students' CR by adding and integrating students' CR ratings from the APTA PT CPI (the performance, or top, level) to the findings of the bottom levels. Since CR cannot be measured independent of pertinent content knowledge,[20] all 4 levels of the CR assessment framework must be measured in the same clinical domain. In other words, the performance, or top, level must come from a clinical education experience that is embedded in the same clinical domain as the bottom 3 levels. The domain-specific and comprehensive (covering all 4 levels of the CR assessment framework) review of CR may provide invaluable inputs to the education programs. For instance, the review may prompt the programs to examine whether their didactic component and clinical education program are sufficient and appropriate in enhancing students' CR, and to contemplate what changes may need to be implemented from a programmatic or curricular viewpoint.

The aggregate results of the 4 levels also provide a 360-degree assessment of students' CR, as the results come from multiple assessors such as the didactic course instructors, the CIs, and the students themselves. If multiple physical therapist education programs adopt the CR assessment framework, the aggregate results can be compared across the programs. Notwithstanding the benefits of applying the CR assessment framework, integrating the CR findings of the 4 levels may not be straightforward. For each clinical education experience, students are likely exposed to patients of more than one clinical domain. In that case, education programs may need to set some criteria to determine the primary clinical domain before matching the clinical domain between the performance level and that of the bottom 3 levels. In addition, while students in the same cohort typically take the didactic course series of the same clinical domain at the same time, they are usually not exposed to patients of the same clinical domains within the same phase of their clinical education. This implies the work of integrating the CR ratings from the APTA PT CPI (the performance level) to those of the bottom 3 levels needs to be done for students on an individual basis.

Future Developments

The CR assessment framework can serve as a roadmap giving us directions to assess student physical therapists' CR. In addition to the map, we need quality vehicles—valid and reliable assessment tools established for specific clinical domains and each level of the framework. There are particular needs at the competency and performance levels in terms of developing assessment tools. TASPE[16] is the only assessment tool established for testing student physical therapists' CR at the competency level. Its application has been tested in the musculoskeletal domain alone. Further testing of the TASPE in other clinical domains is warranted. At the performance level, although we have a standardized and widely used assessment instrument in the APTA PT CPI, the instrument primarily provides a single global rating of students' CR,[18] which may or may not come with rich, descriptive narrative for dissecting out the CR construct variables. It may be time for us to further develop more context-specific measurements that may better reflect, indicate, or imply students' CR at the performance level or ensure that CIs and students understand how to self-assess (see Chapter 3), and diligently provide substantive narrative comments to support their criterion-referenced ratings (see APTA PT/PTA CPI web training module).

The concept of entrustable professional activities (EPAs) has been gaining attention in physical therapist education.[57] An EPA is "a unit of professional practice that can be fully entrusted to a trainee, as soon as he or she has demonstrated the necessary competence to execute this activity unsupervised."[58(p983)] EPAs are characterized by their observable, measurable, and context-specific nature.[58] Examples of EPAs for medical students entering residency include "prioritize a differential diagnosis following a clinical encounter" and "obtain informed consent for tests and/or procedures."[59] While EPAs are not direct measures of the desired qualities of students,[60] the 2 entities are directly related and can be viewed as 2 dimensions of a grid.[58] For instance, it is apparent that CR is one of the desired qualities that a student must possess to be trusted to perform the first example of EPA—prioritize a differential diagnosis following a clinical encounter—without supervision. When a student cannot attain entrustment in one or more EPAs that have CR as a requisite at an expected time, the unsuccessful attainment may imply the student's CR deficiency at the performance level. Future studies should investigate the feasibility, validity, and reliability of the inference when EPAs have been established in physical therapist education.

The CR assessment framework is developed primarily based on Miller's pyramid.[6] Although the framework is theoretically sound, it warrants further testing. Wilkinson and Frampton[61] conducted a before-and-after cohort study with medical students and revealed that the strongest predictive validity of the students' subsequent clinical performance came from a combination of the assessment results from written examinations testing knowledge recall and application, as well as the results from an OSCE. Although the study did not focus on CR, it demonstrated how the bottom 3 levels of Miller's pyramid could predict the top level. Since "prediction is one of the major roles of assessment,"[62(p103)] a study on the predictive validity of the CR assessment framework is warranted. Such a study might find out if the assessment framework could fulfill the role of prediction.

CONCLUSION

CR is a complex, critical, but challenging educational outcome to assess. To overcome the challenge, we need to group and organize our effort from the level of education programs to that of individual courses. More important, we need a roadmap that can help us navigate through the complexity. This chapter describes a 4-level CR assessment framework developed by the author to guide the assessment of student physical therapists' CR in entry-level education. The framework can serve as our roadmap and direct us on how to operationalize the overall assessment, what assessment tools we need, and how to interpret and integrate the assessment findings to gain a more comprehensive understanding of the educational outcome. This, in turn, can help us make informed decisions on students' educational performance outcomes and determine the need for remediation. The framework can also act as a common language for all parties involved to communicate as they share and concert their effort in embracing the challenge.

In designing a new course or revising an existing course with CR as an educational outcome, physical therapy faculty may want to consider using the CR assessment framework to guide the overall assessment plan and the selection of assessment tools. When a student struggles with achieving the expected level of CR in a certain clinical domain, physical therapy faculty may want to review the student's assessment findings at different levels of the assessment framework within the domain to identify any level-specific deficiencies that require remediation. When CR is recognized as a curricular thread, the assessment framework can be used to guide the assessment of the thread with data tracked over time in different clinical domains.

Reflection Moment

How will we—as learners, educators, peers, and faculty—incorporate the new knowledge learned from this chapter to enhance students' CR? What did you find most interesting from your chapter reading, and why?

How can we make use of the CR assessment framework and its assessment findings in designing a new course or revising one with CR as an educational outcome?

Describe how using the CR assessment framework and its assessment findings may be helpful for student remediation and/or self-learning and reflection.

How can we make use of the CR assessment framework and its assessment findings for a programmatic or curricular review?

REFERENCES

1. Edwards I, Jones M, Carr J, Braunack-Mayer A, Jensen GM. Clinical reasoning strategies in physical therapy. *Phys Ther*. 2004;84(4):312-330.
2. American Physical Therapy Association. *A Normative Model of Physical Therapist Professional Education*. Alexandria, VA: American Physical Therapy Association; 2004.
3. Commission on Accreditation in Physical Therapy Education. Standards and required elements for accreditation of physical therapist education programs. http://www.capteonline.org/uploadedfiles/capteorg/about_capte/resources/accreditation_handbook/capte_ptstandardsevidence.pdf. Accessed May 1, 2019.
4. Higgs J, Jones MA. Clinical decision making and multiple problem spaces. In: Higgs J, Jones MA, Loftus S, Christensen N, eds. *Clinical Reasoning in the Health Professions*. 3rd ed. Amsterdam, Netherlands: Butterworth-Heinemann Elsevier; 2008:3-17.
5. Pearce J, Edwards D, Fraillon J, et al. The rationale for and use of assessment frameworks: improving assessment and reporting quality in medical education. *Perspect Med Educ*. 2015;4:110-118.
6. Miller GE. The assessment of clinical skills/competence/performance. *Acad Med*. 1990;65(9):S63-S67.
7. Wiliam D. Assessment: the bridge between teaching and learning. *Voices from the Middle*. 2013;21(2):15-20.
8. Epstein RM. Assessment in medical education. *N Engl J Med*. 2007;356:387-396.
9. Papadakis MA, Teherani A, Banach MA, et al. Disciplinary action by medical boards and prior behavior in medical school. *N Engl J Med*. 2005;353(25):2673-2682.
10. Carr SE, Celenza A, Puddey IB, Lake F. Relationships between academic performance of medical students and their workplace performance as junior doctors. *BMC Med Educ*. 2014;14:157.
11. Epstein RM, Hundert EM. Defining and assessing professional competence. *JAMA*. 2002;287(2):226-235.
12. The American Council of Academic Physical Therapy. Clinical reasoning curricula and assessment consortium. http://www.acapt.org/about/consortium-2/clinical-reasoning-curricula-assessment. Accessed August 13, 2016.
13. American Physical Therapy Association. *Physical Therapist Clinical Performance Instrument*. Alexandria, VA: American Physical Therapy Association. http://www.apta.org/PTCPI/. Published 2006. Accessed December 1, 2016.
14. Roach KE, Frost JS, Francis NJ, et al. Validation of the revised physical therapist clinical performance instrument (PT CPI): version 2006. *Phys Ther*. 2012;92(3):416-428.
15. Middle States Commission on Higher Education. Student learning assessment: options and resources: 2007. http://msche.org/publications/SLA_Book_0808080728085320.pdf. Accessed July 2, 2012.
16. Fu W. Development of an innovative tool to assess student physical therapists' clinical reasoning competency. *J Phys Ther Ed*. 2015;29(4):14-26.
17. Furze J, Gale JR, Black L, Cochran TM, Jensen G. Clinical reasoning: development of a grading rubric for student assessment. *J Phys Ther Ed*. 2015;29(3):34-45.
18. Christensen N, Black L, Furze J, et al. Clinical reasoning: survey of teaching methods, integration, and assessment in entry-level physical therapist academic education. *Phys Ther*. 2017;97(2):175-182.
19. Rethans J-J, Noraini JJ, Barón-Maldonado M, et al. The relationship between competence and performance: implications for assessing practice performance. *Med Educ*. 2002;36:901-909.
20. van der Vleuten CPM, Norman G, Schuwirth L. Assessing clinical reasoning. In: Higgs J, Jones MA, Loftus S, Christensen N, eds. *Clinical Reasoning in the Health Professions*. 3rd ed. Amsterdam, Netherlands: Butterworth-Heinemann Elsevier; 2008:413-421.
21. Brame C. Writing good multiple choice test questions. Vanderbilt University: Center for Teaching. https://cft.vanderbilt.edu/guides-sub-pages/writing-good-multiple-choice-test-questions/. Accessed December 3, 2016.
22. Damjanov I, Fenderson BA, Veloski JJ, Rubin E. Testing of medical students with open-ended, uncued questions. *Hum Pathol*. 1995;26(4):362-365.
23. Watters A. Multiple choice and testing machines: a history. Hack Education. http://hackeducation.com/2015/01/27/multiple-choice-testing-machines. Accessed December 3, 2016.
24. McCoubrie P. Improving the fairness of multiple-choice questions: a literature review. *Med Teach*. 2004;26(8):709-712.
25. Weimer M. Advantages and disadvantages of different types of test questions. Faculty Focus. http://www.facultyfocus.com/articles/educational-assessment/advantages-and-disadvantages-of-different-types-of-test-questions/. Accessed December 5, 2016.
26. Dory V, Gagnon R, Vanpee D, Charlin B. How to construct and implement script concordance tests: insights from a systematic review. *Med Educ*. 2012;46:552-563.
27. Elstein AS. Beyond multiple-choice questions and essays: the need for a new way to assess clinical competence. *Acad Med*. 1993;68(4):244-249.
28. Fournier JP, Demeester A, Charlin B. Script concordance tests: guidelines for construction. *BMC Med Inform Decis Mak*. 2008;8(18):1-7.
29. Page G, Bordage G, Allen T. Developing key-features problems and examinations to assess clinical decision-making skills. *Acad Med*. 1995;70(3):194-201.
30. Farmer EA, Page G. A practical guide to assessing clinical decision-making skills using the key features approach. *Med Educ*. 2005;39(12):1188-1194.
31. Round J, Conrad E, Poulton T. Improving assessment with virtual patients. *Med Teach*. 2009;31:759-763.
32. Harden R. Preparation and presentation of patient-management problems (PMPs). *Med Educ*. 1983;17(4):256-276.
33. Normam G, Feightner J. A comparison of behaviour on simulated patients and patient management problems. *Med Educ*. 1981;15(1):26-32.
34. Groves M, Scott I, Alexander H. Assessing clinical reasoning: a method to monitor its development in a PBL curriculum. *Med Teach*. 2002;24(5):507-515.

35. Lubarsky S, Charlin B, Cook DA, Chalk C, van der Vleuten C. Script concordance testing: a review of published validity evidence. *Med Educ.* 2011;45:329-338.

36. Kelly W, Durning S, Denton G. Comparing a script concordance examination to a multiple-choice examination on a core internal medicine clerkship. *Teach Learn Med.* 2012;24(3):187-193.

37. Dawson T, Comer L, Kossick M, Neubrander J. Can script concordance testing be used in nursing education to accurately assess clinical reasoning skills? *J Nurs Educ.* 2014;53(5):281-286.

38. Page G, Bordage G. The Medical Council of Canada's key features project: a more valid written examination of clinical decision-making skills. *Acad Med.* 1995;70(2):104-110.

39. Guidelines for the development of key feature problems and test cases. Medical Council of Canada. http://mcc.ca/wp-content/uploads/cdm-guidelines.pdf. Accessed December 5, 2016.

40. Hrynchak P, Takahashi SG, Nayer M. Key-feature questions for assessment of clinical reasoning: a literature review. *Med Educ.* 2014;48:870-883.

41. Monnier P, Bédard MJ, Gagnon R, Charlin B. The relationship between script concordance test scores in an obstetrics-gynecology rotation and global performance assessments in the curriculum. *Int J Med Educ.* 2011;2:3-6.

42. Gesundheit N, Brutlag P, Youngblood P, et al. The use of virtual patients to assess the clinical skills and reasoning of medical students: initial insights on student acceptance. *Med Teach.* 2009;31:739-742.

43. Cook DA, Triola MM. Virtual patients: a critical literature review and proposed next steps. *Med Educ.* 2009;43:303-311.

44. VirtualPT Clinician. DxR Development Group. http://www.dxrgroup.com/products/virtualpt-clinician/. Accessed December 10, 2016.

45. VirtualPT Clinician. Instructor manual. DxR Development Group. http://dxrgroup.com/dxronline/downloads/virtualPT_docs/VirtualPTInstrMan.pdf. Accessed December 10, 2016.

46. Huhn K, Deutsch JE. Development and assessment of a web-based patient simulation program. *J Phys Ther Ed.* 2011;25(1):5-10.

47. Huang G, Reynolds R, Candler C. Virtual patient simulation at US and Canadian medical schools. *Acad Med.* 2007;82(5):446-451.

48. Barrows HS. An overview of the uses of standardized patients for teaching and evaluating clinical skills. *Acad Med.* 1993;68(6):443-451.

49. Brender E, Burke A, Glass R. Standardized patients. *JAMA.* 2005;294(9):1172.

50. Elstein AS, Kagan N, Shulman LS, Jason H, Loupe MJ. Methods and theory in the study of medical inquiry. *J Med Educ.* 1972;47:85-92.

51. van Someren MW, Barnard YF, Sandberg JAC. The think aloud method. In: Barnard YF, Sandberg JAC, van Someren MW, eds. *The Think Aloud Method: A Practical Guide to Modelling Cognitive Processes.* London, United Kingdom: Academic Press; 1994:29-40.

52. Higgs J, Trede F, Loftus S, et al. Advancing clinical reasoning: interpretive research perspectives grounded in professional practice, CPEA, occasional paper 4. *Collaborations in Practice and Education Advancement.* Sydney, Australia: The University of Sydney; 2006.

53. Schwartz A, Elstein AS. Clinical reasoning in medicine. In: Higgs J, Jones MA, Loftus S, Christensen N, eds. *Clinical Reasoning in the Health Professions.* 3rd ed. Amsterdam, Netherlands: Butterworth-Heinemann Elsevier; 2008:223-234.

54. Jensen G, Resnik L, Haddad A. Expertise and clinical reasoning. In: Higgs J, Jones MA, Loftus S, Christensen N, eds. *Clinical Reasoning in the Health Professions.* 3rd ed. Amsterdam, Netherlands: Butterworth-Heinemann Elsevier; 2008:123-135.

55. Zayyan M. Objective structured clinical examination: the assessment of choice. *Oman Med J.* 2011;26(4):219-222.

56. Park WB, Kang SH, Lee Y-S, Myung SJ. Does objective structured clinical examination score reflect the clinical reasoning ability of medical students? *Am J Med Sci.* 2015;350(1):64-67.

57. Jensen GM, Nordstrom T, Segal RL, et al. Education research in physical therapy: visions of the possible. *J Phys Ther Ed.* 2016;96(12):1874-1884.

58. Cate OT, Chen HC, Hoff RG, et al. Curriculum development for the workplace using entrustable professional activities (EPAs): AMEE guide no. 99. *Med Teach.* 2015;37(11):983-1002.

59. Englander R, Flynn T, Call S, et al. Toward defining the foundation of the MD degree: core entrustable professional activities for entering residency. *Acad Med.* 2016;91(10):1352-1358.

60. Clardy P, Schwartzstein R. Considering cognition. Current challenges and future directions in pulmonary and critical care fellowship training. *Ann Am Thorac Soc.* 2015;12(4):474-479.

61. Wilkinson TJ, Frampton CM. Comprehensive undergraduate medical assessments improve prediction of clinical performance. *Med Educ.* 2004;38(10):1111-1116.

62. Hamdy H, Prasad K, Anderson M, et al. BEME systematic review: predictive values of measurements obtained in medical schools and future performance in medical practice. *Med Teach.* 2006;28(2):103-106.

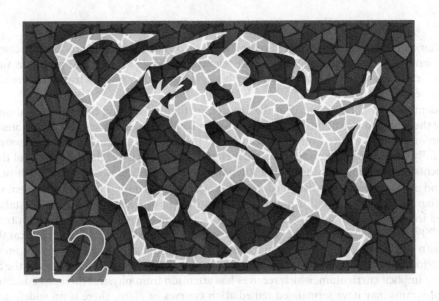

USING A STRUCTURED AND EVIDENCE-BASED APPROACH TO REMEDIATE CLINICAL REASONING:
A Case Report Summary

Wing Fu, PT, PhD, MA

OBJECTIVES

After completing this chapter, you will be able to:

- Describe the educational diagnose-and-treat approach.
- Identify the domains and subdomains in the remediation assessment framework.
- Explain how to use the remediation assessment framework to investigate the specific remediation needs of students with clinical reasoning (CR) deficits.
- Explain how to design and customize an evidence-based educational intervention for students struggling with CR.

INTRODUCTION

Remediation is a critical and challenging undertaking in physical therapist education. Many physical therapist education programs provide remediation to struggling students, as they are required to support student retention and progression through the program[1]; however, little is found in the peer-reviewed literature describing the approaches taken or instructional strategies used for the remediation. The undertaking may be even more challenging when a student needs to be remediated in a hard-to-teach and hard-to-learn area, such as CR.[2]

This chapter describes a case study evaluating and remediating an entry-level doctor of physical therapy (DPT) student who failed a didactic course due to CR deficits. The author used an educational diagnose-and-treat method[3] to assess the needs of

Musolino GM, Jensen GM, eds. *Clinical Reasoning and Decision-Making in Physical Therapy: Facilitation, Assessment, and Implementation* (pp 143-155).
© 2020 Taylor & Francis Group.

the learner and to design and carry out a customized remediation plan. The diagnostic process was composed of an in-depth interview with the student, as well as a thorough review of relevant academic records and pertinent supplemental data. The interview followed a structured assessment framework, which was developed to guide a more comprehensive investigation of the student's specific remediation needs.

Excerpts of the student interview are included in the chapter, further illustrating the educational diagnostic process. The author also shares how she designed a customized remediation plan for the student to address the greatest learning deficit. The remediation plan was informed by evidence from the literature and the data collected following the assessment framework, with practical implications fully considered. To conclude the chapter, the author discusses the limitations of the case study and proposes future developments to help remediate the willing students who need dedicated educators the most.

Physical therapist and physical therapist assistant education programs are required to support student retention and progression throughout the program.[1,4] Remediation[1] is one method identified to provide support for high stakes, professional learners. It has been defined in medical education as "the process of facilitating corrections for physician trainees who are not on course to competence."[5(p787)] The definition applies readily for student physical therapists and physical therapists assistants in need of remediation, with outstanding competency standards to meet,[6] who may struggle along with professional practice and patient management performance development. Despite the ongoing need for providing remediation, the associated policies are recognized as part of the implicit curriculum, which receives less attention from physical therapist education programs.[7] While individual education programs may have formalized remediation courses or plans, there is no widely accepted framework or approach for providing remediation. Often times, remediation is carried out in a customized and individualistic approach based on learners' needs, or by simply repeating material without any customization available in the lock-step curriculum.

CR is a vital component of professional competency for clinicians.[8] The American Physical Therapy Association recognizes the importance of CR and specifies CR as an educational outcome for graduates of physical therapist education programs.[1,9] CR is one of the most common deficiencies noted in medical education.[10,11] It would not be surprising to find a similar pattern in student physical therapist population. The speculation is more convincing taking into account that even novice practicing physical therapists were found to have limited CR skills.[12] CR is a complex and multifaceted phenomenon that permeates throughout clinical practice.[13] The inherent complexity, as well as the breadth and depth of the phenomenon, may make CR difficult to understand and be fully appreciated by students and even educators until called into practice with real-world patients. CR is mostly invisible.[14] The invisibility makes CR not easily accessible to students, and therefore reduces students' chance to learn CR from others. Educators may find CR hard to teach[2] because of the difficulty of professionals in articulating their thought processes, especially when they use pattern recognition—the fast and experience-based CR.[15] Moreover, some CR thought processes may be clinical shortcuts and developmentally inappropriate for students to learn.[16]

According to Healthcare Providers Service Organization, the average indemnity payment for the closed claims involving physical therapists has been on an upward trend from 2001 to 2014 (the latest reported year).[17] The trend was associated with a significant hike of the percentage of costlier claims, which were filed due to severe and irreversible harm to patients. Underperforming physical therapy professionals may lead to consequences that neither our profession nor our patients can afford. Hence, we need to focus on reducing the number of underachieving students in entry-level programs. The advocated reduction is based on the evidence from Carr et al,[18] who performed a descriptive cohort study with 200 research participants and found that academic performance of medical students (both the overall grade point average in an undergraduate 6-year medical program and the score from the emergency medical attachment in the final year of the program) predicted their workplace performance as junior doctors. The workplace performance was measured by a junior doctor assessment tool developed and validated in western Australia to assess junior doctors' performance in the first 2 post-graduate years.[19]

Some may argue that we do not need to worry about the possibility of underachieving students becoming underperforming practitioners because those students are unlikely to graduate from the education programs. Even after they graduate, they would have a hard time passing the National Physical Therapy Examination (NPTE). However, the following data may suggest the opposite. The graduation rate from the Commission on Accreditation in Physical Therapy Education (CAPTE) programs has been high, with the average rate from 91.9% to 96.1% in the 3 most recently reported years (2012 to 2014).[20] Guerrasio et al[21] conducted a survey and discovered an unfortunate "failure to fail" phenomenon. The survey was sent to the student affairs deans or the equivalent at 48 randomly selected health professions schools across the United States. The majority of the respondents agreed that "their institution or other institutions that grant the same degree had graduated students who should not have graduated."[21(p801)] The author speculates that physical therapist education programs might have also experienced the failure to fail phenomenon, especially taking the high graduation rate into account. Similar to the graduation rate, the ultimate pass rate of the NPTE among graduates of the CAPTE-accredited physical therapist education programs has been consistently high, with recently reported graduation years (2011 to 2014) at the 99% level.[22] Given these graduation and ultimate pass rates, it is logical to deduce that once a student is accepted and enrolled into a CAPTE-accredited education program, he or she has a high chance of being a candidate for the NPTE and becoming eligible for obtaining a license, which entitles the individual to manage many patients in his or her career. To protect the public, it is therefore important for physical therapy educators to contemplate on, reflect upon, and make any necessary changes to how we teach, assess, and remediate every critical component of professional competency, including CR.[8] The aim is to minimize the number of underachieving students, who may become underperforming health care professionals after they graduate.

The planned class size and the number of enrolled students among the CAPTE-accredited physical therapist education programs have shown an upward pattern over the past 7 reported years, with a recent drastic rise.[20] The rise heightens the concern of whether we have an adequate number of qualified students to fill the seats in all our programs. For medical education that was projected to have an expansion in enrollment, Cooper stated that "unless a pool of young people who do not now seek medical education materializes, there will be too few applicants in 2015 and the years thereafter to sustain quality as it is now measured."[23(p534)] If the expanded class size in physical therapy leads to an insufficiency of qualified students, we may face an increased absolute number and a higher percentage of weak students enrolled in physical therapy programs. Composite American College Testing score and prerequisite grade point averages were shown to have a positive correlation with academic achievement in physical therapy, NPTE score, and job performance.[24] The job performance was graded by the graduates' supervisors at approximately 6 months after the initial employment date and evaluated in areas including their critical thinking and problem-solving ability. Although American College Testing score is no longer an admission criterion for most, if not all, physical therapist education programs, the study revealed the potential negative impact of enrolling weak students on the quality of future patient care. The upward trend in physical therapy enrollment may therefore require us to put more attention and effort into creating a structured, effective, and efficient system to identify and, more importantly, remediate any struggling students.

The focus of Chapter 12 is on addressing the remediation of student physical therapists' CR within the didactic curriculum. Literature describing how to structure and implement the remediation of CR, regardless of the didactic or clinical setting, is limited.[3,25-28] In addition, the remediation of CR faces barriers for implementation. Guerrasio and colleagues[29] reported that remediation of medical learners' CR required an average of 20 hours of faculty face time, excluding the time for planning, assessment, or preparation. The average face time was the longest among the time spent on the 10 studied types of learner deficits, which included medical knowledge, clinical skills, time management and organization, professionalism, interpersonal skills, communication, practice-based learning and improvement, system-based practice, and mental well-being, in addition to CR.

Aside from time, remediation requires special knowledge and skills. Although educators may be able to reason through patient cases without any difficulties, they may not know how to identify, analyze, and help correct students' CR deficits. They also may not be familiar with the educational theories and literature that provide guidance for the remediation. Even among the individuals responsible for remediation at medical schools, study respondents' answer to the statement, "I am confident in our ability to remediate CR deficits," was, on average, below the Likert scale rating "agree" level.[25] Notwithstanding the barriers, it is time to advocate for and embark on the journey toward establishing an optimal and pragmatic approach to remediate student physical therapists' CR.

The author will now share her case experience in using a structured and practical approach to assess the needs for remediation and to develop a customized remediation plan for a DPT student who struggled with CR. The student provided full authorization and permission to share the de-identified case information. The author used an educational diagnose-and-treat approach, which was inspired and partly guided by the work of Guerrasio.[3]

Case Description

David (a pseudonym) was a student physical therapist attending a CAPTE-accredited physical therapy doctorate program, in which the author worked as a faculty member. David failed a didactic course in the third semester of Year 1 in the 3-year program and was required to "sit out" of the program for a year before retaking the failed course. The didactic course required students to pass a case-based practical examination, which incorporated a think aloud component to test students' CR. The think aloud component required each student, based upon the case description and the patient's medical history (collected from a patient intake form and the supplemental onsite patient interview) to determine if the physical therapy interventions (covered in the didactic course) specified for the case were indicated or not, and verbalize the associated CR thought processes.

The grading rubric of the think aloud component is included in Figure 12-1. The rubric was slightly modified from another think aloud assessment tool that the author developed and examined for testing student physical therapists' CR.[30] The think aloud method was also advocated for teaching and assessing CR in graduate medical education.[31] Students taking the case-based practical examination were graded on the appropriateness of their thought processes and not the determination of indication or contraindication alone. All grading was done by an onsite examiner and consented to by 2 other physical therapy faculty members associated with the didactic course to ensure its consistency and fairness across the entire class of students. David failed the didactic course because he did not pass the practical examination after 3 attempts, with a different patient case of the same content areas and level of challenge each time. He performed particularly poorly on the think aloud, oral CR component during all 3 attempts.

continued

The author reached out to David, one semester prior to his returning to the program. At that time, David had already sat out of the program for 2 semesters, during which he had not prepared for his return. The author met with David and explained the purpose of the remediation: to improve his chance for success in the physical therapist education program. She introduced David to the educational diagnose-and-treat approach[3] that would be adopted in the remediation process, and emphasized the importance of David's taking initiatives and getting involved in the process. David appeared enthusiastic about the opportunity of receiving remediation before retaking the failed course. The meeting ended with a scheduled time between the author and David for an in-depth interview, which was part of the educational diagnose-and-treat method.[3] The author was aware of the general lack of resources for student remediation. She kept track of the resources used, including time spent and monetary compensation, as a means to measure the cost of this individual student remediation process.

Figure 12-1. Grading rubric of the practical examination (think aloud component only).

Scores	Achievement Level	Performance Criteria
5	Complete	Correctly justifies using all available accurate and relevant information. Contains no irrelevant information.
3	Partial	Correctly justifies using mostly all available accurate and relevant information. Contains no irrelevant information.
0	Absent	Incorrectly justifies lacking accuracy in use of available relevant information. Contains irrelevant information.

Activity	Assigned Score (Refer to the above table for the performance criteria)	Comments
Synthesizes Medical History Appropriately: ⅄ Verbalizes and provides rationale why modality IS or IS NOT indicated for the case ⅄ Verbally indicates if treatment will continue with use of modality	5 3 0	

THE REMEDIATION ASSESSMENT FRAMEWORK

The author developed a remediation assessment framework to systematically investigate the remediation needs of individual students who struggle with CR. The author shared the framework with 2 experienced physical therapy faculty members, incorporated feedback from them, and finalized the framework before using it with David. The framework was used to guide an in-depth interview of David, with the interview in turn directing the collection of pertinent information from other sources.

The framework encompasses 4 domains: knowledge, communication, academic skills and support, and personal factors. The first 2 domains are related to the development or presentation of student physical therapists' CR. The last 2 domains are more general and primarily related to academic success and the pursuit of it. Each domain is further divided into subdomains, as shown in Table 12-1. We will review the evidence supporting the inclusion of the 4 domains in the remediation assessment framework and the background information related to the division of each domain into its subdomains.

First, let's look at the knowledge domain. Jensen et al[32] illustrated the importance of knowledge in expert physical therapist practice. Student physical therapists also perceived the application of knowledge as part of CR.[33] The perceived application is consistent with the findings of Anderson,[34] who employed both qualitative and quantitative research methods to investigate the development of undergraduate medical students' CR ability. The qualitative data revealed that the medical students recognized the importance of having knowledge to reason clinically. The quantitative data supported the qualitative finding with a positive statistical correlation shown between the students' knowledge level and their CR ability. The statistical association was again positive and even larger when studying the relationship between the students' CR ability and the level of knowledge they could apply to patient cases.

TABLE 12-1	
THE REMEDIATION ASSESSMENT FRAMEWORK	
DOMAINS	**SUBDOMAINS**
Knowledge	Factual
	Conceptual
	Procedural
	Metacognitive
Communication	Verbal
	Nonverbal
Academic skills and support	Information organization
	Planning processing
	Time management
	Support system
Personal factors	Health (physical and mental)
	Motivation
	Relationship
	Finance

When the author developed the remediation assessment framework, she included the knowledge domain based on the above evidence, and further divided knowledge into 4 subdomains: factual, conceptual, procedural, and metacognitive, according to the revised Bloom's taxonomy.[35] Factual knowledge refers to the basic elements and essential facts of a discipline. Conceptual knowledge covers the interrelationships among the basic elements that allow them to function together within a larger structure. Procedural knowledge includes the knowledge of subject-specific skills and techniques as well as the criteria for determining when to apply them. In the author's point of view, both conceptual knowledge and procedural knowledge encompass not just knowledge, but also include the application of knowledge. Metacognitive knowledge is the knowledge of one's own thinking. Since reflection practice is probably the teaching and learning strategy that has the most evidence supporting its effect in enhancing student physical therapists' CR development,[33,36,37] metacognitive knowledge needs to be evaluated when assessing the remediation needs of students with CR deficits.

Communication is the second domain. As CR is mostly invisible,[14] we cannot fully understand an individual's CR without that person communicating his or her internal thought processes with us. Student physical therapists perceived that through CR, "they could justify their clinical decisions to themselves, their clinical instructors, and their patients."[33(p239)] The justification can be communicated in verbal and/or nonverbal formats. Each format is therefore one subdomain. In David's case, he was expected to use the verbal form of communication to demonstrate his CR during the think aloud component of the practical examination. The author decided to make communication a distinct domain because a student may appear to have CR deficits even when the problem is in communication alone (eg, suffering an expressive deficit, communication fears). The distinction is helpful for any "treatment" purposes and/or identification of other learning, medical, or psychological needs that may or may not have been identified.

The third domain is composed of academic skills and support. In describing characteristics of failing medical students, Mcloughlin[38] identified a few skills more directly associated with the students' efficiency and accuracy in managing academic and clinical tasks. The author decided to incorporate 2 academic skills from the literature—information organization and planning processing—into the domain of academic skills and support as subdomains. Information organization refers to how an individual approaches, arranges, prioritizes, and stores information. It impacts knowledge organization, which is critical to health profession education and at the foundation of CR.[39] Planning processing is defined as how an individual plans and decides to solve problems and the proficiency in solving them.

Other than the 2 identified academic skills, the author selected time management and support system as additional subdomains. Time management was chosen for its potential relationship with student physical therapists' academic performance. College students' self-perceived time management behaviors correlate positively with their self-reported academic performances.[40] Support systems encompass the academic support students have and make use of from faculty, peers, and other resources.

The fourth domain is personal factors, which may impact students' ability and/or desire to pursue academic success and become physical therapists. It has 4 subdomains: health (physical and mental), motivation, relationship, and finance. Health is 1 of the 4 subdomains because of its proven relationship with academic performance. Ansari and Stock[41] studied 380 university students in the United Kingdom and found that those students feeling better general healthwise were more likely to rate their academic performance as being better than their peers. The study also explored the relationships between educational outcomes and factors like health complaints and health behaviors. The health complaint of higher frequency of sleep disorders or insomnia was negatively associated with students' actual achieved grades.[41] Likewise, there was a negative association between alcohol bingeing and the actual achieved grades.[41]

Ruthig et al[42] investigated 203 undergraduate students in the United States and supported the aforementioned association in female students alone. They demonstrated that decreased engagement in binge drinking predicted significantly higher final course grades in the female students (n = 140). Among the male students (n = 63), lower final course grades were predicted by increased tobacco use. With regard to mental health, undergraduate student physical therapists in Turkey were found to have a high prevalence of anxiety (40.5%; n = 64) and depression (18.9%; n = 30) when compared to the general population.[43] It is reasonable to believe that the student physical therapist population in the United States also presents with a high prevalence of mental health issues, especially considering the high academic standards and rigor the student population faces in clinical doctorate programs. Mental health is related to academic performance. Andrews and Wilding[44] showed that depression was significantly related to the subsequent examination performance in university students in the United Kingdom.

Motivation is another subdomain under the domain of personal factors. The selection of motivation is supported by the evidence that there was a significant correlation between school motivation and academic performance (average scores on basic sciences and clinical courses) demonstrated in 344 medical students in Iran.[45]

The final 2 subdomains—relationship and finance—were chosen because both relationship difficulties (eg, separation in steady relationships, serious problems with a close relationship) and financial difficulties (eg, major financial crisis, not being able to afford essential items) experienced by university students were significantly related to their becoming anxious.[44] Financial difficulties were demonstrated to have a significant correlation with the subsequent examination performance.[44]

The author followed the remediation assessment framework to assess and educationally "diagnose" David's case. The significant findings are elaborated in the following section.

THE EDUCATIONAL DIAGNOSTIC PROCESS

The educational diagnostic process was triangulated. It started with an in-depth interview of David, and continued by following the lead of the interview to search and review other relevant records or data. The author carried the roles of a diagnostician, a facilitator, and a helper, but not a grader.

The author followed the approach of Guerrasio[3] and explained to David that she would not share the details from the interview with the physical therapy department chair or other faculty in the department, but would provide them with summarized reports of the remediation process. The goal of the remediation was to "target and fix the greatest deficit"[3(p75)]: the single deficit that is believed to yield the greatest return from the remediation effort. The author also asked David to recognize the interview as a self-assessment and to try to discover more about himself. The interview took 2 hours. It was the first time the author had performed such an interview. The lack of experience from the author's end might have attributed to the length of time of the interview.

Terminologies that might be new to David (eg, factual knowledge and conceptual knowledge) were explained to him prior to asking the related questions. Excerpts of the interview that are deemed helpful in the educational diagnostic process are included below. The author started the interview with questions pertaining to the first domain (knowledge).

Author/Faculty: What do you think about your factual knowledge?

David: For everyone, factual knowledge is the easiest type. Not everyone has the best memory. If you don't use it every day, it's not going to be there.

Author/Faculty: Do you think your factual knowledge has anything to do with the course you failed?

David: Not really. ... I did well on the written tests. ...

The author checked David's written test performances in the course he failed. David did well on the quizzes, with his grades typically well above the mean grades of the class. However, his performances on the midterm and final written examinations were below the class means. The quizzes had more recall-type questions, while the examinations had more questions testing the application of knowledge. Similarly, a review of David's transcript revealed that he did better in courses that rely more on memorization (eg, anatomy), and struggled more in courses that require understanding of concepts (eg, kinesiology).

After asking about the factual knowledge, the author continued the interview.

Author/Faculty: What do you think about your conceptual knowledge?

David: I can always have improvements in making the connections. We went through the massage part very fast in the modalities course [the course David did not pass]. Obviously we didn't have time to go through every single procedure. We were doing stuff on the back and just the back. ... I feel like I need demonstrations on everything. Just like [showing me] what we did on the back to the forearm.

TABLE 12-2
DATA SOURCES EXPLORED UNDER EVERY DOMAIN AND SUBDOMAIN

DOMAINS	SUBDOMAINS	DATA SOURCES					
		Student Interview	Instructor Interview	Exam and Quiz Questions	Exam and Quiz Performances	Transcript	Practical Exam Performances (Videos)
Knowledge	Factual	X		X	X	X	
	Conceptual	X	X	X	X	X	
	Procedural	X					
	Metacognitive	X					
Communication	Verbal	X					
	Nonverbal (not explored)						
Academic skills and support	Information organization	X					X
	Planning processing	X	X				X
	Time management	X					
	Support system	X					
Personal factors	Health (physical and mental)	X					
	Motivation	X					
	Relationship	X					
	Finance	X					

At first glance, the response from David may not sound relevant to the conceptual knowledge. David may even sound as if he were having challenges with the procedural knowledge. However, the author would argue that David was having difficulties with the conceptual knowledge because he was not able to generalize the massage techniques with the associated principles from one body region and translate them to another. That was the reason he felt that he needed demonstrations on everything. The author also interviewed the primary instructor of the course that David failed. The instructor commented that she had no confidence in David's ability to connect knowledge.

[Note: Excerpts of the interview related to the procedural knowledge and metacognitive knowledge are not covered in this chapter, owing to their irrelevance to the educational diagnosis.]

Based on the student interview, the author sought, reviewed, and triangulated various types of data to better understand the first 2 subdomains—the factual and conceptual knowledge—under the knowledge domain. Table 12-2 summarizes the data sources explored under every domain and subdomain.

After completing the first domain, the author went on to the second domain, communication.

Author/Faculty: In 2 of the courses you took, we asked you to verbalize your thought processes. How's the verbalization part to you? Were you comfortable doing it?

David: I think it just depends on the subject. … Some things I am comfortable explaining. Some things I am not.

David did not seem to have any issues with the verbal subdomain of communication. He was able to verbally express himself during the interview without any apparent difficulties. Furthermore, he described that his trouble with the verbalization of his thought processes was content specific. In other words, the trouble should have nothing to do with his verbal communication ability. The communication domain has another subdomain—nonverbal, which was not explored because of its lack of relevance to the student's CR deficits. The deficits were demonstrated in the think aloud component of the practical examination, which was offered in the course he failed. (See Table 12-2 for more on the communication domain data.)

For the third domain—academic skills and support—the author started with questions related to David's academic skills and focused on information organization first.

> *Author/Faculty: When you were taking the annual examination [a comprehensive examination that tests contents from various physical therapy courses] and were reading a question, did you think that was a research question, a kinesiology question, or an anatomy question? Did you recognize the questions by courses or by concepts?*
>
> *David: I think I knew where every question came from. I don't think I said, "Oh, this is an anatomy question." I think you can just tell.*
>
> *Author/Faculty: But in your head, how do you store the information? Do you store per course, or do you store in a different manner?*
>
> *David: Maybe it is by course. … If you want to be sure of something, you can say in your head, "Oh, it is an anatomy question."*

From the author's experience, students who view or store information by courses are the ones who have more trouble connecting the dots. They tend to see information in isolation. They may also have a hard time seeing the bigger picture and forming linkages between the learned materials. David's information organization may lead to his deficit in conceptual knowledge.

Mcloughlin[38] dichotomized students' information-organization skill into successive processing and simultaneous processing. When evaluating David's unsuccessful practical examination performances on videos, the author realized that David would fit the description of the former type of information organization: "When confronted by a patient with diffuse or multiple symptoms, the student fixates on a single element of the presenting symptomatology, misses crucial and 'obvious' clues. … The student engaged in successive processing strategies and does not seek to link data by creating bridges between informational elements."[38(p3)] For instance, during one of his practical examination attempts, when handling a patient case with an open reduction and internal fixation of the left tibial plateau, David focused on the internal fixation component and immediately jumped to the conclusion that it was contraindicated for the patient to receive neuromuscular electrical stimulation. He did not consider the location of the internal fixation component and structural aspects, in relation to the dimensional considerations of the quadriceps muscles, for electrical stimulation.

Reflection Moment

With respect to his clinical problem-solving, how might this be a problem for David as he begins to manage a full caseload of patients?

As the author continued to explore the third domain (academic skills and support), she shifted focus to its planning processing subdomain. The author reviewed David's videorecorded practical examination performances of the 3 unsuccessful attempts. The performances revealed his inability in regulating, modifying, and evaluating his activities. When setting up an ultrasound treatment, David repeatedly turned up the ultrasound intensity without realizing that the intensity was a lot higher than the recommended dosage. At the same time, David did not notice that he never pressed the start button for the ultrasound treatment to initiate. When the examiner (also the primary instructor of the course) was interviewed, she shared her concern about David's lack of organization, preplanning, and planning. She further commented that David seemed to have difficulties managing hands-on skills and information processing at the same time. She noticed that, during the course of the practical examination, David significantly slowed down or paused the psychomotor tasks when the patient asked him a question, which was designed to challenge David's conceptual knowledge and gain insights into his CR.

The interview components pertaining to David's planning processing, time management, and support system (under the third domain) did not yield a lot of helpful information toward making the educational diagnosis. Therefore, most of these components are not discussed in this chapter. A few comments from David about his academic support system are incorporated below to shed light on what he found helpful to his learning. Table 12-2 captures the data sources the author reviewed to understand the third domain (academic skills and support).

> *Author/Faculty: Tell me about your group study. How did that work? Exactly what's the process inside?*
>
> *David: Well, a couple of times when we did group studies, I didn't feel like it was doing anything. We were just going over slides. Just reading them aloud. These were at times kind of wasteful. When we discussed things and answered the "whys," that helped [my learning] more.*

The last (fourth) domain explored was personal factors. Selected interview excerpts are included below to show the probing questions and responses in more private and/or potentially sensitive areas including health and relationships. As shown in Table 12-2, the student interview was the only data source used to understand the fourth domain (personal factors).

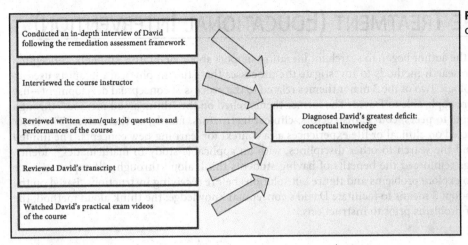

Figure 12-2. The triangulated educational diagnostic process of David's case.

Boxes (top to bottom):
- Conducted an in-depth interview of David following the remediation assessment framework
- Interviewed the course instructor
- Reviewed written exam/quiz job questions and performances of the course
- Reviewed David's transcript
- Watched David's practical exam videos of the course

→ Diagnosed David's greatest deficit: conceptual knowledge

Author/Faculty: Do you have any health concerns? Physical, mental, any concerns?

David: No.

Author/Faculty: Do you have any history of or are you currently taking any substance? Like alcohol or drugs that you rely on?

David: I mean, in the past I took an antidepressant.

Author/Faculty: But you don't need that anymore?

David: No. That was probably 2 years ago. So before [physical therapy] school started.

Author/Faculty: What about any relationship issues?

David: In the summer [the semester in which David failed the didactic course], I was having some problems. It's kind of cleared up, I guess. I mean, it's better.

Author/Faculty: Is it still an issue? Or is it resolved?

David: I think it's resolved.

Author/Faculty: I don't need to know the details. What I want to know is that would that [relationship problem] be a barrier for you to study or return to the [DPT] program?

David: I don't think so.

Wellness Check

Please note, depending upon the contextual situation, a depression screen and/or referral for counseling services may be appropriate for students, or just a reminder that these services are available and the supports provided. It is often helpful to provide the contact information and the success of the student assistance programs available on and off campus, and how to access these resources.

At the end of the interview, the following conversation occurred.

Author/Faculty: So, we covered all the areas. ... Do you have any idea which is your greatest deficit?

David: I would say conceptual knowledge. ... I would like to work on other things, of course, but that one [conceptual knowledge] I would say it's the greatest. ... And, not thinking so linear, but thinking from all different areas.

That was David's "aha" moment. The author had the same thought, too. However, she withheld her judgment and went on to seek and review pertinent academic records and supplemental data. Later, the author triangulated all the related information and concurred that David's greatest deficit was his conceptual knowledge. The triangulated educational diagnostic process of David's case is illustrated in Figure 12-2.

Preparation of the Treatment (Educational Intervention)

After confirming the greatest deficit, the author began to search for literature support about facilitating students' conceptual knowledge. Graham[46] used qualitative research methods to investigate the processes that student physical therapists used to develop conceptual knowledge in kinesiology. Two of the 3 major themes related to the process of conceptual development—use of discussion and use of experience—were applicable to David. The former theme relied on the "think aloud method," through which the subjects verbalized the concepts to peers, course instructors, clinical instructors, family, or themselves. The latter theme focused on how the subjects reflected on clinical or life experiences as a context for learning new concepts. The limited literature prompted the author to expand the search to other disciplines, with an applicable study in mathematics[47] identified. In reviewing the literature, findings reinforced the benefits of having students think aloud through self-explanation or discussion, and advocated for students to explore problems and figure out solutions before receiving instructions. Based on the literature review, the author decided to adopt 3 means to facilitate David's conceptual knowledge: the think aloud method, the use of experience, and the exploration of problems prior to instructions.

Reflection Moment

Do you agree with the diagnose-and-treat approach? Why or why not?

Consider what other possible approaches might be helpful in this case presentation.

Given the time constraints of physical therapy faculty, the author decided to hire and train a tutor to help David develop his conceptual knowledge. The tutor was a near-peer student in the same class with David before he was required to sit out of the DPT program. The author considered several key factors in selecting the tutor. The tutor needed to have solid conceptual knowledge in physical therapy, especially in the subject matter related to the course that David failed. The tutor's ability to articulate his or her own thought processes was essential. More important, the author made sure that the selected tutor not only was approachable and patient, but also was someone David felt comfortable working with. After an appropriate tutor was identified and hired, the author met with the tutor and discussed with her how to structure the tutorial sessions and how to use the aforementioned 3 means to enhance David's conceptual knowledge. The meeting with the tutor alone was held for approximately 1 hour. The author also met with David and the tutor together for roughly half an hour to clarify each one's roles and responsibilities and answer any questions prior to their setting up the tutoring schedule. The tutor was also encouraged to "think out loud" when working with David.

The Treatment (Educational Intervention) Process and Outcome

The educational intervention lasted for 10 weeks with one tutoring session per week. Each session was 2 to 3 hours long. The author lent David a book with many patient cases that were suitable for him to apply the knowledge covered in the course he failed. Prior to each tutoring session, David was required to review several cases from the book and pre-think how to apply the knowledge associated with the course to manage the cases. The tutor was responsible for hearing David out, "thinking out loud," giving him feedback on the proposed case management approach, and guiding his thinking whenever needed. The tutor was asked to hold off sharing her own ways of managing the cases until David was given ample opportunities to determine his own approach. Both David and the tutor were encouraged to pull in their own experiences during the discussions. As the facilitating faculty, the author occasionally sat in on the tutoring sessions for a short amount of time to monitor the educational intervention. The author also maintained open communication with David, the tutor, and the physical therapy department chair during the remediation period.

The remediation effort paid off. David passed the course he once failed and earned a course grade of A-. His practical examination grade went from failing in his first attempt to scoring only slightly below the class mean during the second attempt in the following year. David no longer demonstrated major deficits in the think aloud component (where his CR was tested) of the practical examination. He was allowed to move on to the next semester and continue with the physical therapist education program. The course instructor was interviewed again after David passed the course. (The same instructor had taught the course during David's first and second attempts.) The instructor noted David's big jump in the course grade. She also shared that David had asked more explicit questions related to the course contents and was able to organize his psychomotor skills better during the second attempt of the course.

The author was satisfied with the cost-effectiveness of the remediation. She spent around 5 hours of face time with David and/or the tutor. The time spent is only a quarter of the reported faculty face time used to remediate medical students' CR.[29] The tutor was allowed to have about 2 credits (1.7%) of school tuition waived in exchange for the time she spent tutoring David. The author found the remediation effort meaningful and rewarding, with one of the rewards coming from David's email, in which he stated:

I wouldn't have been so motivated to come back [to the program] if it wasn't for you and the extra help.

LIMITATIONS

This case study has several limitations. As in any other case studies, no causal relationship can be drawn. The educational diagnose-and-treat approach was applied to a student physical therapist who had struggled with CR in the didactic component of the education program. No data are available on using the approach in the clinical education component. Regarding the educational diagnostic process, the remediation assessment framework is new, with its validity and comprehensiveness not proven yet. While the author feels more comfortable with the evidence-based educational intervention, the applicable research evidence is scarce. Moreover, the author finished the case study right after David passed the course and did not keep track of David's long-term performance in the program.

FUTURE DEVELOPMENTS

The author hopes that this case study can serve as a starting point in our journey toward establishing an optimal and widely accepted approach to educationally diagnose and treat student physical therapists' CR deficits. The remediation assessment framework should be further developed with input from experts and with experiential knowledge from users. To promote an evidence-based remediation of CR, more research studies are needed to increase the number of viable and effective educational interventions. Multi-institutional experiments investigating the short-term and long-term outcomes of using the educational diagnose-and-treat approach is also warranted. Short-term outcomes may include retest data and student satisfaction, while long-term outcomes may incorporate effects on students' academic and clinical performances. In addition, the approach should be explored in both didactic and clinical education components of physical therapist education programs.

Finally, the author recognizes that we may need to have a transformation in our institutional assumptions and values toward remediation. As educators, our responsibilities are not only to diligently teach, but also to accurately evaluate and provide remediation to students in need, as part of our role as gatekeepers for the public's protection. The transformation and the implementation of this method may help increase the number of physical therapist educators who are willing and able to identify the struggling students early and customize remediation for them in a timely and appropriate manner.

CONCLUSION

CR is challenging to teach and often times hard to learn.[2] It should not be surprising to find students who struggle with CR as they develop the attribute. While physical therapist education programs are required to support student retention and progression through the program,[1] no literature is available on how to remediate student physical therapists who have CR deficits. In this chapter, the author shares a case study of the remediation using an educational diagnose-and-treat method.[3] The author developed a remediation assessment framework to guide the educational diagnostic process, and incorporated literature support in designing and customizing an educational intervention for the remediation. The remediation process is systematic, practical, and cost-effective. The student, who once failed a didactic course due to CR deficits, succeeded when retaking the course in the following year. Although the case study does not prove any causal relationship between the remediation effort and the student outcome, it may serve as a first step to establish an optimal approach for providing remediation to students struggling with CR. Additional time is also likely a contributing factor for CR development and success, especially in terms of remediation.

In conclusion, physical therapy educators may want to consider adopting an educational diagnosis-and-treat approach when remediating students. The remediation assessment framework is designed for student physical therapists with CR deficits and may be an appropriate framework to help educators carry out a more comprehensive investigation of students' remediation needs and identify the greatest deficit. The remediation plan designed for student physical therapists with CR deficits should be customized to address the greatest deficit first, while maintaining an approach that is practical from both the student's and the educator's perspectives. More attention should be given to develop, assess, and remediate student physical therapists' CR, which is not only a red flag item on the physical therapist clinical performance instrument, but also a must-have for autonomous practitioners.

Reflection Moment

What is considered an educational diagnose-and-treat approach when remediating students?

When using the remediation assessment framework, what are the potential sources of information that may help investigate students' remediation needs?

When a student physical therapist with CR deficits has multiple remediation needs, how do we determine which we should address first?

REFERENCES

1. Commission on Accreditation in Physical Therapy Education. Standards and required element for accreditation of physical therapist education programs. http://www.capteonline.org/uploadedFiles/CAPTEorg/Portal/CAPTEPortal_PTStandardsEvidence.doc. Revised March 4, 2016. Accessed August 10, 2017.
2. Delany C, Golding C. Teaching clinical reasoning by making thinking visible: an action research project with allied health clinical educators. *BMC Med Educ.* 2014;14(20):1-10.
3. Guerrasio J. *Remediation of the Struggling Medical Learner.* LaVergne, TN: Association for Hospital Medical Education; 2013.
4. Commission on Accreditation in Physical Therapy Education. Standards and required element for accreditation of physical therapist assistant education programs. http://www.capteonline.org/uploadedFiles/CAPTEorg/Portal/CAPTEPortal_PTAStandardsEvidence.doc. Revised March 4, 2016. Accessed August 14, 2017.
5. Kalet A, Guerrasio J, Chou CL. Twelve tips for developing and maintaining a remediation program in medical education. *Med Teach.* 2016;38(8):787-792.
6. American Physical Therapy Association. Minimum required skills of physical therapist graduates at entry-level. http://www.apta.org/uploadedFiles/APTAorg/About_Us/Policies/Education/MinimumRequiredSkillsPTGrads.pdf - search=%22minimum%20required%20skills%22. Accessed November 21, 2016.
7. Tippett S. Program impact of student outcome assessment in physical therapy education. *J Phys Ther Ed.* 2006;20(2):38-47.
8. Epstein RM, Hundert EM. Defining and assessing professional competence. *JAMA.* 2002;287(2):226-235.
9. American Physical Therapy Association. *A Normative Model of Physical Therapist Professional Education: Version 2004.* Alexandria, VA: American Physical Therapy Association; 2004.
10. Yao DC, Wright SM. National survey of internal medicine residency program directors regarding problem residents. *JAMA.* 2000;284(9):1099-1104.
11. Guerrasio J. Introduction to identification and diagnosis. *Remediation of the Struggling Medical Learner.* LaVergne, TN: Association for Hospital Medical Education; 2013:11-16.
12. May S, Withers S, Reeve S, Greasley A. Limited clinical reasoning skills used by novice physiotherapists when involved in the assessment and management of patients with shoulder problems: a qualitative study. *J Man Manipulative Ther.* 2010;18(2):84-88.
13. Higgs J, Jones MA. Clinical decision making and multiple problem spaces. In: Higgs J, Jones MA, Loftus S, Christensen N, eds. *Clinical Reasoning in the Health Professions.* 3rd ed. Amsterdam, Netherlands: Butterworth-Heinemann Elsevier; 2008:3-17.
14. Higgs J, Trede F, Loftus S, et al. *Advancing clinical reasoning: interpretive research perspectives grounded in professional practice, CPEA, occasional paper 4. Collaborations in Practice and Education Advancement.* Sydney, Australia: The University of Sydney; 2006.
15. Benner P, Hughes RG, Sutphen M. Clinical reasoning, decision making, and action: thinking critically and clinically. In: Hughes RG, ed. *Patient Safety and Quality: An Evidence-Based Handbook for Nurses.* Rockville, MD: Agency for Healthcare Research and Quality, US Department of Health and Human Services; 2008:1-23.
16. Hauer KE, Teherani A, Kerr KM, O'Sullivan PS, Irby DM. Student performance problems in medical school clinical skills assessment. *Acad Med.* 2007;82(10):s69-s72.
17. CNA and Healthcare Providers Service Organization. Physical therapy professional liability exposure: 2016 claim report update. http://image.exct.net/lib/fe6715707d6d017c7514/m/1/CNA_PT_CS_EXEC_021116p_CF_PROD_ASIZE_LCP+SEC.v2.pdf. Accessed November 30, 2016.
18. Carr SE, Celenza A, Puddey IB, Lake F. Relationships between academic performance of medical students and their workplace performance as junior doctors. *BMC Med Educ.* 2014;14:157.
19. Carr SE, Celenza A, Lake F. Assessment of junior doctor performance: a validation study. *BMC Med Educ.* 2013;13:129.
20. Commission on Accreditation in Physical Therapy Education. Aggregate program data: 2015-2016 physical therapist education programs fact sheets. http://www.capteonline.org/uploadedFiles/CAPTEorg/About_CAPTE/Resources/Aggregate_Program_Data/AggregateProgramData_PTPrograms.pdf. Accessed August 30, 2016.
21. Guerrasio J, Furfari KA, Rosenthal LD, Nogar CL, Wray KW, Aagaard EM. Failure to fail: the institutional perspective. *Med Teach.* 2014;36(9):799-803.
22. Federation of State Boards of Physical Therapy. NPTE graduation year reports. https://www.fsbpt.org/FreeResources/NPTEPassRateReports/NPTEGraduationYearReports.aspx. Accessed August 25, 2016.

23. Cooper RA. It's time to address the problem of physician shortages: graduate medical education is the key. *Ann Surg.* 2007;246(4):527-534.

24. Roberts CM. Relationships among admission variables, professional education outcome measures, and job performance of University of Missouri physical therapy graduates [dissertation]. Columbia, MO: University of Missouri; 1996.

25. Saxena V, O'Sullivan PS, Teherani A, Irby DM, Hauer K. Remediation techniques for student performance problems after a comprehensive clinical skills assessment. *Acad Med.* 2009;84:669-676.

26. Guerrasio J, Aagaard EM. Methods and outcomes for the remediation of clinical reasoning. *J Gen Intern Med.* 2014;29(12):1607-1614.

27. Mutnick A, Barone M. Assessing and remediating clinical reasoning. In: Kalet A, Chou CL, eds. *Remediation in Medical Education: A Mid-Course Correction.* New York, NY: Springer; 2014:85-102.

28. Audétat MC, Laurin S, Dory V, Charlin B, Nendaz MR. Diagnosis and management of clinical reasoning difficulties: part II. Clinical reasoning difficulties: management and remediation strategies. *Med Teach.* 2017;39(8):797-801.

29. Guerrasio J, Garrity MJ, Aagaard EM. Learner deficits and academic outcomes of medical students, residents, fellows, and attending physicians referred to a remediation program, 2006-2012. *Acad Med.* 2014;89(2):352-358.

30. Fu W. Development of an innovative tool to assess student physical therapists' clinical reasoning competency. *J Phys Ther Ed.* 2015;29(4):14-26.

31. Pinnock R, Young L, Spence F, Henning M, Hazell W. Can think aloud be used to teach and assess clinical reasoning in graduate medical education? *J Grad Med Educ.* 2015;7(3):334-337.

32. Jensen GM, Gwyer J, Shepard KF. Expert practice in physical therapy. *Phys Ther.* 2000;80(1):28-43.

33. Christensen N. Development of clinical reasoning capability in student physical therapists [dissertation]. Adelaide, Australia: Division of Health Sciences, University of South Australia; 2009.

34. Anderson KJ. Factors affecting the development of undergraduate medical students' clinical reasoning ability [dissertation]. Adelaide, Australia: Medical Learning and Teaching Unit, University of Adelaide; 2006.

35. Krathwohl DR. A revision of Bloom's taxonomy: an overview. *Theory Pract.* 2002;41(4):212-218.

36. Donaghy M, Morss K. An evaluation of a framework for facilitating and assessing physiotherapy students' reflection on practice. *Physiother Theory Pract.* 2007;23(2):83-94.

37. Roche A, Coote S. Focus group study of student physiotherapists' perceptions of reflection. *Med Educ.* 2008;42:1064-1070.

38. Mcloughlin CS. Characteristics of students failing medical education: an essay of reflections. *Med Educ Online.* 2009;14:1-6.

39. Lubarsky S, Dory V, Audétat M-C, Custers E, Charlin B. Using script theory to cultivate illness script formation and clinical reasoning in the health professions education. *Can Med Educ J.* 2015;6(2):e61-e70.

40. Dipboye RL, Phillips AP. College students' time management: correlations with academic performance and stress. *J Educ Psychol.* 1990;82(4):760-768.

41. Ansari WE, Stock C. Is the health and wellbeing of university students associated with their academic performance? Cross sectional findings from the United Kingdom. *Int J Environ Res Public Health.* 2010;7(2):509-527.

42. Ruthig JC, Marrone S, Hladkyj S, Robinson-Epp N. Changes in college student health: implications for academic performance. *J Coll Stud Dev.* 2011;52(3):307-320.

43. Koçyiğit F, Torun ED, Aslan ÜB. Anxiety, depression, physical activity and quality of life in student physical therapists: a cross sectional study. *Am J Educ Res.* 2015;3(10A):26-29.

44. Andrews B, Wilding JM. The relation of depression and anxiety to life-stress and achievement in students. *Br J Psychol.* 2004;95(4):509-521.

45. Yousefy A, Ghassemi G, Firouznia S. Motivation and academic achievement in medical students. *J Educ Health Promot.* 2012;1:4.

46. Graham CL. Conceptual learning processes in physical therapy students. *Phys Ther.* 1996;76(8):856-865.

47. Rittle-Johnson B, Schneider M. Developing conceptual and procedural knowledge of mathematics. In: Kadosh RC, Dowker A, eds. *The Oxford Handbook of Numerical Cognition.* Oxford, United Kingdom: Oxford University Press; 2015:1102-1118.

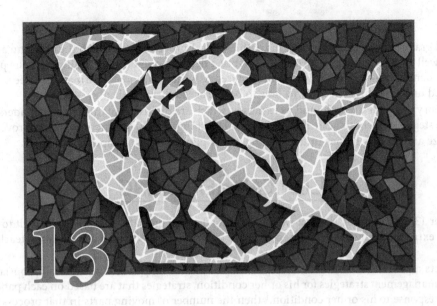

CLINICAL REASONING USING SYSTEM 1 AND SYSTEM 2 MODELING

Chad E. Cook, PT, PhD, MBA, FAPTA, FAAOMPT; Kyle Covington, PT, DPT, PhD; and Yannick Tousignant-Laflamme, PT, PhD

I back away from conscious thought and turn the problem over to my unconscious mind. It will scan a broader array of patterns and find some new close fits from other information stored in my brain. —Arthur Fry, co-creator of the Post-it Note

OBJECTIVES

- Compare and contrast clinical reasoning (CR) using System 1 and System 2 decision-making models.

- Appraise when System 1 or System 2 decision-making is most appropriate.

- Discuss challenges associated with CR using System 1 and System 2 decision-making.

- Evaluate methods to enhance the use of System 1 and System 2 learning in a clinical setting applied with clinical case examples.

- Create a knowledge opportunity for new learners, amalgamating System 1 and System 2 theories applied to a case study.

CR is a multidimensional and complex process involving both nonanalytic and analytic cognitive processes—an exercise identified as dual processing theory. Dual-processing theory encompasses the careful balance of System 1 and System 2 theories. System 1 involves construction of mental maps and patterns, shortcuts, and rules of thumb, or heuristics, as well as "mind-lines." It is developed through experience and repetition, seeing what other people do, talking with local colleagues, and integrating with the personal experiences of one's self and others. System 2 is data-driven, effortful, time-consuming, analytical, and decid-

Musolino GM, Jensen GM, eds. *Clinical Reasoning and Decision-Making in Physical Therapy: Facilitation, Assessment, and Implementation* (pp 157-168).

edly logical. In clinical practice, reasoning often begins with System 1 processing, in which the clinician assesses a patient's presenting symptoms, as well as other clinical evidence, to arrive at a decision point in proceeding with the patient's care. System 2 is often implemented when unknown information is encountered or when additional information is needed, and is continuously assessed, and reassessed until the clinician discerns how to best proceed therapeutically.

Dual processing theory has both strengths and weaknesses, which are discussed in this chapter. Understanding and focus on dual-processing CR strategies, with both academic and clinical teaching, as well as practice, may improve the learner's capacity to further conceptualize and achieve higher-order learning and applications for therapeutic benefit.

CLINICAL REASONING

Let's initiate Chapter 13 with a confession that we are certain all can appreciate. While it is difficult to incorporate good CR into practice, and it is extraordinarily challenging to improve our own CR skills through learning, teaching CR is often even more perplexing.

Indeed, if CR reflects a process in which the therapist interacts with the patient and other appropriate parties to help the patient develop health management strategies for his or her condition, strategies that are based on each patient's unique findings, and the patient's own response to his or her condition,[1] then the number of moving parts in that process is extraordinary. Yet, improving one's CR practices is essential to growth as a clinician. Where does one start?

Presented within this textbook are CR processes, strategies, assessments, and evaluation methods, as well as approaches to improve one's CR skills. All will likely support the assumption that helping trainees develop appropriate CR abilities is a challenging goal in an environment of complexity and unpredictability.[2] We argue that deconstructing the 2 primary domains of CR is beneficial to better understand adept methods for teaching and understanding CR.

One model we advocate is dual processing theory, a careful balance of intuitive, or automatic, thoughts and analytical thoughts.[3] Dual processing theory hypothesizes that both intuitive and analytical systems are simultaneously deployed in most clinical decision-making (CDM) scenarios.[4] We further contend that identifying weaknesses of biases (see Table 3-3) associated with a selected processing model should be a focus of those charged with the responsibility of facilitating CR.

The remaining elements of this chapter are dedicated to dual processing theory and approaches as to how we believe these elements can be incorporated in the learning and teaching of CR through cases. We provide examples of formal teaching strategies implemented that are reflective of dual processing theory applications, to improve the take-home understanding of the concept.

DUAL PROCESSING THEORY

Dual processing theory was first proposed within the psychological literature. It encompasses the idea that there are 2 modes of processing of information, known commonly as System 1 and System 2 thinking.[5,6] The concept was developed in the profession of psychology in 1975 by Evans.[7] Evans[7] suggested that there are 2 types of cognitive processes—heuristic and analytic— and that heuristic processes involve the filtering of information to what is deemed relevant to the current situation. Heuristic process is that of enabling people to discover or learn something for themselves, which is more of a hands-on or interactive heuristic approach to learning. Subsequently, analytic processes are used to make further judgments about the ongoing decision-making scenario or to reprogram heuristic thoughts. Although there are no formal dual processing theories within medicine, the concept instinctively connects to most decision-making processes that clinicians encounter and manage on a daily basis. Table 13-1 outlines an overview of the key features of System 1 and System 2 thinking.

System 1: An Overview

Within the concept of dual processing theory, System 1 assumes that cognition operates automatically and quickly, with little or no effort and no sense of voluntary control.[8] System 1 thinking allows one to jump to conclusions from little evidence, and is not designed to know the size and/or magnitude of the jumps.[9] System 1 involves rapid, emotional, stereotypic, subconscious designs, and includes construction of mental maps and patterns, shortcuts, rules of thumb, or heuristics, and "mind-lines." System 1 is developed through experiences, training, repetition, seeing what other people do, and collaborating with learned colleagues.[10,11]

System 1 is also frequently affiliated with the concept of heurism. Heurism is knowledge derived from empirical study and practical adoption of experience.[12] A hallmark of heurism allows the formulation of quick decisions, often defined as "fast and frugal decision-making" in the absence of complete information through pattern recognition. Norman[13] indicates that most experienced clinicians begin making final management decisions when they have gathered only about 60% to 70% of the available critical data. Although this may suggest a lack of comprehension, there is no known relationship between the amount of data gathered and medically oriented accuracy. If indeed omissions in data gathering are occurring, the outcome does not appear to be influenced.[13] Pattern recognition associated with heurism allows one to make judgments quickly, especially when a patient

	SYSTEM 1	SYSTEM 2
Thought processing	Fast/automatic Unconscious Implicit/tacit Intuitive	Slow Conscious Explicit
Emotional elements	Impulsive Habitual Belief-driven Hot	Reflective Planning Logical Cold
Determinants	Associative factors Experimental	Analytical Systematical
Decision-making drivers	Stimuli	Higher-order rationale
Processes incorporated	Idea generation	Refinement, evaluation, or assessment
Cognition	Pattern association Inductive Heuristic	Deductive Rule-based
Scientific rigor	Low	High
Awareness	Low	High
Bias	High	Low
Reliability	Low	High
Effort	Low	High

TABLE 13-1

THOUGHT PROCESSES

fails to deviate from a recognized pattern. Fast and frugal heuristic actions rely on a small fraction of the available evidence for one to create a management strategy. It is a common method used in emergency room settings or when one is required to think rapidly for health-related and/or safety occurrences and/or immediate situational need.

System 2: An Overview

In contrast to System 1 thinking, System 2 allocates attention to the effortful mental activities that demand it, including complex computations.[8] System 2 thinking stresses conscious attention, thought, and analytical knowledge of tests, measures, outcomes, and other quantitative elements that are used to assimilate a strategy for care. System 2 reflects the analytical values often seen in medical testing (eg, using imaging, clinical tests, test values), or other measuring elements that are a proxy for a construct. Unlike System 1, the deliberate nature of System 2 thinking competes with any other thinking processes and demands full attention. It is well known that many novice learners employ this analytic mode of reasoning more frequently than their experienced counterparts because they lack the mental maps and management patterns that are part of System 1 reasoning.[2] Early aspects of curricular learning are primarily built on System 2 concepts and are considered building blocks of learned expertise. Some early career novices have been able to draw upon minimal experiences and incorporate earlier more of a dual processing approach.[14] Hence, years of experience alone does not preclude one from progressing along the CR strategies continuum.

DECISION-MAKING USING DUAL PROCESSING THEORY

Dual process theory hypothesizes that both systems are simultaneously used in most settings.[4] Croskerry[10] has proposed a model for a decision management process that involves the dual processing system. In the model, during a new clinical encounter, a clinician has the capacity to use either System 1 processing (when a pattern is recognized) or System 2 processing (when a pattern is **not** recognized). Croskerry proposes the use of a cognitive miser calibrator, which attempts to make decisions that use the least amount of cognitive processing. Croskerry also identifies task contextual elements, which are mediators to decision-making that are related to environment, task difficulty, and clarity. Within Croskerry's[10] model, linear and nonlinear processing can occur, allowing one to make decisions using both processes.[3] In a simplified fashion, System 1 processing is used until an unknown encounter occurs during the management process, then System 2 processing is engaged until the pattern is again recognized.

Advantages and Disadvantages of System 1

There are advantages and disadvantages to System 1 decision-making processes. It is important to recognize that through good training, education, and proper patient exposure, the advantages can be maximized, and the disadvantages can be identified and managed. In particular, quality training to increase the number of patient cases, understanding of the role of specific clinical findings, and the ability to reflect on one's own biases are known mediators for maximizing one's System 1 thinking. The postulation that one is "born" with creative, intuitive knowledge in health care is a misassumption.

Advantages

Speed

With respect to advantages, speed of decision-making is certainly a known value. System 1 decision-making is predicated on prior experience and recognition of patterns. System 1 allows one to skip selected steps through formulation of a working hypothesis that is based on logical processes in which multiple premises, all believed true or found true most of the time, are combined to obtain a specific conclusion (inductive reasoning). Inductive reasoning is valuable in settings that require rapid, accurate decisions (eg, emergency room settings) where deliberate, analytical decisions are not plausible.

Creativity

System 1 allows the individual not only to build new patterns but also to identify new, previously unknown situations that were unexplored in System 2 study. System 1 allows for extrapolation and testing of ideas. Further, it allows for each practitioner to develop his or her own reasoning strategies. Kaufman and Singer[6] describe a situation in which one of the wonders of System 1 is its ability to feed creative insights to System 2. This often happens precisely when System 2 thinking is inactive, and System 1 is on autopilot.

Decisions Are Patient Centered

System 1 is built on pattern acknowledgment. It identifies the prevalence of variability in each patient and recognizes that no 2 patients exhibit the exact same profile. Thus, the flexibility built into System 1 thinking allows for patient-centered elements that may be useful and specific for that single patient.

Disadvantages

Cognitive Biases

Cognitive biases involve systematic errors in thinking that directly or indirectly influence decision-making. Often, these biases are related to events from memory or an earlier experience. Examples of errors, as introduced in Chapter 3, may include anchoring bias (focusing on the first piece of evidence), recency bias (focusing on the last piece of evidence), or the availability heuristic (assuming the likelihood of a finding based on prior likelihoods). A tangible example would be the assumption of a meniscal tear for a patient with a knee problem presenting with a positive McMurray's test (performed last-recency bias), despite the fact that 3 other prior test findings were negative or inconclusive.

Information Biases

Information bias arises from measurement error. Information bias is also referred to as observational bias and misclassification. One major challenge associated with information biases is the global acceptance of a special clinical test or clinical interventional assumption based on textbook recommendation, prior use, or training. Understanding System 2 metrics improves one's likelihood of reducing the influence of information biases. A clinical example would be the tendency to use the straight leg raise to confirm the presence of lumbar radiculopathy at the end of the examination, despite the fact that the test does not have the metrics associated with confirmation.

Priming Biases

Priming bias is an implicit memory effect in which exposure to a stimulus (ie, perceptual pattern) influences the response to another stimulus. Priming biases are associated with the tendency to think in a dedicated manner based on experiences and training, or based on prior patient experiences. A clinical example may include the tendency to involve manual techniques such as manipulation in a treatment regimen because previous clinical experience necessitated the need of that intervention, vs something that may be more appropriate for the current population.

EGO BIASES

Ego bias is systematic overestimation of the prognosis of one's own patients compared to the prognosis of patients outside one's clinical management. Ego biases lead to overestimation of one's capability and the increased likelihood of an error in management.[12] Ego biases may also result in a failure to reflect on one's own decisions and the disuse of self-checks through assessment.

EASY STAGNATION

We have all encountered clinicians who have not changed their thought processes, have not read a scientific paper, and address their care patterns the same for all patients. Unfortunately, in the gray world of clinical care, it is far too easy for individuals to lack accountability in their care management options. Yet as a profession we (physical therapists) have guidance[15] and standards that beg otherwise, as well as a code of ethics, often incorporated within state practice acts for the profession of physical therapy.

Reflection Moment

How will you ensure that you do not stagnate as a health care professional?

ADVANTAGES AND DISADVANTAGES OF SYSTEM 2

Advantages

ACCURACY

A hallmark of System 2 is the conscious attention, thought, and analytical knowledge of tests, measures, outcomes, and other quantitative elements of decision-making. Use of known analytical decision-making tools such as imaging, appropriate clinical tests, and evidence should improve the outcomes associated with the management encounter and ought to improve one's CR strategies. The accuracy of System 2 begets improved System 1 processing because the information identified using trustworthy information leads to accurate decisions.

FOUNDATIONAL

System 2 information is the building block of knowledge acquired in a formal educational process. This is why basic science, professional development, and foundational practice management courses are early in most curricula; these are designed to create a roadmap of knowledge and foundational structure to develop professional behaviors for the learner.

Disadvantages

LACK OF ACCURACY

Unfortunately, many of our current tests and measures lack precision and fail to assist us in day-to-day CDM. Further, many of our interventions have variable outcomes for selected patients, demanding the necessity of precision medicine, which is rarely an element of most educational programs. This gray area of knowledge greatly exposes a learner to bad habits in decision-making or information biases in System 1 thinking.

SLOW

A System 2 thinking process is sometimes a slow, deliberate method that rarely fits in a modern, busy clinical practice. Clinicians are rarely capable of evaluating the accuracy of all information sources, and those who do attempt to process all the information may fail to meet the productivity requirements of a facility or may fall behind in their quest for best approaches. Professionals think about their patients/clients all the time; they are continually self-assessing, even in the formative years as a developing professional.[16] CR is ongoing and not time limited, yet time is an impeding factor in many instances.

IMPERSONAL

Although one may argue that the patient encounter likely is associated with a more robust collection of interactions than those simply housed in CR, there is a risk that the strict use of System 2 (by the analytical book) could lead to non–patient-centric care. An increase in the growth of shared decision-making and discrete choice models reflects the necessity of a patient-centered approach that is unique to each individual. By its nature, System 2 may demand a particular care route that the patient opposes.

USING DUAL PROCESSING THEORY IN TRAINING OF CLINICIANS

We are frequently asked by educators, "How can I improve my students' System 1 thinking?" We commonly answer, "You can't feed meat to a baby." By its nature, System 1 learning must occur after a foundational understanding of the contextual elements of patient examination, treatment, and reassessment exist. (However, problem-based learning theorists may argue otherwise.) Inherently, System 1 thinking is created through formal structured learning of foundational knowledge, such as basic anatomy and physiology, exposure to patients, recognition of patterns of clinical symptoms, and knowledge of the underlying meaning of the information gathered through System 2 assessment (ie, a grasp of what tests mean and how interpretation guides decisions).

System 2 knowledge is gained through formal training in which measures and meaning are intertwined. The System 2 elements are the foundation of System 1 thinking. Hence, you should consider how to teach dual processing theory, and how strategies may be best approached by new learners.

Next, let's consider the strategies involved using a dual process theory, active training approach.

TEACHING USING DUAL PROCESSING LEARNING

Dual process learning can be developed and practiced using clinical reasoning learning sessions (CRLSs).[17] CRLSs are case-based learning techniques that focus on patient care. In health care learning environments, these techniques are applied during the preclinical phase of the curriculum. The main objective of CRLSs is to assist in organizing knowledge that is already stored by learners in mental networks, using defined experiences with a goal to improve clinical strategies.

During a typical real or fictitious patient encounter, the learner will use System 1 processes for components he or she recognizes and System 2 processes for new or unrecognized aspects. We will provide a single case that uses CRLSs and dual processing theory. For context, the learner in this case has had only foundation testing and pathophysiology training, and has had no clinical experiences outside seeing faculty and patient exchanges during the course. The learner is engaged in a clinical practice course that emphasizes musculoskeletal training. During the case example, the learner is asked to be the health care provider (performing CR), and the mentor (or another higher-level student) may take the role of the patient who provides information. Generally, several steps in an examination require CDM processes. We will expose and exemplify the 7 steps of the CRLS model (Table 13-2) through a case study application.

THE CASE

- *Context:* A 52-year-old right-handed women seeks your services (self-referred) for shoulder pain of 8 weeks' duration. Her shoulder pain surfaced following a fall, where she fully extended her right arm to protect herself when she fell.

The objective of the first step is to have the learner establish a working diagnosis. This is done by 2 sequential steps.

Step 1A (Identification of Key Elements)

The learner takes a complete history (anamnesis) that leads him or her to formulate a clear problem or identify the most significant or contributing elements for the case (in this case, related to the diagnosis), which will generate a preliminary clinical hypothesis (working diagnosis). The mentor has all the information for the case study, and the learner only has the case contextual information. Following are the findings obtained through the learner's history taking.

BRIEF SUMMARY OF KEY POINTS

- **History:** Shoulder and neck pain were initially present. She then immediately sought the care of her family physician, where she was prescribed plain X-rays (negative) and over-the-counter analgesics for pain (acetaminophen 500 mg every 6 hours). Current and past medical history include type 1 diabetes (controlled with insulin), history of right shoulder

TABLE 13-2

THE SEVEN STEPS OF THE CLINICAL REASONING LEARNING SESSIONS MODEL

STEP	NAME	EXPECTED OUTPUT
1A	Identification of key elements	Formulate clear problem with key elements obtained from history
1B	Preliminary hypothesis	List preliminary diagnosis/hypothesis
2	Clinical testing	Determine strategies to test each working hypothesis
3	Interpretation of results	Interpret the results of clinical testing
4	Final diagnosis	Confirm most likely/probable hypothesis to establish the diagnosis
5	Identification of possible interventions	List interventions addressing deficits in body functions and structures, activity limitations, and restrictions in participation
6	Intervention selection	Select the most appropriate interventions
7	Identification of factors influencing prognosis	Identify factors that will drive the prognosis for the case to establish the overall prognosis

tendinopathy (4 years ago, which completely resolved after 4 weeks of physical therapy). She works full-time as an administrative assistant, is married, and has good support at home; work is another issue. Her employer is not very open to job accommodations. Stiffness and constant pain (2-7/10) are her main complaints. Pain is worst at night but also increased to all shoulder movements above 90 degrees. She has a hard time getting dressed in the morning and doing 100% of her tasks at work, as her symptoms are directly influenced by all upper extremity movements. Because she has good support at home, she reports to minimally use her right arm while performing activities of daily living at home, as her pain symptoms are often closer to 6-7/10 when she returns from work.

- **System 1:** Based on his knowledge, the learner attempts to identify patterns in the patient's history (significant contributing elements). For example, the learner may recognize that a rotator cuff tear or traumatic arthritis both often occur after trauma (the fall), and may also recognize that both conditions may lead to neck or shoulder pain; however, the primary cause of the problem is uncertain. The cognition of a history of diabetes may also suggest a potential competing diagnosis of adhesive capsulitis.

- **System 2:** Implications are minimal during this first step, unless a specific aspect of the case is unknown to the learner (ie, the association between diabetes and adhesive capsulitis) or if the mentor highlights important aspects of the case that the student did not recognize (ie, although the right shoulder was hurt during the fall, the cervical spine might also be implicated, which can create a referred pain pattern to the shoulder). In this scenario, a rational override takes the learner back to System 1, to acquire more knowledge about the specific characteristics with which the patient presents.

Step 1B (Preliminary Hypothesis)

From the results and information obtained during Step 1A, the learner generates a written or oral list of the possible factors that will directly impact or influence the working diagnosis and/or the clinical hypothesis he will be testing. These factors can encompass some biopsychosocial aspects as well, since they can all point to specific aspects to be assessed.

- **System 1:** The learner may identify specific body structures—such as the glenohumeral joint, rotator cuff muscles, glenohumeral ligaments, and subacromial bursa—as the source of the painful symptoms and disability. The learner may recognize the 7/10 pain intensity rating as being of moderate severity. The learner may have already recognized that the symptoms began following a fall (trauma), suggesting intra-articular, tendon, capsular, or ligament injury, since negative X-rays make a fracture or calcification that could explain symptoms improbable. He may also recognize her minimal use of her right arm while at home as a pain avoidance behavior.

- **System 2:** At this step, System 2 is used if the learner requires additional learning to establish a hypothesis and better understand the influence of diabetes on shoulder-related injuries. The learner may also require additional understanding and testing for the neck and shoulder pain distribution, and the mechanism of referred vs radiating pain, to better differentiate the origin of the pain. This is especially true if differentiation of structures has not been previously covered or seen. Lastly, the learner may need to better investigate the role of the social factors. In this case, that is the patient's

	TABLE 13-3	
	EXPECTED HYPOTHESES	
OUTPUT OF STEP 1B	**OUTPUT OF STEP 2**	
Expected Hypothesis	*Test to Challenge the Hypothesis*	*Expected Response to Support the Hypothesis*
Partial rupture of the rotator cuff muscle	Active ROM Manual muscle testing	Full passive ROM Reduced and painful active ROM Decreased strength and pain
Shoulder capsulitis	Active and passive ROM	Symmetrically reduced active and passive ROM Multidirectional reduction of accessory movement of the glenohumeral joint
Subacromial bursitis and/or impingement	Active ROM Supraspinatus test Hawkins-Kennedy	Painful arc in abduction + +
Pain of cervical origin	Neck ROM with overpressures	+

If information or testing is missing or not identified by the learner (by lack of knowledge or failure to recognize which test to use), the mentor or outside information source can facilitate this step by further questioning of the CR process (System 2).

+=positive finding, -=negative finding.

perception or report of her work environment and her employer, since the patient reports low job flexibility and a negative attitude of her immediate supervisor toward adapting her schedule and tasks. These factors could also partly explain the maintenance of symptoms as an overuse injury.

Step 2 (Clinical Testing)

For each working diagnosis, the learner has to plan the objective and/or specific tests he would perform, as well as the expected responses that would support the diagnosis (clinical testing). During Step 2, the learner and mentor can dialogue and exchange ideas on the different assessment strategies and tools or specific tests that can be used to challenge each hypothesis. Furthermore, the learner must speculate on the expected response for each test according to each hypothesis; this step can help enhance future pattern recognition for similar cases. However, it requires prior knowledge of the pathophysiology and objective measures to associate the results of the test and the patient's response (System 2 knowledge). For this case scenario, the output of Step 1B and Step 2 could resemble the expected hypotheses as outlined in Table 13-3.

- **System 1:** The learner may recognize that range of motion (ROM) and strength deficits often are essential findings, based on foundation coursework. The learner may also associate these findings with soft tissue–related injury, which would substantiate the hypotheses regarding soft tissue–related structures. Most likely, since the student is first being exposed to the results of special clinical testing (eg, Hawkins-Kennedy test), he would require System 2 engagement.

- **System 2:** The learner would use System 2 processes to better understand what the findings mean from the results of each specific test. For example, it is well studied that a positive Hawkins-Kennedy is not a valid test to support shoulder impingement, as it lacks specificity. On the other hand, it does suggest that the glenohumeral joint cannot be ruled out as the origin of symptoms. Further investigation or interaction with the mentor may also support that the cervical spine is unlikely the pain generator, since neck range with overpressures was negative.

Step 3 (Interpretation of Results)

Results of the objective physical exam are obtained (via complete physical assessment in clinical settings) or given to the learner (on paper). The mentor and learner can now discuss the repercussions the findings have on the working diagnosis—what supports and confirms the preliminary hypothesis. This truly reflects a dual process approach, where both pattern recognitions and analytical thinking processes occur (with the mentor offering guidance).

TABLE 13-4 **RANGE OF MOTION AND MANUAL MUSCLE TESTING**							
		RANGE OF MOTION			**RESISTED**	**MMT**	
Joint	*Movement*	*Left (A/P)*	*Right (A/P)*	*End-Feel*	*R**	*R*	*L*
Shoulder	Flexion	165 degrees/ 170 degrees	90 degrees/ 90 degrees	Empty	Strong and painless	3-	5
	Extension	40 degrees / 45 degrees	30 degrees/ 35 degrees	Normal	Strong and painless	3-	5
	Abduction	165 degrees/ 170 degree	90 degrees/ 90 degrees	Empty	Strong and painless	3-	5
	Lateral rotation (at 45 degrees abd)	80 degrees/ 85 degrees	40 degrees/ 45 degrees	Empty	Strong and painless	3-	5
	Medial rotation (at 45 degrees abd)	70 degrees/ 75 degrees	55 degrees/ 60 degrees	Normal	Strong and painless*	3-	5
	Scratch test	Can reach T12	Can reach posterior-superior iliac				
Cervical spine	ROM	Full range with no pain	Has full range with no pain with overpressures at end-range				

*Maximal resistance in limited ROM

For objective findings of the clinical assessment for the case scenario (given to the learner), refer to Table 13-4.

- General observations
  - Patient has a hard time removing her coat
  - Right arm maintained in resting position against chest
- Specific observations
  - Reversed scapulohumeral rhythm during shoulder abduction
  - Atrophy of the right deltoid muscle
- Accessory movements of the glenohumeral joint
  - Stiffness and typical pain during glides (all directions)
- Special tests
  - Supraspinatus test (empty can): Negative
  - Hawkins-Kennedy: Cannot tolerate initial position
- Neurological exam
  - Dermatome (C4-T1): Normal
  - Reflexes (C6, C7): Normal
  - Myotome (C4-T1): Normal
- **System 1:** With this additional information, the learner may recognize that general observations are more supportive of a pathology originating from the shoulder vs the cervical spine. He may also acknowledge that the absence of strength deficits eliminates a hypothesis involving rotator cuff muscles, and that since ROM is so limited, an impingement diagnosis is very unlikely.
- **System 2:** Results from the isometric resistive movement findings can be challenging to interpret: Why would strength not be affected while the patient reports moderate pain intensity rating? Furthermore, the learner may not immediately recognize the typical, and in this case important, capsular pattern (major restrictions in shoulder abduction and lateral rotation) associated with adhesive capsulitis. He also might not recognize that the overprotective positioning of her right

TABLE 13-5

DEFICITS, ACTIVITY LIMITATIONS, AND RESTRICTIONS IN PARTICIPATION		
DEFICITS	**ACTIVITY LIMITATIONS**	**RESTRICTIONS IN PARTICIPATION**
Right shoulder pain Decreased ROM Decreased strength Muscle imbalance— scapulothoracic	Getting dressed Housing chores Lifting boxes	Performing 100% of her tasks at work/home/recreation

arm is much more significant than expected, and that he should investigate the nature of this behavior (ie, false beliefs regarding pain vs illness perception). More questioning regarding the patient's perception about work-related beliefs may also be worth exploring (eg, job stress), because the work environment is likely to influence disability levels for the short and long term.

Step 4 (Final Diagnosis)

From the remaining hypotheses (if more than one remains), a hypothesis is confirmed as the final or most probable diagnosis. From all the available data, the most probable clinical diagnosis is determined. For this case, the interpretation of the information presented would point toward a shoulder capsulitis. The complete process for this conclusion mainly involves an analytic approach (System 2), especially for novice learners. At this point, it may be a good opportunity for the learner and mentor to discuss on the CR process, and to identify specific learning objectives or competencies (knowledge or skills) to be acquired by the learner; the mentor can foster this learning process and/or provide lectures and/or resources for the learner.

As this case was built around CR regarding the establishment of a diagnosis, the same process could now be oriented toward the use of dual process CR for intervention selection, to address deficits and limitations, as well as to establish a prognosis.

Step 5 (Identification of Possible Interventions)

Once the diagnosis is established and confirmed, the learner is asked to develop a treatment plan for the identified deficits in body functions and structures, activity limitations, and restrictions in participation. For learning purposes, those can be specified and given to the learner. For this case of right shoulder adhesive capsulitis, interventions should be articulated around the following (Table 13-5).

- **System 1:** With this objective information in mind, the learner could set short-term goals addressing pain and ROM deficits, and list all possible interventions, since these are the 2 main drivers of activity limitation and restriction in participation. He could name that modalities can provide short-term pain relief, activity modification can prevent flare-ups, ROM and stretching exercises could improve ROM, and manual techniques such as low-/high-grade mobilizations can address both pain and ROM deficits.

- **System 2:** Implications are minimal for this step, unless the learner does not know a specific treatment approach related to a deficit or restriction in activity limitation or participation, or if the mentor highlights approaches that the student did not recognize. In this scenario, there is a rational override back to System 1, where the learner needs to acquire more knowledge about the specific treatment approach. Learners may also be challenged here to be more creative and patient centered with interventions and provide additional options.

Step 6 (Intervention Selection)

- **System 1:** As pain and ROM deficits are the patient's main concern, this should guide the learner's treatment priorities. Based on foundation coursework, rehab students are often well trained when it comes to exercise prescription and patient education. Addressing pain in more complex scenarios might be more challenging and refer to System 2.

- **System 2:** The learner could be challenged regarding the type, dose, and timing of all possible interventions for shoulder capsulitis, and might not recognize that this can be facilitated by determining the irritability level and current stage of adhesive capsulitis.[18] Knowing that the patient is in Stage 1 with a moderate irritability would lead the learner to emphasize combining short-duration, active-assisted ROM stretching exercises; adjusting the total end-range time with pain; adding modalities (eg, transcutaneous electrical nerve stimulation [TENS] during the exercises and heat or icing before or after); and including low-grade mobilizations, biomechanical retraining for proper scapulothoracic movement, while educating his patient on the importance of exercising at home on a daily basis. System 2 might also be beneficial when the therapist is asked about more invasive therapy, such as corticosteroid injections or manipulation under anesthesia, with the need for potential referral. Although he could recognize that these are 2 possible medical interventions (System 1), supporting the collaborative CDM process with the patient might suggest more System 2 CR.

Step 7 (Identification of Factors Influencing Prognosis)

- **System 1:** Often, foundation coursework will enable the learner to quickly identify negative prognosis factors. The learner may know that specific causes of secondary adhesive capsulitis, such as type 2 diabetes, may lead to a lengthier and more difficult clinical course, or that patients who had a positive tissue release following a manipulation under anesthesia will have a more rapid and positive prognosis.

- **System 2:** Establishing the prognosis for more nonmusculoskeletal cases (ie, adhesive capsulitis secondary to a stroke or Parkinson's disease) can require a better understanding of the complex clinical picture and entire movement system. System 2 could also be required to compare prognoses between surgical and nonsurgical approaches. For this case scenario, considering that adhesive capsulitis is associated with type 2 diabetes, and the patient is currently in Stage 1, short-term improvements in pain and ROM are reserved.

CONCLUSION

Dual processing theory is a concept associated with the interplay between implicit (automatic), unconscious processes and explicit, conscious processes during CDM. Dual processing theory can be taught to improve CR strategies, specifically those that involve introduction of new knowledge. This chapter provides strategies and examples using CRLS that are designed to be incorporated into formal educational strategies.

Key Take-Home Points

- Dual processing theory is associated with the interplay between implicit, unconscious processes and explicit, conscious processes during decision-making.

- System 1 reasoning is a fast and automatic form of CR based on heuristics and experience. In this form of reasoning, the clinician makes decisions based on patterns of recognition, rules, and experiences built through years of experience or based on the experiences of an expert mentor or teacher.

- System 2 reasoning is a thoughtful and intentional form of reasoning based on the use of quantitative tests and measures that help reveal information the clinician uses to form a plan of care.

- Both systems of reasoning have advantages and disadvantages. Each system is useful in clinical situations that demand its specific qualities. While novice clinicians default more to System 2 reasoning and experts use System 1, dual processing theory recognizes that both systems have advantages and are most effective when used together.

- Awareness of dual processing theory and Systems 1 and 2 reasoning may form an effective framework for educating novice clinicians in how to approach CR and decision-making.

CONCLUDING CONSIDERATIONS

- Decision-making efficiencies improve with greater and more patient exposure.

- Recognition of one's biases is essential to decrease errors in decision-making.

- Correct decision-making with System 1 and System 2 theories involves bidirectional input. In other words, good System 1 training improves System 2 thinking, and good System 2 training improves System 1 thinking.

Reflection Moment

Consider the 2 quotes provided at the beginning and end of the chapter, and discuss how they relate to your thinking about System 1 and System 2 approaches to CR.

Based upon your learning in this chapter, how has your approach to CR-CDM been impacted for your preferred patient care and/or teaching and learning?

The creative mind doesn't have to have the whole pattern—it can have just a little piece and be able to envision the whole picture in completion.   —Arthur Fry

KEY TERMS AND DEFINITIONS

- **Dual processing theory:** A multidimensional form of CR-CDM in which both analytic and nonanalytic processes are used simultaneously to arrive at a decision.

- **System 1 reasoning:** A nonanalytic form of reasoning in which rapid and automatic decision-making is made based on mental maps, lines of thought, stereotypes, and known patterns developed through experience and collaboration with expert colleagues.

- **System 2 reasoning:** An analytic form of reasoning in which effortful and thoughtful decision-making employs quantitative testing and outcome measures to develop a plan of care.

REFERENCES

1. Edwards I, Jones M, Carr J, Braunack-Mayer A, Jensen GM. Clinical reasoning strategies in physical therapy. *Phys Ther.* 2004;84(4):312-330; discussion 331-335.
2. Pennaforte T, Moussa A, Loye N, Charlin B, Audétat MC. Exploring a new simulation approach to improve clinical reasoning teaching and assessment: randomized trial protocol. *JMIR Res Protoc.* 2016;5(1):e26.
3. Marcum JA. An integrated model of clinical reasoning: dual-process theory of cognition and metacognition. *J Eval Clin Pract.* 2012;18(5):954-961.
4. Norman GR, Eva KW. Diagnostic error and clinical reasoning. *Med Educ.* 2010;44(1):94-100.
5. Kahneman D, Frederick S. Representativeness revisited: attribute substitution in intuitive judgement. In: Gilovich T, Griffin D, Kahneman D, eds. *Heuristics and Biases: The Psychology of Intuitive Judgment.* Cambridge, United Kingdom: Cambridge University; 2002:49-81.
6. Kaufman S, Singer J. The creativity of dual process system 1 thinking. https://blogs.scientificamerican.com/guest-blog/the-creativity-of-dual-process-system-1-thinking/. Published January 17, 2012. Accessed December 19, 2016.
7. Evans J. Heuristic and analytic processes in reasoning. *B J Psyc.* 1984;75:451-468.
8. Norman G, Monteiro S, Sherbino J. Is clinical cognition binary or continuous? *Acad Med.* 2013;88(8):1058-1060.
9. Kahneman D, Lovallo D, Sibony O. Before you make that big decision ... *Harv Bus Rev.* 2011;89(6):50-60, 137.
10. Croskerry P. A universal model of diagnostic reasoning. *Acad Med.* 2009;84(8):1022-1028.
11. Croskerry P. Context is everything or how could I have been that stupid? *Healthc Q.* 2009;12:e171-e176.
12. Klein JG. Five pitfalls in decisions about diagnosis and prescribing. *BMJ.* 2005;330(7494):781-783.
13. Norman G. Dual processing and diagnostic errors. *Adv Health Sci Educ Theory Pract.* 2009;14(suppl 1):37-49.
14. Jensen G, Gwyer J, Hack LM, Shepard K, *Expertise in Physical Therapy Practice.* 2nd ed. Salt Lake City, UT: Elsevier; 2007.
15. American Physical Therapy Association. Guide to physical therapist practice. 2nd ed. *Phys Ther.* 2001;81(1):9-746.
16. Musolino GM. Fostering reflective practice: self-assessment abilities of physical therapy students and entry-level graduates. *J Allied Health.* 2006;35(1):30-42.
17. Konopasek L, Kelly KV, Bylund CL, Wenderoth S, Storey-Johnson C. The group objective structured clinical experience: building communication skills in the clinical reasoning context. *Patient Educ Couns.* 2014;96(1):79-85.
18. Kelley MJ, McClure PW, Leggin BG. Frozen shoulder: evidence and a proposed model guiding rehabilitation. *J Orthop Sports Phys Ther.* 2009;39(2):135-148.

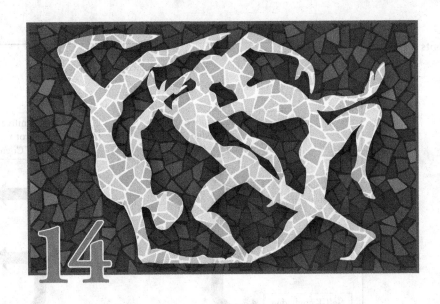

THE RELEVANCE OF METACOGNITION FOR CLINICAL REASONING

Tricia R. Prokop, PT, EdD, MS, CSCS

OBJECTIVES

- Differentiate among the requisite terms and theoretical rationale for incorporating metacognitive training and assessment within physical therapy for enhancing clinical reasoning (CR).
- Construct and deconstruct frameworks for implementing metacognitive objectives to facilitate CR.
- Compare and contrast examples of how to execute metacognitive training for CR.
- Discriminate among metacognitive assessment tools and their use for facilitating CR.

INTRODUCTION

Acquisition of factual, conceptual, and procedural knowledge alone is inadequate for the development of CR. Students must possess effective metacognitive control, so that they may monitor and control their knowledge. Clinical and academic educators are encouraged to establish metacognitive objectives and intentionally incorporate metacognitive training and assessment within a physical therapy curriculum for the development of CR in physical therapy students.

The focus of Chapter 14 is on the relevance of metacognition in the development of CR for physical therapy students. Consider the following situation: 2 students each earn 85% on a recent examination. Typically, that earned grade would not be cause for alarm; however, there may be instances in which a high-performing student will struggle with CR. Now, imagine 2 different students who each earn 65% on the same examination. It is commonly assumed that these students would in turn struggle with CR. The lower-performing students would likely require additional assistance; however, educators must contemplate what type

Musolino GM, Jensen GM, eds. *Clinical Reasoning and Decision-Making in Physical Therapy: Facilitation, Assessment, and Implementation* (pp 169-176).
© 2020 Taylor & Francis Group.

Figure 14-1. Components of meta-cognition.

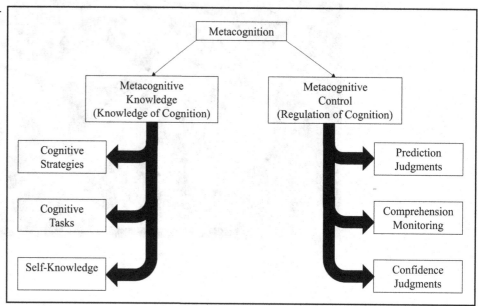

of remediation is most beneficial. In the profession of physical therapy education, consideration needs to be made as to how both high and low examination results may reflect the CR ability of the student, in addition to what types of remediation are necessary for the development of effective CR. Understanding the metacognitive abilities of physical therapy students will provide educators with these insights.

Metacognition can be defined globally as an awareness of the accuracy of one's own thought processes. Pintrich describes 2 components of metacognition: metacognitive knowledge (knowledge of cognition) and metacognitive control (regulation of cognition).[1,2] See Figure 14-1 for an illustration of the components of metacognition.

Knowledge of cognition includes strategic knowledge, knowledge about cognitive tasks, and self-knowledge.[1,2] Regulation of cognition describes those cognitive processes that learners employ to monitor and control their learning. Metacognitive processes include making predictions about how easy something will be to learn, monitoring one's own understanding, and evaluating the accuracy of one's response.[1,2] Development of a physical therapy student's metacognitive knowledge and control will facilitate effective CR.

Metacognitive training has not only been shown to improve student learning in multiple disciplines, including various specialties within medical education,[2-6] but it has also been associated with the development of CR.[7-10] Given CR to be the sum of thinking and deciding during the evaluation, examination, and treatment of patients,[11] it is clear that possession of knowledge is required; however, the ability to monitor thought processes and use accurate judgment is essential to making an appropriate decision. This notion is supported in the literature, which indicates that effective CR is the result of enhanced judgment rather than increased knowledge.[12-14]

Reflection Moment

In the clinical setting, a physical therapy student encounters a patient with an unfamiliar diagnosis. The student proceeds to treat the patient and fails to identify a significant change in status, which jeopardizes the patient's health.

This is clearly a safety concern, and most educators would identify this as a failure in CR. What was the cause for the poor CR? Lack of knowledge, or poor judgment?

There was a lack of knowledge because the patient had a diagnosis that was unfamiliar to the student; however, if we remediate the poor CR by having the student learn about this new diagnosis, have we ensured that this student's CR will be improved in the future?

There was also poor judgment because the student was unable to identify a change in status that was incongruent with his understanding of this patient's care.

If we remediate the poor judgment, how will this impact the student's CR in the future?

TABLE 14-1
REVISED BLOOM'S TAXONOMY

KNOWLEDGE DIMENSION	COGNITIVE PROCESS DIMENSION
Factual	Remember
Conceptual	Understand
Procedural	Apply
Metacognitive	Analyze
	Evaluate
	Create

Adapted from Krathwohl.[19]

As illustrated in Figure 14-1, judgment and monitoring are the components of metacognitive control. Therefore, educators looking to facilitate CR in physical therapy students should strive to improve metacognitive control.

Metacognitive control is essential for effective CR due to the vital role in regulating cognition. Without accurate metacognitive control, students are likely to make errors in CR due to lack of awareness of knowledge gaps or cognitive biases, both of which impact accurate judgment.[8,15] Therefore, CR can be effectively cultivated through strategies intended to develop metacognition, and it has been suggested that metacognitive training be incorporated into the education of all students, including those in medical professions.[1,8,13,14,16] Despite the identified importance in the development of effective CR, metacognition is infrequently taught and assessed.[16] Therefore, the remainder of this chapter is devoted to the practical implementation of metacognitive training within a physical therapy curriculum.

INTEGRATION INTO PHYSICAL THERAPY EDUCATION

Establishing Objectives

As with developing any course curriculum, it is recommended that educators use a backward design to facilitate CR within physical therapy students.[17] A necessary first step in backward design is to identify the desired result, which is accomplished by establishing course outcome.[17] Physical therapy educators are proficient at generating objectives related to the knowledge and skills acquired in the course curriculum. Despite the previously established importance of accurate metacognitive knowledge, minimal attention is typically placed upon metacognitive objectives.[18]

In 2002, Krathwohl[19] recommended that Bloom's taxonomy be revised to include, among other things, a metacognitive knowledge dimension. As seen in Table 14-1, the revised taxonomy includes the traditional cognitive processes to remember, understand, apply, analyze, evaluate, and create, as well as the knowledge dimensions of factual, conceptual, procedural, and the more contemporary inclusion of a metacognitive dimension.[19] The intentional emphasis on metacognitive knowledge in the revised taxonomy only further illustrates the importance of incorporating metacognitive training within physical therapy curricula.

For the sake of clarity and consistency within the cognitive psychology literature, it is important to emphasize that the revised taxonomy only includes the knowledge of cognition component of metacognition, within the knowledge dimensions. Regulation of cognition is not explicitly included. The rationale for this distinction is that objectives written at the higher-order cognitive process dimensions encompass the monitoring and judgment components of metacognitive control[1] (see Figure 14-1). Educators may encounter physical therapy students who, like students of other disciplines, lack metacognitive knowledge.[1] Students must have an awareness of what cognitive strategies are available to them, when to use various strategies, and what they know of their strengths and weaknesses before they are able to regulate their knowledge.[1]

The examples in Table 14-2 illustrate potential metacognitive objectives aimed at development of metacognitive control in physical students. In the first example, students are asked to analyze their practical examination performance, presumably with focused prompts for reflection. The analysis is specific not only to whether the student did or did not possess the requisite knowledge, but also to how the student came to the decisions made during the practical. Because the students are asked to reflect, comprehension monitoring is occurring, which is a component of metacognitive control.

The second and third examples aim to have the students determine the accuracy of their knowledge. These objectives are written at the cognitive process dimension level of evaluate, which is defined as "making judgments based on criteria and standards."[19] The evaluation level objectives incorporate components of metacognitive control, because students are asked to pass judgment on their performance or thought processes. These are just a few examples of the possible objectives that can be written to encourage the development of metacognitive control within physical therapy students' curricula.

TABLE 14-2	
EXAMPLES OF COGNITIVE LEVELS OF METACOGNITIVE KNOWLEDGE OBJECTIVES	
OBJECTIVE EXAMPLES	**COGNITIVE PROCESS DIMENSION**
Students will reflect upon their performance of practical examinations	Analyze
Students will critique their performance of practical examinations	Evaluate
Students will accurately evaluate their own conclusions	Evaluate
Adapted from Krathwohl.[19]	

It is not enough for students to solely possess knowledge; rather, it is the monitoring and control of knowledge that are the necessary components of successful CR. Therefore, it is recommended that physical therapy educators deliberately identify metacognitive objectives, including those at the highest levels of the cognitive process dimension, to facilitate the metacognitive control associated with effective CR. Identification of metacognitive objectives will, in turn, enable the training and assessment of metacognition, in accordance with a backward curriculum design.[17]

Metacognitive Training and Assessment

As with all established objectives, metacognitive objectives must also be assessed. It is not enough for students to engage in metacognitive training without feedback, given that the accuracy of their metacognitive knowledge and control is what is deemed "most crucial for learning."[1] Metacognition can be assessed generally or specifically with regard to the objectives identified. When assessing metacognitive objectives specifically, the types of assessments will vary depending upon the level of cognitive process required to achieve the established objective.[18] Fortunately, metacognitive assessment can also serve as metacognitive training; therefore, they will be discussed concurrently. Various metacognitive training and assessment methods have been described in the literature and in this text, including think aloud protocols, reflection, cognitive debiasing strategies, concept maps, graphic organizers, debriefing interviews, and observations with guided and structured feedback.[2,20]

METACOGNITIVE KNOWLEDGE

Many physical therapy students may lack the requisite metacognitive knowledge to develop effective CR. Students likely believe it is a lack of factual, conceptual, or procedural knowledge, rather than poor judgment, that contributes to ineffective CR. As a result, it is recommended that physical therapy educators incorporate direct teaching of metacognition, and rationalize the curriculum by educating students on the root cause of cognitive error in the clinical setting.

Various cognitive strategies have been recommended to facilitate metacognition and CR. Paramount to CR is that physical therapy students are taught metacognitive strategies, just as they are taught traditional physical therapy content and skills. Strategies that have been identified as effective to enhance metacognitive strategies in medical education, nursing, and other professions include graphic organizers such as concept maps, think aloud techniques, cognitive debiasing strategies, and guided reflection.[15,20] In addition to teaching physical therapy students that such strategies exist, faculty must also encourage students to learn in what context to use various strategies, as well as their individual strengths and weaknesses as a reasoning clinician, because recognizing successful or unsuccessful strategies is a necessary component of developing effective self-knowledge.[1] All 3 of these components—cognitive strategies, tasks, and self-knowledge—are necessary for physical therapy students to develop the metacognitive knowledge required for effective CR.

METACOGNITIVE CONTROL

With the intent to develop effective CR in physical therapy students, physical therapy educators are encouraged to train and assess metacognitive control. To do so, students should be encouraged to regularly monitor their knowledge and pass judgments. Now let's contemplate the scenarios presented in Figure 14-2.

In Figure 14-2, there are 2 students who earned low grades on the assessment. Although both students have knowledge deficits, without additional information, you are unaware of how this will fully impact their CR. With strictly content-based assessment questions, how are you as the educator to discern if the poor performance was due to strictly a lack of content knowledge vs a lack of content knowledge in addition to a lack of metacognitive knowledge and control? The only knowledge that is assessed with traditional quizzes and examinations is the factual, conceptual, or procedural knowledge specific to the content of the assessment. However, if we truly want to examine CR, educators must assess metacognitive awareness as well as content knowledge, because effective CR is the result of enhanced judgment rather than increased knowledge.[12-14]

	High Metacognitive Awareness	Low Metacognitive Awareness
High Grade	Student A No concerns – *student is likely strong in all knowledge dimensions and has effective metacognitive control*	Student C Significant concern – *potential to perpetuate cognitive biases and establish false sense of confidence*
Low Grade	Student B Little concern – *requires remediation of factual, conceptual, or procedural knowledge specific to the assessment*	Student D Significant concern – *likely deficient in factual, conceptual, procedural, and metacognitive knowledge as well as metacognitive control*

Figure 14-2. Metacognitive awareness: possible student scenarios.

Reflection Moment

Let's revisit the clinical scenario presented previously. In the clinical setting, a physical therapy student encounters a patient with an unfamiliar diagnosis. The student proceeds to treat the patient and fails to identify a significant change in status, which jeopardizes the patient's health.

Would a traditional assessment of factual, conceptual, or procedural knowledge have been adequate to identify the lack of effective CR displayed in the clinical setting?

Why or why not?

Now, revisit the example in Figure 14-2. Imagine that Student B earned a low grade, and although you are not privileged to this information, Student B was fully aware that he earned a failing grade. Conversely, Student D also earned a low grade, but Student D left the examination believing that he earned a passing grade. In translating this to the clinical scenario, Student B is likely to realize that he does not possess the necessary knowledge, and is therefore more likely to seek out additional resources and avoid making an error. Student D is unlikely to identify the knowledge deficits, and will in turn rely on assumptions or cognitive biases that will likely result in an error in CR.

The students who earn high grades on examinations are generally not cause for concern. Student A is not only strong in all the knowledge dimensions, but also has adequate metacognitive control. This student is likely to possess the requisite knowledge for effective CR and have the metacognitive control to identify areas of weakness and seek out additional strategies or information as needed. Conversely, Student C may possess the factual, conceptual, and procedural knowledge that is assessed on the examination, but may not have adequate metacognitive control. This is the student who can answer the multiple-choice test correctly or perform the correct call-upon skill in a practical examination, but unfortunately may not know when or why to implement such knowledge in a clinical context. This student possesses content knowledge but not the ability to monitor and judge the knowledge, which can perpetuate biases that would likely present in the clinical setting, resulting in ineffective CR.

These scenarios illustrate how solely relying upon grades on traditional examinations and quizzes may not translate accurately into assessment of a student's CR ability. By encouraging students to pass judgment over their knowledge through self-assessment, the differences between students' cognition and metacognition become even more evident. The scenarios convey the importance of metacognitive control, or accurate awareness of knowledge, in effective CR. Additionally, these scenarios provide the educators with insights as to how best to assist students with remediation as needed. If the intent is to develop accurate CR, educators of physical therapy students must teach and assess not only content knowledge but also the learners' metacognitive control.

Calibration

One method of teaching and assessing metacognitive control is the use of calibration. Calibration is the relationship between judgment of performance and actual performance, and has been studied extensively as a means of quantifying metacognition.[21,22] A prediction judgment of performance is "a monitoring judgment that comes after acquisition and retention but prior to retrieval" in the stages of learning.[22] Post-diction calibration is a retrospective judgment that occurs after retrieval.[22] Both prediction and post-diction calibration are components of metacognitive control.

Calibration assessments can be done throughout a physical therapy curriculum and should be a regular practice for students. This can be accomplished simply by adding prediction and post-diction sections to each assignment or examination. For practical examinations, students can be asked to grade their performance on the grading rubric, such as what was identified in the second objective in Table 14-2. Feedback on the accuracy of their self-reflections would only enhance the evaluative cognitive processes associated with metacognitive control. Once the earned grade has been determined, a calibration score can be assigned by subtracting the estimated score from the actual score.[23] Evidence exists that students who engaged in regular metacognitive training, with appropriate feedback, become significantly more accurate with calibration,[24] which implicates the development of greater metacognitive control.

Response Certitude

Response certitude is a second means of easily facilitating metacognitive control. It is defined as "a subjective estimate of performance expectation."[25] Just as with a calibration assessment, response certitude can be added to existing assignments and examinations in a physical therapy curriculum. See Figure 14-3 for an example of a response certitude assessment on a multiple-choice quiz.

To perform a response certitude assessment on a multiple-choice quiz, students answer the quiz question as they typically would, but are then prompted to make a confidence judgment of their answer by circling "Yes" or "No." Students then rate their confidence in the "Yes" or "No" answer on a scale of 1 to 4, with 1 indicating the lowest level of confidence. See Figure 14-4 for examples of how students will quantify the certitude of their response to the quiz question.

Response certitude scores can be calculated and used as a means of assessing metacognitive objectives, such as the third objective identified in Table 14-2. Positive values are assigned to the confidence scale value (1 to 4) if the "Yes" or "No" answer indicated by the student is consistent with the evaluation made by the instructor. A negative value is assigned to the confidence value if the "Yes" or "No" result is inconsistent with that of the instructor. A response certitude score is calculated by summing the numbers, with a higher positive value indicative of greater metacognitive awareness and a greater negative value revealing poor metacognitive awareness.

Adding assessments such as calibration and response certitude scales allows educators to assess metacognitive objectives and facilitate metacognitive control in physical therapy students. The impact of both these tools lies in the ability for physical therapy educators to gain the insights required to differentiate Student B from Student D in the scenarios identified in Figure 14-2. Student B would presumably be better calibrated and have a higher response certitude score than Student D, which would provide evidence to both the instructor and the student regarding the quality of the student's metacognitive control. The remediation required for Student B would likely be solely acquisition of the factual, conceptual, or procedural knowledge assessed on the examination, whereas remediation for Student D would likely also require development of metacognitive knowledge and control.

Calibration and response certitude also have direct benefits for the students. Accuracy of knowledge is most critical for learning because the opportunity to learn increases as accuracy increases.[1,22] Students are more likely to correct errors in their knowledge base if they are aware that those errors exist. This correction is the necessary step for cognitive debiasing relevant to effective CR. This supports the use of these techniques for not only the development of metacognitive control specifically but also learning in general. Use of calibration and response certitude in conjunction with traditional classroom techniques has the potential to create the meaningful cognitive events required for effective CR through development of metacognitive control in physical therapy students.

General Assessment of Metacognition

In addition to assessment of specific metacognitive objectives, there may be merit in assessment of a student's general metacognitive ability. The Metacognitive Awareness Inventory (MAI) is considered to be a general measure of metacognition rather than a domain-specific instrument.[2] The MAI is a 52-item self-report instrument to assess both metacognitive knowledge and control. Reliability for the subscales of knowledge of cognition and regulation of cognition is reported in the literature as 0.88 and 0.91, respectively.[2] It is worth noting that recent studies have modified the original 100-mm scale to a Likert scale of various ranges, making comparison of raw data across studies unmanageable.[26-29] Regardless of the scale, higher MAI scores are indicative of greater metacognitive awareness. The MAI is an applicable instrument to assess change in metacognition in physical therapy students. The MAI, as well as modifications of the original instrument for use in foreign countries, has been used to assess metacognitive ability of medical and nursing students.[30-32]

Recent studies involving students of health professions have conveyed that the MAI has the capacity to track change in metacognitive awareness over time. When observing metacognition from the beginning to the end of the first year of medical education, authors identify improved metacognitive regulation as measured by an adapted version of the MAI.[31] In an investigation of the metacognitive awareness of medical students, statistically significant differences in the MAI between students

Sample Quiz Question	Did you answer this question correctly?	How confident are you in your Yes/No?
You are examining a patient with elbow pathology and notice swelling in the posterior lateral soft spot between the radius and capitellum. What is the **MOST** likely pathology? a. Ulnar collateral ligament tear b. Lateral epicondylitis c. Triceps tendonitis d. Biceps tendonitis	Yes | No	1 2 3 4

Figure 14-3. Example of a certitude quiz.

Student Response	Did you answer this question correctly?	How confident are you in your Yes/No?
Very confident the question was answered correctly	Yes	4
Took a well-educated guess	Yes	1
Very confident the question was answered incorrectly	No	4

Figure 14-4. Example of student responses.

in the preclinical vs clinical phases of medical education were discovered.[30] Lastly, in a recent study examining the effects of problem-based learning on critical thinking and metacognitive awareness, the authors established statistically significant improvements in the MAI for nursing students engaged in a problem-based learning vs lecture-based curriculum.[32] As physical therapy educators become more aware of the need to teach and assess metacognitive knowledge and control, the MAI can be used as an objective tool to track general changes in the metacognitive knowledge and control of students over time or in response to metacognitive interventions.

The MAI includes items that assess metacognitive monitoring and judgment,[2] akin to the awareness necessary for effective CR. Therefore, a significant, positive change in the MAI would indicate improved metacognitive control, thus the potential to generate effective CR. What are currently unknown are what MAI results indicate effective metacognition, and what values are indicative of meaningful change. More research is needed regarding use of the MAI as a measure of metacognitive awareness in physical therapy students, as well as the relationship between scores on the MAI and effective CR.

CONCLUSION

Educators put forth great effort to establish objectives, create learning opportunities, and develop effective assessment methods to aid students in their ability to acquire the requisite knowledge of their profession. However, in many disciplines, including physical therapy, what is arguably more important than the attainment of knowledge is the ability to accurately monitor and control learners' knowledge acquisition. Therefore, metacognitive control is central to the development of effective CR.

Physical therapy educators and peers should not deemphasize knowledge and skills in the physical therapy curriculum; rather, educators and peers should be encouraged to stress the development of metacognition in addition to requisite content knowledge and skills, with the goal of developing expert CR within physical therapy students. There are various ways to facilitate metacognitive control that are both relevant and practical for implementation within physical therapy curricula. The addition of these methods to traditional physical therapy curricula will provide educators with insights as to how student performance will translate into the clinical setting, as well as what types of remediation may be necessary for the development of effective CR.

References

1. Pintrich PR. The role of metacognitive knowledge in learning, teaching, and assessing. *Theory Pract.* 2002;41:219-225.
2. Pintrich PR, Wolters CA, Baxter GP. Assessing metacognition and self-regulated learning. In: Schraw G, Impara J, eds. *Issues in the Measurement of Metacognition.* Lincoln, NE: Buros Institute of Mental Measurements; 2000:43-97.
3. Lew MD, Schmidt HG. Self-reflection and academic performance: is there a relationship? *Adv Health Sci Educ Theory Pract.* 2011;16(4):529-545.
4. Yusuff KB. Does self-reflection and peer-assessment improve Saudi pharmacy students' academic performance and metacognitive skills? *Saudi Pharm J.* 2016;23(3):266-275.
5. Pai HC. An integrated model for the effects of self-reflection and clinical experiential learning on clinical nursing performance in nursing students: a longitudinal study. *Nurse Educ Today.* 2016;45:156-162.
6. Garrett J, Alman M, Gardner S, Born C. Assessing students' metacognitive skills. *Am J Pharm Educ.* 2007;71(1):14.
7. Kuiper RA, Pesut DJ. Promoting cognitive and metacognitive reflective reasoning skills in nursing practice: self-regulated learning theory. *J Adv Nurs.* 2004;45(4):381-391.
8. Mamede S, van Gog T, van den Berge K, et al. Effect of availability bias and reflective reasoning on diagnostic accuracy among internal medicine residents. *JAMA.* 2010;304(11):1198-1203.
9. Marcum JA. An integrated model of clinical reasoning: dual-process theory of cognition and metacognition. *J Eval Clin Pract.* 2012;18(5):954-961.
10. Cutrer WB, Sullivan WM, Fleming AE. Educational strategies for improving clinical reasoning. *Curr Probl Pediatr Adolesc Health Care.* 2013;43(9):248-257.
11. Higgs J, Jones MA, Loftus S, Christensen N, eds. *Clinical Reasoning in the Health Professions.* 3rd ed. Amsterdam, Netherlands: Butterworth-Heinemann Elsevier; 2008.
12. Croskerry P, Singhal G, Mamede S. Cognitive debiasing 1: origins of bias and theory of debiasing. *BMJ Qual Saf.* 2013;22(suppl 2):ii58-ii64.
13. Mamede S, Schmidt HG, Penaforte JC. Effects of reflective practice on the accuracy of medical diagnoses. *Med Educ.* 2008;42(5):468-475.
14. Mamede S, Splinter TA, van Gog T, Rikers RM, Schmidt HG. Exploring the role of salient distracting clinical features in the emergence of diagnostic errors and the mechanisms through which reflection counteracts mistakes. *BMJ Qual Saf.* 2012;21(4):295-300.
15. Croskerry P. Cognitive forcing strategies in clinical decision making. *Ann Emerg Med.* 2003;41(1):110-120.
16. Burman NJ, Boscardin CK, Van Schaik SM. Career-long learning: relationship between cognitive and metacognitive skills. *Med Teach.* 2014;36(8):715-723.
17. Wiggins G, McTighe J. *Backward Design. Understanding by Design.* 2nd ed. Alexandria, VA: ASCD; 2005:13-34.
18. Airasian PW, Miranda H. The role of assessment in the revised taxonomy. *Theory Pract.* 2002;41(4):249-254.
19. Krathwohl DR. A revision of Bloom's taxonomy: an overview. *Theory Pract.* 2002;41(4):212-218.
20. Colbert CY, Graham L, West C, et al. Teaching metacognitive skills: helping your physician trainees in the quest to "know what they don't know." *Am J Med.* 2015;128(3):318-324.
21. Bol L, Hacker DJ. Calibration research: where do we go from here? *Front Psychol.* 2012;3:229.
22. Hacker DJ, Bol L, Kener MC. Metacognition in education. In: Dunlosky J, Bjork RA, eds. *Handbook of Metamemory and Memory.* New York, NY: Taylor & Francis Group; 2008:429-455.
23. Zabrucky KM, Agler LM, Moore D. Metacognition in Taiwan: students' calibration of comprehension and performance. *Int J Psychol.* 2009;44(4):305-312.
24. Nietfeld JL, Cao L, Osborne JW. The effect of distributed monitoring exercises and feedback on performance, monitoring accuracy, and self-efficacy. *Metacogn Learn.* 2006;1:159-179.
25. Stock WA, Winston KS, Behrens JT, Harper-Marinick M. The effects of performance expectation and question difficulty on text study time, response certitude, and correct responding. *Bull Psychon Soc.* 1989;27:567-569.
26. Schraw G, Dennison RS. Assessing metacognitive awareness. *Contemp Educ Psych.* 1994;19:460-475.
27. Stewart PW, Cooper SS, Moulding LR. Metacognitive development in professional educators. *The Researcher.* 2007;21(1):32-40.
28. Young A, Fry JD. Metacognitive awareness and academic achievement in college students. *J Scholar Teach Learn.* 2008;8(2):1-10.
29. Coutinho SA. The relationship between goals, metacognition, and academic success. *Educate.* 2007;7(1):39-47.
30. Turan S, Demirel O, Sayek I. Metacognitive awareness and self-regulated learning skills of medical students in different medical curricula. *Med Teach.* 2009;31(10):e477-e483.
31. Hong WH, Vadivelu J, Daniel EG, Sim JH. Thinking about thinking: changes in first-year medical students' metacognition and its relation to performance. *Med Educ Online.* 2015;20:27561.
32. Gholami M, Moghadam PK, Mohammadipoor F, et al. Comparing the effects of problem-based learning and the traditional lecture method on critical thinking skills and metacognitive awareness in nursing students in a critical care nursing course. *Nurse Educ Today.* 2016;45:16-21.

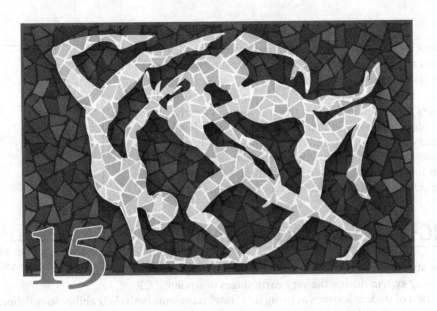

FACILITATION OF CLINICAL REASONING:
Teaching and Learning Strategies
Across the Continuum of Learners

Lisa Black, PT, DPT and Nicole Christensen, PT, PhD, MAppSc

OBJECTIVES

- Examine teaching and learning strategies to facilitate clinical reasoning (CR) at different stages across the professional education continuum.

- Describe the concept of a collaborative patient-centered learning system as the ideal way to facilitate CR development.

- Discuss the importance of strategically integrating considerations of context in the learner's CR as a way to facilitate growth.

INTRODUCTION

Professional growth and development, including the development of clinical expertise, is ideally a career-long endeavor for health professionals; it is an active process and a process that never ends for those who value lifelong learning. For physical therapists, CR and associated experiential learning abilities are the key elements that fuel continuous knowledge and skills development and refinement over the course of their careers.[1-3] Development of CR should begin at the very start of professional education in the academic setting. Ideally, for physical therapist students the learning done in the academic setting lays the foundation for them to engage in experiential learning with their clinical instructors (CIs) and patients in the authentic practice setting.

The practice environment is the most impactful of all learning experiences, as it provides context needed for development and advancement of CR for a learner. Ideally, within the practice environment, the learner (eg, student or resident) and the learning facilitator (eg, CI or residency mentor) work collaboratively with the patient to create a dynamic learning system. In this system,

Musolino GM, Jensen GM, eds. *Clinical Reasoning and Decision-Making in Physical Therapy: Facilitation, Assessment, and Implementation* (pp 177-181).
© 2020 Taylor & Francis Group.

the focus is on the patient and optimal patient outcomes; however, the learner is enabled to engage in trial and error, metacognition, and retrospective reflection to learn and build knowledge from CR experiences.[4,5]

We will frame our discussion of facilitating the learning of CR around the characteristics of learners at 5 key stages across the continuum of early professional development. Three of these stages take place during entry-level education, the fourth is an entry-level clinician, and the final stage involves a learner who is engaged in residency education. We will use the concept of the collaborative learning system formed by the learner, the learning facilitator, and the patient in their care context to frame our discussion for each stage.

BEGINNING-EARLY STUDENT LEARNER

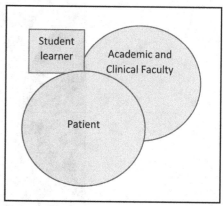

Figure 15-1. The learning system with an early student learner.

The beginning-early student learner is illustrated in Figure 15-1, representing a collaborative learning system during the very early stages of students' CR development. The depiction of student learners as being in a "box" represents both their ability to collaborate while just starting to learn the knowledge and technical skills necessary to interact and collect data, and options for interventions and management. Learners in these very early stages often compartmentalize thinking and decision-making as separate from the performance of the new technical skills. Their focus is on themselves and what is being placed in their box. The sharp "corners" of the box represent the lack of ability to easily integrate into and work "with" the other members of the learning system, including the patient and the academic or clinical facilitator. Many a faculty facilitator has witnessed a student at this stage, gathering information for the sake of checking it off his or her mental list of things he or she needs to do in an interaction, completely disconnected from a reasoning or interpretation process to guide his or her responses to the information received, or to direct the next task he or she chooses to do.

To provide very early learners with the support they need to function in the collaborative learning system, there is a need to give them a framework within which to build their foundations for CR development, even before the student works with real patients in the clinical setting. At this stage of their education, students crave structure (the box) to assist them in paying attention to the important aspects of a clinical situation. To prepare them with a framework to begin to develop CR, students need to develop an understanding of what the concept of CR encompasses. This entails understanding what it includes, how each element relates to the others, and how CR provides a link to their ability to learn from their experiences.[6,7] By focusing on and explicitly developing an understanding of this invisible thing called CR, students are provided with a way to organize their developing understanding, to make sense of what they are learning, and to understand how it all fits together in the context of practice.[6,8]

We know that to facilitate the development of CR, learners need a model and/or language within with which to understand examples of CR.[4,6] By making CR visible in this way early on, learners are able to articulate their questions about CR and clinical decision-making (CDM), receiving and learning to give feedback about the specific elements of their CR performance. Their understanding at this stage will be largely theoretical, as they have not yet put their knowledge into practice.

The more opportunities students are provided for contextualizing this early theoretical understanding of CR within a practice context in the academic setting, the more likely they are to be able to learn about CR in a way that will more directly facilitate their ability to recall and apply their understanding in their clinical experiences. Andragogical strategies that provide students with early opportunities to engage in activities that simulate their clinical experiences work within a collaborative learning system are critical to optimizing development at this early stage.[6,9] Academic faculty can control the number and complexity of contextual factors that students must attend to while learning and practicing aspects of interviewing, conducting physical examinations, and developing plans of care in a progressively challenging way.[10,11] Faculty can work as learning facilitators in the classroom setting by bringing the clinical context to the learning and practice of CR in the academic setting by making use of patient cases, such as paper cases and video cases, and simulations including role-plays, standardized patient simulations, and high-fidelity manikin simulations to stimulate CR and reflection on that reasoning by groups of students.[12] Academic faculty must also facilitate and provide specific guidelines for reflection on these experiences.[6,11] Learners in this setting are most able to reflect retrospectively on their thinking (or lack of thinking) in action, and whether or not their actions were justified by the available clinical data.[13]

Considerations for facilitating the development of very early learners in the clinical setting depend on the level of the learners' development and their preparation before entering the clinical setting for the first time. Learners will be capable of focusing their attention on the patient to varying degrees. As their CIs, learning facilitators can assist students in attending to and processing information in real time by asking questions that shift the student's attention to aspects of the situation they are unable to focus on independently at this stage of their development. The CI often manages how many contextual factors the student has to attend to, often comanaging the more complex aspects of the patient's presentation so that the student can focus on only a few aspects at a time. In these early stages of students' development, the CI has both the challenge and responsibility to make certain that the experience a patient has with the student is worthwhile from that patient's perspective. In essence, CIs must attend to both their own CR as well as that of their students concurrently, so that clinical outcomes are worthwhile, and the students can experience the trial and error necessary to learn from their own CR during patient encounters.

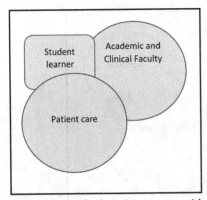

Figure 15-2. The learning system with an intermediate student learner.

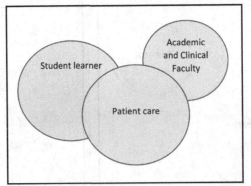

Figure 15-3. The learning system with an advanced student learner.

INTERMEDIATE STUDENT LEARNER

The transition of the learner to an intermediate student level of development is depicted in Figure 15-2. At this stage, intermediate learners have a foundational or basic theoretical understanding of CR and some experiences with reasoning to reflect on; these often include both their own experiences as well as observed experiences of others, or depictions of reasoning via patient cases and simulated experiences. These learners are beginning to understand the gray areas of practice, and the blending of the contextual factors that must be observed and understood in order to reason well.[14] The figure depicts the learner's "sharp corners" having softened a bit; this represents the ability to integrate thinking and actions with those of the CIs and patients. The student's role is still smaller than that of the CI in managing the overall experience of care the patient receives, as CIs still monitor and control the contextual factors the learner must comprehend and integrate into his or her reasoning. CIs often promote focus on these factors retrospectively, after a patient encounter, or help the learner prepare to focus on them prospectively, prior to a patient encounter. Students continue to struggle to think and make sense of information in real time, but have improved in their ability to be more flexible or adaptive in the situation, as dictated by the contextual factors at play. In this stage of development, it is important to allow the learner to experience uncertainty and to struggle with the complexity of actual patient care, or simulated care experiences in the academic and clinical setting.

The facilitation of CR development at this stage is achieved well with peer learning activities in both academic and clinical contexts. Peer learning activities focused on CR development provide opportunities for learners to practice all of the meta-skills required to develop CR and CDM; this is true for real or simulated clinical scenarios providing the context for the peer activity.[15] These meta-skills include[15]:

- Critical thinking, reflective thinking, dialectical (deductive and inductive) reasoning

- Engagement with complexity and exploring interdependencies of all aspects and individuals involved[2]

- Communication, collaboration, and teamwork

Peer learning also promotes intrinsic motivation in the academic setting, for learning and for development of effective collaborative team interactions. This facilitates continued development of the learners' abilities to work effectively within the collaborative system with their CIs, their patients, as well as others in the health care team during clinical experiences.[16,17] There is also the inherent requirement in all peer learning activities of having to collaboratively manage learning by exploring how best to learn together as a team. Reflection as an individual and as a team continue to enhance further CR.[15]

Ten Cate and Durning[17] discuss the importance of developing teaching skills as part of learning in medical education. Because peer learning provides the opportunity for students to learn from teaching their peers, these authors point out the importance of teaching medical students not only to be reflective practitioners[5] but also to be "reflective educators and learn from teaching."[17(p551)]

ADVANCED STUDENT LEARNER

The learning system with the student now able to take on the role of directing the patient encounter, with all of its inherent complexity and relevant contextual factors, is depicted in Figure 15-3. The learning facilitators in both academic and clinical settings step back from the student-patient dyad, and students are able to self-direct their clinical encounters with patients more often than not. Academic and clinical faculty can focus most on helping the learner think and reflect-in-action (as in the Schön reflective practice [RP] model)[5] through strategic questioning in action and retrospectively. The learner can tolerate more probing questioning during reasoning experiences and can succeed in thinking on his or her feet more routinely. At this point, the learner is able to reflect-for-action (Schön RP model)[5] as well in preparation for the patient encounter.

For the advanced learner, the shift in the role of learning facilitator hinges on introduction of focused questioning to promote and develop the learner's critical self-reflection abilities. Questions are the tools used to help learners access their own clinical and theoretical knowledge, and to pull it forward so it can be applied to the situation at hand. The intent is to help the learners realize what they do know, identify what they do not know or have forgotten, and question any underlying assumptions that are leading to unsighted spots in their reasoning and decision-making.[6,11]

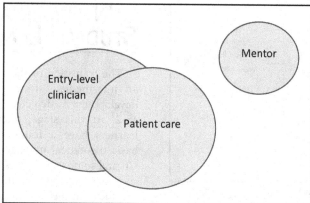
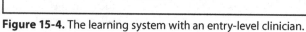

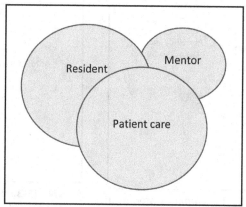

Figure 15-4. The learning system with an entry-level clinician.   **Figure 15-5.** The learning system with a resident.

ENTRY-LEVEL CLINICIAN

Figure 15-4 represents the learning system where the interactions between the entry-level, novice clinicians and their patients are the primary sources of learning facilitation. The entry-level clinician is able to continue learning and facilitating CR independently; however, this is without the presence of the CI for questioning and guiding in practice. As shown in Figure 15-4, entry-level clinicians may be fortunate to have a mentor when they enter independent practice, but in many cases, the mentor does not witness or know the context in specific patient encounters.

The virtuous entry-level clinician continues the practice of critical self-reflection and seeks the opinions of peers for external feedback. Black and colleagues[18] have reported that novice clinicians struggle to continue their development in the absence of mentoring, with learning at this stage primarily the result of social interaction and experience. To continue to facilitate their own CR development, these novice clinicians must actively work to self-assess, to recognize what they do not know, identify their own flaws that may indeed be hidden (very challenging), and take advantage or create new learning opportunities.

While it is possible for the best novices to learn from their own reasoning, it is much easier and arguably more efficient for novices to be helped interactively to further develop their CR abilities. This type of mentoring can be organized between colleagues within a clinic; however, it is becoming progressively more common for novices to consider engaging in post-professional education such as residencies for structured mentoring, in the context of specialty areas of practice for their early career professional development of CR.

RESIDENT

Figure 15-5 illustrates the learning system in residency education; this is in a sense a reunification of the same learning system as exists in entry-level education, but with the learner (resident) now fully capable of managing the patient. Residency education allows for structured mentorship where the mentor can continue to facilitate CR in the resident. Facilitation of CR for this learner is similar to the advanced student learners, but the mentor is typically more advanced in his or her own practice in the specialty practice area and has the ability to facilitate deeper reflection in the resident.

Schön's model of RP,[5] which includes reflection-in-action, or thinking on one's feet, occurs during an experience, and allows for CR that is adaptive and in tune with an emerging understanding of a situation. Novices less commonly use reflection-in-action, and when it is used, it focuses mainly on the patient's performance.[13] In contrast, more experienced clinicians reflect-in-action[5] more often and are focused not only on the patient's performance but also on self-monitoring of their own reasoning in action.[5,13] Hence, facilitation of reflection-in-action[5] and evaluation of one's reasoning are essential to developing expertise in CR.

To enhance their abilities to employ reflection-in-action[5] to modify and enhance CDM in the moment, residents can be helped by their mentors with an explicit focus on strategic gathering of, interpretation of, and decision-making based on contextual clinical data in real time, during a patient encounter. This is achieved through engagement in a dialogue during an encounter in which the mentor questions the resident to encourage critical self-reflection on the resident's thinking in that moment. To employ reflection-in-action to modify CDM in the moment, the mentor must be skilled in creating a collaborative facilitation environment where the resident feels respected and safe in being questioned and engaging in dialogue in the presence of the patient. Ideally, in a true learning system, the patient will be included in the dialogue as appropriate to provide input and feedback to the resident and to the mentor about how successfully they are able to collaboratively reason in real time. We will further discuss residencies and fellowships in Section III.

CONCLUSION

We have framed our discussion of facilitation of CR development within learning stages during professional education and beyond. In addition, we have described the varying roles related to control of the context that academic and clinical faculty serve within the collaborative learning system of learner, learning facilitator, and patient in each stage. Consistent across all levels of learners and all learning settings is the need for an explicit model or framework and a consistent language of CR, shared among the learners and learning facilitators. Facilitation of CR should not end with graduation. The profession needs to continue to develop optimal strategies for teaching and learning CR throughout professional education and practice.

Reflection Moment

Describe 2 teaching and learning strategies that you will implement to challenge CR in your practice setting.

Discuss how you will apply the collaborative patient-centered learning system within your professional practice.

REFERENCES

1. Edwards I, Jones MA. Clinical reasoning and expert practice. In: Jensen GM, Gwyer J, Hack LM, Shepard KF, eds. *Expertise in Physical Therapy Practice*. St. Louis, MO: Elsevier; 2007:192-213.
2. Christensen N, Jones M, Higgs J, Edwards I. Dimensions of clinical reasoning capability. In: Higgs J, Jones M, Loftus S, Christensen N, eds. *Clinical Reasoning in the Health Professions*. 3rd ed. Amsterdam, Netherlands: Butterworth-Heinemann Elsevier; 2008:101-110.
3. Jensen GM. Learning: what matters most. *Phys Ther*. 2011;91(11):1674-1689.
4. Christensen N, Jensen G. Developing clinical reasoning capability. In: Higgs J, Jensen G, Loftus S, Christensen N, eds. *Clinical Reasoning in the Health Professions*. 4th ed. Edinburgh, United Kingdom: Elsevier; 2019:427-434.
5. Schön DA. *Educating the Reflective Practitioner*. San Francisco, CA: Jossey-Bass; 1987.
6. Christensen N, Nordstrom T. Facilitating the teaching and learning of clinical reasoning. In: Jensen GM, Mostrom E, eds. *Handbook of Teaching and Learning for Physical Therapists*. 3rd ed. St. Louis, MO: Butterworth-Heinemann Elsevier; 2013:183-199.
7. Davis B, Sumara D. *Complexity and Education: Inquiries Into Learning, Teaching, and Research*. Mahwah, NJ: Lawrence Erlbaum Associates; 2006.
8. Brookfield SD. *Teaching Critical Thinking: Tools and Techniques to Help Students Question Their Assumptions*. San Francisco, CA: Jossey-Bass Wiley; 2012.
9. Ratcliffe TA, Durning SJ. Theoretical concepts to consider in providing clinical reasoning instruction. In: Trowbridge RL, Rencic JJ, Durning SJ, eds. *Teaching Clinical Reasoning*. Philadelphia, PA: American College of Physicians; 2015:13-30.
10. Irby DM. Excellence in clinical teaching: knowledge transformation and development required. *Med Educ*. 2014;48:776-784.
11. Christensen N, Jones M, Rivett DA. Strategies to facilitate clinical reasoning. In: Jones MA, Rivett DA, eds. *Clinical Reasoning in Musculoskeletal Practice*. 2nd ed. Elsevier; 2018.
12. Christensen N, Villanueva C, Grieve S. Learning reasoning using simulation. In: Higgs J, Jensen G, Loftus S, Christensen N, eds. *Clinical Reasoning in the Health Professions*. 4th ed. Edinburgh, United Kingdom: Elsevier; 2019:455-464.
13. Wainwright SF, Shepard KF, Harman LB, Stephens J. Novice and experienced physical therapist clinicians: a comparison of how reflection is used to inform the clinical decision-making process. *Phys Ther*. 2010;90(1):75-88.
14. Durning S, Artino Jr AR, Pangaro L, van der Vleuten CP, Schuwirth L. Context and clinical reasoning: understanding the perspective of the expert's voice. *Med Educ*. 2011;45(9):927-938.
15. Christensen N, Loftus S, Gwin T. Peer learning to develop clinical reasoning abilities. In: Higgs J, Jensen G, Loftus S, Christensen N, eds. *Clinical Reasoning in the Health Professions*. 4th ed. Edinburgh, United Kingdom: Elsevier; 2019:491-497.
16. Boud D. Introduction: making the move to peer learning. In: Boud D, Cohen R, eds. *Peer Learning in Higher Education*. New York, NY: Routledge; 2013:1-20.
17. Ten Cate O, Durning S. Peer teaching in medical education: twelve reasons to move from theory to practice. *Med Teach*. 2007;29(6):591-599.
18. Black LL, Jensen GM, Mostrom E, et al. The first year of practice: an investigation of the professional learning and development of promising novice physical therapists. *Phys Ther*. 2010;90(12):1758-1773.

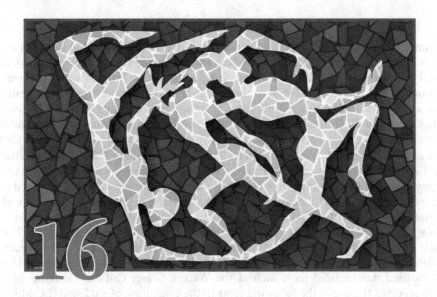

ASSESSMENT OF CLINICAL REASONING:
Strategies Across the Continuum of Professional and Post-Professional Physical Therapy Education

Jennifer Furze, PT, DPT, PCS; Susan Flannery Wainwright, PT, PhD;
Lisa Black, PT, DPT; and Nicole Christensen, PT, PhD, MAppSc

OBJECTIVES

- Describe the complex process of assessing clinical reasoning (CR) skills in physical therapy.
- Discuss the opportunities and pitfalls of existing assessment processes.
- Discover the tools used to assess CR in the didactic setting, clinical setting, and residency and fellowship education.
- Discuss the advantages and disadvantages of various tools in identifying components of CR (knowledge, skills, abilities).

This chapter provides student learners, academic educators, clinical instructors, residency and fellowship directors, mentors, and faculty with effective strategies to assess the CR abilities of students, residents or fellows in both the clinical and didactic setting. CR is a critical component of optimal clinical practice in the health professions. Assessment tools that evaluate and document the progress of the learner across time are described, and application of these tools are illustrated.

IMPORTANCE OF ASSESSMENT

Complexity of the Process

Based upon the definition of CR as described earlier in this text and the factors involved in the dynamic process of CR, challenges for educators in assessing the learner's CR process exist. To begin, it is difficult to objectify something such as a thought

Musolino GM, Jensen GM, eds. *Clinical Reasoning and Decision-Making in Physical Therapy: Facilitation, Assessment, and Implementation* (pp 183-191).
© 2020 Taylor & Francis Group.

or judgment that one cannot see. In addition, CR is not a generic skill that can be learned in isolation and transferred to other settings with different variables.[1] CR remains context dependent and associated with the learner's "working knowledge" about a specific problem, as well as experience with the clinical situation.[2] Thus, novice learners with little working knowledge about particular health conditions, such as cerebral palsy or stroke, will have a limited ability to demonstrate appropriate CR skills when working with a patient with these diagnoses. "Chunking" large amounts of information into an easily accessible memory schema to solve a problem is helpful for clinical problem-solving. Experts in physical therapy have demonstrated the ability to effectively chunk information into illness scripts, and effectively use this information as part of their CR process.[3]

Given the complexity of this CR process, few standardized tests actually evaluate CR abilities specific to physical therapy.[4] Huhn describes standardized assessments for critical thinking, which is one component of CR, in Chapter 17. To gain a better understanding of how physical therapy programs were assessing CR skills, Christensen et al surveyed physical therapist programs in 2015.[5] Results indicated that, to evaluate students' CR abilities, 99% of programs used practical examinations, 94.8% clinical education experiences, 87.5% written examination, and 83% written assignments. In addition to how programs were assessing CR skills, this study also evaluated what tools programs were using for these evaluations. The following tools were identified: 92.7% used the American Physical Therapy Association Physical Therapist Clinical Performance Instrument (APTA PT CPI), while 85.4% designed their own grading rubrics, 43% designed their own grading scale, 43.8% used self-designed grading scales, and 10.4% used standardized tools such as the Watson-Glaser Critical Thinking Appraisal.[5] In a separate survey, clinical educators reported the use of the following tools in the evaluation of students' CR skills in the clinical setting: 54% used the APTA PT CPI, while 15% cited the APTA *Guide to Physical Therapist Practice*, and the remaining respondents indicated other tools including "think aloud/discussion," "faculty-specific tools," and "evidence-based practice such as use of clinical practice guidelines."[6] These results suggest significant variation in the understanding of CR, which leads to an inability to effectively assess the performance of learners (eg, students, residents, fellows) across learning platforms.

The physical therapy profession is not alone in this struggle to understand and evaluate CR. Colleagues in medicine have identified barriers to assessment[7] related to the following key points:

- CR is a collaborative skill that is dependent upon the context of the situation

- A gold standard for the assessment of CR skills does not exist, and thus multiple assessment tools may need to be used to fully capture the true reasoning process

- A variety of tools to assess CR over a time frame, vs a single point in time, is needed to determine competency in CR[2]

ASSESSMENT TOOLS

A majority of the available standardized assessment instruments, such as the Health Science Reasoning Test[8] and the California Critical Thinking Skills Test,[9] evaluate a cognitive component of CR, namely critical thinking, which does not take such things as personal factors and context of the situation into account. In addition, these tests do not pertain specifically to physical therapy practice.[8] Standardized assessment tools to measure CR in medicine are mostly diagnostic in nature and include the following tests:

- Multiple-choice questions

- Script concordance tests (SCTs)

- Concept maps

- CR problem tests

- Standardized patients

Multiple-choice questions based upon case vignettes have limited ability to predict clinical performance. SCTs,[10] which account for expert variance and allow for answers other than "the one right answer,"[11] have also been used in medicine. Essentially, this tool uses cases and aggregate scoring to give credit for potential answers. The disadvantage of this type of test is that it requires an expert panel to provide feedback and initial testing. Concept maps, which help the learner develop illness scripts but take a significant amount of time to grade, have been used in undergraduate medical education and foundational as well as clinical sciences in physical therapy education.[2]

Other tools, including CR problem tests, purport to evaluate the learner's process of CR and not focus on the ultimate outcome.[11] This tool uses a case scenario format to encourage the learner to develop 2 of the most likely diagnoses and then indicate whether clinical features positively or negatively predict the outcome.[11] Standardized patients more closely simulate relevant patient practice; however, the training of standardized patients, as well as training of the assessors, takes time. Traditional classroom assessment methods of CR—such as key feature questions, SCTs,[12] and mind mapping[13]—are limited in that they are more tests of knowledge organization than of true CR.

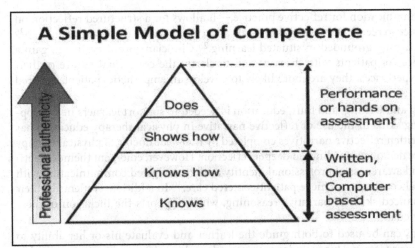

Figure 16-1. Evaluating work-based learning. (Adapted and reprinted with permission from Miller GE. The assessment of clinical skills/competence/performance. *Acad Med.* 1990;65[9)]S63-S67.)

Tools to Assess Clinical Reasoning in Physical Therapy

As we are now aware, meaningful and relevant assessment has moved beyond pen and paper to standardized measures that include think aloud,[14] reflective activities,[15,16] and clinical performance measures. The use of feedback grounded in qualitative judgement made by the evaluator is the way to assess inductive strategies such as a clinical narrative within physical therapy. The following tools could be used to evaluate the CR skills of learners: rubrics; clinical narratives incorporating reflection; and simulations, Objective Structured Clinical Examinations, or virtual cases. Some of these assessments are more applicable at specific points in the curriculum and may be better suited for the didactic curriculum, in preparation for clinical education, and/or residency and fellowship education. The educator's role is to determine the CR tool for the individual circumstances and to meet the situational needs of the learner. The learner may seek to use a variety of tools to gain additional perspective with peer practice and self- and peer assessments.

Clinical Reasoning Grading Rubrics

Recently, rubrics to assess CR have been developed and reported in the physical therapy literature. These represent practice-specific[17,18] as well as broad-practice[19] rubrics to evaluate the CR skills of a learner. The Think Aloud Standardized Patient Examination (TASPE) was developed to assess CR competency in novice physical therapy students during standardized musculoskeletal patient encounters. The TASPE uses the student's performance consistent with Miller's framework for clinical assessment (Figure 16-1).[20]

The Systematic Clinical Reasoning in Physical Therapy (SCRIPT) tool was developed to facilitate and assess deductive reasoning skills for orthopedic manual physical therapists in a post-professional fellowship training program.[18] Novice learners benefit from structure and guidance to organize their thoughts using a deductive approach to reasoning. The SCRIPT assists the learner in this process by guiding the physical therapist in planning and executing a comprehensive physical therapy examination. The tools prompt the physical therapist to identify likely hypotheses as well as alternate hypotheses using a deductive approach, while prioritizing intervention strategies.[18] In addition, when questions remain as to the most appropriate tests and measures to perform or intervention strategies, this tool recommends the therapist generate appropriate diagnostic questions and search the professional, peer-reviewed literature for the best available evidence.[18]

The Clinical Reasoning Grading Rubric (CRGR)[19,21] was developed to evaluate the major constructs of CR in physical therapy practice, and is provided in the chapter appendix. This rubric uses the Dreyfus model of skill acquisition[22] as a foundational component for skill progression as well as constructs of expertise in physical therapy.[23] The purpose of the CRGR was to assess CR skills of physical therapy students over time from low to high performance of knowledge, skills, and attitudes and to evaluate readiness to progress to clinical education experiences. Specifically, the following core components were embedded into the CRGR: learners' use and application of types of knowledge (eg, content and procedural); selection, modification, and performance of skills; identification of relevant context; and reflection. In a pilot study, the CRGR's ability to demonstrate student progress over didactic and clinical components of a professional doctor of physical therapy curriculum was examined.[24] Using the CRGR, 10 assessors evaluated 55 students over 4 points in time in the curriculum. Results revealed the CRGR demonstrated student progress over 4 points in time in both the didactic and clinical curriculum. Few CR tools are structured to identify specific domains within CR and demonstrate the capability of mapping the development and progression of CR across a curriculum in both didactic and clinical components.[24] (Please visit https://www.youtube.com/watch?v=IufH3OO5NKY for the faculty training video.)

Clinical Narratives

Although clinical narratives are used as a teaching tool to facilitate the CR process, they can also be used to assess a student's reasoning process by allowing the educator to see the student's thoughts and thinking process. Narrative is central to human understandings, memory systems, and communication for reflective practice.[25] It allows for a structured reflection on a particular experience using second-order experience to recollect, reexperience, and reflect again on the direct experience.[25,26] Reflection is a process of retelling, reliving, and learning grounded in situated learning.[25] Clinicians use narrative to gain a more holistic understanding of the lived experiences of patients with diseases and to clarify the contextual nature of their functional changes. When reflecting upon these experiences, they are more likely to develop an empathetic, patient-centered relationship.[27,28]

Students demonstrate varying skills in reflecting and writing, and thus, education is needed to support learners in developing these skills.[29] Explicit coursework in developing skills in the use of reflective narrative in physical therapy education has demonstrated a change in abilities and beliefs.[29] Written reflective narratives completed by first-year doctor of physical therapy students on a full-time clinical education experience demonstrated limited deeper reflection. However, emergent themes identified students reflecting on their own confidence and awareness of professional identity as they navigated communication with their clinical instructor and while navigating ethical conflicts to achieve patient-centered care.[30] In addition, students in their final year of physical therapy school reported enhanced skills of narrative reasoning, which supports the inclusion of these strategies within professional physical therapy curricula.[31]

Using the Gibbs reflective cycle, a series of steps can be used to both guide the learner and evaluate his or her ability to adequately reflect upon and describe the steps in this process.[32] This includes accurately describing the case situation, articulating the thoughts and feelings of the learner in the situation, evaluating what went well and what needs improvement, analyzing and interpreting the situation, developing a conclusion about what else could have been implemented, and implementing an action plan for change.[32,33] Including narratives as part of practical examinations or in clinical education could be a powerful assessment tool. Educators are responsible for identifying and correcting students' misconceptions. Narrative can be used as a tool in uncovering these misconceptions. Such narratives may also help track the development of a student's CR skills over time to provide evidence of areas of strength and components needing improvement.

Reflection Moment:
Resources for Clinical Narratives

Please use these guidelines for recording clinical narratives and select an appropriate exemplar to facilitate CR.

First, think of a significant patient situation or event that stands out in your mind. Following are possible prompts:

- An example of good physical therapist practice
- A situation where you made a difference
- A situation that taught you something new
- A memorable interaction in which you learned something
- A situation in which there was a breakdown, error, or moral dilemma

Second, consider the critical components to include in the exemplar:

- What happened, in detail?
- Why was the incident important to you?
- What were you thinking at the time?
- What were you feeling at the time?
- What were your concerns?
- What, if anything, was most challenging about the situation?
- If you encountered these issues again, what would you do differently?
- What did you learn from this interaction?

Third, write the exemplar as noted here:

- Write in the first person.
- Tell your story, and write your key thoughts, feelings, and emotions, not simply a summary of the story.
- Include a reflection on your thoughts and actions at the time.

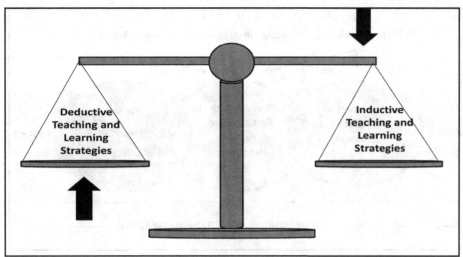

Figure 16-2. Balancing types of teaching and learning strategies. (Reprinted with permission from Furze J, Kenyon L, Jensen G. Connecting classroom, clinic and context: clinical reasoning strategies for clinical instructors and academic faculty. *Pediatr Phys Ther.* 2015;27[4]:368-375.)

Reflection Moment: Clinical Narrative Exemplar

Following the Resources for Clinical Narratives guidelines, let's pause and write an exemplar to facilitate CR:

The educator bears the responsibility of balancing and embedding deductive and inductive teaching and learning strategies across the curriculum depending upon the learner's abilities and need for structure (Figure 16-2).[33,34]

Examples of Assessment Tools Across the Physical Therapy Curriculum

Early (beginning) learner: Employ deductive reasoning skills, TASPE, CRGR, and structured clinical narratives.

Intermediate learner: Deductive strategies continue (as above) with initial integration of inductive strategies such as clinical narratives with less structure.

Prior to graduation: Both deductive and inductive strategies could be used, including CRGR, clinical narratives, and possibly introduction of the SCRIPT.

Residency: Both deductive and inductive tools are used, including the CRGR, SCRIPT, and clinical narratives.

Fellowship: SCRIPT and clinical narratives are used.

Expertise in clinical practice: Clinical narratives are used.

In recent work by the American College of Graduate Medical Education, milestone initiatives are competency based and have focused on the development of a medical resident and fellow from the beginning of education through graduation. Although CR is not 1 of the 6 competencies identified (ie, patient care, medical knowledge, interpersonal and communication skills, professionalism, practice-based learning and improvement, and systems-based practice), one could argue that this skill crosses the 6 competencies.[35]

Figure 16-3. Developing CR Skills. (Adapted with permission from Furze J, Kenyon L, Jensen G. Connecting classroom, clinic and context: clinical reasoning strategies for clinical instructors and academic faculty. *Pediatr Phys Ther.* 2015;27[4]:368-375.)

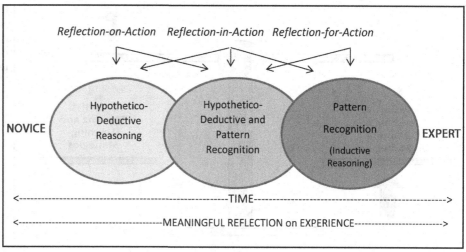

Further, the Association of American Medical Colleges has developed 13 core entrustable professional activities (EPAs) that are units of professional practice, defined as tasks or responsibilities, that all trainees can perform unsupervised once they have attained competence in that area. Core EPAs are the professional activities necessary to begin practice in medicine and are requirements for entering residency education.[34,36] In the assessment process, EPAs serve as measurable outcomes that the resident must achieve at the beginning of residency education.[34,36] The ability to gather a history and perform a physical exam, prioritize a differential diagnosis after a clinical encounter, recommend and interpret common diagnostic tests, and form clinical questions, while retrieving evidence to advance patient care, are 4 of the 13 EPAs.[36] CR could be identified as a component of several of these EPAs. Although not explicitly assessed, there is evidence that medicine is attempting to assess competencies including components of CR based in real-world practice.[35]

The most appropriate CR assessment tool may depend upon the learner's need for structure to facilitate learning. Novice learners typically require more structure for learning to take place. Thus, a CR tool that provides this structure, such as the TASPE or CRGR, may be more appropriate. As the learner requires less structure for learning, more inductive tools, such as clinical narratives and the SCRIPT, may be helpful.

When determining the most appropriate CR assessment tool, the context of the situation and the learner's working knowledge are foundational components for the educator to evaluate. Given the complexity of the CR process, multiple tools may be needed to fully assess the CR skills of the learner.

CONCLUSION

A gold standard for assessing CR skills within the profession of physical therapy does not currently exist. Thus, use of multiple tools, across multiple points in time, will most accurately capture the CR skills of learners. Ultimately, tools that use both qualitative and quantitative methods, and that assess both deductive and inductive aspects of CR, will most likely be needed to fully encompass the complexity of the CR process. As seen in Figure 16-3, CR is a skill that can develop over time when the learner reflects upon a significant experience using various reasoning strategies.[33] The educator's expertise and knowledge of the learner's needs and the context of the environment determines which of the described methods and tools are a best fit for the given situation.

REFERENCES

1. Epstein AS, Shulman LS, Spafka SA. *Medical Problem-Solving: An Analysis of Clinical Reasoning.* Cambridge, MA: Harvard University Press; 1978.
2. Lang V, Schuwirth L, Durning S, Rencic J. Assessment for clinical reasoning. In: Trowbridge R, Rencic J, Durning S, eds. *Teaching Clinical Reasoning.* Philadelphia, PA: American College of Physicians; 2015:122-124.
3. Jensen GM, Gwyer J, Shepard KF, Hack LM. Expert practice in physical therapy. *Phys Ther.* 2000;80(1);28-43.
4. Huhn K, Black L, Jensen G, Deutsch J. Construct validity of the health science reasoning test. *J Allied Health.* 2011;40:181-186.
5. Christensen N, Black L, Furze J, et al. Clinical reasoning: survey of teaching methods, integration, and assessment in entry-level physical therapist academic education. *Phys Ther.* 2017;97(2):175-186.
6. Vendrely A, Huhn K, Black L, et al. Clinical reasoning: survey of teaching methods and assessment in entry level physical therapist clinical education. *J Phys Ther Educ.* 2018;32(3).

7. Ratcliffe T, Durning S. Theoretical concepts to consider in providing clinical reasoning instruction. In: Trowbridge R, Rencic J, Durning S, eds. *Teaching Clinical Reasoning.* Philadelphia, PA: American College of Physicians; 2015:13-20.

8. Facione N, Facione P. *The Health Science Reasoning Test Manual.* Millbrae, CA: Insight Assessment; 2007.

9. Facione P. *The California Critical Thinking Skills Test: Form A and B.* Millbrae, CA: California Academic Press; 1992.

10. Hrynchak P, Takahashi SG, Nayer M. Key feature questions for assessment of clinical reasoning: a literature review. *Med Educ.* 2014;48:870-883.

11. Van der Vleuten CPM, Norman GR, Schuwirth LWT. Assessing clinical reasoning. In: Higgs J, Jones M, Loftus S, Christensen N, eds. *Clinical Reasoning in the Health Professions.* 3rd ed. Amsterdam, Netherlands: Butterworth-Heinemann Elsevier; 2008:418.

12. Charlin B, Roy L, Brailovsky C, Goulet F, Van der Vleuten C. The script concordance test: a tool to assess the reflective clinician. *Teach Learning Med.* 2000;12(4):189-195.

13. Zipp GP, Maher C, D'Antonio AV. Mind mapping: teaching and learning strategy for physical therapy curricula. *J Phys Ther Educ.* 2015;29(1):43-48.

14. Forsberg E, Ziegert K, Hult H, Fors U. Clinical reasoning in nursing, a think aloud study using virtual patients—a base for an innovative assessment. *Nurse Educ Today.* 2014;34:538-542.

15. Plack MM, Driscoll M, Blissett S, MeKenna R, Plack TP. A method for assessing reflective journal writing. *J Allied Health.* 2005;34(4):199-208.

16. Williams RM, Wilkins S. The use of reflective summary writing as a method of obtaining student feedback about entering physical therapy practice. *J Phys Ther Educ.* 1999;13(1):28-35.

17. Fu W. Development of an innovative tool to assess student physical therapists' clinical reasoning competency. *J Phys Ther Educ.* 2015;29(4):14-26.

18. Baker SE, Painter EE, Morgan BC, et al. Systematic clinical reasoning in physical therapy (SCRIPT): tool for the purposeful practice of clinical reasoning in orthopedic manual physical therapy. *Phys Ther.* 2017;97(1):61-70.

19. Furze J, Gale J, Black L, Cochran TM, Jensen GM. Clinical reasoning: development of a grading rubric for student assessment. *J Phys Ther Educ.* 2015;29(3):34-45.

20. Miller GE. The assessment of clinical skills/competence/performance. *Acad Med.* 1990;65(9):S63-S67.

21. Furze J, Black L, Hoffman J. Exploration of students' clinical reasoning development in professional physical therapy education. *J Phys Ther Educ.* 2015;29(3):22-33.

22. Dreyfus HL, Dreyfus SL. The relationship of theory and practice in the acquisition of skill. In: Benner P, Tanner CA, Chelsea CA, eds. *Expertise in Nursing Practice.* New York, NY: Spring; 1986;29-48.

23. Edwards I, Jones MA, Carr J, Brannack-Mayer A, Jensen GM. Clinical reasoning strategies in physical therapy. *Phys Ther.* 2004;84(4):312-335.

24. McDevitt A, Rapport MJ, Furze J. Utilization of a clinical reasoning grading rubric in a physical therapy curriculum: A pilot study. Poster presented at: APTA Academy of Physical Therapy Education, Clinical Reasoning Symposium; July 23, 2017; Omaha, NE.

25. Bolton G. *Reflective Practice: Writing and Professional Development.* 3rd ed. Los Angeles, CA: Sage Publishers; 2010:206.

26. Greenhalgh T, Hurwitz B. Narrative-based medicine: why study narrative? *BMJ.* 1999;318:48-50.

27. Greenfield BH, Jensen GM, Delany CM, et al. Power and promise of narrative for advancing physical therapist education and practice. *Phys Ther.* 2015;95:924-933.

28. Greenfield B, Swisher LL. The role of narratives in the professional formation of students. In: Higgs J, Sheehan D, Currents JB, Letts W, Jensen GM, eds. *Realising Exemplary Practice-Based Education.* Rotterdam, Netherlands: Sense Publishers; 2013:163-170.

29. Kurunsaari M, Tynjälä P, Piirainen A. Students' experiences of reflective writing as a tool for learning in physiotherapy education. In: van Steendam E, Tillema M, Rijlaarsdam G, van Den Bergh H, eds. *Writing for Professional Development.* Leiden, Netherlands: Brill; 2015:129-151.

30. Greenfield B, Bridges P, Phillips T, et al. Reflective narratives by physical therapist students on their early clinical experiences: a deductive and inductive approach. *J Phys Ther Educ.* 2015;29(2):21-31.

31. Caeiro C, Cruz EB, Pereira CM. Arts, literature and reflective writing as educational strategies to promote narrative reasoning capabilities among physiotherapy students. *Physiother Theory Pract.* 2014;30(8):572-580.

32. Gibbs G. *Learning by Doing: A Guide to Teaching and Learning Methods.* Oxford, United Kingdom: Further Education Unit, Oxford Brookes University; 1988.

33. Furze J, Kenyon L, Jensen G. Connecting classroom, clinic and context: clinical reasoning strategies for clinical instructors and academic faculty. *Pediatr Phys Ther.* 2015;27(4):368-375.

34. Ten Cate O, Scheele F. Competency-based postgraduate training: can we bridge the gap between theory and clinical practice? *Acad Med.* 2007; 82:542-547.

35. Accreditation Council for Graduate Medical Education. Milestones overview. http://www.acgme.org/What-We-Do/Accreditation/Milestones/Overview. Accessed October 18, 2017.

36. Association of American Medical Colleges. Core entrustable professional activities for entering residency: curriculum developers' guide. https://members.aamc.org/eweb/upload/Core%20EPA%20Curriculum%20Dev%20Guide.pdf. Accessed June 17, 2018.

APPENDIX
CLINICAL REASONING AND REFLECTION TOOL

Creighton University—Clinical Competence Performance Examination Clinical Reasoning Grading Rubric

Student Name: _____

Content Knowledge—Identifies appropriate foundational knowledge and information related to the *International Classification of Functioning, Disability and Health* (ICF) framework. Content knowledge is the knowledge the student brings to the case, not the knowledge the patient brings/shares. In addition, this is just the identification of the facts and NOT the interpretation of this information.

Sample behaviors to assess:

- Identifies appropriate foundational knowledge integral to patient's health condition, including biological and physical (eg, anatomy, histology, physiology, kinesiology, and neuroscience).
- Determines relevant ICF components as they relate to the patient case (ie, identifies the patient's health condition, body structure and function limitations, activity limitations, participation restrictions, and personal and environmental factors).

RATING SCALE (PLEASE MARK)

BEGINNER	INTERMEDIATE	COMPETENT	PROFICIENT
Limited evidence of content and foundational knowledge and identification of patient-related ICF components.	Moderate evidence of content and foundational knowledge and identification of patient-related ICF components.	Strong evidence of content and foundational knowledge and identification of patient-related ICF components.	Comprehensive evidence of content and foundational knowledge and identification of patient-related ICF components.

Comments:

Procedural Knowledge/Psychomotor Skill—Ability to determine appropriate test/measure/intervention and psychomotor performance of an intervention/test/skill (ie, when to perform skill, what skills to perform, how to perform skill).

Sample behaviors to assess:

- Determines appropriate test/measure/intervention to perform.
- Demonstrates the ability to safely and effectively perform test/measure/intervention (eg, hand placement, patient positioning, palpation, force production, safety, use of equipment).
- Incorporates effective communication strategies including verbal and nonverbal skills (ie, asks the patient the right questions).

RATING SCALE (PLEASE MARK)

BEGINNER	INTERMEDIATE	COMPETENT	PROFICIENT
Limited accuracy in performing test/measures/ interventions, but can safely perform these.	Moderate accuracy in performing test/measures/ interventions, and can safely perform these.	Strong accuracy in performing interventions/test efficiently and effectively using appropriate knowledge base, verbal and manual cues, and equipment to allow the patient to complete test or fully participate in intervention.	Efficiently performs tests and interventions with skill and ease, and able to build patient rapport during the exam and intervention.

Comments:

Conceptual Reasoning (cognitive and metacognitive skills—Data analysis and self-awareness/reflection)— Entails the interrelationship and synthesis of information upon which judgment is made using reflection and self-awareness (making sense out of all of the information).

Sample behaviors to assess and questions to ask include:

- Appropriately justifies, modifies, or adapts test/measure/intervention based upon patient case.
- Interprets exam findings appropriately including interpreting information from the patient (communication).
- Applies and interprets patient information across all aspects of the ICF model to justify test/measure/intervention.
- Listens actively.
- What additional information do you need to make decisions/judgments?
- What would you do differently if you were able to do this examination again?

RATING SCALE (PLEASE MARK)

BEGINNER	INTERMEDIATE	COMPETENT	PROFICIENT
Justifies choice for a few tests/measures/ interventions. Identifies some patient problems. Interprets results of selected tests/measures.	Justifies choice for most tests/measures/ interventions. Identifies relevant patient problems. Generates a working hypothesis and begins to prioritize a patient problem list.	Justifies choice for all tests/ measures/interventions. Prioritizes problem list and incorporates patient goals into plan of care. Confirms/disproves working hypothesis and determines alternate hypothesis. Synthesizes relevant patient data.	Generates a hypothesis, understands patient perspective, and demonstrates reasoning as a fluid, efficient, seamless process (demonstrates reflection-in-action).

Comments:

Student must meet or exceed identified level (eg, intermediate, competent, or proficient) for satisfactory completion in the following areas (please check):

Content Knowledge: _____Satisfactory _____Unsatisfactory
Procedural Knowledge/Psychomotor Skill: _____Satisfactory _____Unsatisfactory
Conceptual Reasoning: _____Satisfactory _____Unsatisfactory

General Comments:

Evaluator: _____   Date: _____

Reprinted with permission from Furze J, Gale J, Black L, Cochran TM, Jensen GM. Clinical reasoning: development of a grading rubric for student assessment. *J Phys Ther Educ.* 2015;29(3):34-45.

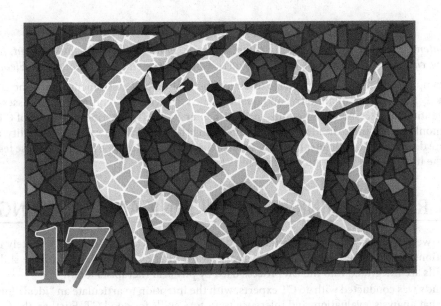

THE ROLE OF STANDARDIZED TESTS IN ASSESSING CLINICAL REASONING AND CRITICAL THINKING

Karen Huhn, PT, PhD

OBJECTIVES

- Compare and contrast critical thinking (CT), clinical reasoning (CR), and the inherent relationship.
- Describe 3 standardized tests: California Critical Thinking Skills Test (CCTST), California Critical Thinking Disposition Inventory (CCTDI), and the Health Sciences Reasoning Test (HSRT) for the assessment of CT.
- Discuss findings related to assessing doctor of physical therapy (DPT) students using CCTST, CCTDI, and HSRT.

INTRODUCTION

CT is an important skill of CR and is one of the few component skills that are amenable to objective assessment. But what is the relationship between CT skills and CR? Does assessing CT mean we are assessing CR? Various standardized tests have been used to assess the CT skills of physical therapy students, and the results support the notion that students entering DPT programs already possess strong CT skills. CT, it is important to remember, is only one component of the highly complex cognitive process of CR. Standardized tests should play a minimal role in assessing CR skills; however, they can play a role in contribution to educational assessment.

Assessing CR is a challenging but necessary task. We have a moral and ethical responsibility to the public to ensure competence and readiness for practice. The Commission on Accreditation in Physical Therapy Education (CAPTE) Standards and Elements (http://www.capteonline.org/AccreditationHandbook/) indicates an accredited curriculum:

Musolino GM, Jensen GM, eds. *Clinical Reasoning and Decision-Making in Physical Therapy: Facilitation, Assessment, and Implementation* (pp 193-197).
© 2020 Taylor & Francis Group.

Must include content and learning experiences in communication, ethics and values, management, finance, teaching and learning, law, clinical reasoning, evidence based practice and applied statistics (Standard 7, Element 7B).[1]

CR, however, is a complex skill that is not amenable to direct observation and assessment. Given the complexity of the skills involved in CR, it is likely that multiple quantitative and qualitative assessments are required to fully assess CR. One component that is amenable to quantitative assessment is the skills of CT. Chapter 17 briefly describes the skills of CT and the relationship to CR. The most commonly used standardized tests of CT—including their derivation, validity, reliability, and research findings related to their use—are described. This chapter concludes with a discussion of how one might use these tests in physical therapy education, as well as the limitation of using standardized tests to assess CR.

CRITICAL THINKING AND CLINICAL REASONING

The relationship between CT and CR is poorly understood, and the terms are often inappropriately used interchangeably. Let's consider the relationship between CT and CR in physical therapy, first by clearly describing the skills of CT, and then by describing how CT skills are integrated into the CR process used by physical therapists today.

In 1998, a Delphi study was conducted with 46 CT experts, with the intention to articulate an "ideal" for CT.[2] The CT experts had a 95% agreement that analysis, evaluation, and inference were core skills for good CT. Further, the CT experts had an 87% agreement that interpretation, explanation, and self-analysis were also core skills. As a result of the Delphi study, a consensus description for CT was determined as follows:

We understand CT to be purposeful, self-regulatory judgment which results in interpretation, analysis, evaluation, and inference, as well as explanation of the evidential, conceptual, methodological, criteriological, or contextual considerations upon which that judgment is based.[2(p2)]

CT skills shape the way in which a clinician approaches, analyzes, and responds to the multiple contexts and variations that occur in everyday practice. Clinicians use the skills of CT within the context of clinical practice. To arrive at a judgment about what to do, clinicians consider signs and symptoms (ie, evidence) in light of the patients' health and life circumstance (ie, context) using the knowledge gained during their health science education and training (ie, domain-specific knowledge) to design an intervention plan, anticipate effects of treatment (ie, judgment), monitor consequences of care (ie, analysis), and modify treatment as appropriate (ie, self-regulation). The component skills of CT are intimately integrated into the CR process but are not comprehensive.

CR in physical therapy involves both cognitive and technical skill. Therapists use technical skill through the use of tests and measures to collect some information, but several parts of clinical decision-making are cognitive: scanning, gathering or interviewing, and appraising. These are cognitive skills and sometimes metacognitive skills that are not considered technical in nature.[3] Appraisal is where CT skills are most frequently applied, while scanning and gathering involve skills beyond the scope and purpose of this chapter. Appraising information involves deciding what is reliable, what should be paid attention to, and what should not; thinking and rethinking about interpretations; and determining what is really happening and what we think is happening. Without these CT skills, a practitioner might travel down an errant path or continue a treatment that is not working, or maybe try something for which there is no evidence.

While CT skills themselves transcend specific subjects or discipline, exercising them successfully in certain contexts demands domain-specific knowledge, some of which may concern specific methods and techniques used to make reasonable judgments in those specific contexts.[2(p5)]

CR in physical therapy can be conceptualized as CT within the domain, or a particular point of view, of the profession of physical therapy. The domain of physical therapy is the set of objects, events, tests, and measures that physical therapists use during examination. Our point of view, or lens, is that we believe we can intervene at the impairment or functional level to impact a change in or restore/repair body systems (Figure 17-1). The relationship between CT and CR becomes somewhat clearer if one pictures it as CT within our domain of practice, and the point of view through which physical therapists approach practice. The skills of CT are inherent in the CR process, and are therefore important for educators and practitioners to consider with the understanding that they do not encompass all the skills of CR.

STANDARDIZED TESTS TO ASSESS CRITICAL THINKING

Many of the component skills of CR are not amenable to objective assessment or measurement; however, the component skills of CT have been objectively assessed using standardized assessments not only in physical therapy, but also across many professions and disciplines, for many years. A thorough understanding of the tests themselves and findings related to them is important to understanding how and if they should be used to assess CT/CR. Two commonly used tests are the CCTST and the more recently developed HSRT.

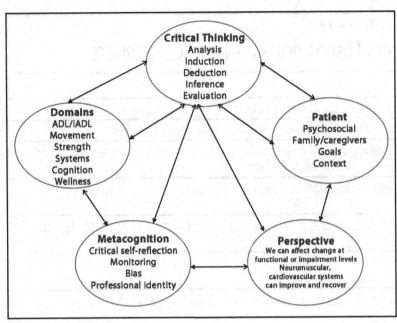

Figure 17-1. Point of view of physical therapists.

The CCTST and the HSRT were created based on the constructs of the Delphi study.[2] Both are multiple-choice tests that provide a total score and subscale scores for inference, deduction, evaluation, analysis, and induction. The tests each have a high correlation with GRE (graduate record examination) scores and have detected changes in CT scores after an educational intervention designed to improve CT.[4] Both tests have high reliability, with the CCTST overall Kuder–Richardson Formula 20 of 0.91, and the HSRT Kuder–Richardson scores ranging from 0.77 to 0.84.[5,6] A score above 0.70 indicates a high level of internal consistency. Construct validity refers to an instrument's ability to measure an abstract concept. Using the known groups method, Huhn et al[7] established construct validity for the HSRT by administering it to a group of physical therapist students and a group of certified clinical specialists. The HSRT differentiated between these 2 groups, thereby supporting construct validity.[7] The most significant difference between the 2 tests is that the CCTST questions are based on everyday scenarios, while the HSRT questions are written in the context of health care scenarios.

CALIFORNIA CRITICAL THINKING SKILLS TEST AND HEALTH SCIENCES REASONING TEST NORMS AND PERFORMANCE BY HEALTH CARE STUDENTS

Established norms indicate that a total CCTST score of 24 is indicative of superior CT skills, and a score between 19 and 23 is indicative of strong skills.[6] In several studies evaluating the CT skills of physical therapy students, all the mean total scores were between 19 and 22, indicative of strong CT skills.[8,9] Of particular interest is that the cohorts in these studies were undergraduate students. A more recent study of graduate-level, DPT students[10] reported an overall mean score of 74, indicating moderate CT skills using an updated 100-point version of the CCTST. In contrast, a study using the older version of the CCTST reported a mean score of 20, again indicating strong strength of CT scores.[11]

On the HSRT, a score of 26 or higher indicates superior skill, while a score between 21 and 25 is considered strong, and 15 to 20 moderate. Huhn et al[7] reported first-year DPT students from 2 geographically different locations had a mean score of 22.49, indicating strong skills at the beginning of the DPT program. In another study, 3 cohorts of entry-level DPT students completed the HSRT again at the beginning of the program as part of correlation study with the national physical therapy exam, and all 3 cohorts had mean HSRT total scores between 21.6 and 23.0, again indicating strong CT skills.[12] The data from studies using either the CCTST or the HSRT indicate that students entering a DPT program already exhibit strong CT skills.

Another aspect of CT is being willing to think critically. One may have the skills of good CT but not be willing to use them in certain situations. A disposition defined as "a characterological attribute of an individual, a person's consistent internal motivation to act toward or respond to persons, events, or circumstances in habitual yet potentially malleable ways."[13(p64)] Teaching CT skills without also fostering the willingness to use those skills is inadequate. Students entering DPT programs already possess strong CT skills. Yet, we also need to consider whether DPT students also possess the drive and willingness to use CT skills in meaningful ways for their patients/clients.

The CCTDI is a 75-item tool in which responders agree or disagree using a 6-point Likert scale ranging from "strongly agree" to "strongly disagree" with statements related to 7 constructs (Table 17-1). Content validity is derived from the same Delphi study on CT. Internal consistency reliability for the 7 individual scales ranges from 0.71 to 0.80.[14] Coefficients of test/retest reliability for the CCTDI have been reported as 0.80, when given 2 weeks apart.[14] A score between 50 and 60 indicates a strong positive disposition toward CT, while a score between 40 and 50 indicates a positive disposition, and a score between 30 and 40 indicates inconsistent or ambivalent feelings toward thinking critically. Several authors have reported scale scores between 40 and 47 for DPT students just beginning their professional education, indicating a positive disposition toward thinking critically.[10,15]

TABLE 17-1	
CALIFORNIA CRITICAL THINKING DISPOSITION INVENTORY CONSTRUCTS	
SCALE	**DEFINITION**
Truth-seeking	The habit of always desiring the best possible understanding of any given situation.
Open-mindedness	The tendency to allow others to voice views with which one may not agree.
Analyticity	The habit of striving to anticipate both the good and the bad potential consequences or outcomes of situations, choices, proposals, and plans.
Systematicity	The tendency or habit of striving to approach problems in a disciplined, orderly, and systematic way.
Confidence in reasoning	The habitual tendency to trust reflective thinking to solve problems and to make decisions.
Inquisitiveness	The tendency to want to know things, even if they are not immediately or obviously useful at the moment.
Maturity of judgment	The habit of seeing the complexity of issues and yet striving to make timely decisions.
Adapted from Insight Assessment.[14]	

CONCLUSION

A fair amount of data indicates students entering DPT programs demonstrate not only strong CT skills, but also a willingness to think critically. Given the limited scope of CR skills these standardized tests assess, and the fact that DPT students already possess strong CT skills, the utility of these standardized tests in assessing DPT students may be quite minimal. They can also be used to assess andragogy related to inductive or deductive thinking, although again, the utility of this is minimal.

These findings should provide some insight for educators that, in most instances, they do not need to focus on the skills of CT, but rather can and should focus on the contextual thinking and CR of a physical therapist, considering reflective skills, integration of knowledge, and clinical contexts. These standardized tests of CT do, however, provide an objective measure that programs are using to assess CT, as a component of meeting CAPTE Standards.

REFERENCES

1. Commission on Accreditation in Physical Therapy Education. *Standards and Required Elements for Accreditation of Physical Therapist Education Programs.* Alexandria, VA: American Physical Therapy Association; 2017.
2. Facione P. *Critical Thinking: A Statement of Expert Consensus for Purposes of Educational Assessment and Instruction.* Millbrae, CA: California Academic Press; 1998.
3. Brookfield S. Clinical reasoning and generic thinking skills. In: Higgs J, Jones M, Loftus S, Christensen N, eds. *Clinical Reasoning in the Health Professions.* 3rd ed. Amsterdam, Netherlands: Butterworth-Heinemann Elsevier; 2008.
4. Huhn K. Effectiveness of a clinical reasoning course on willingness to think critically and skills of self-reflection. *J Phys Ther Educ.* 2017;31(4):59-63.
5. Facione N, Facione P. The Health Sciences Reasoning Test (HSRT): a test of critical thinking skills for health care professionals. Test manual. Insight Assessment. http://www.insightassessment.com/pdf_files/HSRT%20manual.pdf. Accessed March 20, 2018.
6. Facione P. *The California Critical Thinking Skills Test: Form A and B.* Milbrae, CA: California Academic Press; 1992.
7. Huhn K, Black L, Deutsch J, Jensen G. Construct validity of the health science reasoning test. *J Allied Health.* 2011;40(4):181-186.
8. Vendrely A. An investigation of the relationships among academic performance, clinical performance, critical thinking, and success on the physical therapy licensure examination. *J Allied Health.* 2007;36(2):e108-e123.
9. Wessel J, Williams, R. CT and learning styles of students in a problem-based, master's entry-level physical therapy program. *Physiol Theory Pract.* 2004;20(79):79.
10. Domenech M, Watkins P. Critical thinking and disposition toward critical thinking among physical therapy students. *J Allied Health.* 2015;44(4):195-200.
11. Suckow D, Brahler J, Donahoe-Fillmore B, Fisher M, Anloague P. The association between critical thinking and scholastic aptitude on first timepass rate of the national physical therapy examination. *J Stud Phys Ther Res.* 2015;8(3).

12. Huhn K, Parrot S. Exploration of relationships between the Health Science Reasoning Test, the National Physical Therapy Licensing Examination, and cognitive admissions variables. *J Phys Ther Educ.* 2017;31(1):7-13.

13. Facione P. The disposition toward critical thinking: its character, measurement, and relationship to critical thinking skill. *Informal Log.* 2000;20(1):61-84.

14. Insight Assessment. *California Critical Thinking Disposition Inventory Manual.* San Jose, CA: California Academic Press; 2013.

15. Bartlett DJ, Cox PD. Measuring the change in students' critical thinking ability: implications for health care education. *J Allied Health.* 2002;31:64-69.

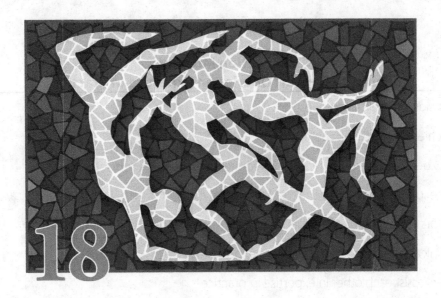

DEVELOPING CLINICAL REASONING AND DECISION-MAKING SKILLS:
Simulations and Debriefing

Karen Huhn, PT, PhD

OBJECTIVES

- Critique theoretical frameworks that support the use of simulations to develop clinical reasoning and clinical decision-making (CR-CDM) skills.

- Examine types of simulations, the role of simulation, and contemporary resources for facilitating CR-CDM skills.

- Appraise Milgram's reality-virtuality continuum.

- Discover the 4 debriefing phases post-simulation: reaction, description, analysis, and application/summary.

- Compare and contrast the plus/delta and advocacy/inquiry, analysis phase methods of debriefing.

- Interpret the role of debriefing in promoting the development of CR-CDM skills.

Musolino GM, Jensen GM, eds. *Clinical Reasoning and Decision-Making in Physical Therapy: Facilitation, Assessment, and Implementation* (pp 199-206).

Reflection Moment
Points to Ponder: Queries on Expertise in Practice

Discuss and consider the following questions:

Is 4.8 years to achieve expertise acceptable?

Is there a way to decrease the amount of time required to achieve expertise?

Do you believe expertise is time dependent? Why or why not?

How do educators expose students to realistic practice without risk of harm to patients?

What role do clinical instructors have in guiding expertise?

How might peers assist each other in expertise in practice?

Must one be an expert to practice?

Would you prefer to be treated by an expert? Why or why not?

INTRODUCTION

This chapter provides an opportunity to continue to consider the theoretical frameworks for CR-CDM through the examination of simulations for learning. The types of simulations for learning are discussed based upon the traditional and contemporary evidence for the enhancement of CR-CDM skills through simulation activities. We will consider Milgram's reality-virtuality continuum and why augmented environments may impact learning and teaching for CR-CDM. Learners will come to appreciate the purpose, phases, and methods of debriefing for CR-CDM. The chapter concludes with resources and discussion of examples pertaining to the promotion of CR-CDM.

Expertise develops through substantial practice in a variety of situations through repeated, deliberate practice.[1] Expertise in CR develops through repeated practice with real patients in clinical settings. Ericsson[1] shares that it takes 10,000 hours of practice to gain expertise. Practicing 40 hours a week, it would take a physical therapist 4.8 years to garner 10,000 hours of experience with patients.

Simulations are used throughout professional education and personnel evaluation.[2] Simulation training reduces error and improves performance in professions such as the airline industry and the military where decision-making is high risk and has the potential to affect lives.[3] In the past 2 decades, educators in medicine and nursing have been increasing dependence on simulations in training, in the hopes of decreasing the incidence of error and improving patient outcomes.[2] Support for the use of simulations is strong, and in fact, the medical licensing examination in Italy and the United States now includes the use of computerized patient case simulations.[4,5] Standards for accreditation of baccalaureate and graduate nursing programs indicate:

> Learning experiences also can occur using simulation designed as a mechanism for verifying early mastery of new levels of practice or designed to create access to data or health care situations that are not readily accessible to the student. These experiences may include simulated mass casualty events, simulated database problems, simulated interpersonal communication scenarios, and other new emerging learning technologies. The simulation is an adjunct to the learning that will occur with direct human interface or human learning experience.[6(p30)]

Although direct evidence indicating simulations are effective at improving CR is sparse, the implications from the literature are substantial. There is strong andragogical support for the use of simulations to improve CR. This chapter focuses primarily on high-fidelity patient simulations and virtual patient simulations as most relevant to the development of CR. The most frequently used approaches for debriefing shall be discussed; however, it cannot begin to promote proficiency in debriefing skills. Training resources for becoming skilled in debriefing are provided in the end of the chapter resources.

SIMULATIONS

What do we mean by simulations? Simulations include "devices, trained persons, life-like virtual environments, and contrived social situations that mimic problems, events, or conditions that arise in professional encounters."[2(p11)] Simulations are described

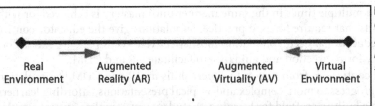

Figure 18-1. Milgram's reality-virtuality continuum. (Reprinted with permission from Milgram P, Kishino F. A taxonomy of mixed reality visual displays. *IEICE Trans Inf Syst.* 1994;77[12]:1321-1329. Copyright © 2016 IEICE, #18RA0094.)

as tools "to replace or amplify real experiences with guided experiences that evoke or replicate substantial aspects of the real world in a fully interactive manner."[3(p126)] Another description is that they "replicate some or nearly all of the essential assets of a clinical situation so that the situation may be more readily understood and managed when it occurs for real in clinical practice"[7(p3)] Fidelity, or the degree of "realness," is an important descriptor when considering simulations. Low-fidelity can be static models often used to learn a discrete skill such as catheterization. Medium-fidelity is often through the use of manikins with software that allow auscultation, breath and bowel sounds, and electrocardiography. High-fidelity typically involves life-sized manikins with a large variety of human physiological responses including responses to pharmacological interventions with adverse events.[8]

Simulations can be conducted with standardized patients (ie, actors trained to portray patients), manikins, or virtually created scenarios. Virtual simulations are "a specific type of computer program that simulates real-life clinical scenarios; learners emulate the role of health care providers to obtain a history, complete a physical exam, and make diagnostic and therapeutic decisions."[9] Milgram and Kishino describe a continuum of virtuality progressing from simple to complex (Figure 18-1).[10]

Virtual worlds portray particular settings, such as a disaster scenario like a plane crash, or natural disaster, or poverty situations. Virtual patients are computerized patient programs that allow the learner to interact with the program to evaluate, diagnose, and manage a patient scenario. Augmented reality (AR) is when a real environment is amplified using computerized graphics.[10] AR is cutting edge, and thus far has not been evaluated for the purpose of improving CR skills. For purposes of this chapter, we will limit the discussion to simulations most frequently used to improve CR: presently, high-fidelity manikins and virtual patient simulations.

WHY SIMULATIONS?

Several theoretical frameworks exist to support the development of competency for CR skills. Constructivism is grounded in the belief that when students have opportunities in which they are required to use prior knowledge in a context in which it is meant to be used and have an experience that creates new awareness or reshapes previous experiences, then meaningful learning can occur. Debriefing after the experience creates an opportunity to examine cognitive representations, misperceptions, and facilitation of linking of old knowledge with new knowledge gained through the experience.

Simulations have the potential to incorporate additional strategies and recommendations for teaching CR. They are clearly experiential in nature, encouraging active engagement, reflection, and deep learning. They lend themselves to Kolb's learning cycle[11] of having an experience, reflecting on that experience, reconceptualizing frames of reference, and then trying out those new frames in another experience. The realism of simulations frequently triggers an emotional response that can influence reflection and retention.[11,12]

Substantial practice with realistic patients is well known to be a key component in facilitating progression from novice to intermediate, and eventually expertise, in CR skill. Simulations are an ideal tool to increase student exposure to realistic patient cases. Virtual patient cases in particular, because they can be completed anytime and anywhere and can substantially increase the number of cases students may experience. Virtual cases can be done outside of class, require no faculty presence, and can be completed as assignments. For example, in one pathology class, students would listen to a lecture on the pathology of stroke and then, as an assignment outside of class, complete 2 virtual cases on patients post-stroke. Each case can depict a different area of infarct and encourage the integration of the pathology with clinical application. The virtual patient can provide immediate feedback on performance and also make the student's thought process visible to the instructor, because it records the student's path through the case. The instructor can later review the student's path and provide more detailed, individualized feedback. In a systematic review of virtual patients, Cook reported, "If expertise in CR is indeed developed through exposure to a large number of cases, then virtual patients are ideally suited to this task."[9(p307)] Upcoming, in Section III of this text, we will examine additional exemplars of technology to facilitate CR for physical therapy learners.

We know CR is situational, in that it depends on context.[13] Learning is intricately tied to thinking and doing, and the environment plays a crucial role. Simulations can be used to expose students to contextual clinical environments such as a school or home, which are not compatible with classroom or laboratory settings. In addition to environment, other contextual factors such as patient and family emotions, body language, and cultural factors can be simulated. Increasing the realism of the experience emphasizes the experience itself as the source of learning and encourages meaningful participation on the part of the learner.

Simulations can be used to expose students to deliberate practice, described as a highly structured activity with the specific goal of improving performance. Deliberate practice involves repetitive, focused practice with an assessment of performance and informative feedback.[14] Simulations can be repeated multiple times in the same manner until mastery is achieved, or with changes implemented designed to focus on areas or skills that require focused practice. Simulations give the educator control to be able to direct the experience to a focused area of educational need. Simulation most effectively keeps patients and clients from harm, and allows errors to occur, with opportunity for redirection and guidance to facilitate CR and CDM.

Illness script formation is known to be a step on the continuum from novice to expert skills in CR and CDM.[15] Simulation scenarios can begin with symbolic representations and progress to more complex and atypical presentations, affording learners an opportunity to build illness scripts and schema, with a built-in scaffold for learning. A student can complete several simulations of patients post-stroke and experience the wide variety of limitations and disabilities that result from cerebral ischemia. As Dewey stated, "For education to be educative, it needs to provide a continuity of experiences."[16]

Through simulations, one can ensure all students are exposed to the same patient experience, thereby ensuring each student gets the chance to work with a particular type of patient or a particular clinical context. Simulations can expose students to infrequently encountered patient diagnoses or novel clinical scenarios. Feedback can be provided during or after the simulation and in many forms, including from the simulator itself. Educators can allow mistakes to play out, providing students an opportunity to experience a negative outcome without harm to a real patient. The same scenario can be practiced multiple times, learning from mistakes and feedback while repeatedly practicing a discrete skill to promote competency in both CR and CDM.

Often, it is difficult for an educator to "see" or understand what a student was thinking or how the student arrived at a decision or action. Through the use of computers and technology, however, many simulations externalize the thought process, making it more visible to the instructor. The instructor then can identify strengths and weaknesses and provide individualized feedback for a student's emerging CR and CDM thought process. The importance of feedback and deliberate practice are well known.[17]

Frequently, students have an "experience" during a simulation, triggering emotional reactions that can then be leveraged through a debriefing process to deepen and reinforce learning. Debriefing, occurring during or, more frequently, upon completion of the experience, is an essential component of any simulation. It is during the debriefing process that the facilitator can, through thoughtful questioning, encourage self-reflection to highlight strengths, weaknesses, or misperceptions in students' CR and CDM.

The experienced debriefer can use the learner's emotional reaction to the experience as a launching point to encourage self-reflection. For example, the facilitator can ask, "Why do you think you reacted that way?" The facilitator can question students related to their frames of reference or understanding of what occurred, or perhaps what should have taken place or been considered. It is during the debriefing that deep learning and changes to reasoning processes can occur, and links can be made between previous knowledge and knowledge gained through the simulation. A deeper exploration of debriefing is appropriate to illustrate its relevance to the development of CR skills.

DEBRIEFING

It has been reported that simulation alone is less effective than simulation with debriefing.[18-21] Debriefing is a teaching and learning strategy through which an instructor facilitates reflection to encourage students to come to terms with clinical issues encountered during simulation.[22] Students and faculty reexamine the simulation to foster the development of CR and decision-making. The intent is to promote a comparison between a trainee's performance and standards or expected outcomes, with the intent to improve student performance.[23] With debriefing processes, 2 assumptions are made: the simulation experience has had some effect on the learner, and a discussion about the experience is necessary to provide insight into the impact of the experience.[20]

Objectives for debriefing sessions are 3-fold and include identifying perceptions, beliefs, and attitudes; linking the experience to prior knowledge, theory, and skill to facilitate transfer of knowledge; and providing the opportunity to receive feedback on one's behavior, thinking, and decision-making thoughts and processes.[24] Reflection, known to be a hallmark of expertise and a critical component of CR, is not inherent in many learners and, therefore, frequently requires facilitation. During the debriefing process, a facilitator encourages reflection to explore emotional reactions to the experience, integration of the simulation encounter with previous knowledge, and reflection on thought processes used.

We have discussed the goals of debriefing, but several elements should be considered when planning a debriefing: Who will do the debriefing? What are the objectives of the encounter? When will the debriefing occur? What environment will the debriefing occur in? And what theoretical framework will support the debrief session? Is it appropriate for peers or near-peers to assist in debriefing?

The people who plan, structure, and present the simulation are most commonly the people who debrief. The facilitator for the debrief session can be an individual or, in the case of an interprofessional simulation, there can be multiple facilitators. When using multiple facilitators, all must understand the objectives of the simulation and work from the same theoretical framework for the debrief session.

The objectives of the debriefing session should be established well before the simulation occurs. *What do you want students to learn from the simulation? What elements of the simulation need to be present to promote that learning?* Ensuring these elements are present involves building the actual patient case itself as well as deciding what type of simulation will be used for the

TABLE 18-1
DEBRIEFING PHASES

PHASE	PURPOSE	GUIDING QUERY EXAMPLE
Reaction	Students share their emotions.	"How are you feeling?"
Description	Students share what they think are the main outcomes of the simulation.	"From your point of view, what were the main factors you had to manage?"
Analysis	Students examine frames and perspectives, self-reflect, and facilitate new frames.	"I noticed you (behavior). What led you to do that?"
Application/ summary	Students summarize discussion.	"What is the take-home message of this experience?"

Adapted from Milgram and Kishino.[10]

experience. *How long will students have to complete the simulation?* As with any educational experience, students should have a clear idea of what is expected of them during the simulation.

Depending on the intended learning outcomes, the debriefing can happen during or after the simulation experience. The simulation can be stopped at any point, and facilitation discussion regarding errors that have been made can occur, if you do not want students to continue down an errant path. Debriefing during the encounter is only recommended when the simulation is drifting too far from the intended outcomes, or when the students are at a complete loss as to how to proceed. Most often, debriefing occurs after the simulation experience is completed.

Participants in the simulation should have a brief period (10 to 20 minutes) to process the emotional experiences of the simulation before beginning the debrief session. The debrief session should occur in an environment in which both students and the facilitator feel comfortable and safe. Often this is not the same room where the simulation occurred. The student learner may also benefit from writing a formal reflection about the debriefing, and/or his or her performance prior to debriefing, to continue the reflection learning for reinforcement as a critical component of CR.

Several frameworks for debriefing exist, and educators with substantial debriefing experience will mix several strategies to be effective. Most facilitation methods share the goal of helping learners explore and externalize their mental models and thought processes, so educators can contribute to making new connections and understandings. In general, most frameworks involve reaction and description phases, followed by analysis, application, and summary (Table 18-1). During the reaction phase, the facilitator invites students to share their feelings and reactions to the simulation. The responses shared in a psychologically "safe" environment often provide the facilitator with a deeper understanding of where to begin the debriefing process. The description phase is when students are asked what they think the simulation was about, what happened, what key events provided insight around major issues, and what errant frames or discrepancies exist between what was expected and what happened.

The analysis phase is when the facilitator encourages self-reflection and begins to examine frames, thoughts processes, and perspectives. While many approaches exist for the analysis phase, experienced facilitators will use a mixture of methods. Two commonly used approaches are the plus/delta and advocacy/inquiry. The plus/delta technique is quick and easy, and works well when there is limited time to debrief. The facilitator creates a table with a plus column and a delta column. The group then discusses what went well during the simulation and places those items in the plus column. Things that could have gone better or things that went wrong would be put in the delta column, for change. As time permits, the items in the delta column can be explored and discussed.[25]

The advocacy/inquiry approach is based on a belief that all learners have a frame of reference from which they approach a problem, and that frame leads to action and ultimately results. By facilitating self-reflection about frames, changes can be made to those frames, which will then in turn change actions and results. The advocacy/inquiry approach focuses on the stance the facilitator takes. In many cases of debriefing and elsewhere in education, the educator is seen as the expert imparting knowledge or indicating what is right and what is wrong. The stance of advocacy/inquiry is one of pure curiosity; the facilitator is a cognitive detective, trying to understand what the learners were thinking and why.[26] The goal is not to tell the students what they learned, but rather to discover what they learned. In advocacy/inquiry, the facilitator would state something he or she noticed during the simulation, and then ask the learners to talk about it. For example, the facilitator could say, "Susan, I noticed you did not place much emphasis on special tests during your examination. I'm curious, how did you view the examination at the time?" This type of questioning is nonjudgmental, and encourages the learners to reflect on how they were feeling and what they were thinking at the time. The advocacy/inquiry process makes the learner's reasoning process visible to the facilitator, making it easier to correct errors in knowledge, perception, and/or process.

The following examples illustrate the advocacy/inquiry debrief process with facilitator queries.

Example 1

Students completed a virtual patient case, and the computer program tracked the tests and measures students completed as part of the examination. The physical examination revealed quadriceps and gluteal strength of 2+/5 bilaterally. The software revealed that 48 students tested ambulation and 17 assessed the patient's ability to do stair elevations. During the debrief session, the facilitator stated, "I noticed many of you either ambulated the patient or assessed stair elevations [advocacy]. Can you tell me what your thought process was in deciding to assess those items [inquiry]?" Students said ambulation was a goal for the patient, so they thought they needed to assess it. The faculty in this program frequently reminded students to ask patients their goals for therapy and direct interventions for those goals. This is an example of an errant frame, perhaps created by faculty not making it clear that physical therapists do need to address the patient's goals, but at the appropriate time. The facilitator then asked what grade of strength one would require in quadriceps and gluteal muscles to transition from sit to stand and to climb stairs. Students reported at least a 3+, and without further input from the facilitator, students started talking about how they now saw that the patient did not have enough strength to properly perform the activities they had attempted to examine. This is also an example of a checklist approach to examination, which is indicative of novice skill level.

Example 2

In a different virtual patient case, students examined a woman in her late 50s who had fallen on a hard floor, landing on her hip and buttock area. Forty students indicated a herniated lumbar disc as a potential diagnosis, yet only 25 included special tests for herniated nucleus pulposis (HNP). The facilitator stated, "I noticed most of you considered HNP as a potential diagnosis [advocacy]. Can you tell me how you ruled HNP in or out?" The ensuing discussion included what signs and symptoms were consistent with HNP and which were not, including what active range of motion might look like if a lumbar disc were herniated, as well as the patterns of pain associated with commonly herniated levels. Special tests and examination items that could have helped rule HNP in or out were also discussed. This allowed the facilitator to help students connect representative signs and symptoms with diagnoses, facilitating the formation of illness scripts.

Debriefing is a key aspect of any type of simulation experience. Learning to be an effective facilitator within a debriefing session takes substantial training and practice. Additional resources for simulation training in debriefing are provided in the resources at the end of this chapter. Despite growing adaptation of simulations, the strength of the evidence related to simulations to promote the development of CR skills remains weak. Two main factors limit the ability to establish a direct correlation between simulations and improved CR skill. One factor is the lack of an objective measure of change in CR skill, and the other is the variety of simulations used in studies. Many studies focus on feasibility and learner satisfaction. Feedback from students is positive, and most feel being able to practice in a real simulation context is beneficial.[27-30] Specific positive feedback includes realism, usage of media to increase realism and actions affecting outcomes (ie, learning from errors), and the ability to work alone.[31,32]

In a systematic review, 11 studies assessed critical thinking either directly or by self-report; 45% reported statistically significantly greater scores for simulation vs control groups.[7] Again, a limitation stated in this review was the variety of simulations used and the use of nonvalidated, or subjective, assessments of reasoning. Comparing virtual cases to paper cases, a simulation group improved on a post-test score by 3.5 points, while the traditional group improved by only one point.[28] A limitation of this study is that the researchers failed to indicate how many cases were completed, and again, the outcome measure used was unfortunately not validated (pre-/post-test).[28] Huhn et al[32] reported no significant differences on Health Sciences Reasoning Test scores between a group that completed group discussion of cases vs virtual cases. There were, however, within-group differences for the simulation group, and they scored higher on all objective measures.[32]

Certainly, there are some drawbacks related to the use of simulations. Simulation scenarios are time consuming to develop, implement, and debrief. Depending on fidelity, the initial costs can be relatively high. Medical educators are addressing some of these issues by creating shared databases of simulation scenarios and virtual patients. Despite the negatives and the lack of strong objective evidence in support of simulations, use of simulations continues to grow. In fact, both the United States and Canada now require all surgical programs to be associated with a simulation center.[33] Simulation use is highest in medical education and nursing, with allied health being the third-most-frequent users. Additional research related to simulations and the development of CR is certainly warranted, but the andragogical support for the use of simulations is substantial.

Reflection Moment:
Additional Web Resources

Now please explore at least one of the additional resources and discuss your findings.

https://www.medbiq.org/
MedBiquitous shares resources for virtual patients and simulation exercises for debriefing in medical education, dedicated to advancing the profession through technology. It includes conferences, blogs, archived discussions, data sharing, research, and resources.

https://harvardmedsim.org/debriefing-assessment-for-simulation-in-healthcare-dash/
The Center for Medical Simulation provides community information on the resources for the *Debriefing Assessment for Simulation in Healthcare* rater handbook and training; simulation training, with scenario development debriefing and assessment; clinical training simulation, with communication and teamwork; crisis resource management, with anesthesia certifications and training; fellowship training; consultation; and more.

http://www.nln.org/professional-development-programs/simulation
The Simulation Innovation and Resource Center provides information related to training and best practices for online simulation courses, vendors, resources, and conferences geared most specifically for nursing educators, with links to grants and research.

https://www.ssih.org/
The Society for Simulation in Healthcare offers courses, congress, certifications, resources, and research tools with links to peer-reviewed journals that publish works germane to the field of simulation in health care, gaming, education, and related industries.

REFERENCES

1. Ericsson KA. An expert-performance perspective of research on medical expertise: the study of clinical performance. *Med Educ.* 2007;41(12):1124-1130.
2. Issenberg B, McGaghie W, Petrusa E, Gordon D, Scalese R. Features and uses of high-fidelity medical simulations that lead to effective learning: a BEME systematic review. *Med Teach.* 2005;27(1):10-28.
3. Gaba D. The future vision of simulation in healthcare. *Simul Healthc.* 2007;2(2):126-135.
4. Guagnano M, Merlitti D, Manigrasso MR, Pace-Palitti V, Sensi S. New medical licensing examination using computer-based case simulations and standardized patients. *Acad Med.* 2002;77(1):87-90.
5. Dillon GF, Boulet J, Hawkins R, et al. Simulations in the United States medical licensing examination (USMLE). *Qual Saf Health Care.* 2004;13(suppl 1):141-145.
6. American Association of Colleges of Nursing. The essentials of master's education in nursing. http://www.aacnnursing.org/portals/42/publications/mastersessentials11.pdf. Published March 21, 2011. Accessed May 2, 2019.
7. Cant R, Cooper S. Simulation-based learning in nurse education: systematic review. *J Adv Nurs.* 2009;66(1):3-15.
8. Lapkin S, Levett-Jones T, Bellchambers H, Fernandez R. Effectiveness of patient simulation manikins in teaching clinical reasoning skills to undergraduate nursing students: a systematic review. *Clin Simul Nurs.* 2010:e1-e16.
9. Cook A, Triolo M. Virtual patients: a critical literature review and proposed next steps. *Med Educ.* 2009;43:303-311.
10. Milgram P, Kishino F. A taxonomy of mixed reality visual displays. *IEICE Trans Inf Syst.* 1994;77(12):1321-1329.
11. Kolb D. Experiential learning: experience as the source of learning and development. Englewood Cliffs, NJ: Prentice-Hall; 1984.
12. Gardner R. Introduction to debriefing. *Seminars in Perinatology.* 2013;37:166-174.
13. Durning S, Artino AR Jr, Pangaro L, van der Vleuten CP, Schuwirth L. Context and clinical reasoning: understanding the perspective of the expert's voice. *Med Educ.* 2011;45(9):927-938.
14. Ericsson KA. Deliberate practice and the acquisition and maintenance of expert performance in medicine and related domains. *Acad Med.* 2004;79:S1-S12.
15. Bordage G. Prototypes and semantic qualifiers: from past to present. *Med Educ.* 2007;41(12):1117-1121.
16. Dewey J. *Experience and Education.* New York, NY: Macmillan; 1929.
17. Ericsson A, Krampe T, Tesch-Romer C. The role of deliberate practice in the acquisition of expert performance. *Psychol Rev.* 1993;100(3):346-406.
18. Shinnick M, Woo M, Horwich T, Steadman R. Debriefing: the most important component in simulation. *Clin Simul Nurs.* 2011;7:e105-e111.

19. Savoldelli G, Naik V, Par J, et al. Value of debriefing during simulated crisis management: oral versus video-assisted oral feedback. *Anesthesiology.* 2006;105:279-285.

20. Lederman L. Debriefing: toward a systematic assessment of theory and practice. *Simul Gaming.* 1992;23.

21. Forneris S, Neal D, Jone T, et al. Enhancing clinical reasoning through simulation debriefing: a multisite study. *Nurs Educ Perspect.* 2015;36(5):304-310.

22. Neill M, Wotton K. High-fidelity simulation debriefing in nursing education: a literature review. *Clin Simul Nurs.* 2011;7(5):161-168.

23. Van De Ridder J, Stokking K, Mcgagie W, Ten Cate O. What is feedback in clinical education? *Med Educ.* 2008;42:189-197.

24. Warrick, Hunsaker P, Cook C, Altman S. Debriefing experiential learning exercises. *J Experiential Learn Simul.* 1979;1:91-100.

25. Motola I, Devine L, Chung H, Sullivan J, Issenberg B. Simulation in healthcare education: a best evidence pracitical guide. AMEE guide no. 82. *Med Teach.* 2013;35:e1511-e1530.

26. Rudolph J, Simon R, Dufresne R, Raemer D. There's no such thing as "nonjudgmental" debriefing: a theory and method for debriefing with good judgment. *Simul Healthc.* 2006;1(1):49-55.

27. Shoemaker M, Riemersma L, Perkins R. Use of high fidelity human simulation to teach physical therapist decision-making skills for intensive care setting. *Caridopulm Phys Ther J.* 2009;20(1):13-18.

28. Aghili R, Khamseh M, Taghavinia M, et al. Virtual patient simulation: promotion of clinical reasoning abilities of medical students. *Knowledge Management and E-Learning: An International Journal.* 2012;4(4).

29. Bearman M. Is virtual the same as real? Medical students' experiences of a virtual patient. *Acad Med.* 2003;78(5):538-545.

30. Bryce DA, King JC, Graebner CF, Myers HJ. Evaluation of a diagnostic reasoning program (DxR): exploring student perceptions and addressing faculty concerns. *Journal of Interactive Media in Education.* 1998;1.

31. Round J, Conradi E, Poulton T. Improving assessment with virtual patients. *Med Teach.* 2009;31(8):759-763.

32. Huhn K, McGinnis P, Wainwright S, Deutsch J. A comparison of 2 case delivery methods: virtual and live. *J Phys Ther Educ.* 2013;27(3):41-48.

33. Qayumi K, Pachev G, Zheng B, et al. Status of simulation in health care education: an international survey. *Adv Med Educ Pract.* 2014;5:457-467.

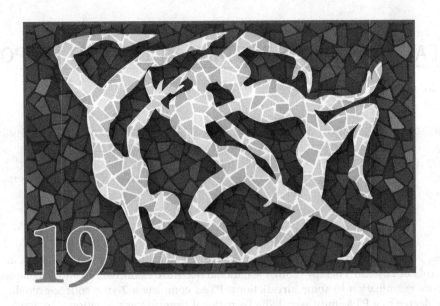

CAPTURING TEACHABLE MOMENTS:
Developing Clinical Problem-Solving of the Physical Therapist Assistant

Peggy DeCelle Newman, PT, MHR

OBJECTIVES

- Delineate the role and scope of work of the physical therapist assistant (PTA) from that of the physical therapist (PT) within the patient/client management (PCM) model.

- Compare the concepts of competence, critical thinking (CT), and clinical problem-solving (CPS) required of the PTA when participating in the PCM model of care with the PT.

- Identify documents specific to PTA education that recognize problem-solving as a foundational element in the clinical work of the PTA within the PT-PTA team.

- Appreciate the developmental nature of acquiring and refining CPS skills.

- Explore realistic methods to explicitly capture teachable moments during the didactic and clinical curriculum to enhance the ability of the PTA to clinically problem solve within the plan of care of the PT of record.

- Offer examples of ways to examine the CPS of the PTA team member in the PT-PTA team.

Musolino GM, Jensen GM, eds. *Clinical Reasoning and Decision-Making in Physical Therapy: Facilitation, Assessment, and Implementation* (pp 207-217).
© 2020 Taylor & Francis Group.

The Physical Therapist Assistant Roles and Responsibilities

Consider this case scenario.

While completing observation hours with a local outpatient PT practice, Cody noticed several framed documents hanging on the wall in the waiting area. Upon closer inspection, he noted several were employees with an associate of applied sciences in PTA degree from the local community college, and 2 were doctor of physical therapy (DPT) degrees from the state university. "Hmm," he thought. "I haven't noticed a difference in what anyone does with the patients. Who can do what here?"

In the United States, PTs now complete a DPT from an accredited education program and must, at a minimum, pass the Federation of State Boards of Physical Therapy (FSBPT)[1] national licensure examination, and may be required to successfully complete a jurisprudence examination in some jurisdictions. PTAs complete a 2-year college-accredited education program to receive an associate degree as a PTA, must pass FSBPT's national licensure examination to practice clinically, and may be required to pass a jurisprudence exam.

So, in the PT and PTA realms of practice, who can do what? What are your thoughts?

Physical Therapists

The PT initiates and manages the provision of all aspects of physical therapy care for each patient/client regardless of the clinical setting. PTs perform the 5 elements of PCM—examination, evaluation, diagnosis, prognosis, and intervention—to maximize functional performance, thereby enhancing quality of life.[2] The essential components of the physical therapy PCM model process help to ensure optimal patient/client outcomes. Findings from the examination process allow the PT to identify a clinical diagnosis, anticipated level of improvement (ie, prognosis), intervention plan (ie, treatment choices), and the frequency and duration of services. The PT clinical decision-making process is recognized as the evaluation and development of the plan of care. The evaluation responsibility is to be borne solely by the PT.[3,4] PTs supervise physical therapy support personnel, which include PTAs, aides, and techs. Additional information specific to responsible supervision of support personnel can be found in Chapter 20, of this text, the FSBPT[1] Model Practice Act, and that of your respective jurisdictions.

Physical Therapist Assistants

PTAs have been making valuable contributions to the provision of efficient and effective physical therapy care since the first PTA graduates entered the job market in 1969. The occupational category was officially created by the American Physical Therapy Association (APTA) House of Delegates in 1967 after nearly 2 decades of discussion over the need for a formally educated worker to assist with treatment. The necessity arose from the physical therapy workforce being unable to adequately meet society's need for care.[5] This deficiency is not unlike what many states and physical therapy practice settings continue to experience today.

Incorporating the PT-PTA team as a viable model of patient/client care delivery amidst the complexities of health care in the 21st century required the 2013 APTA House of Delegates to adopt the APTA Vision Statement and two of the supporting guiding principles around access/equity and collaboration[6]:

Achieving meaningful patient/client outcomes with the fewest resources in the shortest time reigns supreme in today's health care environment. Physical therapist assistants add cost-effective value by contributing their observation, psychomotor, and communication skills to support the physical therapist's clinical judgment toward achieving these outcomes. The Occupational Outlook Handbook *of the US Bureau of Labor Statistics reports that "Physical therapists are expected to increasingly use assistants and aides to reduce the cost of physical therapy services."[7] Unfortunately, recent actions by the federal government may reduce reimbursement when therapy care is provided by the physical therapist assistant (planned implementation in 2022 with Medicare services), waging yet another battle on the value proposition of the fees for the physical therapist–physical therapist assistant service delivery.[8]*

American Physical Therapy Association Vision Statement[6]

Transforming Society by Optimizing Movement to Improve the Human Experience[6]

Excerpt of two of the APTA Vision Statement Guiding Principles:

Access/Equity: The physical therapy profession will recognize health inequities and disparities and work to ameliorate them through innovative models of service delivery, advocacy, attention to the influence of the social determinants of health on the consumer, collaboration with community entities to expand the benefit provided by physical therapy, serving as a point of entry to the health care system, and direct outreach to consumers to educate and increase awareness.[6]

Collaboration: The physical therapy profession will demonstrate the value of collaboration with other health care providers, consumers, community organizations, and other disciplines to solve the health-related challenges that society faces. In clinical practice, doctors of physical therapy, who collaborate across the continuum of care, will ensure that services are coordinated, of value, and consumer centered by referring, comanaging, engaging consultants, and directing and supervising care. Education models will value and foster interprofessional approaches to best meet consumer and population needs and instill team values in physical therapists and physical therapist assistants. Interprofessional research approaches will ensure that evidence translates to practice and is consumer centered.[6]

Reflection Moment

Considering the APTA guiding principles of access/equity and collaboration: How can professionals and patients/clients advocate for PT-PTA services for the benefit of society? What exactly can the PTA perform and do to assist the PT and enhance cost-effective care?

The role of the PTA in patient care activities is to provide designated interventions as directed in the plan of care within the parameters of the patient/client outcomes as written and provided for by the PT of record. More specifically, the PTA's scope of work occurs within the intervention portion of the PCM model of the physical therapy process including coordination, communication, and documentation; patient-related instruction; and procedural interventions.[3]

According to the APTA *Guide to Physical Therapy Practice 3.0*, the consensus document of the APTA, sound clinical judgment of the PTA is necessary to competently carry out the following:

- Determine readiness to participate in the interventions as selected

- Monitor the safety, comfort, and physiologic responses to the interventions being provided

- Perform pertinent tests and measures to collect data to ensure safety and provide information regarding progress toward established goals

- Modify treatments to ensure the greatest efficiency and effectiveness progressing toward goal achievement, and ensuring the safety and comfort of the patient[2]

Every PTA is responsible for accurately understanding their professional scope of work and their ability to make and provide rationales for CPS. The ability to demonstrate CPS is considered an essential skill of an entry-level PTA as documented in the following core documents from the APTA and Commission on Accreditation in Physical Therapy Education (CAPTE):

- APTA Normative Model of Physical Therapist Assistant Education: Version 2007

- CAPTE Standards and Required Elements for Accreditation of Physical Therapist Assistant Education Programs

- APTA Physical Therapist Assistant Clinical Performance Instrument

- APTA Problem-Solving Algorithm Utilized by Physical Therapist Assistants in Patient/Client Intervention[9-12]

Now let's consider the following scenario.

> Shayla, the PTA, observed and documented that her patient presented with increased complaints of tenderness to palpation, redness, local skin, temperature, and edema at the insertion of the Achilles tendon, in addition to the lateral ankle ligaments, which were identified and documented by the PT of record. After reexamining the edema via circumferential measurements consistent with the PT's initial examination, Shayla reviewed the initial measurements for comparison, noted variation, and contacted the therapist of record to confer as to how to proceed.

Shayla observes a considerable change in the patient's condition from the PT's evaluation note. As is the role of the PTA, she collects pertinent data for comparison (eg, circumferential measures) and gets in touch with the PT of record to relay this change in the patient status. As the manager of the patient's care, the PT will determine the necessary next steps. While the psychomotor skills that an observer sees are identical for the intake of data by both the PT and PTA while patient care is occurring, the PT's assessment, analyses, and cognitive interpretation must be different than the requisite problem-solving expectations of the PTA. This difference will be reflected in documentation in the medical records as well. These concepts will be discussed in more detail in Chapter 20.

DEFINITION OF TERMS

To create teaching strategies intended to develop and enhance the thinking and CPS processes of PTA students, as well as to equip clinical instructors (CIs) with ways to capitalize on in-the-moment opportunities, an accurate understanding of related terminology is imperative. Although these terms are often used interchangeably, they are, in fact, not synonymous. For the purpose of this chapter, please use the following definitions relative to the PTA. (See Table 19-1.)

- **Competence:** Possessing requisite knowledge, skills, and behaviors; being able to apply didactic content to novel situations; appreciating the connections among data points; and synthesizing the significance and meaning of information obtained.[10]

- **Clinical problem-solving:** Recognizing a problem exists, identifying and articulating the problem, identifying possible solutions, and understanding the potential consequences of implementing solutions.[10]

- **Critical thinking:** The disciplined, intellectual process of applying skillful reasoning as a guide to belief or action involving the cognitive abilities of analysis, interpretation, inference, evaluation, and explanation.[9-11,13]

Of these terms, competence is arguably the most tangible and familiar. Earning a threshold on a written and/or practical examination and achieving established criteria on the clinical evaluation tool used during student practicums are examples of commonly used ways to determine competence in the skills and behaviors necessary for entry into the profession. CAPTE requires PTA education programs to develop and assess CPS skills.[10] Demonstrating accurate rationale for solutions offered, collecting and comparing data from multiple sources, seeking clarification, determining the need for communicating with the therapist of record regarding changes in patient status, and demonstrating sound clinical judgment about intervention modifications and/or patient progression are examples of essential aspects of CPS for the PTA. In contrast, the clinical decision-making–clinical reasoning skills such as analysis, interpretation, inference, evaluation, and justification are required components of CT and are therefore the role of the PT.[14]

Let's revisit the scenario and apply the terminology.

> Shayla, the PTA, demonstrated competence when she collected the data required to accurately determine an exacerbation in this patient's status. She used CPS skills by recognizing a change in status and pursued follow-up with the PT, who would then employ higher-level diagnostic skills (CT) to properly manage the patient's care. In this example, CPS with reasoning skills would be reflected by both clinicians taking into consideration relevant didactic information regarding the medical condition and physical therapy clinical diagnosis, as well as the uniqueness of this person specifically.

TABLE 19-1

CLINICAL APPLICATION OF TERMS

TERM	EXAMPLE
Competence	Knowledge: Correctly identify an anatomical structure Skills: Safely and effectively operate an ultrasound machine Behaviors: Demonstrate unbiased respect to all
Clinical problem-solving	Recognize patient discomfort requiring positional adjustment Observe cardinal signs of inflammation, requiring data collection to measure pain rating and edema present
Critical thinking	Identify the need for refabricating an effective foot orthosis

Now let's consider perspectives on role delineation of the PT-PTA team, along with matters of practicing at the highest level of your scope of practice and consider matters of efficiency and effectiveness for meeting the needs of society.

ROLE DELINEATION:
WHO DOES WHAT WHEN IT COMES TO DECISION-MAKING?

The most fundamental aspect of CPS by the PTA is comprehending, appreciating, respecting, owning, and exemplifying the role, scope of work, and core values of the PTA as an integral member of the physical therapy profession. PTAs who have been socialized into the physical therapy culture (by reputable faculty who stay abreast, not only of evidence and standards of practice related to the how-to of doing, but also of the essence of being a PTA) recognize the privilege of becoming a part of this amazing profession. It is the rare individual who successfully completes the requisite standards—both CAPTE required and those revered by the PTA faculty and CI role models—without this assimilation of his or her role. Unfortunately, some negative variances do exist. A negative experience by a company and/or PT with a rogue PTA can irreparably damage the ability to trust enough to condone this shared problem-solving and decision-making model of the delivery of physical therapy care.

Clinical Example—Revisited

Howard, the PT, provides the examination/evaluation for Mrs. R., who presents with subacute Grade II anterolateral talofibular ligament sprain. Howard determines Mrs. R. is typically progressing without evidence of active inflammation. Mrs. R. is eager to return to her prior level of function. Howard documents the results of his examination and establishes the physical therapy plan of care designed to achieve functional outcomes, or goals, on which Howard and Mrs. R. have mutually agreed. Howard, as the PT, directs Shayla, the PTA, to begin working with Mrs. R., following introductions, at the subsequent outpatient visit.

At this next visit, Shayla observes and documents that Mrs. R. has significant tenderness to palpation, redness, local skin temperature, and edema at the insertion of the Achilles tendon and around the lateral ankle for which she had been evaluated by Howard. After reexamining the edema via circumferential measurements as done in the PT's initial examination, Shayla reviews the initial measurements that were taken during the evaluation for comparison. She then contacts Howard to report the significant change in Mrs. R.'s condition, which is now acute, and to confer as to how to proceed.

In this example, the PTA, Shayla, demonstrates competence when she recognizes the cardinal signs of inflammation and measures the girth of Mrs. R.'s ankle consistent with how Howard, the PT of record, had originally measured. She uses CPS skills by recognizing a change in status and the need to contact Howard before proceeding with Mrs. R.'s plan of care. Once made aware of the data, Howard is responsible to employ higher-level diagnostic skills (CT) to properly manage the patient's care. In this example, CPS would be reflected by both clinicians taking into consideration relevant information regarding the medical condition and physical therapy clinical diagnosis, as well as the uniqueness of this patient.[15,16]

CAPTE requires PTA education programs to develop and assess CPS skills. The complexity and purpose of the CPS being made vary profoundly with each task performed as a component of physical therapy care, with an intentional skilled action by the PTA. Whenever an option exists, a choice must be made, whether the CPS skill is as basic as using pillows or a wedge to elevate a patient's leg, or more complex such as noting a change in a cardinal sign of inflammation, taking a measurement, noting a discrepancy, and consulting with the PT. The PT is ultimately responsible for decisions regarding discharge planning. However, while it is certainly never the role of the PTA to recommend discharge destination, the PTA must engage in the process of CPS to safely and effectively share the responsibilities of providing patient/client care.[17]

Although PTs and PTAs have been working together for more than 4 decades, confusion continues to exist regarding the scope of work and appropriate involvement of the PTA in the delivery of patient/client care. State practice acts vary considerably in rules and regulations regarding the role, scope of work, and supervision of the PTA and the physical therapy aide. Payers such as Worker's Compensation, Medicare, and Blue Cross/Blue Shield are also inconsistent with their interpretations about the provision of physical therapy services and the value of the PTA.[18]

Reflection Moment

What can a PTA legally and ethically do to assist the PT in patient care?

What are the supervision requirements in a hospital setting?

Does this vary by setting?

How do PTs decide when to include a PTA vs providing the therapy interventions themselves?

In 2007, the APTA's department of education, accreditation, and practice developed 2 algorithms to delineate decision points utilized by PTs to determine whether to include the PTA in assisting with care, and to provide guidance in the appropriate supervision when directing the PTA to perform selected interventions. These algorithms reflect current policies and positions of the profession and are intended to guide the collaborative efforts of the PT-PTA team in achieving patient-centered, functional outcomes in an effective, cost-efficient manner. Figure 19-1 depicts decision considerations, options, and action items by the PT in determining the appropriateness of use and assistance regarding conscientious supervision of the PTA. Figure 19-2 outlines specific steps required of the PTA in every patient/client encounter to provide sound clinical solutions that ensure patient safety while maximizing functional outcomes, effectiveness, and efficiency.[12]

TEACHING STRATEGIES: A DEVELOPMENTAL PROCESS

An ounce of practice is generally worth more than a ton of theory.   —Ernst F. Schumacher, *Small Is Beautiful: A Study of Economics as if People Mattered*

To explore instructional strategies intended to develop CPS skills with PTA students and intentionally prepare DPT students for the crucial legal and ethical responsibility to properly manage the care of the patient/client when choosing to use, and therefore supervise, a PTA, faculty and students all must appreciate what steps are needed for CPS. We must be intentional in the teaching and learning of supervision, direction, and the engagement of the PT-PTA team within the PCM model.

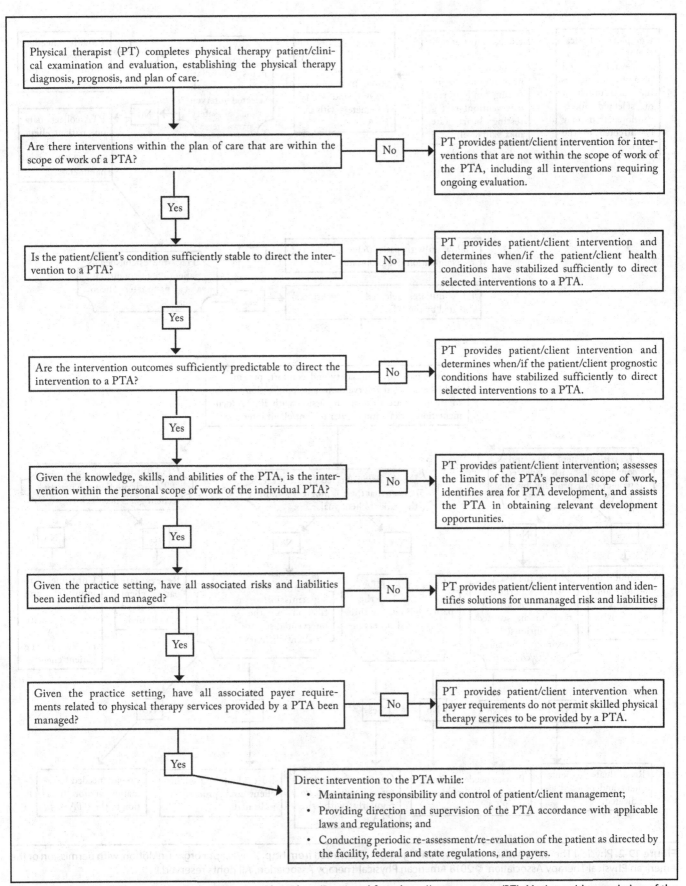

Figure 19-1. Physical Therapist Assistant Direction Algorithm. (Reprinted from http://www.apta.org/PTinMotion, with permission of the American Physical Therapy Association. © 2018 American Physical Therapy Association. All rights reserved.)

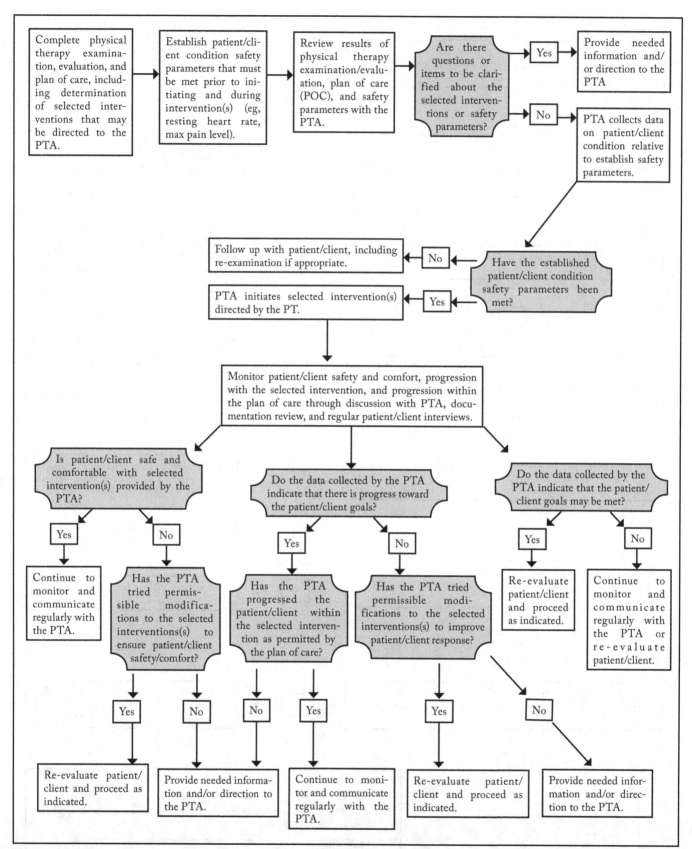

Figure 19-2. Physical Therapist Assistant Supervision Algorithm. (Reprinted from http://www.apta.org/PTinMotion, with permission of the American Physical Therapy Association. © 2018 American Physical Therapy Association. All rights reserved.)

Returning now to the prior example, consider the following.

When and where did Shayla, the PTA, acquire the ability to adeptly identify the cardinal signs of inflammation, collect pertinent data, and immediately contact Howard, the PT of record and manager of the care of this patient?

Are there intentionally prepared didactic experiences that can contribute in the academic curriculum relative to this case scenario?

Or, as is popular belief, does this occur solely because of practice as a student on clinical education experiences with the clinical educator teaching in the moment in a hospital, rehab center, nursing home, school, person's home, or free-standing outpatient clinic? Or is it both?

TABLE 19-2	
DETAILED LOOK AT TERMS—REVISITED	
TERM	**POTENTIAL STRATEGIES FOR DEVELOPMENT**
Competence	Possessing the requisite knowledge, skills, and behaviors for one's role; it begins in the classroom and lab, and is enhanced through opportunities to apply to novel situations to refine and synthesize the significance and meaning of this information.[8] Critical reflection of one's performance and thought processes, or metacognition, is imperative for optimal self-discovery and growth.[19]
Clinical problem-solving	Recognizing that a problem exists, identifying and articulating the problem, identifying viable solutions, and appreciating possible consequences of implementing the solutions.[8] Using a broad body of knowledge to resolve clinical problems followed by intentional consideration, or reflection, of the circumstance to incorporate this experience into an even broader knowledge base.[20]
Critical thinking	Applying skillful reasoning to guide belief or action; includes interpretation, analysis, inference, evaluation, and explanation.[21] This is the role of the PT.

Let's revisit our terms from Table 19-1 in more detail (Table 19-2).

Now let's consider a novice PTA shifting from unconscious incompetence with CPS by the following beginning-level activities:

- Heavily relying on checklists
- Incorrectly applying and interpreting information from the medical record
- Incorrectly interpreting or reporting patient/client cues or responses to care
- Lacking confidence in results of data collected
- Lacking confidence in observations made and reported

Can explicit learning activities be planned to improve the CPS process to move the PTA along the continuum to conscious competence? The answer is yes, absolutely! This begins early on in the didactic portion of the curriculum followed by developmental scaffolding through the entirety of the PTA program. Table 19-3 provides examples. The ability to capture the implicit working knowledge of a seasoned PT or PTA in the moment is an especially powerful way to cultivate the individual learner in how to successfully reason and more confidently become adept with CPS.[22] The PTA is trained to function as an expert observer, recorder, and reporter. As an extender of a PT's reach, the PTA bears the responsibility of being the eyes, ears, and fingertips of the PT when involved in patient/client care.[13] Inherent within this PT-PTA team model of patient care delivery is a shared responsibility requiring a high degree of interdependency between the PT-PTA team members. Consequently, it is essential that both team members understand and respect each other's roles and responsibilities, and are committed to impeccable communication. These need be acquired and honed as do all essential competencies required for successful clinical performance. Examples of such skills can be found in Table 19-3.

TABLE 19-3
TEACHING STRATEGIES TO ENHANCE CLINICAL PROBLEM-SOLVING IN ACADEMIC AND CLINICAL SETTINGS
• Well-written course objectives with correlating content
• Well-designed learning opportunities with explicit performance expectations
• Learning opportunities provided near when the performance/behavior will be assessed
• Ample opportunities to practice the desired performance/behavior
• Timely feedback that is explicit; based on the performance criteria
• Paper patients
• Guided case studies
• Virtual patients
• Peer-to-peer and/or small group problem-solving assignments with oral reports to class
• Thought-provoking, controversial topics for reflection with rationale using citations
• Oral debates over controversial, current topics in health care and the profession
• Establishing clear, realistic, agreed-upon goals consistent with the course syllabus
• Creating a learning partnership between the student and CI based upon respectful, open, honest communication that is patient/client centered
• Asking open-ended questions that encourage exploration of experiences and promote the acceptance of ambiguity and beyond-the-textbook thinking
• Consistent modeling by CI and/or other respected PTAs with timely opportunity for questions, and discussion about solutions being considered throughout sessions
• Conducting student-led patient/client treatment sessions, followed immediately by guided inquiry from the CI about pertinent information gleaned and solutions offered
• Ensuring facilitated reflection following a treatment session, especially when things went awry, so the student can consider what he or she would do differently next time, and why
• Presenting cases in an environment that encourages questions and debate to enhance lifelong learning in the PT-PTA team
• Providing feedback that is specific, based on performance/behaviors (not the student), and in the moment or as soon afterward as is feasible
Adapted from Ladyshewsky,[20] Seif et al,[22] and Foord-May and May.[23]

Strategies for teaching PTA students to connect the dots for CPS must explicitly include the following elements:

- Gleaning pertinent information from the medical record and patient/client
- Competence in data collection, mirroring that obtained by the PT of record for comparison
- Recognizing crucial indicators requiring immediate communication with a PT before proceeding with care, as well as identifying issues that require communication without halting treatment
- Cultivating the ability to accurately assess and intentionally consider one's own thoughts and actions through reflection is critical in developing competence in problem-solving[15,19,20,22]

PATIENT CARE CONSIDERATIONS

Is it expected that every PT will hand off patients/clients to a PTA in the delivery of patient care? In every setting? Is it assumed that once licensed, every PTA is competent and capable to share the responsibility of patient/client care?

Determining whether patient care delivery in a setting or with a specific patient will include the use of the PTA is based upon competence and the PT's trust of the PTA. Each PT is responsible for making the direction decision with each patient/client. To establish the trust needed to confidently share the responsibility of patient care, the PTA minimally must:

- Demonstrate competence in the specific interventions to be provided

- Earn respect and trust by consistently making proper judgments regarding any need for clarification or the need to alert the PT regarding change in status

- Engage in timely, clear, informative communication[4,6]

The nuances of the PT-PTA team in patient care delivery require both partners to understand and respect their roles, responsibilities, and duty of care to patients and to each other. As the manager of the care of the patient, the PT bears the onus of responsibility to ensure the PTA's capability. The only way to build this partnership is for the CPS skills of the PTA partner to earn this privilege through action as patient care unfolds. Working together improves access to physical therapy care and promotes increased efficiency and effectiveness. This not only benefits the patient, but it is also typically rewarding for both the PT and PTA in their own professional growth and development.

REFERENCES

1. Federation of State Boards of Physical Therapy. https://www.fsbpt.org/. Accessed June 2, 2018.
2. American Physical Therapy Association. Guide to physical therapist practice. http://guidetoptpractice.apta.org/. Accessed June 4, 2018.
3. American Physical Therapy Association. Direction and supervision of the PTA. http://www.apta.org/uploadedFiles/APTAorg/About_Us/Policies/HOD/Practice/Direction.pdf. Accessed April 21,2018.
4. Erickson M, McKnight R. *Documentation Basics: A Guide for the PTA.* Thorofare, NJ: SLACK Incorporated; 2012:37.
5. Curtis KA, Newman PD. *The PTA Handbook: Keys to Success in School and Career for the Physical Therapist Assistant.* 2nd ed. Thorofare, NJ: SLACK Incorporated; 2015.
6. American Physical Therapy Association. Vision statement for the physical therapy profession. http://www.apta.org/Vision/. Accessed June 4, 2018.
7. Bureau of Labor and Statistics. Physical therapists and physical therapist assistants job outlook. https://www.bls.gov/ooh/healthcare/physical-therapist-assistants-and-aides.htm. Accessed April 21, 2018.
8. American Physical Therapy Association. Payment under the Medicare therapy cap. http://www.apta.org/PTinMotion/News/2018/02/09/TherapyCapRepeal/. Accessed June 4, 2018.
9. American Physical Therapy Association. *A Normative Model of Physical Therapist Assistant Education: Version 2007.* Alexandria, VA: American Physical Therapy Association; 2007:130-135.
10. Commission on Accreditation in Physical Therapy Education. *Standards and Required Elements for Accreditation of Physical Therapist Assistant Education Programs.* Alexandria, VA: American Physical Therapy Association; 2016.
11. American Physical Therapy Association. *Physical Therapist Assistant Clinical Performance Instrument.* Alexandria, VA: American Physical Therapy Association; 2007.
12. Crosier J. PTA direction and supervision algorithms. *PT in Motion.* 2010;2(8):47-50.
13. Watts NT. Task analysis and division of responsibility in physical therapy. *Phys Ther.* 1971;51:23-25.
14. Commission on Accreditation in Physical Therapy Education. *Standards and Required Elements for Accreditation of Physical Therapist Education Programs.* Alexandria, VA: American Physical Therapy Association; 2016.
15. Hendrick P, Bond C, Duncan E, Hale L. Clinical reasoning in musculoskeletal practice: students' conceptualizations. *Phys Ther.* 2009;89:430-432.
16. Jones M, Jensen G, Edward I. Clinical reasoning in physiotherapy. In: Higgs J, Jones MA, eds. *Clinical Reasoning in the Health Professions.* 2nd ed. Oxford, United Kingdom: Butterworth-Heineman; 2000.
17. Wainright SF, Shepard KF, Harman LB, Stephens J. Factors that influence the clinical decision making of novice and experienced physical therapists. *Phys Ther.* 2011;91(1):87-101.
18. American Physical Therapy Association. PT/PTA teamwork: models in delivering patient care. https://www.apta.org/Supervision Teamwork/Models/. Accessed May 21, 2018.
19. Wruble Hakim E, Moffat M, Becker E, et al. Application of educational theory and evidence in support of an integrated model of clinical education. *J Phys Ther Educ.* 2014;28(1):16.
20. Ladyshewsky RK. Impact of peer-coaching on the clinical reasoning of the novice practitioner. *Physiother Can.* 2004;56;15.
21. Huhn K, McGinnis P, Wainwright S, Deutsch J. A comparison of 2 case delivery methods: virtual and live. *J Phys Ther Educ.* 2013;27(3):41-47.
22. Seif GA, Brown D, Annan-Coultas D. Fostering clinical reasoning skills in physical therapist students through an interactive learning module designed in Moodle learning management system. *J Phys Ther Educ.* 2013;27(3):32-40.
23. Foord-May L, May W. Facilitating professionalism in physical therapy: theoretical foundations for the facilitation process. *J Phys Ther Educ.* 2007;(21):3.

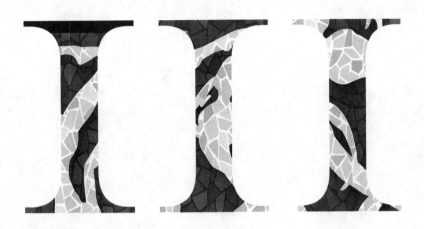

CLINICAL REASONING:
Research, Innovation, and Best Practice Exemplars

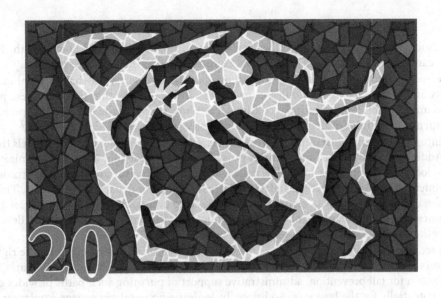

DEVELOPING A SUCCESSFUL CLINICAL APPROACH:
The Collaborative Partnership of the Physical Therapist–Physical Therapist Assistant Team

Peggy DeCelle Newman, PT, MHR and Stephanie A. Weyrauch, PT, DPT, MSCI

OBJECTIVES

- Discuss elements in the clinical environment that affect the physical therapist–physical therapist assistant (PT-PTA) team partnership.
- Appraise the historical perspective of the PTA.
- Review current PT-PTA supervision and direction algorithms.
- Differentiate the educational background, roles, and responsibilities of the PTA.
- Discover core documents that govern the PT-PTA team.
- Apply mentorship principles to maximize the PT-PTA partnership.
- Facilitate effective PT-PTA team-building strategies.

INTRODUCTION

A common denominator for a successful physical therapy practice is a thriving culture. Management establishes the cultural norms of an organization through the values, behaviors, and style of its leadership, which are then reinforced by employees, and subsequently experienced by patients. Team-based cultures are essential in 21st century health care delivery and have been shown to improve employee satisfaction and the patient experience.[1-6] Using a PT-PTA team collaborative for health care is com-

Musolino GM, Jensen GM, eds. *Clinical Reasoning and Decision-Making in Physical Therapy: Facilitation, Assessment, and Implementation* (pp 221-234).
© 2020 Taylor & Francis Group.

mon in many settings, including private practice, skilled nursing facilities, hospitals, and home health. The dynamic between these 2 team members can influence clinic or organizational culture as well as the patient experience.

Using a business perspective, culture is defined as consistent, observable patterns of behavior within an organization—how an organization thinks and feels. A company's culture has norms and standards that define success by outlining behavior deemed acceptable and unacceptable. Organizational culture defines how people in the organization problem-solve, communicate, socialize, treat patients, run clinics or departments administratively, seek knowledge, and react.[7]

To build a strong culture, leadership must establish trust with employees. The leader sets and models the values of the physical therapy practice. Additionally, all flourishing cultures possess an element of cohesiveness. Organizational cohesiveness is defined as each person looking out for his or her fellow colleagues and working toward the same mission and vision. Leaders must create an environment that gives employees a stake in the organization's or department's success. This can include providing monetary incentives, opportunities to lead community or marketing events, or support for professional development. The key for maintaining cohesiveness with team members is communication. Leaders need to coach and develop others, teach and set expectations, keep others accountable, and recognize and reward success.[8,9]

Once the culture is set, efforts to keep it maintained are essential. To do this, leaders must hire the right people and engage staff in the organization's goals to grow business. If an employee demonstrates specific talents in marketing, treating athletic injuries, or having a passion for fall prevention, administrative support of pursuing such paths provides growth opportunities for the employee, and potentially for the business. Additionally, leaders who regularly engage employees in discussions about the vision, mission, and purpose of the organization encourage employee motivation and satisfaction. In organizations, 4 main types of culture exist: customer intimacy, operational excellence, cultivation and collaboration, and competency and expertise.[8,10] While organizations demonstrate all four of these culture types, typically one theme is most predominant.

Organizations with thriving cultures of customer intimacy emphasize relationships with clients and value customer service above all else. Decisions are made collegially, and the environment is highly team oriented. The organization focuses on who will be a good fit for the community when hiring new staff. Some companies exude a culture characteristic of customer intimacy, developing relationships beyond the product with the customer.[10]

Organizational cultures dominant in operational excellence value systems, efficiency, certainty, and order. Decisions are made methodically, and a structured hierarchy is usually followed. Typically, these organizations are power driven, and hire based on a person's fit with the function of the job. This mantra dominates in the service delivery industry.[10]

Organizations strong in cultivation and collaboration emphasize participation and purpose. Decisions regularly involve a group of people who come to a consensus on how their work will advance the organization's mission. Core values and relationships are a centerpiece for this type of organizational culture, and people are hired based on their fit with the vision and purpose of the organization. This culture type is dominant in many nonprofits.[8]

Organizations that have a strong culture of competency and expertise strive to set industry gold standards and value innovation. These organizations are competitive and enjoy challenging the status quo, while often taking steps to recognize creativity and achievements. Hiring is based on merit in a specialty or skill set, as well as fit within the company culture. These organizations are generally responsible to an actively engaged board of directors and found in the top exchanges of the market for their respective industry categories.[10]

When adding a PTA to the existing team, leadership needs to consider how the individual's talents will contribute to improving the organization. Understanding the talents of each team member will optimize the capacity to deliver high-quality patient care and positively contribute to the organizational culture.

Physical Therapist Assistant Education

To optimize the PT-PTA team dynamic, PTs must be aware of the educational preparation, as well as the appropriate role of the PTA within the patient/client management model. The 1964 American Physical Therapy Association (APTA) House of Delegates passed a motion designating a committee to explore the use of a trained assistant to help meet the growing demand to treat patients in need of skilled physical therapy services. The 1967 House of Delegates created the occupational category of physical therapy assistant. In 1969, 15 PTAs graduated from inaugural programs at Miami Dade Community College in Florida and the College of St. Catherine in Minnesota, and the House of Delegates passed the name change to PTA, indicating one who assists the PT,[11] and clearly establishing the PT-PTA partnership. As of 2017, more than 12,000 students are enrolled annually in the more than 350 accredited PTA programs in the United States.[12]

PTA education occurs primarily in community colleges (now referred to as state colleges in many regions), resulting in a 2-year associate's degree. Although PTA program curricular content varies depending on the college's program, all include both general education (eg, English, science, government) and physical therapy content (eg, dynamics of human motion, therapeutic exercise), and all must meet or exceed standards developed and monitored by the Commission on Accreditation in Physical Therapy Education (CAPTE). PTA education (like all health provider education) is focused on the achievement of competencies designed to ensure that graduates acquire the skills, knowledge, judgment, and code of conduct necessary to assist the PT with data collection and interventions within the plan of care to maximize patient/client functional outcomes. Behavioral expectations emphasized throughout the PTA's preparation include self-reflection, diversity, acceptance, effective oral and written communication, and ongoing growth in values-based behaviors such as altruism, caring/compassion, continuing competence, duty, integrity, PT-PTA team collaboration, responsibility and social responsibility,[13] and ethical conduct.[14]

As with PT education, a vital component of PTA education is the real-world application, which occurs during the clinical education components of the curriculum. The average length of terminal, full-time clinical experiences in PTA education is 15 weeks,[12] contrasted with the average of 34 to 36 weeks with doctor of physical therapy clinical education. The clear majority of PTA programs use the APTA Physical Therapist Assistant Clinical Performance Instrument (APTA PTA CPI) to assess students' clinical performance. The clinical education outcomes ultimately determine competency for entry-level performance and readiness for employment. A core document, *Minimum Required Skills of PTA Graduates at Entry-Level*, describing the foundational skills considered indispensable for a new graduate was adopted by the APTA in 2008. It identifies the minimum required skill set that each new graduate PTA is expected to competently perform in the clinical environment. See Table 20-1 for a summary of the PTA skill set and Table 20-2 for those skill requirements exclusive to the PT.[15,16]

Upon program completion, the graduate must successfully pass the Federation of State Boards of Physical Therapy (FSBPT)[17] national licensure examination and meet all state licensure requirements. Nearly all jurisdictions in the United States require licensure for PTA practice. Regardless of state regulatory requirements, Medicare and other payers require PTA licensure to participate in providing care to beneficiaries.[18,19]

Regardless of practice setting, the determination to use a PTA in the delivery of therapy care requires the education, expertise, and professional judgment of a PT as defined in the profession's Standards of Practice and Code of Ethics. The PT remains responsible for the management of the care of the patient/client directing the PTA to assist with selected interventions toward achieving established goals via a written plan of care. This means it is never acceptable for the PTA to treat a patient until the PT has conducted an initial examination and evaluation, established functional goals, and set forth the plan of care to be followed. It is never acceptable for the PTA to be supervised or directed to provide physical therapy care by anyone other than a licensed PT. It is never acceptable for anyone other than the PT who conducted the examination and evaluation to determine if participation by a PTA is prudent (ie, it is not to be determined carte blanche by administrators). Most jurisdictional physical therapy practice acts specifically delineate appropriate supervision, direction, roles, and responsibilities. To see the actual wording of your state's practice act, visit https://www.fsbpt.org/. Regardless of the specificity of wording in state statutes, it is inconsistent with the profession of physical therapy's standards of care and ethical practice to participate in deviations from the above.[18,20]

THE PHYSICAL THERAPIST ASSISTANT'S ROLE IN PATIENT/CLIENT MANAGEMENT

In the 50 years that the PT-PTA team has collaborated to provide physical therapy services, differences of opinion regarding the proper role and use of support personnel have existed among PTs. Practice guidelines and the scope of work—specifically the boundaries for what a PTA is permitted to do with regard to patient care–related tasks—remain under discussion even today. Foundational constructs initially defining the direction of responsibilities in physical therapy came from a 1971 *Physical Therapy* article in which Nancy Watts proposed a process based upon the doing or deciding aspects of practice (eg, clinical decision-making regarding directing the PTA). Within this taxonomy, Watts distinguished the components of what is to be accomplished, how, and by when, as the process of decision-making that includes using best available evidence, comparing rationales for alternatives, and weighing the choices accordingly in the best interest of the patient/client within a given situation.

The role of decision-making is solely borne by the PT. Effectively implementing the psychomotor skills—the how-to—is the process of doing. The mixture of doing and decision-making in the delivery of patient care appropriately varies depending upon the circumstances. Specifically, the doer and decision-maker need be one person (the PT) when the circumstances are uncertain or unpredictable, or the results of actions being taken are unclear and/or are changing rapidly. These landmark concepts are the basis from which the determinants of clinical decision-making, task responsibility, and delegation in physical therapy are derived.[21]

PTAs provide physical therapy care under the direction and supervision of a licensed PT. Responsibilities of the PTA include collecting data (eg, patient-/client-related information, tests, measures) necessary to implement the plan of care and determine progress toward patient/client goals as established by the PT; implementing and modifying selected components of interventions consistent with the plan of care to ensure patient/client safety and comfort; and progressing the patient/client and providing pertinent documentation within the medical record. PTAs communicate, educate, and interact with all members of the health care team, as well as with patients/clients and families/caregivers. PTAs respond to patient/client and environmental emergencies; participate in administration, teaching, and research; and may supervise therapy aides, techs, or volunteers consistent with state law. Licensed PTAs may serve as clinical instructors for student PTAs, yet the assistant is ultimately, inextricably tied to the PT. The PT is ultimately responsible for the physical therapy services provided with the PTA.[18,22] Both PTs and PTAs are highly encouraged to become APTA credentialed CIs, if taking on the clinical teaching responsibility.

TABLE 20-1
MINIMUM REQUIRED SKILLS FOR
PHYSICAL THERAPIST ASSISTANT GRADUATES AT ENTRY-LEVEL

- Plan of care review
- Provisional interventions
  - Therapeutic exercise
  - Electrotherapeutic modalities
  - Functional training
  - Manual therapy techniques (eg, massage, soft tissue mobilization, passive range of motion)
  - Application and adjustment of devices and equipment
  - Airway clearance techniques
  - Integumentary repair and protection techniques
  - Physical agents
  - Mechanical modalities
- Patient instruction
- Patient progression (identify need to progress via data collection within the PT's plan of care)
- Communication of pertinent information in a timely manner
- Relationship of psychosocial factors to progress
- Clinical problem-solving
- Data collection
  - Interview skills
  - Ability to modify techniques
  - Documentation and communication
  - Competent data collection
    - Anthropometric characteristics; arousal, attention, and cognition; assistive and adaptive devices; body mechanics; environmental barriers, self-care, and home management; gait, locomotion, and balance; integumentary integrity; muscle function; neuromotor function; orthotic and prosthetic devices and equipment; pain; posture; range of motion; sensory response; vital signs
- Documentation (including relevancy, accuracy, and ability to adapt)
- Safety, CPR, and emergency procedures
- Health care literature
- Education (including colleagues, students, and community)
- Resource management (human, fiscal, systems)
- Behavioral expectations (values-based behaviors, guide to ethical conduct)
- Communication (interpersonal and conflict management/negotiation)
- Promotion of health, wellness, and prevention
- Career development (self-assessment, maintaining/enhancing competency)

TABLE 20-2

EXCLUSIVE RESPONSIBILITIES OF THE PHYSICAL THERAPIST

- Interpretation of referrals when available
- Initial examination, evaluation, diagnosis, and prognosis
- Development and/or modification of a plan of care that is based on the initial examination or reexamination and includes the goals and expected outcomes
- Determination of when the expertise and decision-making capability of the PT requires the PT to personally render physical therapy interventions, and when it may be appropriate to use the PTA. A PT shall determine the most appropriate use of the PTA that provides for the delivery of service that is safe, effective, and efficient.
- Reexamination of patients/clients, considering their goals and revising the plan of care as needed
- Establishment of the discharge plan and documentation of discharge summary/status
- Oversight of all documentation for services rendered to each patient/client

Note: These are not comprehensive. Adapted from the Direction and Supervision of the Physical Therapist Assistant. [HOD P06-05-18-26] APTA, 2006. Reprinted from http://www.apta.org/PTinMotion, with permission of the American Physical Therapy Association. © 2018 American Physical Therapy Association. All rights reserved.

PHYSICAL THERAPIST–PHYSICAL THERAPIST ASSISTANT TEAM RESPONSIBILITIES

A successful PT-PTA team relies on many elements, including but not limited to:

- Mutual respect
- Confidence and trust in each other
- Accurate understanding of and appreciation for educational preparation
- Steadfast adherence to standards of practice and pertinent laws and regulations
- Shared enthusiasm and commitment toward patient-/client-centered goals
- Dedication to clear communication, self-reflection, and lifelong learning[18]

PTs and educators also foster the enhancement of the PTA's clinical problem-solving (CPS) skills. Bloom's taxonomy[23] is a useful framework for facilitating deeper critical thinking for this purpose, and clinical educators and supervising PTs, as well as PTA peers, may find the following queries helpful to facilitate CPS by the PTA:

To **promote** knowledge acquisition (lower level on Bloom's taxonomy[23]):

- Are you able to repeat the information you just gathered?
- Did you memorize the information?

To **encourage** understanding:

- Can you explain what the information means?
- Does it make sense to you?
- Do you know why the information is important?

To **apply** concepts (higher level):

- Is there an example you can give to tie this idea to a real-world situation?
- How does this information relate to your professional experiences?

To **evaluate** pertinent information:

- Can you critique this idea on its intellectual merit?
- Can you differentiate what is important and what is nonessential regarding this topic?

To **stimulate** creative problem-solving:

- Are there other ways to think about or interpret this information?

- Can you generate a new idea by combining elements of the topic or applying the information to a new problem?

These questions may help PTs, PTAs, CIs, and educators to provide thoughtful direction to the PTA during development of CPS skills. Additionally, PTs should thoroughly communicate expectations to the PTA for optimal patient care. Communication can be achieved through written, oral, digital, or electronic means. ***Consider the following scenario.***

Scenario 1

Gerald is a PT in an inpatient rehabilitation facility. He frequently works with Francine, a PTA. Gerald plans to spend the following few days at a conference and asks if Francine would take on his caseload while he is gone. Francine regularly works with Gerald's patients and thoroughly understands both their goals and plans of care. The day before Gerald leaves, he sends Francine a secure email highlighting each patient's physical therapy clinical diagnosis, progress, and planned focus of treatment for the remainder of the week.

Francine checks her email. A paragraph regarding one patient draws her attention. "Mrs. S. is here with a chief complaint of weakness following hospitalization for sepsis as a complication of right hip arthroscopy. I have seen her twice. We have been working primarily on hip range of motion, bed mobility, and strength. Please continue with treatment to address improving these impairments." Because Mrs. S. is a relatively new patient, Francine has not yet interacted with her. She decides to check Mrs. S.'s medical record and notices that the patient has been performing base-level strengthening exercises for her home program. She knows Gerald will be at the conference for 3 days and wonders if it is safe to begin transitioning Mrs. S. to resistive exercise. She walks over to Gerald's office.

"I received your email," she says to Gerald. "I have a question about Mrs. S."

Gerald looks up from his computer. "Sure. What's up?" he says, pausing his documentation.

"It looks like you have been performing a lot of base-level activities such as active hip rotation with knee flexion in side-lying, passive hip range of motion, and bed mobility activities such as rolling. How is she doing with those?"

"She is doing fairly well. She requires supervision for rolling, and she still needs some help transferring from supine to sitting."

"How much assistance does she need?" asks Francine.

"Minimal assistance. Mostly, she has difficulty moving her right leg where she had surgery. Her wheelchair-to-mat transfer is a different story."

"How so?"

"She has a lot of pain when standing, and she requires moderate assistance of one person for initiation of the transfer and for successful completion, with guarding, and facilitatory tapping, along with verbal cues and instructions."

"But no pain at rest, right?" Francine clarifies.

"Correct."

Francine and Gerald discuss Mrs. S. for a few more minutes before she asks about progressing the patient to resistive hip exercise. Gerald agrees it would be good to add low-level TheraBand exercises including supine bridging progressing to light resistance, side-lying hip rotation with knee flexion, and prone hip extension with assist as needed, to Mrs. S.'s regimen.

continued

The first 2 days of Gerald's absence are smooth for Francine. She assesses Gerald's patients as needed and continues with his plan of care for each patient. On the third day of his absence, however, Francine notices Mrs. S. is in significantly more pain than usual. Prior to this visit, Francine had been progressing Mrs. S.'s resistive exercises, and she is now able to transfer wheelchair to mat with minimal to moderate assist and no pain. On this day, Mrs. S. complains of right calf pain at rest. She rates her pain as a constant 7/10. Francine examines her bilateral lower extremities. There is noticeable erythema and swelling in Mrs. S.'s right leg. Palpation reveals calf tenderness. Additionally, Francine measures the circumference of both lower extremities 10 cm below the tibial tuberosity and notes the right leg is 3 cm greater than the left leg. Francine is concerned about the patient's presentation, so she calls Gerald on the phone.

"Hey, Francine," answers Gerald.

Francine explains the findings of her assessment and the change in Mrs. S's symptoms. "Should I still treat her, Gerald?"

Based on the information Francine relays, Gerald knows Mrs. S. is at high risk for a blood clot and recommends referral to the emergency department for further medical evaluation.

When Gerald returns from his conference the following Monday, Francine conveys that Mrs. S. has been diagnosed with a deep vein thrombosis.

Reflection Moment

Do you believe this is appropriate communication for the PT-PTA team? Why or why not?

What aspects of the PT-PTA team effort could have been improved? Why?

This scenario is a good example of proper communication for the PT-PTA team. Gerald communicated his expectations to Francine through email, establishing directions for continuing range of motion, strengthening, and bed mobility activities for Mrs. S. However, Gerald did not include other pertinent information that would have provided more comprehensive instruction. Francine decided to gather more information by talking to Gerald directly. The dialogue gave Francine additional knowledge about the patient's pain status, tolerance to treatment, amount of assistance needed, and appropriate progressions of exercise—information that was lacking in Gerald's original email. Finally, when Francine noticed a change in status with Mrs. S., she collected the necessary data for Gerald to make an informed clinical decision as to whether Mrs. S. was appropriate for physical therapy intervention. Francine conveyed the data to Gerald via telephone.

Communication between the PT and PTA can be affected by factors including state laws, practice location, clinical setting, and experiences with both professionals and personal relationships. The PT needs to be cognizant of the authority differential and foster an alliance that facilitates mentorship, trust, and open communication. Mentorship provided by the PT may enhance the PTA's CPS. *Consider the following scenario.*

Scenario 2

Carl is a new graduate from the local PTA program, and Jenny has been an outpatient orthopedic PT for 5 years. Jenny and Carl have been assigned to work together as a PT-PTA team. Jenny wants Carl to feel comfortable discussing patient management and treatment, and also desires to facilitate his growth as a clinician. She decides to implement a weekly journal club to help both team members apply the evidence to their patient caseload. Their first journal club examines a randomized controlled trial of Mechanical Diagnosis and Therapy/McKenzie Method (MDT) in people with low back pain. Jenny is certified in MDT and uses this form of classification and treatment for most of her patients with low back pain. Carl learned basic interventions for MDT in class as well as during a previous clinical experience; however, he is unfamiliar with proper assessment and application of MDT theory and technique.

continued

Through Jenny's recommendation, Carl uses the PEDro[24] scale to evaluate the quality of the study for this week's journal club. He determines that the study had an appropriate specification of eligibility, randomization, concealed allocation, baseline characteristics, assessor masking, follow-up, and statistical analysis, but poor participant and therapist masking of procedure. Based on this, he concludes the study is of high quality.

"What were the conclusions of the study?" Jenny asks.

"Pain and disability scores decreased significantly in both groups treated with MDT intervention and standard intervention," replies Carl. "Within the MDT intervention group, participants who experienced centralization of symptoms responded faster to treatment than those who did not experience centralization."

"And what was the population?"

"Males and females with acute and chronic low back pain."

Jenny asks Carl to apply the results of the study to their current cases.

"Well, I know Mr. P. had less leg pain when I assessed his lumbar extension range of motion today. I could have communicated that to you, and we could have tried MDT extension exercises to decrease his leg and back pain," Carl suggests.

Satisfied with their discussion, Jenny proceeds to educate Carl on proper MDT techniques, exercise progression, and prognostic factors to note when treating a patient with low back pain. Carl is impressed with how eager Jenny seems to be when teaching and mentoring.

Reflection Moment

How did this example illustrate, or not, the PT-PTA teamwork for patient/client management?

Where would you go from here to further facilitate CPS?

This scenario is an example of Jenny facilitating Carl's learning by helping him recognize patterns so he can better treat patients with low back pain. She uses research to promote evidenced-based practice and CPS. While the literature provides clinicians with treatment guidelines, CPS is required to apply and customize that evidence to particular patients with particular conditions and life experiences.[25]

Learning and growth are the ultimate goals for both mentor and mentee. In clinical practice, much of this learning comes from experience. A PT mentor can facilitate a PTA's experiential learning by encouraging reflection, interaction with others, and "purposeful attention to and critical evaluation of one's own thinking and past learning in light of new clinical experience."[25]

Experiential learning occurs before, during, and after a clinical experience. In our scenario, Jenny promoted experiential learning before a patient interaction by helping Carl plan how he would proceed in working with a patient with low back pain who presented with certain prognostic signs. Jenny could further facilitate CPS by having Carl reflect on his knowledge and skill in treating people with low back pain. This may assist Carl in better asking for help with developing his ability to treat future patients. Because Carl is a new graduate, he is still working toward Schön's reflective practice (RP) capabilities.[26] Carl has not yet developed his experiential learning during a clinical encounter, termed reflection-in-action. Reflection-in-action thinking can influence delivery of care in the moment an intervention or assessment as performed.[26] As a clinician gains more experience, reflection-in-action becomes easier and more natural. As Jenny continues to mentor Carl, his ability to apply experiential learning during a clinical encounter (ie, reflection-in-action cognition) will improve. However, Jenny's encouragement of Carl to apply the journal club article to a current patient is an example of applying experiential learning after a clinical experience, termed reflection-on-action.[26]

Recalling Schön's model of RP, reflection-on-action occurs by recalling the details and reflecting on an experience in more depth after the experience occurs.[26] This type of experiential learning allows PTs to assist PTAs in identifying errors in their CPS.[26] In our scenario, Carl recalled that Mr. P.'s leg pain decreased when he extended his lumbar spine, which, after reflection, he realized could have been communicated to the PT to help gain a better patient outcome. Emotions can influence experiential learning, and it is therefore essential that mentors, supervisors, and educators consider the range of possible feelings and emotional reactions associated with a particular learning experience, and understand how this may affect PTAs and their learning process. In Scenario 2, Jenny's outward and apparent eagerness to teach Carl, in itself, enhanced his learning experience with a positive impact on his self-efficacy.

PTs must be readily available and open to the PTA who wants to question, clarify, and report changes in patient status. Likewise, the PTA must promptly communicate when patient re-evaluation is required. ***Let's reflect on the following scenario.***

Scenario 3

Kim, a PT, has worked with Alicia, a PTA, in a private practice for the last 5 years. Kim had evaluated Mrs. G. for left-sided neck and shoulder pain a few weeks ago, and determined her symptoms were originating from her cervical spine. After 3 treatments, Mrs. G.'s neck pain had resolved, but her shoulder pain was still present. Alicia had been tasked with treating Mrs. G. per Kim's plan of care for the past 2 visits. On Mrs. G.'s sixth therapy visit, she again states her shoulder is painful with lifting of her arm above her head.

"I haven't really noticed much change in my shoulder. I still have pain reaching for things in my cupboard and when doing my hair," Mrs. G. says. "But my neck feels great."

Alicia assesses Mrs. G.'s neck range of motion, which is normal in all directions. Her shoulder is strong. She has pain during supraspinatus testing. Active and passive range of motion produce pain at end-range of shoulder abduction.

Based on her assessment, Alicia suspects Mrs. G. has separate shoulder involvement and expresses her impression to Kim. "Perhaps you should reassess her to see if she would benefit from a scapular strengthening program," Alicia suggests. "Mrs. G. has not made much progress with her shoulder over the last week, so maybe we need to change our approach."

Kim reassesses Mrs. G. and finds poor scapular upward rotation and posterior tilt with overhead movements. This finding prompts activation and strengthening exercises of the serratus anterior and lower trapezius muscles. Mrs. G. continues to see Alicia for another 3 visits. On her 10th visit, Mrs. G. reports that her shoulder pain has resolved, and Kim discharges her from therapy.

This scenario is a good illustration of collaborative reasoning between the PTA and the PT. Collaborative reasoning is defined as cultivating a "consensual approach to working with patients in the interpretation of examinations, setting and prioritization of goals, and choice of intervention strategies."[25] In our example, this strategy is demonstrated between both the patient and the PT-PTA team. Mrs. G. expresses to Alicia that her shoulder pain has not improved, and her neck pain seems resolved. Alicia interprets this as Mrs. G. informing her that it is time for a reassessment. Alicia obliges and, after reassessing Mrs. G., suspects shoulder involvement, for which she then informs Kim, the supervising PT. After performing her examination and confirming Alicia's findings, Kim concludes that scapular dysfunction is affecting Mrs. G.'s shoulder mechanics, and updates their plan of care.

There are 4 reasoning strategies involved with collaborative reasoning[25(p10)]:

1. **Reasoning about the procedure** allows the clinician to choose and administer interventions based on available data.

2. **Reasoning about teaching** helps patients understand their condition, which influences self-efficacy and recovery.

3. **Predictive reasoning** involves prognosis and addressing the potential ramifications of the prognosis on patients' thoughts and behaviors.

4. **Ethical reasoning** encompasses the ideas and decisions made in attempts to resolve moral and ethical dilemmas that occur in the practice of physical therapy.

In our example, Kim specifically employs reasoning about procedure[25] when deciding to change the plan of care by having Alicia administer new interventions (ie, serratus anterior and lower trapezius recruitment exercises). Clinicians very commonly employ a combination of these strategies when completing CPS.

TABLE 20-3
LEVELS OF SUPERVISION

The American Physical Therapy Association (APTA) supports the following levels of supervision within the context of physical therapist practice. The following levels of supervision are the minimum required for safe and effective physical therapist services. The application of a higher level of supervision may occur at the discretion of the physical therapist based on jurisdictional law regarding supervision, patient or client factors, the skills and abilities of the personnel being supervised, facility requirements, or other factors.

Further information regarding supervision is available in the APTA Direction and Supervision of the Physical Therapist Assistant, Student Physical Therapist and Physical Therapist Assistant Provision of Services, and The Role of Aides in a Physical Therapy Service (www.apta.org).[30]

- **General Supervision:** General supervision applies to the physical therapist assistant. The physical therapist is not required to be on site for supervision but must be available at least by telecommunications. The ability of the physical therapist assistant to provide services shall be assessed on an ongoing basis by the supervising physical therapist.

- **Direct Supervision:** Direct supervision applies to supervision of the student physical therapist and student physical therapist assistant. The physical therapist, or the physical therapist assistant when supervising a student physical therapist assistant, is physically present and immediately available for supervision. In both cases, the physical therapist, or physical therapist assistant will have direct contact with the patient/ or client on each date of service. Telecommunications does not meet the requirement of direct supervision.

- **Direct Personal Supervision:** Direct personal supervision applies to supervision of a physical therapy aide. The physical therapist, or where allowable by law the physical therapist assistant, is physically present and immediately available to supervise tasks that are related to patient/and client services. The physical therapist maintains responsibility for patient and client management at all times.

PHYSICAL THERAPIST CONSIDERATIONS WHEN DIRECTING AND SUPERVISING A PHYSICAL THERAPIST ASSISTANT

Determining the proper use of a PTA in a setting with a specific patient or client is essential to ensure safe, ethical, legal, and outstanding patient care. Supervision is defined as "having the direction and oversight of others."[18] The PT and PTA share responsibility to adhere to laws and regulations and participate in clinical care models that promote the best interest and safety of patients. State and/or jurisdictional physical therapy practice acts delineate the minimally acceptable level of supervision required for any practice setting and often address the maximum number of PTAs a PT may supervise at a time. Table 20-3 lists the levels of supervision as defined by the APTA. Every PT and PTA must know, understand, and remain current with his or her state and/or jurisdictional practice act. Failure to do so can lead to fines and ethical and legal ramifications, the need to appear before a board of PT practice of peers, and the loss of the privilege to practice.[18]

Regardless of freedoms allowed by state law, it is the PT's responsibility to always engage in an active decision-making process about the level of supervision required for a specific patient/client with a specific PTA. See the algorithms depicted in Figures 19-1 and 19-2, which identify key decision points for consideration by the PT when supervising PTAs.

The PT decides who will perform which parts of care. To confidently share the responsibility of patient care with a PTA, the PT must be confident in his or her competence of the skill set needed for the patient or client, make proper clinical judgments, and be vigilant about timely and pertinent communication. The degree and amount of supervision necessary to ensure quality physical therapy care depend upon many factors. Table 20-4 lists key care considerations regarding use of a PTA; state and federal guidelines must also be considered.

The nuances and complexities of the responsibilities, roles, and decisions that the PT-PTA team must make in patient care delivery to provide cost-effective, quality physical therapy are complex and extensive. Resources exist in the form of algorithms to provide guidance with managing the responsibility of supervision and decisions to direct patient care delivery (see Figures 19-1 and 19-2).

TABLE 20-4

KEY FACTORS AFFECTING PHYSICAL THERAPIST SUPERVISION AND DIRECTION OF A PHYSICAL THERAPIST ASSISTANT

The PTA's education, training, experience, and skill level: New graduate or years of experience? New setting? Worked with this patient type/mix?

Patient/client criticality, acuity, stability, and complexity: How much and how rapidly is a change in status likely? How grave may be the consequences if a poor decision is made or an intervention is performed poorly?

The predictability of the consequences: How uncertain is this situation? How confidently can the consequences be predicted?

The setting in which the care is being delivered: Will the PT be onsite? Are other health care providers on the premises?

Federal and state statutes: Who can do what? How often?

Liability and risk management concerns: What do company policy and job descriptions state? Has there been a recent incident or lawsuit?

The mission of physical therapy services for the setting: What do therapy services primarily consist of? Consultation? Education? Treatment?

The needed frequency of reexamination: How often is examination or assessment anticipated? Is it prudent for the PT to be the caregiver?

BUILDING A STRONG MENTORING RELATIONSHIP

To build a successful PT-PTA team, it is imperative for the PT to both mentor and be collaborative with the PTA. Mentorship is defined as a one-to-one relationship in which an expert or senior person voluntarily gives time to teach, support, and encourage another.[27] More recent literature examines mentoring through the lens of individual career development, with the mentor serving as confidant, career guide, and information source.[3-5,28,29] The PT-PTA team ought to embody peer mentoring, where participants are colleagues. Both members have something valuable to contribute and to gain from the relationship.

Mentorship programs in an organization can be formal or informal. Development of formal mentorship programs shows investment and desire to maximize employee growth. Formal mentorships are typically developed by the organization and identify specific guidelines and structure for the relationship. These programs have official objectives with scheduled meeting times to discuss progress of the mentee. Formal programs are often shorter term, and the relationship may be assigned (as opposed to created spontaneously). These relationships are usually less emotionally intense compared to informal mentorship relationships, but facilitate a good foundation for the PT-PTA team to be effective. Sometimes, formal programs can catalyze informal mentorship.[28]

Compared to formal mentorship programs, informal mentorships are less structured and develop out of personal and/or professional respect and admiration, making the relationship collegial. Typically, informal programs emerge voluntarily as the mentor and mentee readily identify with each other. The relationship is frequently more emotionally intense when compared to formal mentorship relationships, facilitating depth and richness of a lifelong connection.[27]

Significant evidence supports mentorship in physical therapy. Peer-to-peer mentorship improves the confidence and competence of a novel learner[3] and promotes deeper learning for both the mentee and mentor.[27] Mentorship between a PT and PTA improves PT knowledge of PTA capabilities, which helps to avoid underuse and negative misperceptions. These relationships foster enthusiasm, camaraderie, and professionalism, positively impacting organizational culture.[4] The mentor-mentee partnership builds passion in both parties and strengthens our profession.[28]

To enhance the mentorship culture of the PT-PTA team, PTs need to prioritize mentoring their PTA counterparts and be open to learning from them as well. Getting to know one another at a personal and professional level is encouraged.[5,29] Sharing professional goals, personal goals, family, and experiences promotes a deeper level of understanding and compatibility, which may result in a more unified approach to high-quality and cost-effective care delivery. Peer development can occur both inside and outside the clinical environment, enhancing trust, communication,[4] and collaboration. Both parties should engage in dialogue about skill set, ethical practice, expectations, and shared goals.

Pressure to maximize productivity and misconceptions about educational preparation, roles, responsibilities, and/or supervision may lead to overuse or underuse of the PTA. Overuse occurs when a PT provides inadequate direction and supervision, is not readily available to discuss or reexamine when requested, and/or fails to complete timely documentation needed by the PTA to safely treat the patient or client.

For example, the PT performs evaluations, then routinely turns over most patients to be seen by the PTA until discharge. This behavior is inconsistent with practice standards and the code of ethics, and very likely against state law, as the PT is expected to be involved in the ongoing management of the care of each patient. Underuse occurs when the PT does not involve the PTA at all, or only with aide-level duties, in providing clinical care. For example, solely allowing a competent PTA to set up equipment or provide modalities represents underuse.[18,20,30] By utilizing PTAs to their fullest capacity, the PT's time is freed up to provide evaluations to more efficiently meet societal needs or to perform other responsibilities such as documentation.

TEAM-BUILDING STRATEGIES

A compatible PT-PTA team results in a more unified approach to the delivery of high-quality, cost-effective care, which enhances optimal patient and client outcomes. Successful collaboration depends on one's perspectives and actions toward others and a staunch commitment to effective communication. Stereotypes, biases, and pre-conceived ideas about others are natural human tendencies; however, such thoughts can significantly obstruct development of an alliance or any semblance of a high-functioning team.

Identify Assumptions and Break Down Barriers

The first step in developing competency toward partnering in a collaborative relationship is identifying one's own biases. What preconceived notions do you have about working with a PTA? What shaped these? Have these ideas evolved with more exposure to working with a PTA in the clinic, or by considering information after reading this text? Is partnering with this physical therapy extender even desirable?

It is helpful to examine one's confidence in and the difference between the roles and responsibilities of the PT and the PTA. One's belief about roles determines expectations and interaction with others. Professional behaviors such as communication, interpersonal skills, effective use of constructive feedback, and the ability to function effectively on a team are considered foundational requirements for success in a health care career in the 21st century. Regardless of whether collaborating within the PT-PTA partnership or as a member of an interprofessional team in a rehabilitation hospital, one's collaboration quotient is expected in today's health care environment.[18,31] Collaboration is a problem-solving approach that fully acknowledges the interests of all involved parties. Communication skills, patience, and unconditional positive regard are essential to effective partnering. Collaboration involves team-building. Developing a thriving PT-PTA team depends on many factors, including:

- **Mutual respect:** Do I truly value what my team member has to offer? Am I open to hearing his or her input and ideas? Do I actively listen to the whole message when interacting?

- **Confidence and trust in one another:** Demonstrating competent clinical intervention, proper judgment, and effective communication is how confidence and trust are earned by each partner.

- **Role responsibility:** Accuracy and appreciation for educational preparation, role delineation, applicable laws, and practice standards of each partner are critical.

- **Patient-/client-centered care:** Enthusiasm and commitment toward patient/client outcomes, and placing the patient/client ahead of one's own interests, are mandatory.

- **Commitment:** Demonstrating a desire toward excellence, lifelong learning, and fidelity to each other are crucial components to a successful team.[18]

Cost-cutting measures often result in fewer therapists seeing more patients. Documentation requirements change frequently and are sometimes seemingly cumbersome and complex. Risk management, accountability, and attaining value-based outcomes are demands of current clinical practice, regardless of practice setting. Practice management demands can strain the PT-PTA team's working relationship, unless team members follow vigilant strategies to develop and uphold uncompromising mutual respect, collaboration, and effective communication. Although specific strategies will depend upon the individuals and unique circumstances involved, coming to consensus using a communication strategies checklist may minimize unintended conflicts due to miscommunication or missed expectations for the PT-PTA team.

Physical Therapist–Physical Therapist Assistant Team Communication Strategies Checklist

DIRECTIONS

Place a ✓ if you feel it is positive on your team, or an X if you believe it needs work.

___ 1. Determine strategies for timely, efficient transfer of pertinent information

___ 2. Identify mutually agreeable times and methods to communicate

___ 3. Clarify expectations including confusion, illegible or unknown wording, and abbreviations

___ 4. Mutually agree to this mantra: If in doubt, check it out!

___ 5. Actively listen; hear the whole message, ignore distractions, and ask for clarification

___ 6. Be genuine; treat others as you wish to be treated

___ 7. Be willing to give and receive honest feedback

___ 8. Be humble

___ 9. Display empathy

___ 10. Be loyal, and have each other's back, in line with the basic ethical principle of "fidelity to colleagues"

DEBRIEF

After the PT-PTA team members have completed the ratings, have a debriefing meeting to compare impressions and discuss how to improve communication strategies.

CONCLUSION

Although obstacles exist, developing a high-functioning PT-PTA partnership can positively affect the quality of care and enhance the overall delivery of efficient physical therapy services. It is up to each PT-PTA team member to follow these guidelines:

- Maintain a clear understanding of the state practice act regarding supervision and provision of services by a PTA.

- Stay connected to mentors and supportive colleagues who strive to provide legal, ethical, and superior patient/client care.

- Stay up-to-date about reimbursement regulations pertaining to the supervision and provision of services by a PTA.

- Maintain membership and actively participate in the APTA. Having easily attainable access to the most current and credible information regarding practice standards is the most prudent way to protect yourself from unnecessary liability risk and stay up-to-date with the complexities of health care delivery.

- Finally, never compromise your ethics or character—no matter how tempting it is or who is urging you to do so. Listen to your instincts.

It remains the duty and ethical obligation of each PT-PTA team member to accomplish and uphold the teamwork in daily practice to ensure appropriate CPS for patient/client management for the benefit of society and those we serve.

REFERENCES

1. Robinson AJ, McCall M, DePalma MT, et al. Physical therapist' perceptions of the roles of the physical therapist assistant. *Phys Ther.* 1994;74:571-582.

2. Robinson AJ, DePalma MT, McCall M. Physical therapist assistants' perceptions of the documented roles of the physical therapist assistant. *Phys Ther.* 1995;75:1054-1064.

3. Solomon P, Miller PA. Qualitative study of the novice physical therapists' experiences in private practice. *Physiother Can.* 2005;57:190-198.

4. Plack MM, Williams S, Miller D, et al. Collaboration between physical therapists and physical therapist assistants: fostering the development of the preferred relationship within a classroom setting. *J Phys Ther Educ.* 2006;20(1):3-11.

5. Plack MM. The learning triad: potential barriers and supports to learning in the physical therapy clinical environment. *J Phys Ther Educ.* 2008;22(3):7-18.

6. Jelley W, Larocque N, Borghese M. Perceptions on the essential competencies for intraprofessional practice. *Physiother Can.* 2013;65(2):148-151.

7. Dauber D, Fink G, Yolles M. A configuration model of organizational culture. *SAGE Open.* 2012;2(1):1-16.

8. Lockwood T, Papke E. *Innovation by Design: How Any Organization Can Leverage Design Thinking to Produce Change, Drive New Ideas, and Deliver Meaningful Solutions.* Wayne, NJ: Career Press, Inc; 2017.

9. Bolman LG, Deal TE. *Reframinig Organizations: Artistry, Choice, and Leadership.* 5th ed. San Francisco, CA: Jossey-Bass; 2013.

10. Treacy M, Wiersema F. Customer intimacy and other value disciplines. *Harv Bus Rev.* 1993;71:83-93.

11. Carpenter-Davis CA. Physical therapist assistant education over the decades. *J Phys Ther Educ.* 2003;17(3):80-85.

12. Commission on Accreditation in Physical Therapy Education. Aggregate program data: 2017-2018 physical therapist education programs fact sheets. http://www.capteonline.org/uploadedFiles/CAPTEorg/About_CAPTE/Resources/Aggregate_Program_Data/AggregateProgramData_PTPrograms.pdf. Accessed June 6, 2018.

13. American Physical Therapy Association. Values-based behaviors for the physical aherapist assistant. http://www.apta.org/uploadedFiles/APTAorg/PTAs/Careers/Values/ValuesBasedBehaviorsforPTA.pdf. Accessed June 3, 2018.

14. American Physical Therapy Association. APTA guide for conduct of the physical therapist assistant. http://www.apta.org/uploadedFiles/APTAorg/Practice_and_Patient_Care/Ethics/Guidefor ConductofthePTA.pdf. Accessed June 3, 2018.

15. American Physical Therapy Association. Physical therapist assistant clinical performance instrument. http://www.apta.org/PTACPI/. Accessed June 3, 2018.

16. American Physical Therapy Association. *Minimum Required Skills of the Physical Therapist Assistant Graduates at Entry-Level.* [HOD G11-08-09-18.] Alexandria, VA: American Physical Therapy Association; 2009.

17. Federation of State Boards of Physical Therapy. https://www.fsbpt.org/. Accessed June 3, 2018.

18. Curtis KA, Newman PD. *The PTA Handbook: Keys to Success in School and Career for the Physical Therapist Assistant.* 2nd ed. Thorofare, NJ: SLACK Incorporated; 2015.

19. Ball J, DeCelle Newman P. *PTA program handbook.* Oklahoma City Community College 2017. Unpublished document.

20. Pagliarulo MA. *Introduction to Physical Therapy.* 5th ed. St. Louis, MO: Mosby; 2015.

21. Watts NT. Task analysis and division of responsibility in physical therapy. *Phys Ther.* 1971;51:23-25.

22. American Physical Therapy Association. *A Normative Model of Physical Therapist Assistant Education: Version 2007.*

23. Anderson LW, Krathwohl DR, Airasian PW, et al. *A Taxonomy for Learning, Teaching, and Assessing: A Revision of Bloom's Taxonomy of Educational Objectives.* New York, NY: Pearson, Allyn & Bacon; 2001.

24. PEDro scale. https://www.pedro.org.au/wp-content/uploads/PEDro_scale.pdf. Accessed June 3, 2018.

25. Christensen N, Jones MA. Current concepts of orthopedic physical therapy: clinical reasoning and evidence-based practice. 2nd ed. *American Physical Therapy Association Independent Study Course* 16.2.1; 2006.

26. Schön D. *Educating the Reflective Practitioner: Toward a New Design for Teaching and Learning in the Professions.* San Francisco, CA: Jossey-Bass; 1987.

27. Inzer LD. A review of formal and informal mentoring: processes, problems and design. *J Leadersh Educ.* 2005;4(1):31-50.

28. Ezzat AM, Maly MR. Building passion develops meaningful mentoring relationships among Canadian physiotherapists. *Physiother Can.* 2012;64(1):77-85.

29. Black LL, Jensen FM, Mostrom E, et al. The first year of practice: an investigation of the professional learning and development of promising novice physical therapists. *Phys Ther.* 2010;90(12):1758-1773.

30. American Physical Therapy Association. Direction and supervision of the physical therapist assistant. [HOD P06-05-18-26.] http://www.apta.org/Policies/Practice/. Updated 2012. Accessed June 3, 2018.

31. Interprofessional Education Collaborative Expert Panel. *Core Competencies for Interprofessional Collaborative Practice: Report of an Expert Panel.* Washington, DC; 2011.

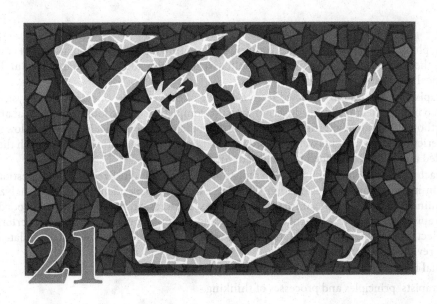

A THREE-DIMENSIONAL MODEL FOR DEVELOPING CLINICAL REASONING ACROSS THE CONTINUUM OF PHYSICAL THERAPIST EDUCATION

N. Beth Collier, PT, DPT, OCS, FAAOMPT;
Margaret M. Gebhardt, PT, DPT, OCS, FAAOMPT; and Leslie F. Taylor, PT, PhD, MS

OBJECTIVES

- Differentiate among the 3 core constructs and their associated subconstructs of clinical reasoning (CR) within the 3-dimensional (3D) model.

- Articulate the trajectory of development of CR from novice to expert across the constructs of logic, performance, and presence.

- Use the 3D CR model (3D CRM) as a guide to design learning opportunities in classroom and clinical settings to develop CR across levels of training within the constructs of logic, performance, and presence.

- Facilitate the progression of reflective practice across levels of training to develop CR within the constructs of logic, performance, and presence.

INTRODUCTION

Physical therapists strive to optimize the quality of life of patients and clients by providing efficient and effective care. Using a formal CR strategy is one mechanism therapists may employ to achieve this goal. A pilot study that was implemented to identify CR development trajectories across levels of formal training within physical therapy is discussed in this chapter, presenting a theoretical model of CR development that emerged with application to entry-level, residency, and fellowship education. A mixed-methods, multiple case study design, following a concurrent nested approach, was used to identify and explore common

Musolino GM, Jensen GM, eds. *Clinical Reasoning and Decision-Making in Physical Therapy: Facilitation, Assessment, and Implementation* (pp 235-244).
© 2020 Taylor & Francis Group.

constructs exist among physical therapists of various training levels within a patient examination in a controlled environment. Principles of grounded theory guided the analysis of the qualitative data, with additional quantitative and qualitative data integrated into the theoretical model in the interpretation phase.

Three physical therapists were randomly selected from a sample of convenience: one doctor of physical therapy (DPT) student (intern) in the last 6 months of entry-level education with the completion of one long-term clinical affiliation, one resident in the last month of orthopedic residency training, and one orthopedic manual physical therapist fellow with less than 5 years of clinical practice experience. Three patients were selected to undergo an initial examination with each therapist. The examinations were videorecorded and audiotranscribed by a masked third party.

Immediately after each examination, the physical therapists answered a standardized series of questions to investigate their CR and clinical decision-making from each evaluation. Three researchers independently read and analyzed the transcriptions of the 9 subjective examinations and 9 post-examination interviews. Each researcher identified and coded common constructs and trends of each therapist's approach to a patient examination and CR. Subsequently, researchers performed video reviews of the 9 subjective and objective examinations. Qualitative data from the transcript reviews were triangulated with qualitative and quantitative data from review of the examination videos.

A working conceptual framework of CR emerged consisting of 3 main constructs:

1. Logic, the therapists' principles and processes of thinking

2. Presence, the therapists' state of being, encompassing verbal and nonverbal communication

3. Performance, the therapists' execution of the examinations

Within each construct, 3 subconstructs demonstrated development across training levels. Within the Logic dimension, subconstructs included diagnostic, contextual, and management thinking. Subconstructs identified within the Presence dimension included rapport, confidence, and therapist identity. Subconstructs in Performance included skill, time, and process. Further, intersections among the constructs and subconstructs demonstrated the complexity of the CR process and its multidimensional development across levels of formal training. The 3D CRM that emerged articulates specific trajectories that should be considered across and within entry-level, residency, and fellowship curricula for physical therapy. The 3D CRM serves as the foundation for further exploration of a comprehensive CR approach.

Physical therapists strive to optimize the quality of life of patients/clients by providing efficient and effective care. Using a formal CR strategy is one mechanism therapists may employ to achieve this goal. Within the health professions literature, definitions of CR differ, and there are disagreements as to the required constructs.[1,2] CR entails internal mental processes used by clinicians when approaching clinical situations, while incorporating the situational contexts and acknowledging the role of experience.[3,4]

CR may be taught and fostered, in whole or in part, in entry-level or post-professional programs, continuing education courses, and/or through work and life experiences. The nonlinearity of CR suggests that there is not one direct path to the development of CR expertise, but rather multiple routes that fall within an acceptable range.[5] The Commission on Accreditation in Physical Therapy Education (CAPTE) requires that all entry-level physical therapist education programs develop and assess CR skills.[6] Further, the American Board of Physical Therapy Residency and Fellowship Education includes CR as 1 of 7 core competencies that must be monitored and measured over the course of a residency program.[7] Despite these mandates, best practice standards of teaching CR and its subsequent assessments are lacking.

The goal of incorporating CR into physical therapy education programs is to produce clinically effective and efficient therapists. To determine the success of a learned CR process, researchers have explored patient outcomes of therapists who have completed residency training compared to therapists who have not. While the literature is somewhat limited in the profession of physical therapy, current evidence suggests that therapists with residency training produce no greater improvements in patient outcomes than therapists with orthopedic-certified specialist credentials, those with manual therapy certification, or those with no advanced specialty training.[8,9] Fellowship-trained therapists demonstrate greater efficiency and achieve better patient outcomes compared to non–residency- or non–fellowship-trained therapists, or those who were residency-trained only.[9] Current literature exploring patient outcomes demonstrates inconsistent effects of formal post-graduate training. In each of these studies, rather than matching residency- and fellowship-trained therapist groups with physical therapists with a similar number of years of experience, the outcomes of advanced-trained therapists were compared to therapists with a broad range of years of experience. Also, group size varied significantly, with the smaller group sizes generally being the residency- and/or fellowship-trained groups, which may have skewed outcome data. Though limitations in methods may limit the generalizability of findings from most of the published studies, the advantages of completing formal post-professional training remain unclear.

Teaching CR is required across entry-level and post-professional curricula to ultimately improve physical therapists' efficiency and effectiveness in patient care. Although residency and fellowship programs provide intentional, mentored development of CR, the limited research to date has not demonstrated improved patient outcomes in these groups. These apparent inconsistencies and the lack of identifiable constructs of CR led us to explore characteristics of a patient examination as performed by physical therapists across the educational continuum. A pilot study was implemented to identify CR development trajectories across levels of formal training. A theoretical model of CR development emerged with application to entry-level, residency, and fellowship education.

METHODS

Based on principles of grounded theory, the pilot study used a mixed-methods, multiple-case study design following a concurrent nested approach.[10-12] Study subjects included one DPT student (intern) in the last 6 months of entry-level education with completion of one long-term orthopedic clinical affiliation, one resident with 1 year of clinical practice experience in the last month of formal orthopedic residency training, and one fellow of orthopedic manual physical therapy with 4 years of clinical practice experience. Participants were randomly selected from 1 of 3 samples of convenience corresponding to level of training. All participants were associated with a local university and were located within the metro-Atlanta area during the time of the study.

Three patients were recruited to participate. Patients were eligible to participate if they had a current active pain complaint, they had not sought examination or treatment from another health care provider before the beginning of the study, and their condition was not hyperacute or hyperirritable, so as to be able to tolerate 3 examinations. We specifically sought self-referred patients in an effort to limit any preconceived ideas that might exist from receipt of a prior diagnosis. The 3 patients selected presented with complaints of acute low back pain (pain exacerbation of less than 2 weeks), chronic low back pain, and chronic elbow pain.

Data collection began with all 3 therapists being asked to perform an initial examination of each patient and gather enough information to be able to establish a physical therapy clinical diagnosis and plan of care. All examinations occurred in a small, private treatment room at a private practice clinic outside of the clinic's regular patient hours. No time limit was imposed. Each therapist was asked to avoid providing the patient with information or education of their findings, diagnosis, or treatment to limit bias of patient perceptions in subsequent examinations. The order of examinations was intentionally scheduled such that each therapist was the first to perform an initial examination once. All 3 examinations of each patient were performed within 5 days, with no more than 2 examinations occurring within 24 hours. Each examination was videorecorded and then audiotranscribed by a masked third party. Immediately after each examination, the therapist proceeded to a separate private treatment room with a third-party interviewer who asked a series of predetermined questions to ascertain the therapist's CR and clinical decision-making processes. These interviews were also audiorecorded and transcribed by a masked third party.

Data analysis began with consideration of 9 audiotranscribed narratives of examinations and 9 audiotranscribed interviews with the therapists. The narratives were de-identified, and the reviewers were masked to the identity of the therapist (T1, T2, or T3) and the patient (P1, P2, or P3). The 3 researchers met to discuss the analysis plan and review the principles of systematic research procedures founded in the inductive methodology of grounded theory. Initial coding required 1 month, in which each researcher engaged in the line-by-line analysis of the 18 transcriptions (9 examinations and 9 post-examination therapist interviews), identifying and coding common constructs and trends of each therapist's approach to the patient examination and his or her CR. The research team met to compare and discuss the coded data and developed an initial schema of 5 dimensions. The team separated again to further consider the data, and over 2 additional meetings, the researchers reached intercoder agreement of the 3 main constructs. Through the constant-comparative method, 3 subconstructs emerged for the logic and presence dimensions, and 1 for the performance dimension. Subsequently, researchers performed video reviews including qualitative and quantitative analysis of the 9 examinations. Per the concurrent nested mixed-methods design, some aspects of the video data were subject to quantitizing, such that qualitative data were transformed into quantitative data and analyzed.[10] Three aspects of the data were calculated and considered:

1. Time spent in the subjective examination, time spent in the objective examination, and total time to complete the examination (Figure 21-1)

2. Total number of tests that each therapist performed, including the number of special tests and the percentage of special tests that were functional movement tests vs pathoanatomical/diagnostic tests (Figure 21-2)

3. The number of body regions considered during objective testing (Figure 21-3)

The findings of the quantitized data analysis were integrated with findings from the qualitative analysis. Two additional subconstructs for the performance dimension emerged, and the intersecting relationships among primary constructs were evident.

RESULTS

Core Constructs

The conceptualization of a 3D CRM emerged and included 3 main dimensions of CR during an examination: logic, presence, and performance. Logic encompassed the therapists' principles and processes of thinking. Presence encompassed the therapists' state of being as seen through verbal and nonverbal communication. Performance comprised the execution of the examination (Figure 21-4).

Figure 21-1. The sub-construct, time, as demonstrated by total time to perform an examination, time to perform a subjective examination, and time to perform an objective examination. Total time to perform an examination and time to perform an objective examination trended down as levels of training increased.

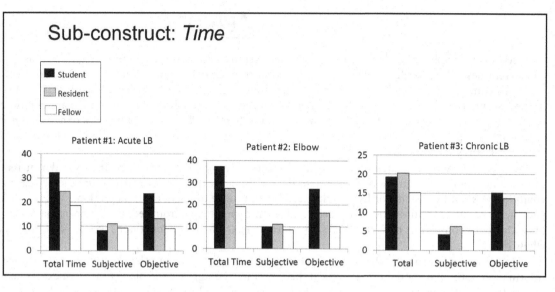

Figure 21-2. The first graph under each patient shows the total number of clinical tests and measures, as well as the number of special tests performed in each examination. The second graph shows the percentage of special tests that were functional or movement-based (black) vs diagnostic in nature (grey).

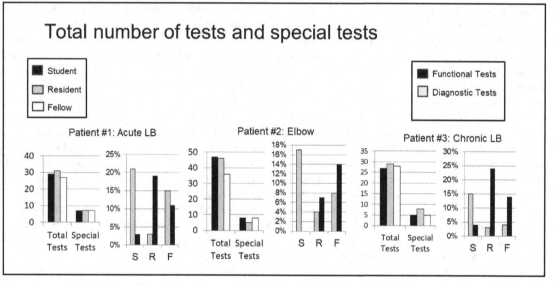

Subconstructs

Within each dimension, 3 subconstructs emerged, which demonstrated development across training levels (Figure 21-5).

The first dimension we will explore is the **logic theme,** with subconstructs identified as *diagnostic thinking, contextual thinking,* and *management thinking.* Diagnostic thinking was the way in which the therapist processed information to obtain a diagnosis. The DPT intern used a pathoanatomical process. For example, when asked what might cause the patient's elbow pain, the intern responded:

> … *The ulnar or median nerve into tissues of the arm. … I guess (it could be) for the medial elbow the UCL [ulnar collateral ligament] could be an issue. However, it wasn't lax from the start.*

The resident used a biopsychosocial approach, with an emphasis on psychosocial factors. When asked about the likely pain mechanisms of a patient's back pain complaints, the resident responded:

> *Nociceptive. It sounds like there are clear-cut aggravating factors. I did ask when things start to get busy and does the back pain get worse? I think there are just so many more physical factors. I just don't think her emotional factors affect her pain.*

The fellow employed an integrated approach of the biopsychosocial model that considered pathoanatomical and psychosocial variables and weighted each based on the patient's complaints. For example, when discussing the interpretation of a patient's elbow complaints the fellow stated:

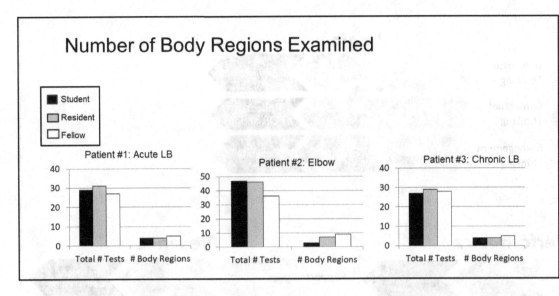

Figure 21-3. Total number of tests and measures performed, as well as total number of body regions examined, during each patient examination. Generally, the fellow performed fewer tests and measures while considering more body regions.

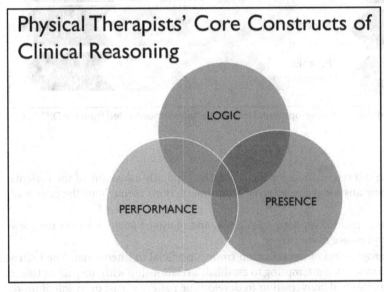

Figure 21-4. The 3 dimensions of CR as demonstrated by all 3 therapists within each patient examination. This model demonstrates the relationship among all of the individual dimensions.

I think he just thought of it as no big deal, so he let it go. Like he had shoulder issues for 3 years and then his elbow problem for about 3 months now. He is definitely in a chronic inflammatory state. Just his indifference to the tissue has caused the chronic inflammatory state.

The next subconstruct of the logic dimension is contextual thinking, the process by which the therapist interpreted and weighted the importance of the information obtained throughout the examination. The intern primarily employed reflection-on-action—that is, thinking back on an action that had already occurred.[13] The intern's reflection-on-action strategy[13] became apparent in the interview after completion of each examination, in which the intern was verbally processing events that had transpired during the examination and was trying to make sense of the information collected while talking to the interviewer. The resident primarily used a reflection-in-action approach, responding to information as it presented during the examination.[13] The fellow primarily used a reflection-for-action approach,[13] which encompassed the ability to plan ahead while in the moment. Using a reflection-for-action strategy,[13] the fellow's examination appeared more thoughtful and intentional. The fellow's examination was streamlined and demonstrated the ability to gather multiple pieces of information within a single objective test.

Finally, within the logic dimension, management thinking highlighted the interventional strategies identified by each therapist to address the concerns of the patients. The intern identified managing the patient as fixing the problems at hand. In response to an interview question, "What does the patient expect from the physical therapist?" the intern answered, "He just wants to know if I can help him relieve any pain." To the same question, the resident responded with, "It looks like he wants to learn how to manage it better" and "She [the patient] wants to learn what's going on," thus highlighting an emphasis on the therapist's role in patient education. The fellow's mindset was one of patient facilitation. In response to the same question, he responded, *"To be able to give her the appropriate exercises to help decrease or change the pain,"* or *"She [the patient] wants exercises and stretching to help change her pain and to prevent it from returning."* While the question of patient expectations of

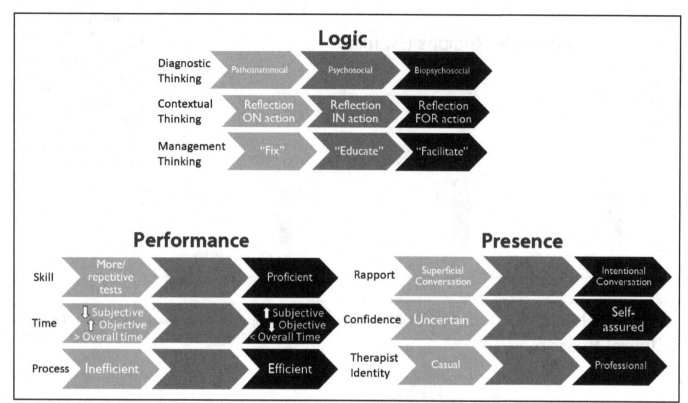

Figure 21-5. Subconstructs within each core construct are identified and developmental trajectories are demonstrated from the DPT intern (light colors) to the fellow (dark colors).

the physical therapist was asked in the post-examination interviews, none of the therapists explicitly asked any of the patients about their expectations for physical therapy; rather, their answers were inferred from interactions throughout the course of the examination.

Subconstructs of the second main dimension, **presence,** include *rapport, confidence,* and *therapist identity.* In the next few paragraphs, we will explore each of the subconstructs of presence more closely.

First, within rapport, the researchers identified the progression of conversation from superficial to intentional. The intern tended to engage in superficial conversation with the patients, often attempting to establish a relationship with the patient based on commonalities or shared interests. The fellow used intentional conversation to develop the patient's trust or to solicit more information. In all 3 examinations, the patient with acute low back pain reported that bending forward and lifting caused an increase in her back pain. The DPT intern asked the patient if picking up something light, like her purse, would exacerbate her pain. She then remarked jokingly with the patient about how her purse may not actually be very light. The fellow, given the same information, asked the patient to set up a work environment using the high-low table and to simulate her job function, asking specific questions about how often each task was performed and how her pain responded.

Confidence, the second subconstruct of presence, spanned from the uncertainty of the intern to the self-assuredness of the fellow. The confidence subconstruct was apparent in the therapist's observed demeanor, patient interactions, and other non-verbal communication. Verbally, the intern seemed uncertain and almost awkward at times in conversations with the patient. Throughout the course of the examination, the intern turned many statements into questions and used filler words in times of silence between questions. The fellow had command of the conversations and appeared poised in his interactions.

Finally, within presence, the subconstruct of therapist identity described how the therapists viewed themselves and their role as a physical therapist. Each of the therapists was given the same broad instructions before beginning the study: that he or she would be participating in a research project performing initial patient examinations. The intern and resident both presented to the examinations in casual workout attire, demonstrating an egocentric perspective, prioritizing their desire to be comfortable rather than accounting for the visual impression they would be making with the patient. The fellow presented to the examinations in a button-down shirt and khakis, demonstrating a patient-centered perspective, with the intention to establish a more professional relationship with the patients. The fellow projected professionalism in the delivery of physical therapy through all interactions.

The third dimension identified was **performance,** with identified subconstructs of *skill, time,* and *process.*

The first subconstruct of performance, skill, referred to the ability to do something well. The intern used a greater number of objective tests and performed more repetitions of the same or similar tests. The progression of the resident to the fellow during the examinations demonstrated increased proficiency in the performance of objective tests and measures.

The second subconstruct of performance, time, included the quantitative measurement of time spent on the entire examination, as well as the time spent in subjective and objective portions of the examination. Time also was measured qualitatively based on the use of open-ended questions and the observation of the examination flow. Overall, the intern required more time to complete the entire examination, while the fellow had overall shorter examinations. The intern generally spent more time on the objective examination, while the fellow consistently spent less time on the objective examination. In the subjective examination, the resident and fellow consistently spent more time than the intern. Qualitatively, the intern tended to ask more narrow and closed questions, while the fellow engaged the patients in dialogue to allow them to tell their story while still guiding the conversation to collect specific intentional information.

The third subconstruct of performance, process, referred to the manner in which the examinations were conducted. The intern was less efficient, while the fellow demonstrated more efficiency, as demonstrated by the management of patient positioning and flow of the examination, as well as environmental awareness. The DPT intern required the patient to change positions multiple times in a seemingly disorganized fashion, whereas the fellow had a streamlined flow to the examination in which each position was exhausted of necessary tests before asking the patient to change positions. The resident was mindful of the surrounding environment, showing conscious effort to be sure the entire examination was captured by the camera placed in the corner of the room.

TRIANGULATION OF VIDEO DATA

Intersection of Logic and Performance Constructs

As we explored the intersection between the logic and performance dimensions, we discovered the relationship between diagnostic thinking and time. The intern's thinking encompassed a pathoanatomical approach, and more time was spent in the objective portion of the examinations. Using a pathoanatomical approach within diagnostic thinking would support spending more time in the objective portion of an examination, as most information relating to pathoanatomy would be obtained from clinical tests and measures. The influence of a pathoanatomical approach to diagnostic thinking on performance was confirmed by calculating the percentage of clinical tests chosen by the intern that were diagnostic special tests, which was consistently greater than those of the resident or fellow. The increased use of diagnostic special tests by the intern showed that the intern's focus was to collect information regarding tissue pathology. The fellow integrated pathoanatomical and biopsychosocial thinking, and spent more time in the subjective portion of the examinations. The fellow's blended way of thinking supported spending more time in a subjective examination, in which the therapist would obtain more information from the patient's narrative to decide what information was required from objective tests and measures. The fellow's percentage of special tests varied depending on the presentation of the patient, but ultimately integrated functional and diagnostic special tests with each patient. Employing such an integrated approach allowed the fellow to determine a structural cause when needed, while also identifying contributing factors.

Within the number of total tests performed during each examination, we counted the number of body regions that the therapists chose to investigate. The intern performed a prescriptive examination that encompassed all the elements taught within an entry-level curriculum. These tests were limited in the number of regions included in the examination. It seemed that many of the tests were performed, not necessarily because they would provide specific valuable information, but because they were expected in a given patient presentation. The intern's somewhat scripted approach demonstrated a lack of reflection-in-action.[13] Rather than processing the information obtained during the examination to select particular tests and measures, the DPT intern completed clinical tests commonly associated with pathology to a local region and reflected on the meaning of information gained after the examination during the interview. Because hypotheses were not reevaluated during the course of an examination, the intern was required to perform more tests overall. Consistently, the fellow performed fewer tests than the intern and resident while investigating more body regions. Purposeful selection of clinical tests and measures allowed the fellow to choose fewer tests while investigating more regions. The fellow's reflection-for-action[13] allowed for more salient information from the tests used and improved efficiency.

Intersection of Presence and Performance Constructs

Within observation and quantization of skill, the DPT intern demonstrated more episodes of repeating the same clinical test within the course of a patient examination. The uncertainty of the DPT intern in the presence dimension supported the need to repeat the same clinical test multiple times to corroborate perceived findings. Further, the DPT intern required all 3 patients to change positions multiple times during the course of the examinations. The intern's uncertainty led to the performance of an inefficient examination process. The self-assuredness of the fellow allowed for the performance of fewer tests overall in each patient examination, and ultimately allowed for a more efficient examination.

Intersection of Presence and Logic Constructs

Therapist identity guided management thinking. With an egocentric view of her professional identity, the intern perceived that it was the duty of the therapist to fix the problems the patients presented. Therefore, the reported management strategies of the DPT intern included interventions that largely focused on what the physical therapist could do for the patient, rather than how participation in physical therapy could affect the patient. The intern often used the terms *physical therapist* and *physical therapy* interchangeably, showing an inability to differentiate between the role of a therapist and the action of providing physical therapy.

In contrast, the fellow had a patient-centered approach, which correlated with a facilitatory management thinking strategy. The fellow kept the best interest and long-term goals of each patient in mind in determining a management strategy. The fellow's rationale for choosing a postural intervention for one patient directly showed the relationship between these 2 dimensions: *"I feel like if I could get her some positive wins at work, then I'll be able to build rapport with the patient too."*

DISCUSSION

A proposed model of constructs specific to physical therapists within an examination was developed. The 3D CRM includes Logic, Performance, and Presence as core constructs that influence CR.

Logic, as the representative thinking dimension, is well discussed within critical thinking literature in nursing.[14-17] Expert physical therapists tend to use a patient-collaborative, problem-solving approach to diagnostic reasoning,[18,19] similar to the integrated biopsychosocial diagnostic reasoning employed by the fellow in this current study. Literature also supports that expert clinicians use patient education and facilitation as a primary management strategy,[19,20] which was also demonstrated by the fellow. These characteristics were less evident in the intern, who demonstrated emphasis on pathoanatomical considerations, similar to previously identified compartmentalized or procedural thinking seen in clinicians with less experience or situational exposure.[21,22] The resident demonstrated an interesting strategy that heavily weighted psychosocial variables while still considering pathoanatomy, yet struggled to integrate the 2 processes fully, illustrating the progression of the development of diagnostic reasoning from the novice intern to the expert fellow.

Performance, as representative of the doing or psychomotor dimension, is also well supported in the literature. Prior research in physical therapy has shown that the expert clinician uses a narrative reasoning approach to capture the patient's story,[19] has a central focus on movement linked to patient function,[18] and more efficiently manages the environment and extraneous variables that may occur within a patient's session.[20] The efficiency of the fellow's examination—spending more time in the subjective portion of the examinations and using more functional or movement-based special tests based on patient reports—exemplified these characteristics. The procedurally focused performance exhibited by the intern has been previously identified in a study of students' CR during straightforward patient case-based competencies.[22] Skill development from novice to proficient has also been supported in the literature,[23,24] though other studies recognize levels beyond proficiency, such as expertise and mastery.[24] Attributes of performance as demonstrated by the resident were found to be between the identifiable characteristics of the intern and the fellow.

Aspects of Presence, as representative of the being dimension identified in the 3D CRM, is referred to in the literature.[25-27] Characteristics of intentionality and virtue have been identified,[18,20] but evidence of these qualities and their effects on CR and patient outcomes remains unclear. Confidence, awareness, and acceptance of professional identity have been shown to increase in novice therapists with more experience and over time.[28] The 3D CRM labels attributes of presence as rapport, confidence, and professional identity, and demonstrates the relationship of these attributes with the other constructs of CR, logic and performance. As with each dimension within the 3D CRM, we do not believe this is a comprehensive list of attributes, but rather a proposal of characteristics to continue exploring.

CONCLUSION

The 3D CRM serves as a guiding framework for educators of physical therapists across the continuum. In working with students, peers, residents, and fellows, educators and mentors should make an explicit effort to address each of the dimensions of the 3D CRM: logic, presence, and performance. Specific attributes of each of the 3 dimensions are often the focus of individual physical therapy courses and/or post-professional continuing education training. Integration of the 3 constructs, whether entry-level or after, may not be obvious to the learner. For instance, psychomotor skills that are associated with performance and their application within the context of an examination (ie, logic) are the focus of clinical courses. Professionalism skills, such as those associated with presence, usually are taught in professional development courses in DPT curricula and are often only implicitly addressed and demonstrated in other DPT or post-professional courses. Presentation of content in silos leaves the learner with the expectation to connect concepts from each dimension, which may further impede CR progression. The 3D CRM demonstrates the complexity of the relationship among each of the 3 dimensions and the importance of explicit threading of attributes across and among courses to facilitate the learners' understanding and development.

Previous studies in physical therapy literature have captured the nonlinear development of CR and professional behaviors over time.[22,28,29] The 3D CRM posits that CR is not only nonlinear, but also 3D, and can be likened to an image of a triple helix with a component of interconnectedness among each strand or dimension (refer to Section II, Chapters 8 and 9). The 3D CRM builds on research demonstrating trajectories of development with formal training and provides a framework for integration of specific attributes. The trajectories identified in the 3D CRM can serve as guidelines for assessment of physical therapist development, with the awareness that characteristics within dimensions may develop at different rates.

We recognize that a sample of 3 therapists, with only one from each stage of formal training, may not have allowed for saturation, a potential inherent study limitation. Similarly, we recognize that randomly selecting therapists from samples of convenience lacks variety of educational background, knowledge, and clinical biases. However, we propose that the consistency in educational background knowledge and clinical training may have offset the smaller sample size. Nonetheless, we submit that the 3D CRM is a working conceptual framework and should be tested on a larger scale with students and physical therapists of varying levels of experience and clinical training. In an effort to limit patient knowledge bias, we removed the ability of the therapist to provide education to the patient. Omitting patient education is not true to clinical practice, and we recognize that some therapists may rely on patient education to build on other factors, such as rapport. By controlling the environment and asking each therapist to examine the same patient, we were able to analyze factors specific to the therapist. However, many other factors pertaining to the clinical environment and to the patients themselves may affect how a clinician practices. Future research should include exploration of all these factors independently (eg, patient factors and practice factors),[5] as well as exploration of the relationships and interactions among each of the factors. Further, the investigation of these factors should focus on their effect on patient outcomes, as our goal is to develop smart, clinically reasoning therapists who provide effective and efficient patient care. Variables associated with good patient outcomes should help guide curricular development for professional education and post-professional training programs.

The 3D CRM identifies dimensions of logic, presence, and performance, as well as subconstructs within each dimension and trajectories of these subconstructs across levels of physical therapy training. The trajectories of the characteristics in the 3D CRM should serve as a guiding framework for the development and assessment of physical therapists' CR abilities. The 3D CRM articulates the interconnectedness among logic, presence, and performance, and underscores the necessity to cultivate the attributes within each dimension to foster the development of a comprehensive CR approach.

REFERENCES

1. Schuwirth LWT. Is assessment of clinical reasoning still the Holy Grail? *Med Educ.* 2009;43:298-299.
2. Gruppen L. Clinical reasoning: defining it, teaching it, assessing it, studying it. *West J Emerg Med.* 2017;18(1):4-7.
3. Christensen N, Black L, Furze J, et al. Clinical reasoning: survey of teaching methods, integration, and assessment in entry-level physical therapist academic education. *Phys Ther.* 2017;97(2):175-185.
4. Durning SJ, Artino AR. Situativity theory: a perspective on how participants and the environment can interact. *Med Teach.* 2011;44:85-93.
5. Durning SJ, Artino AR, Schuwirth L, van der Vleuten C. Clarifying assumptions to enhance our understanding and assessment of clinical reasoning. *Acad Med.* 2013;88(4):442-448.
6. Commission on Accreditation in Physical Therapy Education. Standards and required elements for accreditation of physical therapist education programs. http://www.capteonline.org/AccreditationHandbook/. Accessed July 2016.
7. American Board of Physical Therapy Residency and Fellowship Education. Quality standards for clinical physical therapist residency and fellowship programs. http://www.abptrfe.org/uploadedFiles/ABPTRFEorg/About_ABPTRFE/ABPTRFEQualityStandardsCallForComments.pdf. Accessed July 2017.
8. Resnik L, Jensen G. Using clinical outcomes to explore the theory of expert practice in physical therapy. *Phys Ther.* 2003;83(12):1090-1106.
9. Rodeghero J, Wang Y, Flynn T, et al. The impact of physical therapy residency or fellowship education on clinical outcomes for patients with musculoskeletal conditions. *J Orthop Sports Phys Ther.* 2015;45(2):86-96.
10. Vankatesh V, Brown S, Bala H. Bridging the qualitative-quantitative divide: guidelines for conducting mixed methods research in information systems. *MIS Quart.* 2013;37(1):21-54.
11. Vankatesh V, Brown S, Sullivan Y. Guidelines for conducting mixed-methods research: an extension and illustration. *J Assoc Inf Sys.* 2016;17(7):535-594.
12. Strauss A, Corbin J. Grounded theory methodology: an overview. In: Denzin NK, Lincoln YS, eds. *Handbook of Qualitative Research.* Newbury Park, CA: Sage Publications Inc; 1994:271-285.
13. Schön DA, DeSanctis V. *The Reflective Practitioner: How Professionals Think in Action.* New York, NY: Basic Books; 1983.
14. Holdsworth N. On laying the foundations for an empiricological model of mental health nursing. *J Adv Nurs.* 1992;17:1095-1105.
15. Kataoka-Yahiro M, Saylor C. A critical thinking model for nursing judgment. *J Nurs Educ.* 1994;33:351-356.
16. Scheffer BK, Rubenfeld MG. A consensus statement on critical thinking. *J Nurs Educ.* 2000;39:352-358.
17. Forneris SG. Exploring the attributes of critical thinking: a conceptual basis. *Int J Nurs Educ Scholarsh.* 2004;1:1-18
18. Jensen G, Gwyer J, Shepard K, Hack L. Expert practice in physical therapy. *Phys Ther.* 2000;80(1):28-43.

19. Edwards I, Jones M, Carr J, Braunack-Mayer A, Jensen G. Clinical reasoning strategies in physical therapy. *Phys Ther.* 2004;84(4):312-340.

20. Jensen G, Shepard K, Hack L. The novice versus experienced clinician: insights into the work of physical therapists. *Phys Ther.* 1990;70(5):314-323.

21. Eva K. What every teacher needs to know about clinical reasoning. *Med Educ.* 2004;39:98-106.

22. Furze J, Black L, Hoffman J, et al. Exploration of students' clinical reasoning development in professional physical therapy education. *J Phys Ther Educ.* 2015;29(3):22-33.

23. Carraccio C, Benson B, Nixon J, Derstine P. From the educational bench to the clinical bedside: translating the Dreyfus developmental model to the learning of clinical skills. *Clin Teach.* 2008;83(8):761-767.

24. Dreyfus HL, Dreyfus SE. *Mind Over Machine.* New York, NY: Free Press; 1988.

25. Jensen G. Wisdom of practice. *Adv Physiother.* 2004;6:97-98.

26. Greenfield BH. The meaning of caring in five experienced physical therapists. *Physiother Theory Pract.* 2006;22:175-187.

27. Greenfield J. Understanding lived experiences of patients: application of a phenomenological approach to ethics. *Phys Ther.* 2010;90(8):1185-1197.

28. Hayward L, Black L, Mostrom E, et al. The first 2 years of practice: a longitudinal perspective on the learning and professional development of promising novice physical therapists. *Phys Ther.* 2012;93(3):369-383.

29. Black LL, Jensen GM, Mostrom E, et al. The first year of practice: an investigation of the professional learning and development of promising novice physical therapists. *Phys Ther.* 2010;90(12):1758-1771.

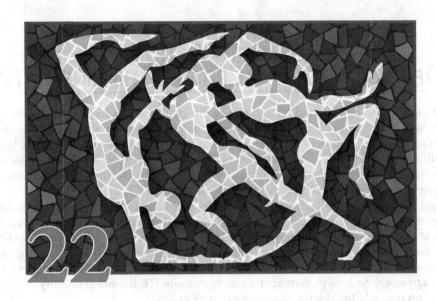

RESPONDING TO THE CALL:
Measuring Critical Thinking in Physical Therapist Education

Anita S. Campbell, PT, MPT, NCS, ATP and Brad W. Willis, PT, MPT, GCS

OBJECTIVES

- Identify a method for systematically collecting critical thinking (CT) data within a physical therapy program.

- Recognize the effectiveness of identifying shared CT challenges within a physical therapy program, and analyze how systematic evaluation impacts teaching strategies.

- Compare and contrast how mixed curricular models influence CT skill development.

- Outline strategies for implementing curricular change, and discuss results of a targeted, explicit mixed-model approach for CT development, providing lessons learned.

In an ongoing longitudinal study, one institution began to explore and challenge assumptions about CT. The California Critical Thinking Skills Test (CCTST) was used to examine the impact of CT in combination with a historically implicit immersion curricular model. The researchers identified both limitations and gaps in the education design. Specific interventions, including a mixed curricular model, were implemented to increase the impact on CT. This chapter looks at the insights gained, the lessons learned, and recommendations for additional research opportunities in response to the profession's need for increased exploration of CT and CR.

Musolino GM, Jensen GM, eds. *Clinical Reasoning and Decision-Making in Physical Therapy: Facilitation, Assessment, and Implementation* (pp 245-254).

A CALL TO ACTION:
THE DEVELOPMENT OF A CRITICAL THINKING INITIATIVE

The promotion of clinical reasoning (CR) and CT skills in health care providers has gained significant attention in recent years and is understood to be a significant component of success as a practicing physical therapist.[1-3] Specifically, the ability of health care providers to integrate CT skills into their daily practice has been correlated with, but not limited to, the improvement of diagnostics skills, increased efficiency, and reduction of medical errors.[4,5] The American Physical Therapy Association (APTA) has called for advances in physical therapist curricular design that target learning domains with cognitive, psychomotor, and affective behavior skills, which may contribute to the advancement of CT and CR.[6-10]

As previously outlined in this text, there has been no universally accepted definition or assessment tool for CR, despite the importance and relevance for daily physical therapy practice.[11] Validated measures do exist, however, for CT, a consistently identified key component of CR, defined by the American Philosophical Association as "the process of purposeful, self-regulatory judgement ... [giving] reasoned consideration to evidence, contexts, conceptualizations, methods, and criteria."[3,9,11-14] Readers may refer to Section II regarding valid and reliable tools for assessment of CT. Previous challenges in CT investigations have included a lack of agreement on how to most appropriately measure CT, limited continuity of educational intervention strategies, and, in education research, the absence of a proper control group.[15]

In this chapter, we will describe an ongoing longitudinal study to explore the understanding of students' CT development within physical therapy education. Our aims included collecting CT data on first-, second-, and third-year doctor of physical therapy (DPT) students who received an implicit, immersive CT curricular approach; identifying shared challenges from CT results to guide intervention strategies; discussing the methodology to implement an explicit, mixed-model CT approach across the curriculum in a first-year cohort; and, finally, examining the effects of an explicit mixed-model CT approach on standardized CT performance, as compared to an implicit model.[16]

INSTRUMENT SELECTION

Although the investigators support the additional use of qualitative methods as described elsewhere in this text, previous studies examining physical therapy CT development have used a quantitative approach.[1,16,17] The investigators selected the CCTST due to its established content validity by the American Philosophical Association, the instrument's reliability, its recognized use in health profession curriculum, and its suggested ability to measure change among multiple cohorts of physical therapy students.[1,11,14,17] Since the initiation of this study, other instruments, namely the Health Sciences Reasoning Test, have also demonstrated promise as assessment tools in this area.[11,18] As the role of standardized tests in assessing students' CT skills, including the use of the CCTST, were outlined in Section II, the discussion of the specifics of the CCTST will be limited in this chapter.

CRITICAL THINKING DEVELOPMENT:
MEASURING AN IMMERSION MODEL

CT development among first-, second-, and third-year DPT students within a single program was measured. A total of 149 students volunteered, including 50 first-, 57 second-, and 42 third-year students, approximately 93% of the physical therapy student body. All students had undergone the immersion approach of CT instruction throughout the DPT program, in which CT concepts and procedures were not made explicit to them.[19] The immersion model asserts that CT maturation will occur through time, experience, and practice with subject-specific instruction without defining the skills themselves. Refer to Table 22-1 for definitions of CT development curricular models.[19,20] The CCTST was administered to all 3 cohorts simultaneously at the end of the academic year.

The performance of each cohort was analyzed using descriptive statistics and a one-way analysis of variance. Although all 3 cohorts fell into the "strong" category on the CCTST, no significant difference was observed in overall CCTST, percentile, and/or subscale scores among the first-, second-, and third-year students, despite a maturation of academic and clinical experience. Following these results, educational research questions began to emerge:

- Why were no differences detected?

- Could any shared challenges be identified among the groups?

- Could first-year CCTST outcomes be improved with a different CT model instead of an immersion approach, and how might this model be implemented?

TABLE 22-1
ENNIS CRITICAL THINKING DEVELOPMENT—CURRICULAR MODELS
Definitions of curricular approaches and studies regarding the efficacy of each approach guided the investigators to move from an immersion approach to a mixed approach in development of the curricular intervention model.
• **General:** Teaches critical thinking separately from the presentation of the content of existing subject matter. • **Infusion:** Attempts to integrate critical thinking instruction in standard subject matter instruction and makes general principles of critical thinking explicit to students. In this approach, students are encouraged to acquire and explicitly practice critical thinking skills through deep and well-structured subject matter instruction. • **Immersion:** Attempts to integrate critical thinking within standard subject matter instruction. However general critical thinking principles and procedures are not made explicit to students, with the assumption that they will acquire the thinking skills as a result of engaging in the subject matter instruction. • **Mixed:** Consists of a combination of the general approach with either the infusion or immersion approach. In the mixed approach, there is a separate thread or course aimed at teaching general principles of critical thinking, but students are involved in subject-specific critical thinking instruction where the objectives of critical thinking are either explicit or implicit.
Adapted from Ennis[13,20,31] and Tiruneh et al.[19]

- Was the CCTST sensitive enough to detect changes within a physical therapy graduate program, especially with all participants scoring high overall?
- What other additional factors influence early development of CT skills?

Influences on CT skill development may include that early exposure leads to increased self-reflection, repetitive exposure reinforces CT concepts, or increased consciousness of strengths and weaknesses motivates learning. Likely, a multitude of additional relevant factors may warrant investigation beyond the scope of this pilot work. While the CCTST has been shown to be sensitive to changes in CT, and there are norms for graduate-level health science students, the researchers were concerned with a ceiling effect.[12] Although some studies have demonstrated change, there is concern for the test's ability to detect growth within physical therapy programs due to the strong performance of these students at baseline.[1,17,21]

SAME ISSUES, DIFFERENT CLASS: SHARED CHALLENGES AMONG COHORTS

Following the discovery of no significant differences among cohorts on CCTST performance, the existence of commonalities in subscale performance among the groups was investigated. The CCTST provides 5 domain subscores as follows: analysis, inference, evaluation, induction, and deduction.[12] See Table 22-2 for definitions of CCTST domains as defined by Facione and the CCTST *User Manual and Resource Guide*.[12] Subscores are interpreted as not manifested, moderate, or strong, and were correspondingly ranked 1, 2, or 3, for statistical purposes.[12] Friedman's test was used to determine the presence of significant differences among the 5 domains. To determine differences between domains, pairwise comparisons were performed.

Despite variance in academic progress, the first-, second-, and third-year students demonstrated shared deficits in the CT domain of evaluation, and the first- and third-year students demonstrated shared deficits in the domain of deduction. Analysis and induction scores were consistently higher for all cohorts (Figure 22-1). A hypothesis arose regarding targeted curricular intervention with a mixed-model approach and its impact on CT skills.

INFORMED INTERVENTIONS: ESTABLISHING AN EDUCATIONAL FRAMEWORK

Previous chapters within this text provide background on the multiple proposed theoretical frameworks for CT development. The initial educational framework for CT development stemmed from Benjamin Bloom[22] and associates, considering their taxonomy for information processing skills and applications for higher-order thinking. Bloom's taxonomy transitions from knowledge and remembering at the lowest level of learning, with evaluation and creating at the highest.[22-24] See Table 22-3 for

---

TABLE 22-2

FACIONE DEFINITIONS OF CRITICAL THINKING DOMAINS AND THE CALIFORNIA CRITICAL THINKING SKILLS TEST USER MANUAL AND RESOURCE GUIDE

Domain-specific interventions focused on the areas of evaluation and deduction.

- **Analysis:** Analytical reasoning skills enable people to identify assumptions, reasons, and claims, and to examine how they interact in the formation of arguments. We use analysis to gather information from charts, graphs, diagrams, spoken language, and documents.

- **Inference:** Inference skills enable us to draw conclusions from reasons and evidence. We use inference when we offer thoughtful suggestions and hypotheses. Inference skills indicate the necessary or the very probable consequences of a given set of facts and conditions.

- **Evaluation:** Evaluative reasoning skills enable us to assess the credibility of sources of information and the claims they make. We use these skills to determine the strength or weakness of arguments.

- **Induction:** Decision-making in contexts of uncertainty relies on inductive reasoning. We use inductive reasoning skills when we draw inferences about what we think is probably true based on analogies, case studies, experience, statistical analyses, simulations, hypotheticals, and patterns recognized in familiar objects, events, experiences, and behaviors.

- **Deduction:** Decision-making in precisely defined contexts—where rules, operating conditions, core beliefs, values, policies, principles, procedures, and terminology completely determine the outcome—depends on strong deductive reasoning skills. Deductive reasoning moves with exacting precision from the assumed truth of a set of beliefs to a conclusion that cannot be false if those beliefs are true. Deductive validity is rigorously logical and clear-cut.

Adapted from Facione et al.[12,14]

---

the revised taxonomy.[23] Bloom[25] identified 3 domains of learning: cognitive (the mental skills), affective (the attitudes or feelings), and psychomotor (the physical skills or doing). This model associates the ability to analyze, synthesize, and evaluate findings with CT.[24]

Influenced by the work of Ennis,[20] who outlined 4 instructional models for CT curricular development including general, infusion, immersion, and mixed approaches, this chapter focuses exclusively on the immersion and mixed curricular models. Multiple investigators support the acquisition of CT skills through the subject-specific immersion or infusion models.[26-28] The immersion approach attempts to integrate CT within standard instruction; however, general CT concepts and procedures are not made explicit to students.[19] The immersion

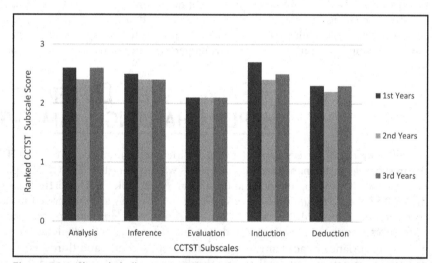

Figure 22-1. Shared challenges in CCTST subscales: Immersion approach raw CCTST subscale scores were ranked 1 = not manifested, 2 = moderate, and 3 = strong for the purpose of statistical analysis.[12]

approach asserts that students will acquire these cognitive skills as a result of engagement in subject-specific instruction, with maturation occurring through time, experience, and practice.[19] Other investigators suggest CT is general in nature, relying on fundamental criteria that are applied across subjects and that can be explicitly taught separately from the subject matter.[24,29]

Instead of a binary approach, multiple researchers support the notion of CT development being both subject specific and general, essentially blending the 2 curricular models.[14,19,20,30,31] In contrast to the immersion or general approaches, the mixed approach involves the addition of explicitly taught principles of CT prior to and alongside immersion into the subject matter.[31] Abrami and colleagues performed a meta-analysis of 117 empirical studies on the effectiveness of these 4 models, showing that the mixed approach had the greatest effect on students' CT skills and disposition, while the immersion approach had the

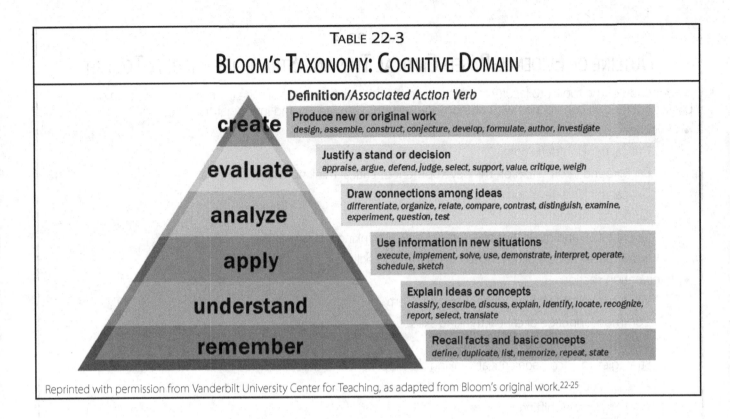

TABLE 22-3

BLOOM'S TAXONOMY: COGNITIVE DOMAIN

Definition/Associated Action Verb

create — Produce new or original work
design, assemble, construct, conjecture, develop, formulate, author, investigate

evaluate — Justify a stand or decision
appraise, argue, defend, judge, select, support, value, critique, weigh

analyze — Draw connections among ideas
differentiate, organize, relate, compare, contrast, distinguish, examine, experiment, question, test

apply — Use information in new situations
execute, implement, solve, use, demonstrate, interpret, operate, schedule, sketch

understand — Explain ideas or concepts
classify, describe, discuss, explain, identify, locate, recognize, report, select, translate

remember — Recall facts and basic concepts
define, duplicate, list, memorize, repeat, state

Reprinted with permission from Vanderbilt University Center for Teaching, as adapted from Bloom's original work.[22-25]

smallest.[24,30] Building upon our pilot study data, the available evidence in the peer-reviewed literature, and following the call to action from educational leaders, the curriculum was transitioned from an immersion model to a mixed model to enhance CT performance within the incoming first-year cohort.[6-10]

ROOT CAUSE ANALYSIS:
TRANSITIONING TO AN EXPLICIT MIXED MODEL

Educators are called to engage in an important role in promoting CT skills.[32,33] Developing a shared language between students and faculty regarding CT skill and acquisition is critical.[9] To this end and as a result of this investigation, chapter authors developed an Evidence-Based Critical Thinking Strategies Faculty Toolkit to provide support and resources to the other educators involved in the curricular changes (Table 22-4).

The toolkit was divided into overview and intervention sections. The overview section contained CT definitions, background information, and evidence-based CT development goals; supported curricular models; and proposed quantitative and qualitative measures, and individual characteristics of progressively advancing CT skills.[3,10,14,19,20,31] The intervention section discussed the value of explicit CT teaching within the curriculum, review of cognitive biases, type I/II errors, and multiple evidence-based CT strategies.[33-41] Evidence-based strategies included structured Socratic questioning, perspective shifting, reflective writing/narratives, case-based learning, small group classroom huddles, simulated learning, and the use of concept mapping.[3,33-36,38-41]

To enhance faculty readiness, individual one-on-one faculty development coaching sessions were performed with all physical therapy faculty who taught within the first year of the program. The sessions included review of the handbook details and discussed specific activities to implement a mixed CT curricular model. Faculty were encouraged to choose and implement the evidence-based strategies that best fit their current first-year courses. Although their choices increased variability, it greatly enhanced faculty buy-in and compliance.

Several instructional changes were implemented during the transition to a mixed-model approach. Key modifications in the early courses of the program included the explicit introduction of CT definitions and subsections, relevance to CR in patient care, and a review of cognitive biases and type I/II errors.[3,12,37] Instructional changes were applied within lectures as well as through online learning. Initial comprehension was gauged with foundational in-class quizzes, oral discussions on basic concepts, and reflection assignments. Additional case-based scenarios were presented, illustrating the domains of evaluative, analytical, inferential, inductive, and deductive reasoning processes. Also, an online module was developed to review basic CT concepts, including an example of each domains' relevance to clinical practice, and questions aimed to review these foun-

TABLE 22-4
OUTLINE OF EVIDENCE-BASED CRITICAL THINKING STRATEGIES FACULTY TOOLKIT

Introduction of the toolkit to faculty teaching courses within the first year of the DPT program consisted of a paper packet outlined, in conjunction with one-on-one sessions with faculty and investigators.[3,33-35,38-42]

- Overview section
  - Critical thinking definition
  - Background information on the development of critical thinking within curricula
  - Critical thinking development goals
  - Curricular models
  - Quantitative and qualitative measures of critical thinking
  - Individual behaviors of advanced critical thinking skills
- Intervention section
  - Value of explicit teaching within the curriculum
  - Common language of critical thinking skills
  - Cognitive biases and common errors
  - Strategies to encourage critical thinking development and utilization
    - Socratic questioning
    - Perspective shifting
    - Reflective writing
    - Case-based learning
    - Small group classroom huddles
    - Simulated learning
    - Concept mapping

dational concepts. (See Table 22-5 for further details regarding the online module.) While all aspects of CT were addressed, emphasis was given to classroom content focused on evaluative and deductive reasoning skills, due to the shared challenges found in the baseline data.

Additional changes by faculty members included an increase in group activities at the beginning of class to foster small classroom huddles, discussion, and encourage problem-solving and self-reflection. Participating faculty also reported increased use of Socratic questioning with students during patient lab activities.

CHANGING THE WAY THEY THINK: EXAMINING THE MIXED-MODEL IMPACT

Two successive first-year cohorts were examined, comparing those who received an immersion approach (n = 50) and a mixed approach (n = 19). Both cohorts completed the CCTST at the end of their first academic year. The mixed-model first-year cohort also completed the CCTST at the beginning of the academic year. Both groups completed the same core didactic coursework and participated in similar levels of cumulative clinical experience within the departments' community physical therapy clinic. Paired t-tests compared differences between pre- and post-CCTST performance in the mixed-model group, examining CT maturation over the first year, as well as comparisons between the immersion and mixed-model cohorts at the end of the first year.

The mixed-model cohorts showed significant CT maturation over the course of the year when comparing pre- and post-CCTST performance. Specifically, overall CT score, percentile rank against other health science graduate students, inference, and deductive reasoning were improved (Figure 22-2). This is consistent with earlier studies showing the CCTST is sensitive to detecting change, and an explicit approach can impact CT skills.[1,11,17] Comparing end-of-year CCTST performance between the mixed-model and immersion cohorts, the mixed approach demonstrated a significant increase in evaluation. Results of the mixed-model curricular approach are useful in facilitating advancement of CT skills during early didactic instruction.

TABLE 22-5

ONLINE CRITICAL THINKING MODULE FOR FIRST-YEAR DOCTOR OF PHYSICAL THERAPY STUDENTS

The online module consisted of a voiceover PowerPoint presentation, followed by completion of a critical thinking quiz and self-reflection.[3-5,12,34,42]

I. Critical thinking within physical therapy practice

II. Stages of critical thinking development

   a. Definitions of novice, intermediate, and expert

   b. Knowledge level, skills used, and attitudes related to each stage

III. Critical thinking foundations

   a. Definitions of each domain

     • Induction, deduction, analysis, inference, evaluation

   b. Examples of each domain used within physical therapy

   c. Self-assessment strategies to improve skills

IV. Individual behaviors of advanced critical thinking

   a. Truth-seeking, open-mindedness, analyticity, systematic critical thinking, self-confidence, inquisitiveness, maturity, intellectual humility

V. Critical thinking quiz

   a. Use of critical thinking skills within the context of first year curricular information

   b. Multiple-choice questions

   c. Answers with rationale for reasoning and potential errors

VI. Self-reflection: Areas of strength and weakness

   a. Self-identification of focus areas for addressing weaknesses

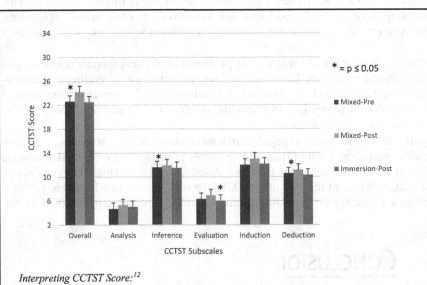

Interpreting CCTST Score:[12]
Overall: 0-7=Not Manifested; 8-12=Weak; 13-18=Moderate; 19-23=Strong; ≥ 24=Superior.
Analysis: 0-2=Not Manifested; 3-4=Moderate; ≥ 5=Strong
Inference: 0-5=Not Manifested; 6-11=Moderate; ≥ 12=Strong
Evaluation: 0-3=Not Manifested; 4-7=Moderate; ≥ 8=Strong
Induction: 0-5=Not Manifested; 6-11=Moderate; ≥ 12=Strong
Deduction: 0-5=Not Manifested; 6-11=Moderate; ≥ 12=Strong.

Figure 22-2. Comparison of first-year mixed and immersion approaches on CCTST performance. Significant differences are denoted with an asterisk. The mixed curricular model group demonstrated significant improvements in overall critical thinking score, inference, and deduction during pre- to post-testing. A significant improvement in percentile rank (as compared to health science graduate students) was also seen in pre- and post-testing for the mixed-model group, although this is not depicted. As compared to the immersion group, the mixed-model group demonstrated improvements in evaluation.

Specifically, targeted instructional changes aimed at areas of previously identified shared challenges offer opportunities for educational intervention. The CCTST domains of evaluation and deduction were identified as areas of weakness across multiple cohorts and were emphasized during the first-year mixed-model approach. Examining the impact of the targeted approach, the mixed-model group increased deduction during the first year of study as compared to the pretest. When comparing the mixed and immersion cohorts at the end of the first year, evaluation scores were significantly higher in the mixed-model group. The investigators suggest that by implementing regular longitudinal assessment of CT skills, educators may effectively determine the impact of such andragogical changes aimed at CT development.

Summary of Findings

Insights gained by this preliminary work suggest the following findings: (1) an immersion approach may not facilitate change in general CT skills as measured by the CCTST; (2) shared challenges exist among cohorts in the domains of evaluation and deduction, while analysis and induction are strengths; (3) the CCTST can detect change in CT skills during the first year of didactic training; (4) a mixed-model approach is superior to an implicit, immersion model in the CCTST's evaluation domain; and (5) domain-specific curricular interventions can target and improve areas of identified weakness in CT development. Knowledge gained from this work shows CT can be improved through curricular change and potentially impact CR.

Limitations and Further Considerations

Limitations included small sample sizes and a drop in CCTST participation in our mixed-model cohort. There was a sharp decline in participation during the intervention year, with approximately 69% (n = 40) of the mixed-model cohort beginning the study and only 38% (n = 19) completing it, as compared to 86% (n = 50) in the immersion cohort. Descriptive statistics and a series of Wilcoxon rank sum tests were run. No significant differences were noted that impacted the results of this study. Notably, the CCTST is only one of many assessment tools to measure CT. Applicability concerns of the normative data on the CCTST could be improved if graduate physical therapy programs were identified, instead of general health science graduates. An additional limitation of this investigation was that the CCTST performance was not compared to psychomotor ability (eg, laboratory skills, checkouts, direct patient care), a critical aspect of physical therapy education.

With limitations identified, the investigators turned to specific areas of future study grounded in our initial findings. Quantifying the impact of the mixed-model curricular approach during the second and third year of doctoral training, as compared to the implicit immersion approach on CCTST scores, is warranted. Educators should examine which faculty-wide curricular implementation strategy is most effective, employing a mixed-model approach to assess faculty buy-in and engagement. Furthermore, scrutinizing which curricular interventions demonstrate the greatest improvement within each CT domains is key.

Future investigations should also examine the development of CT within post-professional physical therapy residency and fellowship programs, as well with board-certified clinical specialists. Likewise, the development of tools blending subject-specific and general CT assessment within physical therapy education is recommended. By advancing CT research among physical therapy graduates, educators may shed light on more definitive methods to assess and enhance CR. In addition, because CT is only one facet of CR, other components need to continue to be explored.

The completion of work such as this requires an invested and engaged department chair, faculty, students, and staff. Therefore, consideration must be given to the additional investment of time and resources to implement such curricular-wide changes. Investments included the increased time and effort to develop the Evidence-Based Critical Thinking Strategies Faculty Toolkit, weekly meetings with core faculty and staff, department funding of the CCTST, a willingness of co-faculty to be available for one-on-one instructional sessions, the time necessary for providing feedback, and the intermittent use of class and student time to complete testing.

Conclusion

Educators, be it clinical or academic, have experienced frustration with the breakdown of process in CR we expect from a student. During these mentoring opportunities, we try to ascertain the reason for these roadblocks/detours and hope to offer solutions to bridge this gap. The exploration of the breakdown is grounded in assumptions that we understand what defines advanced CR, how it is measured, and how it is positively impacted. This single institution's longitudinal study leans on the advancement of CT performance, hoping that it provides further insights about a student's CR ability.

As in clinical practice, without a defined outcome, it is difficult to establish goals, make those goals measurable, and establish interventions to meet those goals. CT has been consistently defined as an essential component of CR, with the CCTST demonstrating precedent as a useful tool to quantify this domain within physical therapy education.[1,12,21] Ongoing assessment of CT within physical therapy education programs can lay the groundwork for establishing positive curricular change.[16,17,21] Importantly, the mixed-model approach to teaching CT continues to be confirmed as more effective than an implicit immersion model. Furthermore, the identification of shared challenges provides insights for targeted, domain-specific interventions that may improve CT skills.

Based on the study findings, a single institution has engaged in an andragogical shift to develop CT skills using a mixed-model approach throughout the curriculum, including specific emphasis on the learning domains of evaluation and deduction. This has since been deemed a strategic initiative for the institution, with unanimous support by departmental faculty. Ongoing interventions encompass both the foundational science and clinical application courses. Additionally, department faculty are receiving ongoing training in the mixed-model approach and implementation strategies, both generally and for application within the specific content areas. These activities are in concert with longitudinal use of the CCTST, aimed at evaluating the impact of targeted interventions. Methods for continued support of both faculty and student success are being explored. Moreover, it is expected that additional insights into other aspects of CR will continue to shape the initiative.

Beyond the initial results, the dialogues and insights generated from this study have been especially rewarding. More students are seeking advice on how to enhance domain-specific CT skills, and peer faculty are engaging in additional one-on-one dialogues to discuss educational best practice. Furthermore, the development of a shared language to approach CT has been constructive. Following faculty training, educators are now able to more easily define which domain of CT a student and/or cohort may require additional attention.

It is clear to the authors that the mixed-model approach was superior in the development of CT skills over the previously established immersion model. The transition in models stemmed from a preliminary objective to identify strengths and weaknesses of the program in the development of CT skills. Following the results, the authors were able to focus interventions and demonstrate significant improvements in targeted areas. This highlights the importance of systematic examination of CT skills across a curriculum. Likewise, the use of institutional self-reflection and assessment, aimed to enhance learning outcomes, is crucial. Through this process, institutions may effectively identify which curricular model may best serve their students and empower faculty to implement change. Moreover, providing a unified initiative and common language was beneficial in programmatic development.

Within physical therapy professional education, there is a lack of reported department-wide initiatives assessing CT skills development. Nationally, the call for advancements in CT acquisition has been sounded, especially as the educational requirements, professional autonomy, and societal needs of physical therapists grow.[6-10] As a result, the authors' institution has deemed this to be a strategic initiative, with a commitment to ongoing longitudinal assessment and faculty training.

When it comes to assessing and quantifying CR within physical therapy, there are more questions than answers. Clinicians regularly identify the importance of CR abilities in providing optimum and efficient patient care.[1,10,11] Although the findings of this study offer only limited insight into the complexity of this challenge, systematic assessments are recommended to inform faculty on the effectiveness of curricula for the development of skills necessary to practice.[1,2,17,18]

ACKNOWLEDGMENTS

The authors wish to acknowledge several co-investigators and their instrumental help with this project. We thank our department chair, Dr. Kyle Gibson, PT, PhD, OCS, for his consistent encouragement, insights, support, and leadership. We also thank co-investigator Dr. Stephen Sayers, PhD, for his mentorship, as well as editorial and statistical support. Additionally, we graciously thank co-investigator and staff member Elizabeth Beal, who completed the consenting process, performed masking procedures, administered the tests, and emailed personalized CCTST performance reports to students. Finally, we thank all the wonderful staff, faculty, and students at the University of Missouri department of physical therapy program for their support and daily demonstration of excellence.

REFERENCES

1. Bartlett DJ, Cox PD. Measuring change in students' critical thinking ability: implications for health care education. *J Allied Health.* 2002;31(2):64-69.
2. Behar-Horenstein L, Niu L. Teaching critical thinking skills in higher education: a review of the literature. *J Coll Teach Learn.* 2011;8(2): 25-41.
3. Huang G, Lindell D, Jaffe L, Sullivan A. A multi-site study of strategies to teach critical thinking: "why do you think that?" *Med Educ.* 2016;50:236-249.
4. Chang MJ, Chang YJ, Kuo SH, Yang YH, Chou FH. Relationships between critical thinking ability and nursing competence in clinical nurses. *J Clin Nurs.* 2011;20(21-22):3224-3232.
5. Harasym PH, Tsai TC, Hemmati P. Current trends in developing medical students' critical thinking abilities. *Kaohsiung J Med Sci.* 2008;24:341-355.

6. American Physical Therapy Association. Vision statement for the physical therapy profession and guiding principles to achieve the vision. www.apta.org/Vision/. Updated September 9, 2015. Accessed May 15, 2017.

7. American Physical Therapy Association. Guide to physical therapist practice. 2nd ed. *Phys Ther.* 2001;81:9-744.

8. Gwyer, J, Hack LM. The continuing conversation on educational research in physical therapy. *J Phys Ther Educ.* 2016;30(2):5.

9. Huang G, Newman LR, Schwartzstein RM. Critical thinking in health professions education: summary consensus statements of the millennium conference 2011. *Teach Learn Med.* 2014;26(1):95-102.

10. Brudvig TJ, Dirkes A, Dutta P, Rane K. Critical thinking skills in health care professional students: a systematic review. *J Phys Ther Educ.* 2013;27(3):12-25.

11. Brudvig TJ, Mattson DJ, Guarino AJ. Critical thinking skills and learning styles in entry-level doctor of physical therapy students. *J Phys Ther Educ.* 2016;30(4):3-10.

12. Facione N, Blohm S, Howard K, Giancarlo C. *California Critical Thinking Skills Test: User Manual and Resource Guide (Revised).* Millbrae, CA: California Academic Press; 2016:1-85.

13. Ennis RH. A logical basis for measuring critical thinking skills. *Ed Leadersh.* 1985;43(2):44-48.

14. Facione PA. *Critical Thinking: A Statement of Expert Consensus for the Purposes of Educational Assessment and Instruction. Research Findings and Recommendations.* Newark, DE: American Philosophy Society; 1990:3.

15. Ross D, Loeffler K, Schipper S, et al. Do scores on three commonly used measures of critical thinking correlate with academic success of health professions trainees? A systematic review and meta-analysis. *Acad Med.* 2013;88:724-734.

16. Wessel J, William R. Critical thinking and learning styles in a problem-based, master's entry-level physical therapy program. *Physiother Theory Pract.* 2004;20(2):79-89.

17. Zettergren KK. Changes in critical thinking scores: an examination of one group of physical therapist students. *J Phys Ther Educ.* 2004;18(2):73-79.

18. Huhn K, Black L, Jensen G, et al. Tracking change in critical thinking skills. *J Phys Ther Educ.* 2013;27(3):26-31.

19. Tiruneh D, Verburgh A, Elen J. Effectiveness of critical thinking instruction in higher education: a systematic review of intervention studies. *Higher Education Studies.* 2014;4(1):2-3.

20. Ennis RH. Critical thinking and subject specificity: clarification and needed research. *Educational Researcher.* 1989;18(3):4-10.

21. Vendrely AM. An investigation of the relationships among academic performance, clinical performance, critical thinking, and success on the physical therapy licensure examination. *J Allied Health.* 2007;36(2):108-123.

22. Adams NE. Bloom's taxonomy of cognitive learning objectives. *J Med Libr Assoc.* 2015;103(3):152-153.

23. Vanderbilt University Center for Teaching. https://cft.vanderbilt.edu/guides-sub-pages/blooms-taxonomy/. Accessed October 2017.

24. Lai E. Critical thinking: a literature review: research report. Pearson: always learning. http://images.pearsonassessments.com/images/tmrs/CriticalThinkingReviewFINAL.pdf. Accessed July 25, 2017.

25. Bloom BS. Foreword. *Taxonomy of Educational Objectives, Handbook Book 1: Cognitive Domain.* Longman, NY: Longman; 1956:6-8.

26. Bailin S, Case R, Coombs JR, Daniels LB. Conceptualizing critical thinking. *J Curric Stud.* 1999;31(2):285-302.

27. Case R. Moving critical thinking to the main stage. *Ed Canada.* 2005;45(2):45-49.

28. Willingham DT. Critical thinking: why is it so hard to teach? *Am Ed.* 2007;31:8-19.

29. Van Gelder T. Teaching critical thinking: some lessons from cognitive science. *College Teach.* 2005;53(1):41-48.

30. Abrami PC, Bernard RM, Borokhovski E, et al. Instructional interventions affecting critical thinking skills and dispositions: a stage 1 meta-analysis. *Rev Educ Res.* 2008;78(4):1102-1134.

31. Ennis RH. Critical thinking and subject specificity: clarification and needed research. *Educational Researcher.* 1989;18(3):4-10.

32. Kawashima A. Critical thinking integration into nursing education and practice in Japan: views on its reception from foreign-trained Japanese nursing educators. *Contemp Nurs.* 2003;15(3):199-208.

33. Myrick F, Yonge O. Enhancing critical thinking in the preceptorship experience in nursing education. *J Adv Nurs.* 2004;45(4):371-380.

34. Chang Z. A systematic review of critical thinking in nursing education. *Nurs Educ Today.* 2013;33:236-240.

35. Kaya H, Sen H, Kececi A. Critical thinking in nursing education: anatomy of a course. *New Ed Rev.* 2011;23(1):1159-1173.

36. Raymond CL, Profetto-McGrath J. Nurse educators' critical thinking: reflection and measurement. *J Nurs Educ Pract.* 2005;5(4):209-217.

37. Wilke A, Mata R. Cognitive bias. In: Ramachandran VS, ed. *The Encyclopedia of Human Behavior.* Cambridge, MA: Academic Press; 2012:531-535.

38. Mun MS. An analysis of narratives to identify critical thinking contexts in psychiatric clinical practice. *Int J Nurs Pract.* 2010;16(1):75-80.

39. Jenkins SD. Cross-cultural perspectives on critical thinking. *J Nurs Educ.* 2011;50(5):268-274.

40. Hsu L, Suh-Ing H. Concept maps as an assessment tool in a nursing course. *J Prof Nurs.* 2005;21(3):141-149.

41. Pottier P, Hardouin JB, Hodges BD, et al. Exploring how students think: a new method combining think-aloud and concept mapping protocols. *Med Educ.* 2010;44(9):926-935.

42. O'Sullivan SB, Siegelman RP. Introduction. In: *National Physical Therapy Examination: Review and Study Guide.* 18th ed. Evanston, IL: TherapyEd; 2015:1-19.

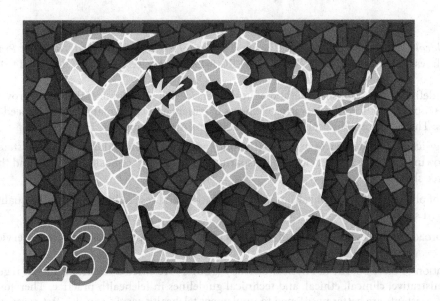

TELEHEALTH:
An Innovative Educational and Instructional Strategy to Develop Clinical Decision-Making in Physical Therapist Practice

Alan Chong W. Lee, PT, PhD, DPT, CWS, GCS; Daryl Lawson, PT, DSc;
Ken Randall, PT, PhD, MHR; Trevor Russell, BPhty, PhD; and
Steven L. Wolf, PT, PhD, FAPTA, FAHA, FASNR

OBJECTIVES

- Provide the historical view of Frontiers in Rehabilitation Science and Technology (FiRST) with physical therapy perspectives.
- Provide a historical view of telehealth in physical therapy.
- Discuss models of telehealth education in current academia that facilitate and promote clinical decision-making (CDM).
- Explore future implications for telehealth in research, practice, and education.

INTRODUCTION

As telehealth is implemented in clinical practice to allow practitioners to interact with patients and clients, collaborating for sound CDM using telecommunication technologies becomes an imperative. More important, students, residents, and practitioners need to develop clinical problem-solving skills using telehealth to provide competent care in the digital age. This chapter discusses innovative telehealth models in physical therapy curricula to augment effective CDM in physical therapist practice, research, and education.

The American Physical Therapy Association (APTA) 2014 House of Delegates[1] endorsed telehealth as an appropriate model of service delivery for the profession of physical therapy, when provided in a manner consistent with the Association's positions, standards, guidelines, policies, procedures, *Standards of Practice for Physical Therapy*,[2] the *Code of Ethics* for the physical thera-

Musolino GM, Jensen GM, eds. *Clinical Reasoning and Decision-Making in Physical Therapy: Facilitation, Assessment, and Implementation* (pp 255-266).

pist,[3] *Standards of Ethical Conduct for the Physical Therapist Assistant,*[4] *Guide to Physical Therapist Practice,*[4] and telehealth definitions and guidelines.[5,6] During the 2019 APTA HOD RC 8-19 Amend: Telehealth HOD (P06/14-07-07) was adopted by consent as follows:

Telehealth is a well-defined and established method of health service delivery. Physical therapists provide services using telehealth as part of their scope of practice, incorporating elements of patient and client management as needed, to enhance patient and client interactions. The American Physical Therapy Association (APTA) supports:

- Inclusion of physical therapist services in telehealth policy and regulation on the national and state levels to help society address the growing cost of health services, the disparity in accessibility of health services, and the potential impact of health workforce shortages

- Advancement of physical therapy telehealth practice, education, and research to enhance the quality and accessibility of physical therapist services

- Expansion of broadband access to provide all members of society the opportunity to receive services delivered via electronic means

In 2015, the Federation of State Boards of Physical Therapy (FSBPT)[7] released a telehealth model regulation recommendation addressing administrative, clinical, ethical, and technical guidelines in telehealth practice. Therefore, physical therapists and physical therapist assistants are better positioned to implement telehealth services in the 21st century. However, telehealth practice and regulation come with new challenges for physical therapist practice, research, and education.

Physical therapy professionals must be cognizant of the latest developments in the innovative arena of telehealth for the patients/clients we serve. We need to be prepared to deliver telehealth services in all aspects of practice, research, and education. To fully prepare physical therapy practitioners and students to use telehealth as a means of delivering care, it is important to educate developing practitioners and seasoned professionals regarding the key factors that influence academic and clinical success, based on evidence and CDM principles.

The purpose of this chapter is 3-fold: to provide a brief history of FiRST and telehealth and describe applications related to rehabilitation; to discuss models of telehealth education in current academia to promote CDM; and to explore implications of telehealth in practice, research, and education for rehabilitation.

HISTORICAL VIEW OF FRONTIERS IN REHABILITATION SCIENCE AND TECHNOLOGY

In 2006, the APTA House of Delegates developed Vision 2020, a remarkable effort directed at informing the public that physical therapists will be professional practitioners of choice for whom consumers should have direct access to be evaluated for the treatment or prevention of impairments, or for improving upon limitations in activity or restrictions in participation as they pertain to movement function.[8] The elements embedded within the 2006 APTA Vision included the need to operationally define autonomous physical therapist practice; direct access; doctor of physical therapy and lifelong education; evidence-based practice; practitioner of choice; and professionalism. Subsequently, the 2006 House of Delegates sought a strategic plan that would enact this plan and would include these elements.[9] The plan incorporated new knowledge for the education of physical therapists and physical therapist assistants.[10]

Hence, it was determined that a summit be convened to solicit input from a variety of disciplines instructed to focus on how physical therapists would meet current health care needs as well as future societal needs. That summit served as the foundation for the actions that followed. To this end, the House of Delegates passed a second motion in 2006:

> *That APTA convene a summit in or by 2010 with annual reports to the HOD that shall focus on how physical therapists can meet current, evolving, and future societal health care needs. The consideration of innovative process, technology, or practice models by this Summit on Physical Therapy and Society shall not be constrained by existing law, regulation, education, or reimbursement.*[11]

The gathering of experts who represented clinical specialties within and outside physical therapy, biotechnologies, multiple aspects of scientific exploration including genomics and regenerative processes, telecommunications, and health care policy was to be the modus operandi of this initiative. The specific charge was as follows:

- Bring together leaders and conceptual thinkers from physical therapy with visionaries from other medical professions, engineering, health information technology, industry, academia, government, and caregivers to focus on how physical therapists can meet current, evolving, and future societal health care needs

- Provide an environment for discussion that was not constrained by today's realities in physical therapist education, practice, and research

Moreover, the potential innovations offered by these external experts was to be undertaken in the absence of any constraints from legal, regulatory, educational or reimbursement components. Those members and guests who contributed to what became known as the Physical Therapy and Society Summit (PASS), convened in February 2009, were instructed to present their opinions and recommendations with due deliberation and in the context of their individual perceptions of the profession and after contemplating aspects they felt were lacking and required attention in rapidly changing health care, scientific, and technological arenas.[9] A steering committee assembled by the APTA was to assist in the organization of PASS and was charged with providing a report to the 2009 House of Delegates. This last task was achieved and the report to the 2009 House was approved unanimously.

While many recommendations emerged from this most successful "thought-producing" initiative and meeting,[12,13] aside from the profession becoming far more consumer-centric, the most urgent needs were directed toward ensuring that clinicians and students alike become attuned to and educated about the exponential accumulation of base knowledge within science and technology. Specifically, contemporary and evolving areas most often cited included sensing technologies such as robotics, virtual environments, and wearables with data transmission capability; genomic-rehabilitation interfaces; regenerative rehabilitation; and telehealth, primarily in the form of telerehabilitation. Moreover, while the last of these important content elements could easily be perceived as a stand-alone component, the ability to use telecommunications to educate clinicians and students in the other 3 content areas became immediately obvious. In addition, there was an emerging sense that today's students and tomorrow's therapists would expect, if not demand, the use of telecommunication technologies, as they have experienced firsthand within many social contexts (eg, media, gaming) as part of their own everyday lives.

THE BIRTH OF FRONTIERS IN REHABILITATION SCIENCE AND TECHNOLOGY

One outcome, on which the PASS steering committee insisted, was ensuring they would be granted total control of information dissemination resulting from the PASS experience. To achieve this control, members of the PASS steering committee worked with the education and research departments of the APTA to determine a configuration for perpetuating this effort and disseminating existing and future information. A collective decision was then rendered to recognize the need to create a leadership continuum that would bring together experts in the fields of biotechnology, genomics, regenerative rehabilitation, and telehealth. This solidified that all areas identified at PASS are important arenas for future science and technology, directly relevant to future practice and growth of the profession. Furthermore, we recognized that the configuration of these teams would require the collaborative input from both physical therapists and non–physical therapists who were invested and committed to the FiRST mission.[14] With that promise in hand, committee members promptly engaged APTA components resulting in presentations[14-18] given at the 2011 and 2013 educational leadership conferences, the 2013 student conclave, and section and component meetings. At each meeting, the response from the physical therapy community was overwhelmingly favorable. Remarkably, among the entirety of our educational leaders, there was no opposition to the notion of including this content within existing curricula. The obvious issue was one of counterbalance: how to best incorporate emerging concepts, and what content to compromise or remove.

The notion that the APTA would continue to support FiRST was not sustainable, and clearly a new and dynamic mechanism needed to emerge. In concert with APTA leadership, a proposal to create a FiRST council was generated and approved by the APTA Board of Directors in February 2016. The purpose of the council is to provide leadership in advancing science and technology that will favorably impact education, research, and practice of the physical therapy profession in collaboration with other health care, health services, engineering, and scientists and professionals who are committed to this purpose.

The FiRST council's objectives are as follows:

- Provide leadership and a convening of thought leaders to enhance discovery and information flow to the profession in areas of rehabilitation science and technology innovation pertinent to the education, practice, and research of the profession of physical therapy

- Be a vehicle for innovation in rehabilitation science and technology to promote and assist in the achievement of the APTA vision, including all principles, and the strategic plan

- Serve as a resource for development and adoption of the movement system as a core element of the profession

- Provide a supportive and collaborative environment for the profession, including true collaboration with the APTA components, to engage and advance rehabilitation science and technology with critical and engaged health care providers, researchers, and engineers who hold the same vision and passion for the future practice of health care as outlined in the APTA vision

- Be a resource to provide increased visibility of the advances recognized and adopted by the profession that transform society, optimize movement, and improve the human experience[8]

- Advance 4 areas of focus: genomics, regenerative rehabilitation, sensing and robotics technology, and telehealth, with scoping for the recognition of new areas that would be valuable to pursue as discovery occurs, such as imaging

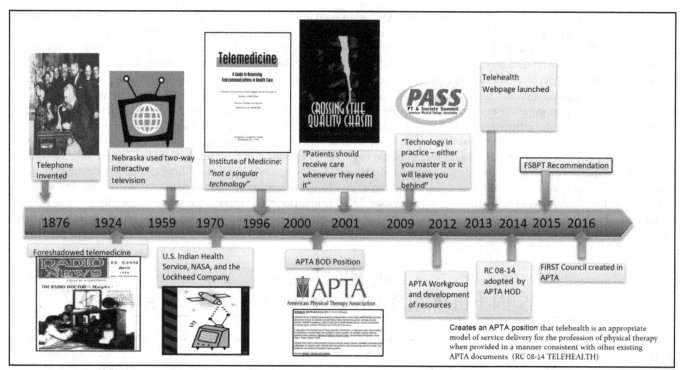

Figure 23-1. Telehealth history. (© 2019 American Physical Therapy Association. All rights reserved. Adapted with permission.)

The executive committee comprising the initial council membership is the same leadership that built the 4 pillars that defined FiRST. Added to that leadership and to the physical therapist and non–physical therapist members of each pillar (approximately 10 per group) were:

- Individual(s) designated by each of the supporting section and academy leaders to proactively advance this effort (6 APTA sections and academies to date)

- APTA members involved in the focus areas

- APTA members involved in components who wished to be included

- Other health care professionals involved with the effort at a leadership level

- Non–physical therapist scientists, engineers, and health-related professionals committed to ensure that the FiRST council will advance its purpose and objectives

- Designation of an APTA board liaison and staff members to support the council's work

The FiRST configuration permits proactive involvement and investment on the part of APTA academies and sections, many of which are eager to be an instrumental part and catalysts for how emerging aspects of science, technology, and health care will impact their specialties. The intent is to construct a FiRST council that meets the needs of clinicians and educators while providing direct input and structure to foster a self-sustaining profile. The investment of resources should ensure a prolonged and active effort at inquiry and discovery of relevant new information, configured by therapists along with their clinical and scientific partners. The extent of this mutual collaboration is expected to grow and is based upon perceived needs of the profession to address health care reimbursement, deliver service, and assist in embracing novel learning approaches, economics of scale, and the yet-undefined territories of technology that will become unveiled with time, along with revelations with current and emerging genomics and robotics.

HISTORICAL VIEW OF TELEHEALTH

The evolution of telehealth, along with the FiRST council, is relevant for the physical therapy profession. The concept of telehealth in the United States was introduced in the 1924 issue of *Radio News* (Figure 23-1). This newspaper edition featured a futuristic drawing of a physician auscultating his patient with a stethoscope through a radio, displaying an early, surreal version of telemedicine.[19] In reality, a clinical case report in the *Lancet* described a physician interacting with a caretaker and a child via telephone to diagnose a child's cough in the late 1890s. In the late 1950s, Albert Jutras in Canada established telemedicine implementation programs in teleradiology, while the Nebraska Psychiatric Institute initiated a telepsychiatry program in conjunction with the University of Nebraska in the United States. By the 1960s, the National Aeronautics and Space Administration had established a telehealth program to monitor its astronauts and assisted in international emergency earthquake disaster relief telemedicine efforts. Throughout the 1970s and 1980s, in the Boston International Airport, the first telehealth remote kiosk program was established to triage airport travelers encountering medical emergencies. In the current era, health care professionals use secured telecommunication technologies from one site to another to improve a patient's clinical health status and monitor progress.[20]

Telehealth was first mentioned as "virtual care" and seen as an opportunity for the physical therapy profession to collaborate with other health care professionals and policy stakeholders in 2000.[21] For example, licensure concerns in telehealth were viewed as an opportunity for physical therapists to collaborate with other health care professionals and policy stakeholders.

The APTA defines telehealth as "the use of secure electronic communications to provide and deliver a host of health-related information and health care services; including physical therapy–related information and services for patients and clients."[5] In rehabilitation, speech therapists in the United States define telehealth applications as telepractice.[6] Internationally, physiotherapists and occupational therapists use telerehabilitation[6] as the common term for telehealth applications. In practice, telecommunication technologies that deliver real-time audio- and videoconferencing between providers and patients is described as synchronous telehealth. Other telehealth applications include secure electronic transmission of clinical information and medical data, described as asynchronous, store-and-forward telehealth.

Remote patient monitoring in telehealth has emerged alongside the advent of biotechnology and virtual environments. Overall, telehealth practice and research may enhance patient and client interactions, overcome barriers of access to physical therapy services, and improve care where health disparities might exist addressing cost and travel. For example, telehealth physical therapy services between a physical therapist in Dillingham, Alaska, and a patient with a musculoskeletal injury located in rural southwestern Alaska occurs using a secured, real-time audio and video telehealth system.[5] Furthermore, research in asynchronous telehealth physical therapy services for rehabilitation of patients after total knee arthroplasty is emerging.[22]

In a randomized trial,[22] clinical outcomes with asynchronous telehealth were compared to usual care with 51 patients following total knee arthroplasty using a video-based software platform supervised by physical therapists. After a pre- and postoperative visit with patients receiving in-home physical therapy visits for 2 weeks, the patients were randomized to either the traditional care or asynchronous telehealth group (TG). Patients in the asynchronous TG were taught how to use Apple's iPod Touch or their own mobile device with an uploaded application, with videos illustrating the same exercises taught in the traditional outpatient clinic care. The videos were each less than 3 minutes in length with both subscript text instruction and audio in English. The physical therapist would send instructional videos to the TG patients in a secure platform, and the patients would respond with recordings of themselves completing their exercises. The physical therapist would be notified, review the video, compare the patient's progress to previous videos, make any necessary change to the plan of care, and upload more advanced exercise videos as necessary.

Each patient's home exercise program was personalized, while at any time patients in the TG could request additional in-person visits or return to using traditional clinic follow up. All patients completed the patient-reported outcomes questionnaire including 3 validated scores in a 10-point visual analogue scale, the Veterans RAND 12-item health survey, and the Knee Injury and Osteoarthritis Outcome Score Physical Function Short Form. In addition, the TG completed a 5-point Likert scale to evaluate the experience with the asynchronous telehealth platform. After 3 months, the usual care group exercised a mean of 60 minutes per day, compared to the TG with a mean of 47 minutes per day. However, the mean travel time to the clinic was 75 minutes for the usual care, while no travel was necessary for the TG intervention, except for the postoperative in-home visits and telehealth set-up.

After 3 months, both groups showed equivalent clinical outcomes. Most important, a large drop in the number of in-person visits to the outpatient physical therapy clinic from the TG intervention was noted, even though patients were allowed access to clinic visits as deemed necessary. Therefore, emerging telehealth practice and research present new opportunities for physical therapy educators and practitioners to address proper CDM with telecommunication technologies, since some patients may prefer connecting with physical therapists with telehealth encounters, based on lifestyle or occupational demands. In addition, telehealth practitioners and educators need to model competent care using telecommunication technologies for novice practitioners and students in physical therapy, since use of computers and digital mobile devices in clinical practice may require enhanced telerapport with digital devices for proficient patient/client interaction with technology that is unique for effective communication and efficient practice.

According to Richard Frankel, PhD,[23] of Regenstrief Institute, the Center for Healthcare Information and Communication, the challenge is to find the best ways to incorporate computers in the examination room without losing the heart and soul of health care: the patient–practitioner relationship. Dr. Frankel suggests a framework based on evidence and describes the POISED mnemonic: prepare, orient, information-gathering, share, educate, and debrief with patients during an office visit, using digital media or computers at the bedside.[23]

Similarly, telehealth applications present new opportunities for practitioners and students to develop sound CDM when incorporating telecommunication technologies. For example, Miller reports interpersonal aspects of patient–practitioner communication are affected by telehealth encounters.[24] During a consultation, a third-party provider and/or a caregiver may be involved in a telehealth encounter. Thus, sound CDM with common vocabulary for all participants during telehealth information gathering and sharing are necessary for high-quality care. In addition, physical distance between a patient and practitioner with telehealth may introduce social and professional distancing. A patient and practitioner should, if possible, prepare in person with clear CDM for a telehealth encounter to assist with concerns that may arise, to establish a trusting and respectful patient–practitioner relationship.

Furthermore, as strong evidence and new clinical practice guidelines[25] continue to emerge in the digital age, physical therapists have a responsibility to implement appropriate telehealth services. For example, when in-person assessment is impractical, both the American Heart Association and American Stroke Association scientific statements report Class I recommendations for assessment of physical disability in stroke care by physical therapist professionals via high-quality video teleconferencing (HQ-VTC) systems using specific standardized assessments. The standardized rating instruments have been validated for HQ-VTC use and administration by trained personnel using structured interview (Class I, Level of Evidence B).[25] Physical therapist providers need to be able to recognize the need for HQ-VTC, problem-solve when HQ-VTC is an appropriate course of action, and advocate for the assessment when in-person presentation is prohibited or improbable.

Based on recent national surveys of physical therapy program directors and faculty, the vast majority of respondents deemed telehealth education as important and necessary, agreeing on the need for students to be educated on the risks and benefits of telehealth, and the ethical, legal, and social implications related to telehealth implementation and availability. However, faculty and program directors lament that telehealth education is lacking in physical therapist education.

On the contrary, in a recent survey of nursing program directors, 88% of the program directors agreed that telehealth education should be included in nursing curricula, and 42% of the surveyed nursing programs had some form of telehealth educational experience that used a remote telehealth system, with 63% of telehealth learning experiences using synchronous telehealth communication.[26] Erickson and colleagues reported a significant change for nurse practitioner students to mold their education with telehealth to prepare for technology-related services in practice after a telehealth classroom course.[27]

In academic medicine, the University of Iowa began incorporating telemedicine into its health sciences curriculum in 1999. In addition, University of Texas Medical School added a telehealth elective for medical students in their fourth year to address primary care with telehealth delivery, while the University of Texas physician assistant program reported the use of telehealth in clinical education.[28] Nursing and academic medicine are forging ahead with telehealth education. Physical therapy professionals and educators may benefit from collaborating with telehealth health care practitioners to address CDM and clinical reasoning (CR) in the digital age.

TELEHEALTH EDUCATION SUPPORTING CLINICAL DECISION-MAKING

Shifting focus now, we will connect the classroom to the clinic, presenting telehealth physical therapy education curricular examples that promote CR and CDM.

Interprofessional Decision-Making With Telehealth Education

The use of audio, video, and other technologies to exchange information and provide care to patients who are geographically remote is becoming a more-routine part of practice, making it imperative to prepare health care program students in its use.[29] Incorporating telehealth into patient management introduces unique factors that health care practitioners will want to consider in the CDM process. For example, should all providers use telehealth? Is it appropriate for all providers to incorporate audio and video technology for all patients? Or are there criteria and key questions that guide one in the most appropriate approach for technology implementation?

One key consideration in using telehealth is the influence of the technology on interactions with patients and among members of the interprofessional team who may be involved with their care.[30] For example, communication between doctors and nurses is challenging because of philosophical differences on what information is required and who should share this information with patients.[24] In addition, usual differences between generalists and specialists are further complicated by distance and traditional community practice in rural and urban settings. Thus, interprofessional respect for each other is key to working with CDM with technology interfaces.

Educational models exist to prepare students in the health care professions to practically apply and implement telehealth in academia for real-world preparations.[26-28] Curricular strategies include traditional classroom presentations, online learning, simulation experiences, and clinical practice encounters.[31,32] At Oklahoma University, an educational telehealth model for teaching students in physical and occupational therapy, as well as nurse practitioners, incorporated elements of web-based learning, simulated patient encounters, and application with true-to-life patients in the clinic setting, within the context of interprofessional team building and CDM. This 3-year grant-funded program expanded telehealth infusion into 3 semesters in the classroom, as well as telehealth encounters in the clinic.[33]

The first of the 3 semesters of the telehealth curriculum consisted of online modules in which the students in their respective health disciplines learned about interprofessional core competencies, received an introduction to telehealth technology, and formed interprofessional groups to address issues and solve problems using case-based patient scenarios. The second semester

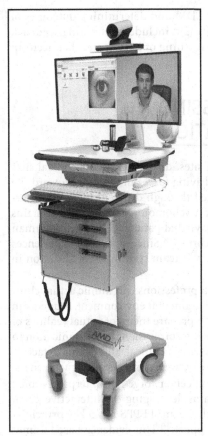

Figure 23-2. AMD Global Telemedicine cart. (Reprinted with permission from AMD Global Telemedicine.)

consisted of the same teams using a telehealth technology cart with peripheral stethoscope attachment, linked with a remote student to assess a standardized patient in a simulated clinical environment. The third semester entailed the teams delivering synchronous telehealth care to patients, remotely interacting with students exchanging secured examination information, using CDM for the peripheral attachments on a telehealth cart (eg, stethoscope, otoscope, hand-held high-definition camera) in an ambulatory care clinic (Figure 23-2).

The outcomes of student knowledge and attitudes toward telehealth technology were measured in this program using both quantitative and qualitative methods at various times during each of the 3 semesters.[32] The findings of this study revealed student knowledge of telehealth improved significantly after the online learning modules. Of interest, student attitudes regarding the perceived usefulness of telehealth, although remaining positive overall, declined from their baseline perceptions measured prior to using telehealth technology in the clinic environment. This may be due to the fact when encountering novel tasks including technologies, as one learns how much more there is to learn, one goes through a period of becoming less confident, then with more practice trials, more confident. Qualitative data shed light on this decline in the perception of the utility of telehealth. The students reflected that the telehealth technology created a barrier to communicating with patients, as well as with one another, as members of the interprofessional team. The students reported that their ability to establish rapport with the patient was hindered by not being physically present in the room, as well as by sometimes having difficulty seeing nonverbal elements such as facial expressions, body positioning, and gestures, as has been noted in other telehealth studies.[34,35]

An international example of telehealth education and training is notable with the University of Queensland, Australia, physical therapy curriculum, where a state-of-the-art telerehabilitation clinic has been established. The clinic uses telerehabilitation technologies to provide clinical rehabilitation services to the public. The services are provided by physical and occupational therapy, speech pathology, and audiology students under the supervision of clinical educators. Students are placed in the clinic in the clinical education components of their respective degrees, and the clinic provides the students with hands-on skills and experience in delivering services via telehealth. Prior to placement in the telerehabilitation clinic, students are introduced to the theory and practical aspects of telerehabilitation service delivery through an introductory education unit.

The education unit consists of self-directed online learning modules, quizzes, and practical hands-on experience with telerehabilitation technology. The units positively impact knowledge, confidence, and perceptions on the use of telehealth for clinical service provision.[36] The modules cover both general information about telerehabilitation practice and also discipline-specific information that addresses the unique considerations for each discipline with respect to delivering care via technology. More specifically, the general modules cover information such as history, definitions, nature of services provided, drivers and barriers to practice, privacy, confidentiality, security, technologies and technology selection, research, legal considerations, reimbursement, and practical considerations for implementing telerehabilitation. For each discipline, 4 modules are presented, which cover assessment and treatment, client selection, safety and risk, technology functionality, clinical scenarios, and the evidence base. CR is addressed specifically in the clinical scenarios presented in the modules and in the hands-on practicum where students work through clinical cases.

As the use of telehealth technology becomes more mainstream in practice, current and future practitioners will find it helpful to attend to the potential barriers and advantages during a patient encounter. Key considerations include implementing methods to optimize communication and intentionally establishing rapport with patients. Structured and scaffolded learning experiences that introduce progressively greater demands on students to address challenges of using telehealth will enhance their CDM, reasoning, and problem-solving abilities, which they can apply in any practice setting.

Educators can develop teaching strategies to address the potential barriers that telehealth technology might introduce to patient care and interprofessional teams, beginning with questions that challenge students to develop their own strategies, based on evidence, for enhancing patient rapport when using telehealth technology. Students' creativity and familiarity with technology may produce a wealth of approaches, including using the zoom feature of the telehealth camera to facilitate a more connected view of both sites and the users. Adopting nonverbal postures of openness and receptiveness are needed to enhance rapport. Further, students can verbally express to patients or other members of the team at a remote location how the technology might interfere with the communication process and users' empowerment to provide feedback, if they perceive any barriers during the informed consent process. In fact, the telehealth clinic space should maintain the privacy and security of a clinical environment between the patient and provider. Given that telehealth technology typically has the capacity to record patient visits, having students review and discuss video captures of the telehealth encounter can provide opportunities for reflection, self-assessment, and peer feedback for promoting CR and CDM and determining outcomes of competing care approaches and interventions. Finally, clinical encounters with patients might include a debriefing/feedback session that explicitly addresses perceived barriers and offers the same type of reflective learning opportunities that occur in the classroom to ultimately enhance clinical care.

TELEHEALTH SIMULATION ADDRESSING INTERPROFESSIONAL COMMUNICATION

Initiatives for increased patient safety, shorter hospital stays, competition for clinical sites, disparities across clinical sites with student placements, and faculty shortages in the clinical settings have been strong driving forces in the move toward the use of simulation in the classroom and the clinic.[37] Clinical experiences can be simulated through different methods, offering learners and practitioners a safer environment to practice their skills in the cognitive, psychomotor, and affective domains with less risk for harm to patients. Simulation includes case studies, partial task trainers, virtual patients, low-fidelity human patient simulators, high-fidelity human patient simulators, standardized patients, and hybrids.[38] Since simulated experiences can stimulate critical thinking and judgment, this simulation has become an integral part of team training and education in the health professions.[39]

For example, a high-fidelity scenario with code blue cardiac arrest simulation in health professions can mimic actual clinical encounters, requiring the health care team's critical thinking and CDM in a safe, nonjudgmental environment. Students in health professions reflecting on the aftermath of high-risk simulation indicate it may better prepare them for actual realities of clinical practice. A key consideration in using telehealth simulation is the opportunity for interprofessional communication to facilitate team collaboration using telehealth technology.[34,35] However, telehealth administrative, clinical, and technical factors must be addressed to mitigate potential barriers and perceptions in telecommunication use between patients and practitioners.

At Mount Saint Mary's University in Los Angeles, California, the experiential learning center forged an interprofessional collaboration for telehealth simulation between the nursing and physical therapy programs, leveraging the interactive Team Strategies and Tools to Enhance Performance and Patient Safety (TeamSTEPPS) approach. TeamSTEPPS has 5 key principles based on team structure, communication, leadership, situation monitoring, and mutual support.[40] This evidence-based framework thrives on interprofessional collaboration.

After several team-based meetings between faculty in both programs, the learning objectives of this interprofessional simulation included incorporating aspects of TeamSTEPPS[40]; integrating key telehealth practices[6]; and establishing patient-centered outcomes, with telecommunication implementation.

Physical therapist students at the end of their first academic year and nursing students in the second year had several opportunities to meet in a group with both faculty prior to the telehealth simulation. This was completed during the summer semester, with actions decided upon early in curriculum development. During the meetings, the students introduced themselves to each other and learned about academic and clinical experiences in their respective programs. In addition, a case study based on integumentary, mixed arterial and venous wound management was provided for student learning and opportunity for telehealth consultation with a wound care specialist. Lastly, the student groups decided that telehealth simulation could address cultural linguistic communication based on their past clinical encounters. Thus, the simulation would address patient-centered outcomes with a Spanish-speaking patient.

To conduct a telehealth simulation, key practice standards were established for students to follow as telehealth competencies. First, students needed to conduct the informed consent process with the patient for telehealth consultation. Second, the students needed to log into a patient privacy compliant telehealth portal (VSee)[41] for real-time audio and videoconferencing between students in the simulation lab and with a wound care specialist in the remote central simulation center. Third, the students needed to take a wound image with a Canon digital camera with minimum of preferred resolution of 1024 x 768 pixels. This wound image would be stored and forwarded to the wound care specialist during the telehealth session, while all consultation activity would be documented as a telehealth encounter by the students. These telehealth competencies were modeled to students by a faculty member familiar with telehealth clinical practice during 2 to 3 brief presimulation meetings. CDM is stimulated by querying if the need for specialty consult is warranted and if telehealth visits offer a viable opportunity for the patient needs and outcomes. Students also compare/contrast their clinical impressions and rehabilitation potentials with that of the specialist.

In the simulation, students interacted at the bedside using the TeamSTEPPS recommendations. Thus, all students at the bedside communicated situation, background, assessment, and recommendation methods for patient hand-off discussions between nursing and physical therapy students. The telehealth simulation required a translating nursing student who was fluent in lay and medical Spanish at the bedside to conduct the teleconsultation with a high-fidelity simulator who spoke only in Spanish during the patient encounter. Once the patient interview concluded, physical therapist students conducted a secured telehealth encounter using an iPad[42] with the telehealth portal (VSee)[41]) and requested a teleconsultation with a wound care specialist. After telehealth wound consultation, nursing and physical therapist students discussed proper bedside wound management.

After the simulation, debriefing sessions occurred with nursing and physical therapy students, with the nursing faculty member guiding the discussion for formative assessment. The simulation debriefing elements addressed what went well and what could be improved for a patient encounter with telehealth consultation. In reflection, all students appreciated the ability to learn about the other disciplines' roles and responsibilities. For example, nursing students did not realize that physical therapist students, with supervision from clinical instructors, can perform wound management in various settings. On the other hand, physical therapist students did not realize specialized communication techniques for interprofessional interactions were taught in the nursing program. Most interestingly, both nursing and physical therapist students did not realize telehealth consultation was a possibility prior to this simulation experience, as the students had not observed telehealth clinic practice in the community.

Students agreed that additional telehealth education would be beneficial in the curriculum. They also agreed that moving the simulation experience during or after the integumentary coursework in the physical therapy curriculum would align the students in the same year of academic training. As for faculty reflection, the ability for nursing and physical therapist students to focus on patient-centered care with cultural awareness and interprofessional collegiality were quite remarkable to observe after brief meetings among students, nursing, and physical therapy faculty. Most important, all participants agreed to place the need of the patient over individual autonomy.

Interprofessional communication and collaboration are required to make informed CDM with sound CR in practice. Academic faculty in health professions should expose students to early opportunities for potential collaboration and communication between disciplines to improve patient-centered outcomes. Telehealth simulation presents a unique opportunity to collaborate as a team and standardize communication between health professions. With scarce resources in academia, combining faculty resources and expertise with the use of smart technology can improve interprofessional communication and prepare students for clinical practice in the digital age.

TELEHEALTH DISTANCE EDUCATION USING CLINICAL OBSERVATION FROM THE CLINIC TO CLASSROOM

Finding clinical observation opportunities for physical therapist students in an integumentary course can be challenging. Since integumentary care includes wound management with wound images, a distance learning physical therapy course that blends both traditional classroom activities with actual telehealth clinical observations performed by a wound care practitioner may facilitate clinical learning and reasoning in learners. A distance learning telehealth education was implemented using clinical observation from a wound care clinic to university classroom to facilitate students' satisfaction with learning.

At Elon University in North Carolina, physical therapist students in their third year observed 3 synchronous telehealth sessions, approximately 45 minutes each, from an outpatient wound center in Reno, Nevada, once a week for 4 weeks during an integumentary course. The telehealth education used a LifeSize 220 system[43] connected to a hardwire line, allowing synchronous audio and video teleconferencing. Students viewed the teleconference on seven 32-inch flat screen monitors in the classroom with Shure wireless microphones that were routed through a Creston DMPS300 system to foster interactive conversations among physical therapists, students, and the patient with wounds. At the wound center, a telehealth treatment room with fixed focal lens camera mounted on a television was used by a physical therapist who had 14 years of wound management service, including credentials as an advanced wound care specialist.

The 3 telehealth sessions complemented the classroom coursework by addressing student satisfaction and CDM during wound evaluation and examination assessed with a practical exam (Session 1), wound interventions including mechanical and sharp debridement (Session 2), and total contact casting (Session 3) performed on an actual patient. Students described, then performed, specific interventions based on patient scenarios. The student satisfaction with telehealth education was assessed with a validated survey previously reported in academic medicine literature.[44] In a group of 43 physical therapist students in a wound management course, telehealth education was perceived as high-quality experience with time spent learning/teaching wound management rated at 3.28 ± 0.67 on a scale of 1 = poor, 2 = satisfactory, 3 = good, and 4 = excellent. The ability for the students to ask questions to both the physical therapist and patient was rated at 3.79 ± 0.47, with good sound quality at 3.42 ± 0.63. However, satisfactory visual image of the procedures was rated at 2.98 ± 0.60, while watching the sessions was rated at 2.70 ± 0.74.

Other wound care interventions were introduced via distance education with asynchronous video recordings from Duke University's Women's Health residency program.[45] A physical therapist resident and the director of Duke University's Women's Health residency program provided an online lecture on lymphedema, along with a recording of specific interventions for a patient with lymphedema. The students viewed the online videos posted on the e-Learning platform. The CDM was evaluated by short quizzes after the videos, as well as ability to ask questions from residency program therapists via email communication.

Telehealth distance education is an alternative to traditional 1:1 or 1:2 clinician/student ratio interaction for clinical encounters that provide more students an opportunity to observe and discuss complex and unique practice patterns in physical therapy. In physical therapy education, the use of online videos served as an effective method of instruction of advanced clinical psychomotor skills and a relatively time-efficient instructional method to enhance traditional classroom experiences.[46] Telehealth distance education from clinic to classroom and/or asynchronous video recordings can create an active learning environment among students, practitioners, and/or patients. For example, dynamic learning and CR for proper evaluation, examination, and interventions can be discussed, and patient preference can be addressed via telehealth distance education. However, educators need to be mindful of telehealth limitations and barriers with technology. For example, some students had difficulty visualizing telehealth sessions due to limited technology in the clinic. Other clinical barriers need to be addressed for effective teaching and learning in the classroom. Telehealth delivery of clinical content in the classroom may be one method to present clinical evaluation, examination, and interventions, with sound CR and with evidence-based discussions.

FUTURE IMPLICATIONS IN PRACTICE, RESEARCH, AND EDUCATION

Telecommunication technologies provide an opportunity to connect the classroom to the clinic with learners in physical therapy. Since progression to advanced clinical practice requires development of a CR process linked with the evolution of practitioners' knowledge,[47] having students, residents, and practitioners collaborate via telehealth, and developing complex thought processes in patient management, would be helpful. With well-established clinical residency programs in large academic centers, an opportunity is available for using existing telehealth networks within the academic centers to develop clinical and interprofessional partnerships. With clinical residency faculty addressing CR and CDM with residents, including telehealth education in post-professional clinical education would be a useful consideration. Incorporating residents/fellows-in-training with entry-level telehealth education is a viable model to also enhance CR for all and use nearer-peers to build confidence.

In research, active telerehabilitation clinical trials are registered in the international registry to study the impact of telehealth research on rehabilitation. Although evidence is building, translating this knowledge into broader, large-scale implementation in physical therapist practice is premature. To illustrate this point, a quality assessment of systematic reviews on telerehabilitation noted that 50% of evidence was high quality for mental health care of patients with spinal cord injuries in the short term, cardiorespiratory conditions such as asthma affecting children and adolescents, and chronic conditions in rural communities using telerehabilitation.[48] Insufficient evidence for stroke care and cost-savings with telerehabilitation was noted and attributed to lack of analysis of the grey literature, lack of documented exclusions, potential bias or likelihood, and heterogeneity of research.

Other systematic reviews resonate with a lack of health care use and cost associated with telerehabilitation that require further study.[49] In addition, academic education requires key ethical consideration with technology use.[50] Therefore, there should be investigation of health services research based on Assessment of Multiple Systematic Reviews quality methodology (an 11-item instrument used to assess the methodological rigor of systematic reviews) for future studies, as well as the impact of telehealth on cost savings, work flow, and ethical practice with technology use in physical therapy.

Distance education with telehealth is becoming mainstream and enables rural health care providers to manage complex diseases within their communities. The University of New Mexico's Project ECHO (Extension for Community Healthcare Outcomes) has demonstrated effective use of telehealth to equip rural health care providers with additional training and to address patient care in their communities.[51] Recent US legislation, the 21st Century Cures Act, will require study of how telehealth enables distance learning for medical providers, with a specific focus on rare diseases. Therefore, physical therapy educators and practitioners should use telehealth services to address health disparities and timely access to physical therapy care for the underserved in society. Overall, the success of telehealth in physical therapy will be judged by the ability to address CDM and CR with evidence developed from practice, research, and education.

CONCLUSION

This chapter introduced aspects of telehealth initiatives within the physical therapy profession. In addition, 4 physical therapy telehealth curricular models addressing sound CDM and CR were presented. Overall, physical therapist practice, research, and education require evidence from researchers, educators, and practitioners to facilitate CDM in the digital age.

Reflection Moment

Identify the perspectives on telehealth from the American Physical Therapy Association, Federation of State Boards of Physical Therapy, and your state physical therapy board after reading the article "Skype's the Limit in Ethics in Practice" (http://www.apta.org/PTinMotion/2016/4/EthicsinPractice/).

Discuss some of the current US and global telerehabilitation research trials related to telehealth and telerehabilitation from the clinical trials website (https://clinicaltrials.gov/).

Justify the necessary administrative, clinical, ethical, and technical factors for telehealth use and implementation in your physical therapist practice; consider the reference list in this chapter as part of your justification.

ACKNOWLEDGMENTS

The authors would like to thank Matt Elrod, PT, DPT, for his contribution in the figure illustration. In addition, sincere gratitude to Marco Milano, PT, DPT, who assisted with survey research on telehealth education, and Lindsey Brunner, PT, DPT, for the telehealth simulation at Mount Saint Mary's University, Los Angeles, California.

REFERENCES

1. American Physical Therapy Association. 2014 House of Delegates minutes. http://www.apta.org/HOD/Minutes/2014/. Accessed April 7, 2018.
2. American Physical Therapy Association. Standards of practice for physical therapy. http://www.apta.org/uploadedFiles/APTAorg/About_Us/Policies/Practice/StandardsPractice.pdf#search=%22standards%20of%20physical%20therapy%20practice%22. Accessed April 7, 2018.
3. American Physical Therapy Association. Core ethics documents. http://www.apta.org/Ethics/Core/. Accessed April 7, 2018.
4. American Physical Therapy Association. Guide to physical therapist practice 3.0. http://guidetoptpractice.apta.org/. Accessed April 7, 2018.
5. American Physical Therapy Association. Definitions and guidelines on telehealth. http://www.apta.org/Telehealth/. Accessed April 7, 2018.
6. Brennan D, Tindall L, Theodoros D, et al. A blueprint for telerehabilitation guidelines. *Int J Telerehabil*. 2010;2(2):31-34.
7. Federation of State Boards of Physical Therapy. Telehealth in physical therapy policy recommendations for appropriate regulation. https://www.fsbpt.org/FreeResources/RegulatoryResources/TelehealthinPhysicalTherapy.aspx. Accessed April 7, 2018.
8. American Physical Therapy Association. Vision 2020. http://www.apta.org/vision2020/. Accessed April 7, 2018.
9. Kigin C, Rodgers M, Wolf SL. The Physical Therapy and Society Summit (PASS): observations and opportunities. *Phys Ther*. 2010;90:1555-1567.
10. The evolution of autonomous practice and vision 2020. http://www.apta.org/PTinMotion/2006/5/BoardPerspective/. Accessed April 7, 2018.
11. RC 23–06 Summit on Physical Therapy and Society. In: *Minutes of the 2006 American Physical Therapy Association House of Delegates meeting*. Alexandria, VA: American Physical Therapy Association; 2006:23.
12. PASS graphic recordings. American Physical Therapy Association website. http://www.apta.org/PASS/GraphicRecordings/. Accessed April 7, 2018.
13. Physical therapy and society summit (PASS). American Physical Therapy Association website. http://www.apta.org/PASS/. Accessed April 7, 2018.
14. Wolf SL. FiRST and foremost: advances in science and technology impacting neurologic physical therapy. *J Neurol Phys Ther*. 2013;37(4):147-148.
15. Wolf SL. Correspondence: home based therapy can be of, at least, short term value. *Int J Ther Rehabil*. 2011;18(2):116-117.
16. Ambrosio F, Trumbower R, Wolf SL, Wagner W. *Regenerative medicine and the role of physical therapy (an independent study course)*, 2013:38. American Physical Therapy Association, Alexandria, VA.
17. Wolf SL. Exploring the future of neurologic physical therapy. *J Neurol Phys Ther*. 2015;39(1):1-2.
18. Wolf SL. A changing landscape for science and technology: potential impact on PT practice and health policy. *Phys Ther J Policy Adm Leadersh*. 2014;14(8):31.
19. Bashshur RL, Shannon GW. *History of Telemedicine: Evolution, Context, and Transformation*. New Rochelle, NY: Mary Ann Liebert, Inc. Publishers; 2009.
20. About telemedicine. http://www.americantelemed.org/main/about/about-telemedicine#. Accessed April 7, 2018.
21. Richardson JK. Tipping the scales of time. *Phys Ther*. 2000;80(11):1121-1124.
22. Bini SA, Mahajan J. Clinical outcomes of remote asynchronous telerehabilitation are equivalent to traditional therapy following total knee arthroplasty: a randomized control study. *J Telemed Telecare*. 2017;23(2):239-247.
23. Physician computer use affects patient's perception of care. http://www.medscape.com/viewarticle/855282. Accessed November 26, 2016.
24. Miller EA. The technical and interpersonal aspects of telemedicine: effects on doctor-patient communication. *J Telemed Telecare*. 2003;9:1-7.
25. Schwamm LH, Holloway RG, Amarenco P, et al. A review of the evidence for the use of telemedicine within stroke systems of care. *Stroke*. 2009;40:2616-2634.
26. Ali NS, Carlton KH, Ali OS. Telehealth education in nursing curricula. *Nurs Educ*. 2015;40(5):266-269.
27. Erickson CE, Fauchald S, Ideker M. Integrating telehealth into the graduate nursing curriculum. *J Nurs Pract*. 2015;31(11): e1-e5.
28. Asprey DP, Zollo S, Kienzle M. Implementation and evaluation of a telemedicine course for physician assistants. *Acad Med*. 2001;76(6):652-655.
29. Koch S. Home telehealth—current state and future trends. *Int J Med Info*. 2006;75:565-576.
30. Randall KE, Steinheider B, Isaacson M, et al. Measuring knowledge, acceptance, and perceptions of telehealth in an interprofessional curriculum for student nurse practitioners, occupational therapists, and physical therapists. *J Interact Learn Res*. 2016;27(4):339-353.
31. Freeth D, Reeves S, Koppel I, Hammick M, Barr H. Evaluating interprofessional education: a self-help guide. *High Educ Acad*. 2005.

32. Shortridge AM, Stienheider B, Ciro C, et al. Simulating interprofessional geriatric patient care using telehealth: a team-based learning activity. *MedEdPORTAL Publications.* 2016;12:10415.

33. Shortridge AM, Ross HM, Randall KE, Ciro, CA, Loving GL. Telehealth technology as e-learning: learning and practicing interprofessional patient care. *Int J E-Learn.* 2018;17:95-110.

34. Gratch J, Morency L, Scherer S, et al. User-state sensing for virtual health agents and telehealth applications. *Stud Health Tech Inf.* 2013;184:151-157.

35. Tanis MA. Cues to Identity in CMC. The impact on person perception and subsequent interaction outcomes. [PhD thesis]. Amsterdam, Netherlands: University of Amsterdam; 2003.

36. Theodoros D, Jeffery L, Russell T. Evaluation of a telerehabilitation education program for allied health students: a pilot study. Successes and failures in telehealth. 7th Annual Meeting of the Australian Telehealth Society; October 31 to November 3, 2016; Auckland, New Zealand.

37. Hayden JK, Smiley RA, Alexander M, Kardong-Edgren S, Jeffries PR. The NCSBN national simulation study: a longitudinal, randomized, controlled study replacing clinical hours with simulation in prelicensure nursing education. *J Nurs Regul.* 2014;5:2.

38. Cannon-Diehl MR. Simulation in health care and nursing: state of science. *Crit Care Nurs Q.* 2009;32(2):128-136.

39. Yudkowsky R, Vlades W, Raja S, Kiser R. Assessing residents' telehealth communication skills using standardized patients. *Med Educ.* 2011;45:1155.

40. Agency for Healthcare Research and Quality. TeamSTEPPS 2.0 pocket guide. AHRQ Pub. No. 14-0001-2. 2013.

41. HIPAA messenger + video telehealth. https://vsee.com/. Accessed April 7, 2018.

42. iPad pro. http://www.apple.com/ipad/. Accessed April 7, 2018.

43. Lifesize makes any meeting better. https://www.lifesize.com/. Accessed April 7, 2018.

44. Gul YA, Wan AC, Darzi A. Use of telemedicine in undergraduate teaching of surgery. *J Telemed Telecare.* 1999;5(4):246-248.

45. Duke University Women's Health Residency. https://sites.duke.edu/ptot/physical-occupational-therapy-residencies/womens-health-residency/. Accessed April 7, 2018.

46. van Duijn AJ, Swanick K, Donald E Kroog. Student learning of cervical psychomotor skills via online video instruction versus traditional face-to-face instruction. *J Phys Ther Educ.* 2014;28(1):94-102.

47. Tichenor CJ, Davidson JM. Post-professional clinical residency education. In: Shepard KF, Jensen GM, eds. *Handbook of Teaching for Physical Therapists.* Woburn, MA: Butterworth-Heinemann; 2002.

48. Rogante M, Kairy D, Giacomozzi C, Grigioni M. A quality assessment of systematic reviews on telerehabilitation: what does the evidence tell us? *Ann 1st Super Sanita.* 2015;51(1):11-18.

49. Kairy D, Lehoux P, Vincent C, Visintin M. A systematic review of clinical outcomes, clinical process, healthcare utilization and costs associated with telerehabilitation. *Disabil Rehabil.* 2009;31(6):427-447.

50. Greenfield B, Musolino GM. Technology in rehabilitation: ethical and curricular implications for physical therapist education. *J Phys Ther Educ.* 2012;26(2):81-90.

51. American Telemedicine Association's resource and buyer's guide. http://telemedicineresourcecenter.org/getProducts.cfm?searchmode=home&dir=251DAE&expCats=&abid=2816AB1F1B0F&pid=2118AD141903&ncol=1. Accessed April 7, 2018.

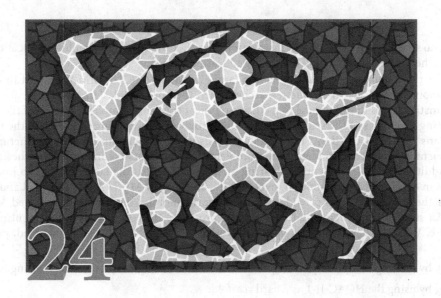

MOBILE-BASED INSTRUCTIONAL SCAFFOLDING:
A Developmental Tool for Facilitating Physical Therapist Student Clinical Reasoning

Nancy Smith, PT, DPT, PhD, GCS; A. Daniel Johnson, PhD; and
Andrew S. Bartlett, PT, PhD, MPA

OBJECTIVES

- Describe the current uses of computer-based technology to facilitate scaffolding of clinical reasoning (CR) in physical therapy and other professions.

- Identify scaffolding strategies from education literature that may facilitate complex clinical problem-solving (CPS) and hypothetico-deductive reasoning.

- Illustrate the technical design and development process of a researcher-generated mobile application to facilitate CR.

- Examine the educational impacts of a researcher-generated mobile application on an investigation for needed scaffolding to facilitate CR.

- Compare and contrast the current evidence with the results of a novel investigation of a clinical reasoning mobile-based instructional media application (CR-MBIMA).

INTRODUCTION

Computer-based instructional media (CBIM) scaffolding can assist learners in developing the critical skills and practices of CR and ill-defined problem-solving, as results are germane to health professions education and research studies. However, there is a paucity of research in the profession of physical therapist education on utilizing CBIM scaffolding principles to

Musolino GM, Jensen GM, eds. *Clinical Reasoning and Decision-Making in Physical Therapy: Facilitation, Assessment, and Implementation* (pp 267-298).
© 2020 Taylor & Francis Group.

facilitate CR. Further, no studies exist on the use of instructional scaffolding employing mobile applications (eg, CR-MBIMA) to facilitate CR within the profession of physical therapist education.

Chapter 24 describes the development, implementation, and evaluation of CR-MBIMA to assist in learning for physical therapist CR. In developing the CR-MBIMA, the researchers used the analysis, design, development, implementation, and evaluation (ADDIE)[1] instructional design model to facilitate physical therapists' implementation of the sequence and strategies of CR, incorporating principles of the scientific reasoning framework scaffolding model[2] and the Hypothesis-Oriented Algorithm for Clinicians II—Part 1 or HOAC II-1.[3] First, analysis was conducted using physical therapist CR research and the researchers' experiential knowledge to identify the problems that students commonly have when engaging in CR and ill-defined CPS. An additional problem, identified during analysis, related to the lack of access to just-in-time knowledge support in the classroom or clinic. Next, a solution involving the use of a CR-MBIMA was designed and developed by defining the major goal of the CR-MBIMA: to provide a cross-platform mobile solution that employed MBIM scaffolding to assist physical therapist students in structuring the decisional processes that occur while implementing CR with an actual patient or practice case. With the development of this application, 5 major scaffolds were included, providing support for the CR-MBIMA:

1. Sense-making by making disciplinary strategies for CR evident through expert guidance using hard scaffolding;

2. Sense-making by using the HOAC-II-1 as a hard scaffold;

3. Sense-making by using soft scaffolds that provide help for the reasoning process through cueing;

4. Sense-making by providing support for discipline specific knowledge; and

5. Reflection, articulation, and process management through the use of hard scaffolds (application structure).

Preliminary results from a singular case, using a qualitative narrative a-priori deductive and inductive coding analysis of pre-and post-test think aloud interview, indicate changes in the CR process evoked by the application. Notable changes in CR included more time spent in collecting subjective information, more directed subjective questioning and gathering of objective data, better problem prioritization, and use of higher order reasoning strategies such as pattern recognition. Further data from student feedback supports that the application-enhanced knowledge and acquisition of a CR strategy . Initial data analysis of other participant cases supports that the mobile application facilitated the use of effective higher order reasoning strategies and improved sequencing efficiencies.

Congruent with previous research in education and medical education, CR-MBIMA results in development of practices and knowledge that support the process of CR in physical therapist students. Further research should focus upon a larger cohort of students, students at different levels of physical therapist education, and whether changes produced by the CR-MBIMA transfer to practice in clinical settings, to fully support its use in physical therapist education.

The practice of the physical therapist requires individuals to act autonomously and to make effective decisions that are in the best interest of their patients, all within an ever-changing, complex health care environment. Therefore, physical therapist students and practitioners must develop the capability to reason clinically. Definitions of CR may include multiple processes, including clinical decisions reached based upon the data collected, cognitive processes of deliberation about an appropriate course of action within a specified clinical context, reflection on activities used by the clinician to arrive at a diagnosis, or strategies used to manage patient care based upon knowledge, patient goals, patient belief systems, and professional judgment.[4-7]

To facilitate student competence in CR, educators have been challenged with providing andragogy that focuses on the domains and processes associated with CR. This chapter addresses the need by describing the development of a researcher-generated, case-based mobile application that provides decisional scaffolds based upon the scientific reasoning framework scaffolding model[2] and HOAC II-1.[3] Further described is the ability for the CR-MBIMA to cultivate the sequence and process of first-year physical therapist students' CR.

LITERATURE REVIEW

In considering how to develop CR through educational interventions in physical therapy, it is important to first understand that CR and hypothesis-generation develop on a continuum as knowledge and skills are developed; for this reason, these faculties differ between novice and expert practitioners.[6,8-10] Within physical therapy, studies have demonstrated that compared to novices, experts tend to use more succinct reasoning schemata such as pattern generation, revert to hypothetico-deductive reasoning strategies when confronted with challenging problems, make better and more correct clinical decisions, and use reflection during and after their evaluation processes to shape clinical decisions.[6,11] In contrast, novice physical therapists and physical therapist students often have difficulty formulating and evaluating hypotheses and making correct and/or accurate clinical decisions once they have gathered subjective and objective sources of information from the patient; they also tend to use less reflection during the course of examination and treatment.[6,12,13]

CR and hypothesis-generation develop on a continuum; hence, educators in physical therapy and medicine have identified key constructs essential to facilitating CR and hypothesis generation in students within the cognitive learning domain, and less directed toward the development of psychomotor skills.[5] However, other competencies within CR also need to be developed and focused on to promote sound CR and hypothesis generation.[5,14,15] Focusing on the CR competencies, multiple authors have cited the need for increased andragogical focus on competencies situated within the cognitive domain, including teaching students how to process data using decisional pathways or algorithmic frameworks, form hypotheses including alternatives, recall and organize knowledge in more than one way, and reflect on decisions made, setting aside potentials with inherent bias.[3,6,14,16]

Within physical therapist education, researchers have explored the use of algorithmic frameworks[17] to support the development of CR. However, limited research has occurred within physical therapy that employs technology-based strategies to facilitate CR, using either case-based approaches or scaffolding built from a reasoning framework. Currently, scant studies exist within the physical therapy literature that support the use of CBIM to specifically facilitate CR using a case-based approach.[18-20] No study has examined the use of CBIM in combination with the HOAC II-1, specifically, to provide a scaffolded, algorithmic, reasoning framework-based approach to CR. A gap exists within the physical therapy literature on the use of mobile technology to scaffold the sequence or process of CR, either using case-based methods or case-based methods in combination with an algorithmic framework.

In contrast, the professions of education and medical education provide a rich body of research on the effectiveness of CBIM to scaffold the scientific reasoning process, assist learners in solving ill-defined scientific problems, and present learners with case-based andragogy.[21,22] Scaffolding within education has been described as "expert support for a novice's learning,"[23(p2)] defined as a means to move a learner who is developing certain problem-solving skills such as CR, to a higher level of CPS, initially by providing explicit instruction, followed by decreasing supports, or scaffolds, as the learner becomes more independent.[24] Within technology-enhanced environments such as CBIM, the technology functions to provide scaffolding based upon expert or disciplinary strategy guidance, facilitating cognitive tasks such as managing cognitive load or assisting with metacognitive processing.[23] The CBIM scaffolds may be provided in a fixed or non-negotiable manner (hard), or in a contextually sensitive or on-demand manner (soft), similar to the supports provided by an instructor at the point of care or key intersections with reasoning processes.[23]

Within education, a guideline for CBIM to facilitate complex CPS using a hypothetico-deductive strategy[2] advocates for a methodological design to scaffold CBIM to best manage learning the complex process of decision-making. Within this guideline, the hypothetico-deductive process of scientific reasoning is defined by 3 domains: sense-making, process management, and reflection and articulation.

Sense-making within the model directly relates to the steps the learner goes through in hypothetical reasoning—specifically, generating hypotheses, making comparisons, collecting observations, analyzing data, and interpreting data. The second domain, process management, relates to the cognitive load tasks that the learner must perform when making decisions such as keeping track of hypotheses, data, and results. Process management further relates to the organizational strategies that the learner employs to manage data, such as using algorithmic frameworks or following protocols. Finally, the last domain, articulation and reflection, relates to the process of providing metacognitive support for helping learners convey their thought processes, guide the thought process, and reflect upon decisions. CBIM scaffolding supports these 3 domains of hypothetico-deductive reasoning. Studies within education have shown positive effects, primarily in structuring the learning process of solving ill-defined problems and helping learners successfully engage in more efficient and effective discipline-related decision-making.[2,25,26] While CBIM has been successful in scaffolding CR, it is not always available at the point of care. Therefore, MBIMA has been suggested as an appropriate media to inform and support the process of CR, due to its ability to provide easily accessible information at the point of care.[27]

In recent years, researchers within medicine and physical therapy have begun to advocate for the use of mobile technology, such as with smartphones and tablets, within the classroom and clinical environment to facilitate learning.[28-30] Justification for this position is found in Kozma,[31] who argued that if the media interacts with the environment around it, or with the cognitive and social processes by which knowledge is constructed, learning may be enhanced.[31(p7)] While building on Kozma's[31] argument, researchers within medicine have explicated the features that are unique to mobile devices to extend learning of CR tasks.

First, mobile technology may lead to increased interaction with the patient and learning opportunities provided[29,32] due to its portability and accessibility. Second, mobile technology also provides contextual, situated learning, which the student constructs in the clinic or laboratory, by providing supports for both just-in-time knowledge (knowledge supports needed during the reasoning process),[33] and scaffolds for the sequence of the student's diagnostic process.[27,32,34] As the knowledge and supports are situated within the learning environment of the laboratory or clinic, knowledge may be extended, and thus, students' abilities to reason from their own experience may be increased.[27,35] Third, mobile technology may also provide flexibility in assessment,[34] which is "matched to the ability of the learner, offering diagnosis and formative guidance that builds on success."[35(p3)] Further, while not extensively studied in medical disciplines, mobile technology may provide a medium from which to facilitate the social and emotional domains of reasoning, due to the pervasiveness of this technology.[32] Therefore, it is reasonable to explore whether or not mobile technology that scaffolds a hypothetico-deductive CR process, using patient cases, provides physical therapist students with the ability to acquire skills within the cognitive domain of CR.

Study Method: Application Design, Development, and Scaffolds

The CR-MBIMA was developed using an iterative design model, the ADDIE framework, which consists of analysis, design, development, implementation, and evaluation.[1(p54)] Initially, analysis was conducted using the researchers' experiential knowledge to identify the problems that students commonly have when reasoning clinically. Three problems were identified related to cognitive CR, which consisted of students' inability to organize data into a framework that allows hypotheses to be developed, generate hypotheses from data collected, and select appropriate tests to confirm or deny hypotheses (ie, knowledge base). A correlate problem identified related to the lack of access to just-in-time (situated) knowledge support that could be accessed while working with a patient in the clinic, or, alternatively, when working with a partner in the classroom during laboratory sessions consisting of tests and measures, pathologies, and treatment strategies. Therefore, considering the capabilities of mobile devices and computer-based algorithms, a solution involving the use of a CR-MBIMA was proposed.

The solution was derived by defining the major goal of the CR-MBIMA: to provide a cross-platform mobile solution that employed scaffolding to assist physical therapist students in structuring the decision processes that occur while contemplating CR with an actual patient or practice case. Based upon the articulated goal, a CR-MBIMA was designed using HTML-5 (hypertext markup language) and the JQuery Mobile database that had the capabilities to be used with an actual patient or practice case. HTML-5 and JQuery Mobile were selected in programming the application to allow the application to have a responsive design and, therefore, be used on all mobile devices and laptop computers.

In considering the application design, the use of scaffolds to support learning was of prime importance. Following the recommendation that learners be provided an intentional learning framework that encourages them to "articulate their understandings through structured discourse,"[2(p339)] a method of reasoning was identified to structure the cognitive processes of CR, using the HOAC II-1 framework. In addition, learner-centered design[2] was employed to provide scaffolds for the tasks commonly performed by physical therapist students when they are clinically reasoning. The scaffolds (Table 24-1) used in the application are detailed with the application feature (in Column 1) that provides the details of the scaffolding features built into the CR-MBIMA. The application features are classified and explicated further by scientific inquiry (see Table 24-1, Column 2), which describes a broad category of actions taken by learners during hypothetico-deductive reasoning or complex CPS (eg, process management, sense-making, articulation, reflection) as previously defined. The third column of Table 24-1, the scaffolding strategy, provides the specific example of what the CR-MBIMA does to facilitate the CPS process. In the final column of Table 24-1, the type of scaffold used (hard or soft) is provided.[2,23]

From this design process and based upon the scaffolding guidelines, the application wireframes were completed, as demonstrated in an exemplar provided in Figure 24-1.

After the wireframes were developed, an Excel database was created to form the basis for a JQuery database to underpin the application. The use of a database for this project was framed by 3 goals: the database was structured to contain a limited condition set of objective tests, results, and subjective responses related to the diagnosis of lower-extremity vascular disorders to limit access to data choices during sense-making; the database was structured for the linkages among the objective tests, results, and subjective responses, and to return them to the user to manage nonsalient tasks during the reasoning process; and the database was structured to provide a back-end administrative panel that allowed modifications of the application by adding or deleting cases, conditions, tests, expert recommendations for tests, help resources, and reports of background analytics to quantify time on-screen and steps taken by the user, which provided data for later, follow-up analysis.

In addition to the database being created, 9 clinical cases were developed and reviewed by 2 content experts. Following the review, cases were modified, and then a request for bid quotes was sent to application developers and selected. From this initial development process, a CR-MBIMA mobile application was developed based upon the wireframes, expert-reviewed cases, and database provided.

Five figures provide a description of the scaffolding features incorporated, the administrative panels, and the database. The application's scaffolds and screenshots are depicted in Figures 24-2A through E. Figure 24-2C gives examples of scaffolds for articulation and reflection. An exemplar of the administrative panels is depicted in Figure 24-3, and finally, a database exemplar is illustrated in Figure 24-4.

	TABLE 24-1		
	SCAFFOLDS USED WITHIN THE CR-MBIMA		
APPLICATION FEATURE	**SCIENTIFIC INQUIRY COMPONENT**	**SCAFFOLDING STRATEGY**	**TYPE OF SCAFFOLD**[23]
Buttons consistently identifying steps in the HOAC II-1 framework process	Process management	Facilitate navigation among tools and activities Decompose a complex task into its constituents using unordered task decompositions	Hard
Cues to indicate out-of-order steps in the framework through pop-up when HOAC II-1 sequence is not followed	Sense-making	Make disciplinary strategies explicit in the learner's interactions with the tool	Soft
Reflection on steps taken out of order	Articulation and reflection	Provide reminders and guidance to facilitate productive monitoring	Soft
Hint button	Sense-making	Embed expert guidance to help learners use and apply content Make disciplinary strategies explicit in the learner's interactions with the tool	Soft
Consistent application format	Process management	Facilitate navigation among tools and activities	Hard
Help feature for Patient History	Sense-making	Embed expert guidance to help learners use and apply content	Soft
Help feature for About HOAC	Sense-making	Embed expert guidance to help learners use and apply content	Soft
Help feature for About Tests	Sense-making	Embed expert guidance to help learners use and apply content	Soft
Limited condition set with data queries including subjective questions, tests, patient problems, and diagnoses	Sense-making	Make disciplinary strategies explicit in the learner's interaction with the tool (access to relevant data choices)	Hard
Help feature for About Conditions	Sense-making	Embed expert guidance to help learners use and apply content	Soft
Arrows beside tests in objective examination screen that, when tapped, links the user to information about that test	Sense-making	Embed expert guidance to help learners use and apply content	Soft
Opportunity to provide reflections on given result on (last) debriefing screen: "How can you improve for next time?"	Articulation and reflection	Provide reminders and guidance to facilitate articulation during sense-making	Hard
Textual instructions that explain the scientific practice in each step	Sense-making	Embed expert guidance to clarify characteristics of scientific practices	Hard

continued

TABLE 24-1 (CONTINUED) SCAFFOLDS USED WITHIN THE CR-MBIMA			
APPLICATION FEATURE	**SCIENTIFIC INQUIRY COMPONENT**	**SCAFFOLDING STRATEGY**	**TYPE OF SCAFFOLD**[23]
Opportunity to provide rationales/justify decisions offered during different points in the HOAC framework, including identifying their hypotheses and alternate hypotheses, formulating a strategy	Articulation and reflection	Provide reminders and guidance to facilitate productive monitoring	Hard
Opportunity to provide notes on thoughts with data collection screen as evaluation is being planned, identifying other questions to ask after articulating the hypothesis, and identifying other symptoms for which they are looking during the examination	Articulation and reflection	Provide reminders and guidance to facilitate productive planning	Hard
Opportunity to provide a rationale for the final diagnostic hypothesis achieved and treatment decision	Articulation and reflection	Provide reminders and guidance to facilitate articulation during sense-making	Hard
Debriefing provided using expert guidance	Sense-making	Embed expert guidance to clarify characteristics of scientific practices	Hard
Data management for cognitive load or management of memory tasks. Facilitated with previous data returned at decision points. User-entered data is returned to user during process steps of initial identification of patient problems, problem identification after objective exam performed, determining final hypothesis, and debriefing.	Process management	Facilitate the organization of work products	Hard

IMPLEMENTATION PHASE

After the completion of the CBIM application design process, the CR application was tested with first-year, second semester doctor of physical therapy (DPT) graduate-level students, from a medium-sized, 4-year, public, Level V Carnegie-classed[36] institution in the southeastern US. Six students were selected for participation using purposive sampling,[37] allowing the sample to be representative of the currently enrolled student population with respect to gender (50% male, 50% female) and minority status (30%).

The selection of first-year DPT students was important because previous studies have demonstrated that these students have relative inexperience with CR in physical therapy, and, therefore, use faulty reasoning strategies, collect too much data, and make more errors as they are first beginning CDM.[3,12,13] Because of the relative inexperience that DPT student participants bring to the challenges of CR, the use of scaffolds as noted previously, was able to give guidance for sense-making, support process management, and assist with articulation and reflection, thereby facilitating a more cohesive reasoning strategy.

To evaluate the utility of the CR-MBIMA in facilitating learning of CR strategies, an intervention-based, sequential, qualitative research design was used.[38,39] This design was employed to discover how the CR-MBIMA affected the strategies and sequence of CR employed thorough the use of a qualitative pre-intervention task-based interview, a set of 4 experiences with the intervention (CR-MBIMA), and, finally, a qualitative post-intervention task-based interview.

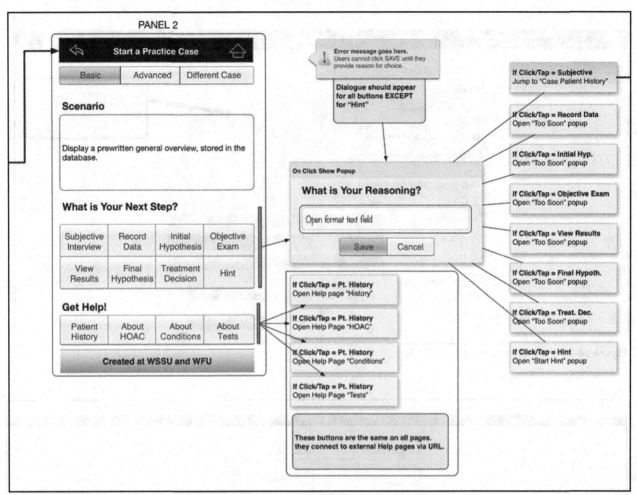

Figure 24-1. Wireframe exemplar.

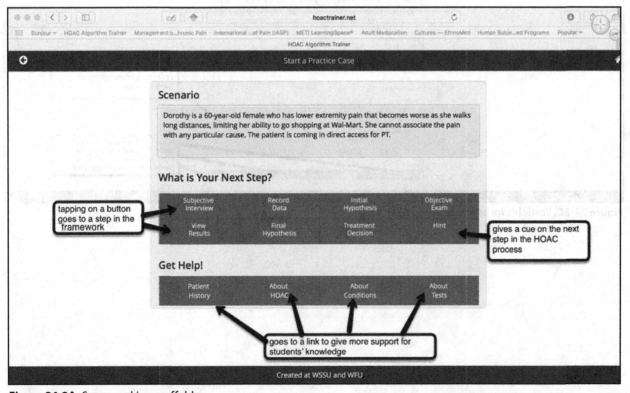

Figure 24-2A. Sense-making scaffolds.

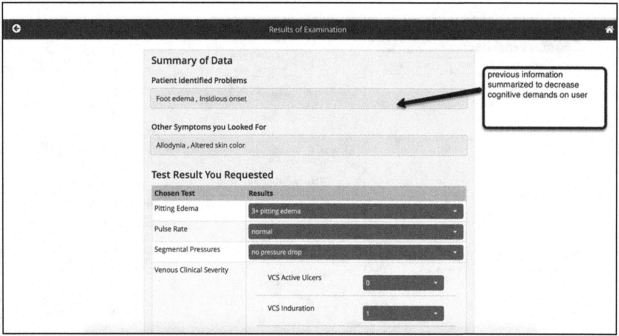

Figure 24-2B. Process management scaffolds.

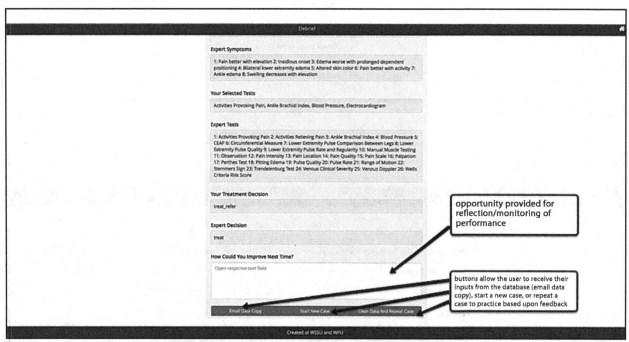

Figure 24-2C. Scaffolds for articulation and reflection.

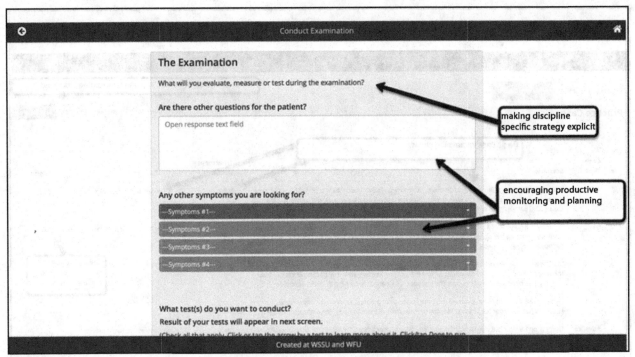

Figure 24-2D. Collecting tests and measures: scaffolds for sense-making and articulation and reflection.

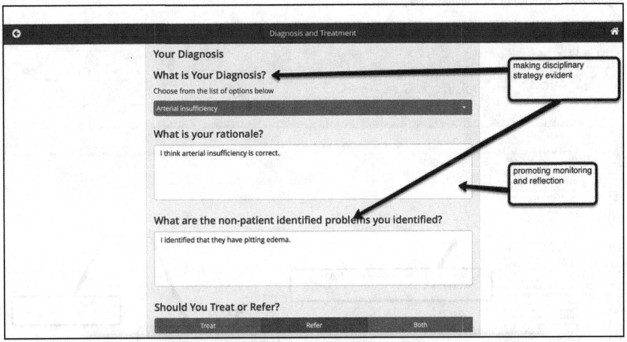

Figure 24-2E. Final hypothesis: scaffolds for sense-making and articulation and reflection.

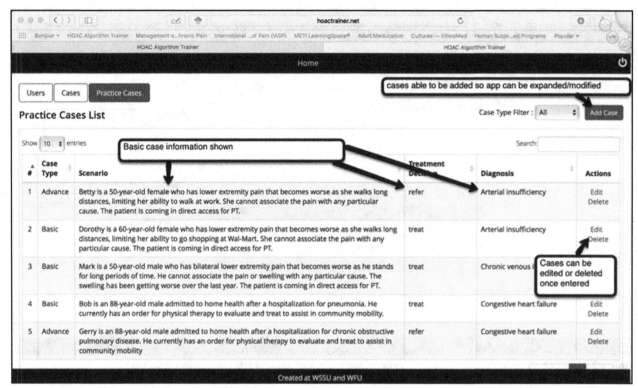

Figure 24-3. Exemplar of the administrative panels.

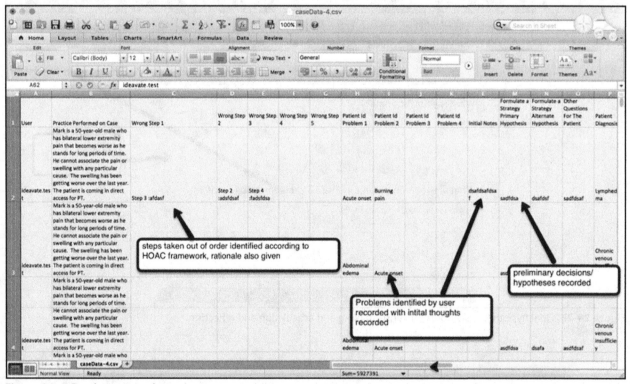

Figure 24-4. Database exemplar.

PRE-INTERVENTION PHASE

After completion of informed consent documents, each participant completed a semistructured task-based interview (think aloud) that was audio recorded. The purpose of the interview was to elicit hypothesis generation and CR strategies that students used prior to interacting with the CR-MBIMA, as well as perceived factors influencing CR. At the start of this interview, participants were instructed in the expectations and process of the interview.

Next, participants were given a sheet of paper with an introduction to the clinical case used during the task-based interview process, on which they were asked to write any thoughts that they had regarding the case or any information that they needed to help them in the reasoning process (participant form). This form was collected at the end of the interview. During the interviews, the researcher verbally provided information to the participants to assist them in gaining data necessary to solve the patient problem, as participants solicited information about the case by questioning the interviewer. As data were provided to the participants, the researcher asked participants to describe the rationale for both the CR strategies they used and the hypotheses that they generated toward diagnosis and appropriate treatment, as well as perceived factors that may influence CR. Further data were collected during task-based interviews using researcher field notes to document researcher impressions of CR strategies and the sequential order of examination and evaluation used during the task-based interview.

INTERVENTION PHASE

After the pre–task-based interview, participants had 4 intervention sessions (1 hour each) with the CR-MBIMA. The first intervention session consisted of an instructional session in the application's features and use. After logging in with a unique, de-identified login, the participant selected a randomized practice scenario case specific to lower-extremity vascular disorders. Following case selection, a set of standardized buttons that were present on each subsequent screen, except for the diagnosis/treatment and debriefing screens, was presented with the case information. Within the application, the buttons allowed the participant to either select a step in the HOAC II-1 or seek help. Within the application, help was provided to participants to explain the steps in the patient history, the HOAC II-1 framework, the conditions represented within the cases, and the physical therapy examination measures commonly used to attain a physical therapist diagnosis for the conditions covered in the cases. The participant was able to obtain a hint about what step to pursue in the framework if he or she needed assistance. Further, if a participant selected an incorrect next step in the framework, the participant was asked for a rationale for the step selected, and that was recorded into a database for post-session analysis.

As the research participant-user moved through the case, subsequent screen layouts were varied and scaffolded for instructional guidance (sense-making) according to the HOAC II-1 framework. Table 24-2 illustrates the steps and links within the application to the HOAC II-1.

The CR-MBIMA layouts allowed for the collection of initial data, the identification of patient-identified problems, the generation of an initial and alternate hypotheses, and the collection of examination data. Links were provided to resources for knowledge support. After the collection of examination data, the database returned the initial patient-identified problems, test results, and other entries or notes that the participant entered, so that evaluation was possible.

At this point, the participant was able to choose to go back and collect more data by returning to the examination page, or could proceed to form a final diagnostic hypothesis; make a clinical decision whether to treat, refer, or treat and refer; and provide rationales. Participant data from this interaction was recorded to the database for post-session analysis. Following this data entry, a debriefing screen was presented to the participant-user, consisting of the diagnoses and tests that the participant selected, and information from an expert practitioner listing the true diagnosis, the tests that should have been selected (if they were not), the most appropriate treatment decision, and the rationale for the treatment or referral decision. Also contained within the debriefing screen was an open-ended text box that allowed the user, after he or she reviewed his or her performance with the case, to enter a reflection/self-assessment on performance and any improvements needed for the next time. After participant-users entered their reflections, they could choose to select another case, receive the case data by email, or save their data and exit. After an option was selected, the reflection data was recorded to the database for post-session analysis.

Following the initial intervention session, consisting of instruction on the CR-MBIMA, participants underwent 3 intervention sessions. During each session, the participant used the application to practice CR using a single expert-reviewed case that focused on lower-extremity vascular disorders, and that was varied from time to time, to limit practice effects as a confounding variable. Following the first practice and 3 intervention sessions, a second post-semistructured task-based interview was collected, following the same procedures as the initial task-based interview, except for the addition of questions pertaining to the CR-MBIMA to use as an additional component in the debriefing session.

TABLE 24-2		
APPLICATION FEATURES AND HOAC II-1 FRAMEWORK SUPPORTED		
APPLICATION SUPPORT	**APPLICATION FEATURE**	**FRAMEWORK SUPPORTED**
Scenario (pre-built)	Application provides initial data to student	Collecting initial data
Application pop-ups: "What is your rationale?"	HOAC not followed in order	Sequence of HOAC II process
Patient History	Application provides a link to information about data to be gathered within the patient history	Knowledge needed for CR
About HOAC	Application provides a link to information about the HOAC II framework	Knowledge about the HOAC II framework
About Conditions	Application provides a link to information about conditions covered by the application	Knowledge needed for CR
About Tests	Application provides a link to information about tests needed to evaluate the patient problem	Knowledge needed for CR
Hint	Application gives a hint about the next step in the evaluative process	Process implementation of the stepwise framework of the HOAC II
Subjective Interview Button	Enter data from referral, case information given, observation, and subjective interview	Collecting initial data
Record Data Button	Application asks the user to create a list of patient problems/symptoms to which the student can refer later, with an open text box for notes or problems/other items the student finds significant	Generating patient-identified problems list
Initial Hypothesis	Application asks the user to input an initial working hypothesis and other hypotheses under consideration to be evaluated	Formulating examination strategy
Objective Examination	Application provides a list of possible tests based upon symptoms; help will be provided for knowing what the tests are, alternate symptoms, or other questions to which they want to know the answer	Formulating examination strategy and conducting the examination
View Results	Application lists positive and negative tests in summative form, symptoms that they looked for, patient-identified problems, and hypotheses	Refining hypotheses and carrying out additional tests as needed
Generate Problem List	Application provides a list of patient and non–patient-identified problems from tests, and allows user input of other detected problems	Adding non–patient-identified problems
Final Hypothesis	Application gives a list of possible patient diagnoses; user will provide a rationale for selecting the diagnosis, and ask for further non–patient-identified problems and for a treatment/referral decision and rationale	Generating a hypothesis, and refining problem list

DATA ANALYSIS METHODS

All qualitative data from the interview sessions—including pre– and post–task-based interview transcriptions, researcher field notes, and participant-users' student work—were analyzed, aided by Atlas TI (a software program that assists in qualitative analysis by helping visualize linkages in data). In analyzing data, a within- and across-case approach allowed the researcher to "develop an in-depth description and analysis of a single case or multiple cases to provide an in-depth understanding."[38(p104)]

Data Collected During Interview Sessions

Data obtained from task-based interview transcriptions, researcher field notes, and student work were analyzed using an a priori code manual (Table 24-3) to guide the data analysis process.[40]

The CR-MBIMA code manual used information from the steps in the HOAC II-1[3] and themes from the CDM frameworks[12] to provide the codes (a priori) for analyzing the narrative process of the think aloud interviews related to the order and types of reasoning used, respectively. The reliability of the code manual was tested using peer debriefing from the pre-intervention phase (first task-based interview) and was revised based upon an inductive coding process to ensure that all participant statements were adequately represented, and their essence maintained.[38,40] Descriptions and definitions of inductive codes related to the CR process that were added are described in Table 24-4.

After the CR-CBIM code manual for the application was revised, Atlas TI was used to collapse codes into higher-level categories, to split codes into more representative categories, and to redefine categories. From this process, an additional inductive theme (reasoning about patient factors) was added to the reasoning framework, relating to the consideration of non–patient-identified and patient-identified problems during the reasoning process. Once data were coded according to the CR process and the HOAC II-1 framework, they were analyzed using a narrative analysis approach. The narrative analysis approach allowed the researcher to provide an explanation for the "complexity of human action with its relationship of temporal sequences and motivations."[41(p7)] Within this analysis, the HOAC II-1 and reasoning strategies expressed by Gilliland[12] were used as a comparative framework to analyze the CR sequence and strategies, respectively, expressed by the student in pre– and post–task-based interviews. Once these data were analyzed, a further analysis looked at the interplay between the sequence and types of reasoning employed to describe the integration between the types and order of reasoning strategies used, and the resultant outcomes from the selection of a reasoning strategy. By analyzing data in this way, the researchers were able to elicit data on the changes produced by the CR-MBIMA to the sequential orientation to the HOAC II-1 or in the types of CR strategies used.

A further analysis was conducted on post questions contained within the first and second interviews related to the participant's attitudes toward perceived factors that may influence CR and decision-making, and on questions that were solely found in the second interview related to CR-MBIMA's utility and effects. These were analyzed using inductive coding, collapsing into axial codes, and then generating themes,[38] aided by Atlas TI. The derived codes used are noted in Table 24-5.

VALIDITY/RELIABILITY

To address validity and reliability of the qualitative findings, several methods were used.[38] First, triangulation occurred among sources of qualitative data (ie, task-based interview session data such as field notes, student worksheets, transcriptions) so that corroborating evidence was located and findings were supported.[38] Second, the reliability of the code manual was tested using peer debriefing, and revised based upon an inductive coding process to ensure that all participant statements were adequately represented and their essence maintained.[38,40] Finally, member checking occurred with the participants, first on the transcription to ensure accuracy, and second to ascertain whether the participants agreed with the themes derived from task-based interviews and researcher field notes. Both peer debriefing and member checking revealed agreement with the subsequent findings.

PRELIMINARY FINDINGS

In total, 6 participants from a medium-sized, Level V Carnegie–classed institution[36] who were enrolled in their first year in a DPT program participated in the study. The research participants constitute a representative sample of their class, being composed of 33% male and 66% female (cohort: 30% male, 70% female), 50% majority and 50% minority (cohort: 60% majority, 40% minority), and an average age of 24.33 (cohort average age: 23 years). However, for this chapter, we will focus on an in-depth analysis of a singular representative case from the study, as remaining data are still being analyzed. Preliminary data analysis from these remaining cases, however, demonstrates that all participants were able to progress using higher-order reasoning strategies as a result of their interactions with the mobile application.

	TABLE 24-3	
THE CODING MANUAL AND RELATIONSHIP TO THE FRAMEWORK		
CODE	**PURPOSE**	**CONNECTION TO A STEP IN THE HOAC II-I OR GILLILAND[12] CR MODEL**
Acquiring patient subjective information	Eliciting information about the patient subjectively	Collecting initial data in the HOAC II framework
Acquiring objective tests and measures	Asking about objective tests	Conducting the examination and analyzing data; seeking data about objective measures (HOAC II step: conduct the initial examination)
Making an assessment (multiple hypotheses)	Proposing multiple hypotheses about the patient problem	Generating a hypothesis about why the problem exists, or used in the initial examination strategy where an initial set of hypotheses are generated from available data and from the patient-identified problems (HOAC II step: generating initial hypothesis in formulating examination strategy)
Cues acquired (summarizing information)	Summarizing information about the patient either subjectively or objectively	Generating a patient-identified or non–patient-identified problem list from data collected (HOAC II step: patient-identified/non-identified problems)
Hypothesis generated	Representing a physical therapy diagnosis	Generating a hypothesis as to why the problem exists (HOAC II step: conduct the examination, generate a hypothesis)
Clinical decision generated	Representing a physical therapy clinical decision toward treatment appropriateness	Deciding if referral or consultation is necessary from the hypothesis generated from the refined list of problems generated from the hypotheses generated or from the test performed (HOAC step: refine problem list, referral if necessary)
Hypothesis reconsideration	Proposing reconsideration of the first diagnosis suggested	Refining hypotheses from conducting the examination, analyzing data, and carrying out additional tests (HOAC step: conduct the examination, generate hypothesis)
Clinical decision reconsideration	Proposing reconsideration of the clinical decision made	Refining the clinical decision made based upon the need for consultation or referral
Strategies employed	Ordering and organizing the evaluative process	Relating to the logical progression of following the HOAC II framework or other CR strategy to progress toward a diagnosis
Missing information	Realizing the information is not enough to generate a diagnosis	Relates to the diagnostic phase of the HOAC II framework; may trigger a return to the collection of further subjective or objective data
Difficulty with hypothesis generation (error made or unable)	Realizing any faulty determination of the patient problem based upon information gathered	Generating a hypothesis as to why the problem exists or a rationale for the hypothesis
Difficulty with CDM (error made or unable)	Realizing any faulty determination of the appropriateness of physical therapy treatment based upon information gathered	Generating a rationale for consultation or referral based upon available data
Reasoning strategies used	Reasoning about pain, trial and error, following protocol, rule in/out, hypothetico-deductive, pattern recognition	Relating to the types of strategies employed during reasoning

continued

	TABLE 24-3 (CONTINUED)	
	THE CODING MANUAL AND RELATIONSHIP TO THE FRAMEWORK	
CODE	PURPOSE	CONNECTION TO A STEP IN THE HOAC II-I OR GILLILAND[12] CR MODEL
Reasoning about pain	Notating the type of reasoning strategy used; using the pain description and aggravating/relieving factors to guide reasoning; and considering chronicity, severity, and irritability	Relating to the CR strategy types
Trial and error	Notating the type of reasoning strategy used, no plan for reasoning or hypothesis from the beginning, reasoning appears randomly generated, no clear movement from one structure to another	Relating to the CR strategy types
Following protocol	Notating the type of reasoning strategy used, following a standard protocol (reference to a protocol to guide evaluation)	Relates to the CR strategy types
Rule in/out	Notating the type of reasoning strategy used, beginning with one or more hypotheses, reasoning about that hypothesis, and moving on to another hypothesis	Relating to the CR strategy types
Hypothetico-deductive	Notating the type of reasoning strategy used, generating hypotheses, and using an organized plan of testing to rule out or rule in; demonstrates ability to shift hypotheses with contradictory information	Relating to the CR strategy types
Pattern recognition	Notating the type of reasoning strategy used, making a primary hypothesis to a matching patient description from prior experience, and using examination to confirm a hypothesis and explaining data findings considering diagnosis	Relating to the CR strategy types
Strategies employed (in HOAC order)	Ordering and organizing the evaluative process, relating to the discourses of the students as they are reasoning through the clinical case	Following the sequence and strategy of the HOAC framework
Strategies employed (out of HOAC order)	Ordering and organizing the evaluative process, relating to the discourses of the students as they are reasoning through the clinical case	Not following the sequence and strategy of the HOAC framework

PARTICIPANT DESCRIPTION—SINGULAR CASE

Sara is a 25-year-old white woman who majored in exercise, sports science, and athletic training. She is a licensed and certified athletic trainer who states that she has some experience with reasoning clinically for the orthopedic population, but does not have experience with other patient populations.

Findings: Themes and Narratives

The following section first thematically illustrates the types of reasoning strategies used pre-and post-intervention using the constructs proposed by Gilliland,[12] and the added inductive CR theme, reasoning about patient-related factors, such as patient-identified and non–patient-identified problems, as a theoretical basis for analysis. Second, it focuses on the narrative related to the order of the reasoning process generated, as related to the HOAC II-1 framework.[3] Third, the interplay between the sequence and types of reasoning employed is related, which integrates the types and order of reasoning strategies used, and the resultant outcomes from the selection of strategy and order of the reasoning process from an inductive coding methodology. Finally, themes related to the participant's perceptions regarding influential constructs that facilitate CR, gleaned pre- and post-intervention from inductive coding, are presented.

TABLE 24-4
INDUCTIVE CODES RELATED TO THE CLINICAL REASONING PROCESS ADDED FROM FIRST- AND SECOND-PASS CODING AND PEER DEBRIEFING

CODE	DEFINITION
0 to 5 minutes spent to collect patient subjective. 5 to 10 minutes spent to collect patient subjective. > 10 minutes spent to collect patient subjective.	Relates to the amount of time spent collecting data
Certainty in clinical decision	Demonstrates confidence in the clinical decision to treat or refer
Clarifying physical therapist role	Clarifies scope of practice or role of a physical therapist
Considering non–patient-identified problems	Uses information gained from steps in the HOAC framework to guide reasoning, hypothesis generation, or treatment rationales that were detected by the physical therapist and not identified by the patient
Considering patient-identified problems	Uses information gained from steps in the HOAC framework to guide reasoning, hypothesis generation, or treatment rationale that were stated by the patient
Cued for HOAC order by interview	Shows interview prompted order of evaluation flow during think aloud
Cues acquired (knowledge support)	Highlights cues used by the student to support the reasoning process through knowledge (sense-making cues)
Diagnosis correct	Recognizes correct diagnosis achieved
Diagnosis correct but not specific	Notes diagnosis was in the right system, but not articulated as a specific diagnosis
External factors influencing hypothesis generation, diagnosis decision, or clinical decision	Recognizes external factors such as scope of practice or participant background influence hypotheses, diagnoses, or clinical decisions
Generating problem list	Generates problem list from patient- or therapist-identified problems
Hypothesis correct	Formulates correct hypothesis
Hypothesis correct but not specific	Formulates hypothesis for correct system, but not specific to a diagnosis
Reasoning about patient factors	Uses factors in the medical history, patient-identified, or non–patient-identified problems in the reasoning process
Treat and refer for physical therapy	Decides to treat and refer (HOAC)
Treatments not best evidenced for condition	Recommends treatment that is not the best evidenced for the condition; in this case, arterial insufficiency, should be graded aerobic exercise
Treatments proposed	Proposes possible treatments for the patient condition
Uncertainty in diagnosis	Expresses uncertainty in diagnosis obtained

TABLE 24-5

INDUCTIVE CODES RELATED TO THE CR-MBIMA'S UTILITY/EFFECT ADDED FROM FIRST AND SECOND PASS CODING AND PEER DEBRIEFING

INDUCTIVE CODE	CODE DEFINITION
Participant liked application	Participant indicated positive feelings toward the application
Mobile application needs changes	Any changes participants recommended to the mobile application
Mobile application increases comprehensiveness of objective tests	Mobile app affected type or amount of objective information collected
Mobile application increases/changes subjective questioning	Mobile app increased subjective information collected or changes noted in questioning (new inductive code)
Mobile application narrows problem focus	Problem list or reasoning more focused from app
Mobile application structures diagnostic process	Structure was provided for diagnostic process from app
Mobile application supports knowledge acquisition	Mobile app helped gain knowledge
Mobile application increases focus/specificity to the objective exam	App helped focus reasoning process by giving different objective tests and questions and focusing the exam (new inductive code)
Disliked about app: debriefing screen not functional	The debriefing screen at the end did not work
Knowledge supports CR	Statements that alluded to gains in knowledge supporting CR, a need for knowledge to support CR
Lack of knowledge as a reason for error or influencing reasoning	Statements that alluded to a lack of knowledge as a cause of error or faulty CR
Need for knowledge to support treatment decisions	Participant cited need for increased knowledge about treatment
Need to collect more objective data to confirm diagnosis	Participant stated need for more objective data to support reasoning
Need to collect more subjective or health history information	Participant stated a need for more subjective information to support CR
Knowledge from coursework supports CR	Participant stated that new knowledge from classwork influenced CR or treatment rationale
Previous experience influencing diagnostic reasoning	Interview stated that previous experience affected the diagnostic process
Previous experience influencing treatment rationale	Participant stated that treatment rationale was influenced by experience

Types of Reasoning Employed and Supports Needed Pre-Intervention

In evaluating the types of reasoning employed initially, there was not a clear, focused strategy for CR. Instead, Sara used a combination of strategies including trial and error, reasoning about pain, following protocol, reasoning about patient-related factors such as patient-identified and non–patient-identified problems, and a rule-in/rule-out strategy. Table 24-6 relates evidence of the types of strategies used during the think aloud.

To generate CR during the first task-based interview, Sara required 3 scaffolds (supports), provided by the facilitating interviewer. The first support was for sense-making related to knowledge support, as exemplified by the following exchanges:

Sara (S): What was that last one?

Interviewer (I): Hyperlipidemia.

	TABLE 24-6
	REASONING STRATEGIES USED PRE- AND POST-INTERVENTION
TYPE OF REASONING	**PITHY QUOTES**
Trial and error	**Pre-** *Only Homan's. I don't think that it has very good reliability. I don't know if that's right.* *I'm still going to go with blood clot just because I don't know enough about the vascular system. Especially the hyperlipidemia, I don't know what that can influence with the vascular system because we haven't gone in that kind of detail with that. I don't think it's an orthopedic problem at this point.* *My diagnosis, I'm still not sure what it is.*
Reasoning about pain	**Pre-** *Just reading the history form, the first thing that popped in mind was what kind of pain she's having, because in here it just says she has lower extremity pain. It's very vague. It also says she walks long distances, so for me, I want to take the vague words that a patient has and try to be more specific with what I want to know to determine what could be the cause of this pain.* **Post-** *All it says is lower extremity pain, so pain can mean a lot of things. So, I need to know what type of pain it is, and then lower extremity could be anywhere in the lower extremity ... Then just knowing what makes it (the pain) worse and better can help you decide if she's tried things on her own or knowing what aggravates her symptoms as well could give you a better idea of what might be precipitating the cause.*
Rule-in/ rule-out	**Pre-** *Only: Because I wanted to look at palpation first to just see generally where her pain is located, so palpating over the musculature structures, some of the vascular structures, some of the neural structures, and even connective tissue just to see if that elicits pain, because then that may make me be surer of what the diagnosis might be. The manual muscle tests could obviously help me decide if it's something going on muscular. The range of motion, that's going to help me look and see how much either the joint is moving or how much tension she's got within a tendon or even ligamentous structures. The special tests can help me decide orthopedically if there's something going on.* *Then checking her range of motion as well, so looking at her knee range of motion, looking at her ankle range of motion, even looking at toe range of motion. If I want to throw in the hip a little bit farther up, if I'm not really seeing any discrepancies down lower I might want to look a little bit farther up as well.*
Following protocol	**Pre-** *Only: Student work page: Writing data in SOAP note format.* *I'd still do a special test even though they all came back negative. I would still want to rule that out. I think they're just as effective in helping you determining what's wrong, as well as the palpation. I wouldn't want to leave out any of those parts of my testing procedures.*
Reasoning about patient-related factors such as patient identified, and non–patient-identified problems	**Pre-** *But I also haven't really evaluated an elderly population, so I think that's something different to look at because their problem list can be different, their health history can be different.* *I'm sure she's seeing a physician for these things or has seen somebody at some point for them. I would recommend her following up to make sure the diabetes is still under control, the hyperlipidemia is under control. I would want to make the doctor aware of the hypertensive reading that I had for her blood pressure. I'm also finding things that I can help her with, so I think that's the reason that I would still suggest, "You can come see me because I can help you work on these things," and it might even be more preventive care than it is to help with the pain right now, which might be more of a vascular issue that can be helped by a physician.* **Post-** *S: Her diabetes, her high blood pressure, her high cholesterol, then her diminished sensation can lead to other problems 'cause then she could have sores or something like that.* *I: Okay, so she could develop wounds.* *S: Yeah, and infections and all that good stuff. Then the ABI [ankle brachial index] just means that she's not really getting the blood flow where she needs to, so it could lead to even more problems. Kidney problems.*

continued

	TABLE 24-6 (CONTINUED)
	REASONING STRATEGIES USED PRE- AND POST-INTERVENTION
TYPE OF REASONING	**PITHY QUOTES**
Pattern recognition	**Post-** Only: *One thing that I'm thinking is there could be something with the arterial system, especially being high cholesterol, high blood pressure, and diabetic, that's going to put more strain on the arterial system. ... Yes, arterial, and then again, we haven't gotten in the stuff with the venous and the arterial system, but the fact that being in a dependent position makes it feel better, in my mind, that makes me think that it's not a venous issue.* *Then also, the cyanosis of the toes means she's not getting the blood flow down there. So that could mean that the arterial system just isn't getting where it needs to be to give you that oxygen and blood.* *Because I was leaning toward something wrong with the vascular system given her medical history and what makes it better and what makes it worse and the type of pain. The only thing that came back as abnormal would be her ABI.* *Meds and comorbidities will kind of go together.*

S: *What's that?*

I: *High lipid levels in her blood.*

S: *I mean, if they're... I guess this is just a question. If they're coming to see us, aren't we supposed to treat them?*

I: *It really depends on the patient case presentation.*

The second support was related to process management for acquiring cues (summarizing information), where Sara states:

Yeah, I think that says on here that yeah, the pain is not associated with a cause.

The third and final support was related to sense-making for cueing related to the sequence of the reasoning process, which will be exemplified in the upcoming discussion of the sequence used.

Types of Reasoning Employed and Supports Needed Post-Intervention

After the 4 sessions with the mobile application, Sara primarily used 2 strategies for reasoning: reasoning about pain and pattern recognition. Interspersed with this were examples of reasoning about patient factors. In contrast to her initial think aloud interview, Sara mainly used process management scaffolding supports during her interview: acquiring cues, summarizing information that she had collected from her initial examination in the objective measure's session to manage cognitive load. An example of this is when she states:

Yes, arterial ... but the fact that being in a dependent position makes it feel better, in my mind, that makes me think that it's not a venous issue. ... But in my mindset, if you're in a dependent position, your veins should be okay if it feels okay to be in that position, if that makes sense.

This was also supported by participant form, where she recorded collected data in a systematic manner to manage her cognitive load. A final support that she used was knowledge support for sense-making; however, there were only 2 instances of this during the interview. One instance is exemplified by the following conversation:

I: *Heart auscultation, you hear an S1 and S2.*

S: *Is that good?*

I: *Lub dub.*

S: *Okay.*

I: *So, it's normal.*

S: *Okay, so no murmur.*

Sequence of the Reasoning Process Employed Pre-Application Use

Sara's reasoning process during the initial interview was frequently out of congruence with the HOAC II-1 algorithmic framework, which resulted in difficulty in data-gathering and generating hypotheses to accurately diagnose the patient's problem. For this reason, Sara was frequently cued by the interviewer to reason within a hypothetico-deductive process for sense-making. This process of reasoning, and the scaffolding provided by the interviewer, is illustrated by describing the narrative process she undertook during the first task-based interview, also illustrated in Figure 24-5, including the prompts offered by the interviewer.

Sara's first decision in her reasoning sequence was when she initiated the interview to collect objective data, as captured in her statement:

I want to know what distances she is walking [walking time to claudication].

Sara's second move was to collect initial data, in the form of patient subjective information:

I would want to know the type of pain she's experiencing, if it's aching, if it's numbness, sharp, shooting, anything like that. I would want to know the pain levels on a scale of 0 to 10, how bad is her pain, and then also how long does her pain last, so does it go away after she's done walking, or does it persist.

Sara's decision to begin by collecting objective data was incongruent with the HOAC II-1 framework in that initial, subjective data should be collected before objective data. Next, after receiving the answers to her subjective questioning, Sara proceeded to collect data from "an objective exam." This decision conflicted with the HOAC II-1 process, which recommends that practitioners first generate a patient-identified problem list, and then form some initial hypotheses (the "formulate exam strategy" step). For these 2 steps in the HOAC II-1 process, the interviewer provided cues to elicit these responses. Specifically, prior to allowing Sara to collect objective data, the interviewer asked Sara to state the patient problems and hypotheses. Her responses were exemplified by the following 2 quotes, respectively:

The biggest thing is her restriction of activity because she can only walk 100 feet before having pain, and it becomes an 8 out of 10, so that's a huge limitation for her, and then any sort of exercise is causing pain.

I am wondering if she has a blood clot.

The fourth step in Sara's reasoning sequence was to collect objective measures, in alignment with the HOAC II-1 framework step of "Conduct the examination, analyze data, refine hypotheses, and carry out additional examination procedures needed to confirm or deny hypotheses."[3(pp459-460)] Sara did this by asking for palpation, manual muscle testing, Homan's sign, range of motion, and strength.

Fifth, after receiving the results of the objective examination, Sara required cues to complete the next 2 steps in the HOAC II-1 process: to state a physical therapist diagnosis ("Generate a hypothesis as to why the problem exists"), and to generate 2 problem lists, one patient-identified and the other non–patient-identified ("Identify the rationale for believing anticipated problems are likely"). During this process, Sara performed hypothesis reconsideration, but her hypothesis was nonspecific (ie, *"All of the orthopedic tests came back negative, so I'm thinking this is more of like a vascular issue because, especially with the paleness of the skin and the blue toes."*) Once further cued, Sara subsequently generated a problem list for anticipated problems or problems that needed to be addressed by the physical therapist:

I think one of the biggest things now that I see is she is hypertensive. I think that's a problem for her. The other problem list is her range of motion. She has no dorsiflexion, and her strength within her gastroc and soleus, and yeah, dorsiflexion as well, so anterior tib and things like that.

Following articulation of her problem list, Sara was cued by the interviewer to identify a more formal diagnosis, to which she stated, *"I'm still going to go with blood clot."* At this point, she was asked by the interviewer what her next step was, and she stated that she would refer, which represents a possible next step in the HOAC II-1 framework. When the interviewer asked for a rationale for this decision to refer rather than treat, she reconsidered:

You (the patient) can come see me because I can help you work on these things, and it might even be more preventive care than it is to help with the pain right now, which might be more of a vascular issue that can be helped by a physician. … I could state to the patient there's a few exercises that I would like you to start doing (for range of motion deficits and strength).

When making this reconsideration, however, Sara neglected the last step in the framework, establishing goals. She made no statements toward goals, even when prompted by the interviewer.

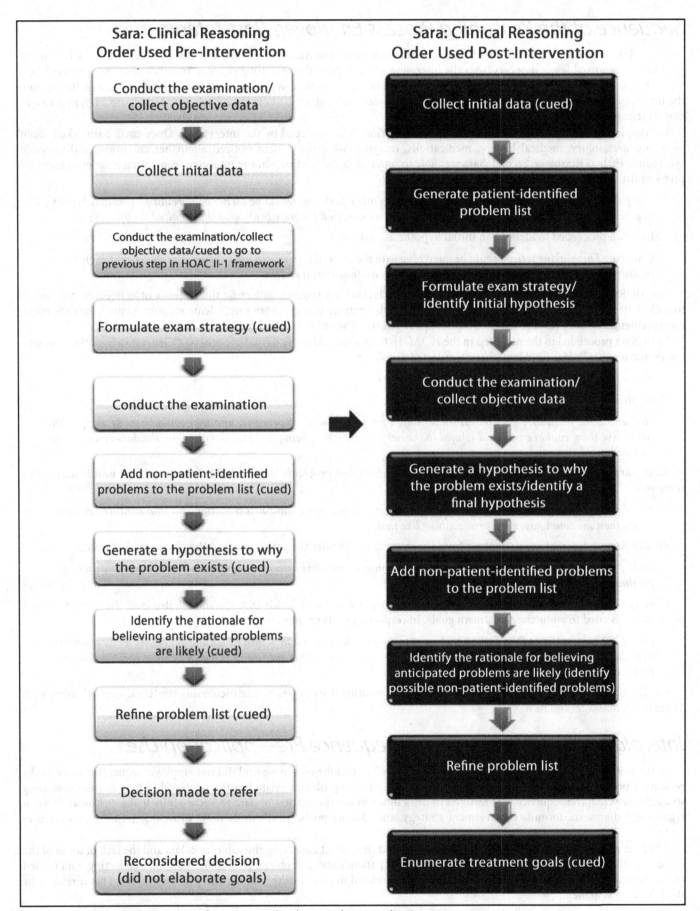

Figure 24-5. Participant's sequence of reasoning utilized pre- and post-application use.

Sequence of the Reasoning Process Employed Post-Intervention

Overall, in Sara's second think aloud interview that occurred post-intervention, she was more sequentially ordered in her process and required fewer supports from the interviewer to complete the reasoning process. In Sara's post-intervention interview, she used pattern recognition, demonstrated by generating a singular hypothesis and testing that hypothesis throughout the interview. Therefore, congruence with the HOAC II-1 was demonstrated, as explained below and in Figure 24-5, in relationship to the singular hypothesis generated.

In completing the first step, collecting initial information, Sara was cued by the interviewer. Once cued, Sara asked about pain, previous injury, medical history, medications, imaging, what the patient noticed about her condition, and systemic symptoms, such as dizziness. Second, Sara was able to proceed to the next step in the interview, generating a patient-identified problem list, where she stated:

> The patient has cramping and aching of the calf, with other problems would be all her comorbidities, previous history of a heart attack, and then her integumentary issues as well, and the muscle atrophy she's noticed.

Third, Sara proceeded to identify an initial hypothesis, stating:

> One thing I'm thinking is there could be something with the arterial system, especially being high cholesterol, high blood pressure, and diabetic, that's going to put more strain on the arterial system.

Fourth, Sara asked to move on to the next step in the HOAC II-1 process, collecting the patient's objective data. She asked to collect 10 pieces of data: blood pressure, heart rate, pulse oximetry, respiratory rate, edema measurements, circumferential measurements, sensory testing, range of motion, strength, and the ankle brachial index.

Fifth, Sara proceeded to the next step in the HOAC II-1 algorithm, identify a final hypothesis ("Generate a hypothesis to why the problem exists"). Her final hypothesis was stated as follows:

> To me it seems like there's insufficiency in her arteries.

Sixth, she proceeded to generate a problem list, stating:

> Her sensation, yeah, she's got diminished sensation for touch and deep pressure, and that could be going along with the … like there could be ischemia related to the nervous system … being diabetic, dorsiflexion, she doesn't have any, and decreased strength.

Next, Sara was cued to identify possible non–patient-identified problems that could lead to diminished health status. Her reply was:

> Her diabetes, her high blood pressure, her high cholesterol, and her diminished sensation can lead to other problems 'cause then she could have sores or something like that.

Finally, Sara chose, without prompting from the interviewer, to refer the patient back to the physician. She stated:

> Well, I'm not really sure really what I would do for someone who has arterial insufficiency or what our guidelines are for that, but I'd probably send her back to the doctor.

However, after making this statement, Sara did change her mind and decide that she should also treat the patient. At this point, she was cued to enumerate treatment goals. In response to this prompt, she stated:

> One of the biggest things would probably be increasing circulation, and then also educating her on her medical history that she has and making sure that she's eating properly and taking her meds and is aware of what can happen with these issues.

Finally, once asked a probing query, Sara listed some treatment strategies of gastrocnemius stretches, strengthening with TheraBand, massage, and heat.

Interplay Between Strategy and Sequence Pre-Application Use

In the initial think aloud interview, Sara used several strategies for reasoning and did not employ a sequential order in the reasoning process. The lack of strategy and order contributed to problems related to the relationship between the reasoning strategies selected and sequence that resulted in difficulties in the integration of data to successfully make a clinical decision regarding a diagnosis, formulate a treatment strategy, and identify goals. To illustrate these difficulties, 4 examples are presented.

The first problem noted in the process related to limited time spent collecting the subjective data and the lack of focus of the subjective questions when analyzed in relationship to the patient's stated problem. Sara spent 3 minutes collecting data related to the patient problem, and only asked general questions related to pain, health history, and previous injury. This is relayed by the following statement:

I would want to know the type of pain she's experiencing, if it's aching, if it's numbness, sharp, shooting, anything like that. I would want to know the pain levels on a scale of zero to 10, how bad is her pain, and then also how long does her pain last, so does it go away after she's done walking, or does it persist. I want to know her previous health history, so if she has any underlying factors that could be causing this. Another thing that I would be interested in is ... any previous injury that she might've had to that lower extremity as well.

After receiving the answers to these questions, she did not follow up to receive more information from the patient to further elicit information that could help direct the evaluation process.

A second issue during the process related to Sara's limited linkage of the subjective data to the articulation of the initial hypothesis and the problem list, therefore creating difficulties with identifying a correct hypothesis and creating an error that persisted throughout the reasoning process. During the problem identification step, Sara only identified and considered one problem in her generating a patient-identified problem list step (the activity limitation) by stating:

The biggest thing is her restriction of activity because she can only walk 100 feet before having pain, and it becomes an 8 out of 10, so that's a huge limitation for her.

Within this step, she did not consider the types of pain the patient experienced, or the patient health history in formulating her problem list, leading to difficulties in articulating a correct hypothesis. Thus, she subsequently identified a blood clot as her initial hypothesis, which did not relate to the patient identified symptoms of:

I: Her pain is relieved by rest, and the pain worsens with exercise. She describes the pain as cramping and aching. Her pain, she rates it at 8 out of 10 with activity, a zero out of 10 with rest. The pain is in both calves. She's able to walk 2 minutes until the onset of pain, which is about 100 feet. The pain resolves after 5 minutes of rest. She can't remember any injury.

The third problem in the reasoning process was the lack of any relationship of the tests selected in the objective examination to the initial: data collected, problems identified, and hypotheses generated, resulting in difficulty with integration of data to formulate a diagnosis and a diagnostic error. This can be best exemplified by Sara's selection of nonspecific and nonconfirmatory tests for her hypothesis of a blood clot, such as blood pressure, orthopedic special tests, range of motion in the knee, ankle, and hip manual muscle testing, palpation, Homan's sign, and visual observation. After receiving results of these tests, Sara proposed a nonspecific diagnosis, stating:

All of the orthopedic tests came back negative, so I'm thinking this is more of like a vascular issue because, especially with the paleness of the skin and the blue toes, it basically means she's not really getting circulation that she needs there, and then with the blood pressure being high, I'm thinking this isn't a muscular or a ligamentous issue or something like that. It's going to be more vascular.

When asked to be more specific about her final diagnosis, she identified her diagnosis (blood clot) without having substantiated data to support her conclusion. Later, Sara expressed:

My diagnosis, I'm still not sure what it is.

Fourth, and finally, Sara demonstrated difficulty in formulating a treatment decision and failed to articulate goals related her diagnostic error. She stated:

I would want to refer for that purpose and see what's going on there, especially since she has the history of the heart attack, the diabetes, and the hyperlipidemia, and then I'm getting a high blood pressure reading on her. In the meantime, I would say, "I think this is very serious. You need to go see your physician, but here's a few exercises that I would like you to start doing."

However, when asked why she made this decision she stated:

I mean, if they're ... I guess this is just a question. If they're coming to see us, aren't we supposed to treat them?

When further probed, Sara decided to refer to the physician, and did not articulate goals, due to uncertainty about the diagnosis.

Interplay Between Strategy and Sequence Post-Application Use

In contrast to the pre-intervention interview, Sara's relationship between strategy and sequence was much more refined, resulting in a more focused subjective questioning, more time spent in the collection of initial data, and a better relationship among the patient-identified problems, subjective information collected, initial problems and hypothesis identified, objective tests selected, problem reconsideration, and final hypothesis generated.

Herein are discussion points of why the themes are supported through Sara's data. First, within her reasoning process, there was more focus in the collection of subjective data related to the amount of time spent collecting subjective data and the questions selected to identify the patient problem. Within the step of collecting initial information, Sara spent more time (8 minutes) collecting data from the interviewer to gain a more detailed subjective description from the patient. Further evident in her collection of data was the process used, moving from less specific questioning to more specific questioning, keeping the patient problems in mind. In her initial questioning, Sara once again asked general questions such as the presence of previous injury, location and type of pain, pain intensity, and aggravating and alleviating factors for pain. In contrast to the initial exam, however, Sara also asked for medications the patient was on to correlate for comorbidities, for any systemic symptoms such as dizziness the patient was having, and for comorbid medical conditions. Her rationale for asking these questions is summarized when she stated:

> Then with this being insidious onset, you want to think about what else she might be having going on in her medical history that could pertain to this issue.

After receiving these answers, she asked for any changes the patient had noticed regarding the condition of her legs, consultations with physicians, and for imaging studies done to "give [me] a better idea of what might be precipitating the cause."

Second, illustrated subsequently is Sara's improvement in her ability to identify relationships among patient-identified problems, subjective information collected, initial problems and hypothesis identified, objective tests selected, problem reconsideration, and final hypothesis generation. As she transitioned from collecting her initial data, Sara was first able to use the answers to the subjective questioning to identify a problem list, stating:

> The cramping and aching of the calf, all her comorbidities, previous history of a heart attack, and then her integumentary issues as well … and the muscle atrophy.

Next, she was able to perform integration of the subjective information into her hypothesis-generation process by stating,

> One thing that I'm thinking is there could be something with the arterial system, especially being high cholesterol, high blood pressure, and diabetic, that's going to put more strain on the arterial system … but the fact that being in a dependent position makes it feel better, in my mind, that makes me think that it's not a venous issue. But I'm not sure if that's correct. But in my mindset, if you're in a dependent position, your veins should be okay if it feels okay to be in that position, if that makes sense … then worse with exercise makes me think that you're having to pump more out so that increases the blood pressure, so that's going to put more strain on the arterial system. Then also, the cyanosis of the toes means she's not getting the blood flow down there. So that could mean that the arterial system just isn't getting where it needs to be to give you that oxygen and blood.

Based upon this reasoning process of identifying a hypothesis and some patient problems, Sara articulated objective measures that addressed 3 areas: comorbidities, nonspecific information, and hypothesis-specific information. In addressing the contribution of comorbidities to patient problems, Sara asked for objective measures of vital signs, checking for sensation and edema, and heart auscultation. Nonspecific information was addressed by asking for information such as range of motion and strength testing. Sara finally tested her hypothesis (an arterial issue) by selecting to receive the results of the ABI. Her rationale for selecting this focus for the tests selected included the following 2 statements:

> I would want to do sensory testing, especially with diabetes.

> Because I was leaning toward something wrong with the vascular system given her medical history and what makes it better and what makes it worse and the type of pain.

Next, Sara used data (ABI) from the objective measures to identify her final hypothesis of arterial insufficiency, stating that the test confirmed "that she's getting decreased blood flow to the lower extremity." Later she also demonstrated integration of all data collected during the interview process when she presented her rationale, stating the following:

> 'Cause in the subjective, she talked about the dependent position being better … Then taking her comorbidities into factor, what are they likely to cause? So, she could be having atherosclerosis and things like that that could then lead to the decreased oxygenation and blood flow through the arterial system.

After identifying this as her patient diagnosis, Sara demonstrated better ability to identify and incorporate patient-identified and non–patient-identified problems into her problem list, stating:

> Her artery isn't working, her sensation, yeah, she's got diminished sensation … like there could be ischemia related to the nervous system with her being a diabetic, her dorsiflexion, she doesn't have any so that could present problems with walking.

Despite the improvements noted above, however, Sara continued to have difficulty with generation of a treatment decision and articulation of goals for treatment. She also made errors during this process, deciding to refer and then to treat using strategies that were not the best evidenced according to the expert-recommended treatment plan of a graded exercise program. When asked, Sara alluded to having difficulty with making the decision to treat or refer and formulating goals, relating it to a lack of knowledge, stating:

> Well, I'm not really sure really what I would do for someone who has arterial insufficiency or what our guidelines are for that, but I'd probably send her back to the doctor … I can't remember [what to do].

	TABLE 24-7A
	PERCEIVED INFLUENCES ON CLINICAL REASONING
	PRE-APPLICATION USE

THEME	SUPPORTING STATEMENTS
Need to collect more information to support CR	*I think maybe asking more about the health history stuff, because I mean, me personally, I don't know much about the hyperlipidemia. I didn't ask the type of diabetes that she has or if she's on the medication for that. So, just a little bit more detailed about her health history. I'd want to add that in there.*
Knowledge is impactful for supporting the CR process	*I need to learn more about the vascular system.*
	We haven't really gotten into detail with SOAP notes or gone over what's included in a subjective and objective and the assessment and the plan components. We have done the objective measurements or parts of them. We've done the range of motion, so being able to know what's normal and abnormal is helpful in this portion of diagnosing this patient.
	I think in anatomy, I've become more aware of the vascular system and the nervous system as well, so keeping those in mind when I'm looking at patients, because I used to be very homed in to the orthopedic side of things, so thinking more like muscular and ligamentous and bone injuries, as opposed to something that could be going on neurovascularly.
Previous experience is impactful for supporting the CR process	*I've worked as an athletic trainer now for 3 years, so I've seen a lot of orthopedic injuries. That's what I'm used to dealing with, and especially on an outpatient basis. I think having a lot of previous experience evaluating individuals is helpful, but I also haven't really evaluated an elderly population, so I think that's something different to look at because their problem list can be different.*
	Working in athletic training, I treat them. It's my athlete, so if they're coming to see me, it's … like my obligation to treat them, as well as when I worked in the physical therapy clinic. We had referrals from a physician, so we didn't have patients just coming in to see us without referrals … I've never had a patient that I've said no to before, so it's kind of a new idea that I can say, "Nope, not going to treat you." I've never done that. I've had to refer a lot of my past people as well because we have a sports med physician that works with every team. If I felt like it was out of my control or out of my scope of practice, then I'd refer to our physician.

Perceived Influences on Clinical Reasoning Pre- and Post-Application Use

In Sara's initial reflection upon the case, and upon experiences that could influence CR, several themes emerged. After using the application, Sara was once again asked to reflect upon the case used in the post-test interview and on experiences that could influence CR. From this reflection, slightly different themes emerged. These themes and supporting statements are in Table 24-7A (pre) and 24-7B (post).

Summary of Themes Related to Clinical Reasoning Pre- and Post-Intervention

From the pre-intervention interview to the post-intervention interview, most themes were congruent, with 2 exceptions. From pre- to post-, Sara continued to identify that knowledge and previous experience were impactful for influencing the reasoning process. However, her perspective changed from needing to collect more subjective information from the patient to the importance of selecting appropriate examination measures for assessment. This change in perspective could be related to the changes in the reasoning process produced by the CR-MBIMA. Another perspective change noted was the influence of external factors such as role definition or scope of practice on the reasoning process, which was possibly related to knowledge gained within the DPT education program, since this was a topic within class during the study period.

TABLE 24-7B
PERCEIVED INFLUENCES ON CLINICAL REASONING POST-APPLICATION USE

THEME	SUPPORTING STATEMENTS
Knowledge is impactful for supporting the CR process	*[I need to] learn more about the vascular system.* *'Cause especially with direct access and people with so many comorbidities knowing what I can and can't do.* *I think pathophys has made you think of all of the complications that can arise.*
Collecting appropriate tests and measures supports the CR process	*I think that also getting more specific for the lower extremity because I didn't ask about the pulse rate and everything for the lower extremity and checking dorsal pedal pulse. I just asked heart rate, which is only regular pulse, which could be different. So, I have to keep that in mind and checking segmentally.* *Oh, crap. I didn't think of the lower extremity as a segment. I was just looking at the body as a whole.*
Previous experience is impactful for supporting the CR process	*Outside of physical therapy school. My background's all musculoskeletal, and I was very positive this was not a musculoskeletal issue, so I was able to rule out musculoskeletal from my experience as an athlete trainer.* *To be honest, we haven't even done SOAP notes and talked about bringing in the subjective and the objective into making an assessment in a plan. That's more from my previous experience bringing all that together.*
External factors like scope of practice and physical therapist role definition are involved in CR	*I can't do anything with her meds and things like that, so she needs to see the doctor for those type of things. I can help with the range of motion since she doesn't have that.* *There are things on … within my scope of practice, like treating the musculoskeletal, and helping with the circulation, and patient education. But … if the meds need to be adjusted or if there's something more going on with her heart, like maybe she needs some other imaging … to make sure there's nothing going on up in there since she does have a history of a heart attack, I can't do that.*

CR-MBIMA Themes Emerging Post-Intervention

During the post-interview, feedback about the CR-MBIMA was sought to determine its possible impact on the CR process and to determine what changes, if any, needed to be made. Sara identified that the CR-MBIMA was impactful in 3 ways: structuring the process of examination, increasing the problem focus, and increasing knowledge. Supporting statements for these themes are found in Table 24-8.

DISCUSSION

In considering the effects of the CR-MBIMA, 3 key areas of the CR process were impacted. These areas were changes in the types of reasoning strategies used and supports needed, sequence of the reasoning process, and interplay between strategy and sequence, which resulted in refinements in the amounts and types of information collected, better integration of information during the CR process, and better problem identification (ie, more correct diagnoses) with decreased error. Despite these impacts, CR-CBIM mobile application, in this one instance, with a novice DPT student learner, did not seem to appear to impact the process of making a treatment decision. Each of these outcomes is now considered with respect to the CR literature.

THEMES	**SUPPORTING STATEMENTS**

TABLE 24-8

CR-MBIMA—FOCUSED THEMES

THEMES	SUPPORTING STATEMENTS
The mobile application structures the process of examination	*I tried to think in the line of here was your questions that you asked, then all of the, not just special tests, but vital signs and things like that, that's what reminded me at the end like, "Oh, crap. I didn't think of the lower extremity as a segment. I was just looking at the body as a whole." That's what reminded me of that. I was like, "Oh, oops."* *S: I think it moreso changed the questions that I asked and the objective information that I gathered.* *I: Okay. So, more kind of structured your diagnostic process.* *S: Mmm-hmmm [affirmative].* *I would ask the objective stuff that I thought was more important first, and then I could go through it and I could get those answers, then that could help me decide if I wanted to ask something more in-depth, and I could go back and say, "Okay, now I want to look at this subjectively," rather than giving me all the information.*
The mobile application supports knowledge	*Because there was a couple I was like, "I don't know what this is," but then you can flip directly to it.* *I liked that you could go through and see what those tests were.*
The mobile application increases problem focus	*The mobile application helps me to consider different segments, 'cause in my mind I normally just think of it as a whole, and sometimes I don't take in the segments unless I'm doing a special test, and that's about it.* *There's the one screen where you put the 4 things that you think are the biggest problems … I think a couple of pages after that, it's like, "Are there any more problems?" But I didn't write anything down there because I felt like I had sufficient enough information within the 4 problems.*

REASONING STRATEGIES USED AND SUPPORTS NEEDED

Reasoning Strategies Used Pre- and Post-Intervention

From the initial interview to the subsequent interview, changes in the reasoning strategies used were observed from the narrative analysis. From this analysis, it appears that the CR-MBIMA facilitated the use of higher-order reasoning strategies, which presents the first evidence for CR-CBIM mobile technology's ability to influence and improve the types of CR strategies used with DPT students. This improvement is best illustrated by comparing Sara's initial and subsequent strategies used for CR. Based upon the thematic coding of the initial interview, Sara's initial strategy for CR was to use a combination of strategies including trial and error, rule-in/rule-out, and following protocol. The use of these types of unsophisticated strategies in the initial interview is congruent with the literature regarding the development of reasoning in DPT students.[12]

However, subsequent to the use of the CR-MBIMA, Sara demonstrated the use of a more sophisticated, higher-order reasoning strategy within her interview—namely, pattern recognition. This gain in the ability to use a higher-order strategy to clinically reason may be attributable to the use of hard scaffolds for sense-making (making the disciplinary strategy evident) and process management (consistent identification of the steps in the process) to support the reasoning process.[2] This progression of reasoning is congruent with Gilliland,[12] who found that students can progress in their reasoning strategies through practice and the use of reasoning frameworks, resulting in more sophisticated (higher-order) strategies of CR. Congruent also with Gilliland[12] is the maintained use of the strategy of reasoning about pain, both pre-and post-intervention.

A second finding related to the progression of CR fostered by the CR-MBIMA is related to the consideration of patient-identified and non–patient-identified problems. While Sara's use and development of CR strategies was mainly congruent with Gilliland's conjectures about the development of CR, Sara's ability to consider patient-identified and non–patient-identified problems during the pre-interview session from a limited standpoint, and post-interview session using an integrative approach, was in contrast to Gilliland's findings that an advancement of CR comes with the ability to consider patient-identified and non–patient-identified problems during the reasoning process.[12] The ability to consider these problems in both Sara's initial and subsequent sessions may be due to the fact that Sara is an athletic trainer, and therefore may have some experience with CR. This may have caused her to initially and subsequently integrate her experiences to inform her thought process, congruent with previous studies on CR.[9,10]

Scaffolds Needed for the Reasoning Process Pre- and Post-Intervention

In congruence with Sara's development of CR fostered by the CR-MBIMA was the decreased use of needed supports (scaffolds) from the pre- to post-intervention interviews for sense-making. During her pre-intervention interview, Sara required scaffolding to support sense-making (ie, knowledge support and sequencing of the reasoning process). The use of sense-making types of scaffolds for both knowledge supports and sequencing pre-intervention is consistent with the literature that states that novice practitioners and students who are developing CR skills need to be supported with educational approaches that allow students to process data using decisional pathways or algorithmic frameworks, form hypotheses, and recall and organize knowledge.[5,14] Post-intervention, Sara required fewer sense-making supports (ie, 2 instances of knowledge support) to facilitate the reasoning process, albeit lower levels of cognition processing. This decrease could be attributable to the use of the CR-MBIMA in that it may have increased Sara's organization of knowledge and depth of knowledge, consistent with Patel et al,[9] who found that algorithmic frameworks when used with CBIM increased knowledge and the ability to organize that knowledge to inform hypothesis generation.

In spite of the decreased use of sense-making cues during the reasoning process, Sara continued to need process management supports to summarize information, thereby mitigating cognitive load, which has been posited to improve decision processes and decrease error.[42] Therefore, the sustained use of this scaffold by the learner could present an identified need for teaching methodologies to teach students to better manage the information collected during reasoning process, for synthesis and application, or use a CR-MBIMA such as the one under study, which returns information at key decision points to manage cognitive load while students are learning to reason.

ORDER OF THE CLINICAL REASONING PROCESS

In evaluating the narrative organization of the CR process, Sara's initial reasoning strategy was less focused and less organized, which is congruent with previous research.[43] Subsequent to application use, it is apparent that Sara used a more organized process for the collection of data. This organization could have been facilitated by the hard scaffolds present in the CR-MBIMA related to sense-making and process management, namely using an algorithmic framework to make the disciplinary strategy for CR evident, and breaking down the task into its component parts using ordered task decompositions.[2] Practitioners are better able to organize knowledge when algorithmic processes using CBI, based upon the hypothetico-deductive model of reasoning, are used to structure the CR process.[44] The challenge occurs with the deconstruction and reconstruction of making meaning of the data with the novice DPT.

Similar findings were noted using the HOAC I framework to support CR, which uses a similar structure for CR to the HOAC II.[45] The HOAC I model, when used with DPT students on a first clinical rotation, helped students "think about what they were doing and why they were doing it."[45(p5)] The model also assisted them in "identifying omissions in their assessment, treatment, or reasoning."[45(p8)] Finally, research by Gilliland[12] found that the integration of external frameworks in DPT curricula with first-year students, similar to the HOAC II, allowed them to better scaffold the reasoning process, resulting in a more organized and sequential process.

INTERPLAY BETWEEN STRATEGIES AND SEQUENCE

While Sara was able to consider patient-identified and non–patient-identified problems prior to using the CR-MBIMA, her process was not refined. In contrast, during the post–think aloud interview, the influence of the CR-MBIMA is demonstrated by better problem prioritization and improved integration of the patient problems to shape the reasoning process. Her enhancements in problem prioritization could be due to the hard scaffolds present in the application, resulting in development of CR.[11,12,46] These scaffolds, provided throughout the reasoning process, focus on 2 areas: sense-making, and articulation and reflection.

First, sense-making was scaffolded by providing textual information in the manner of embedding expert guidance to clarify characteristics of scientific practices.[2] This scaffold was used for assisting the learner to perform problem prioritization and identification. Second, the articulation and reflection process for providing reminders and guidance to facilitate productive monitoring[2] was scaffolded via text entry boxes. These boxes prompted the learner to articulate his or her thought processes.

In summary, these scaffolds asked the learner to prioritize, articulate, and then subsequently refine problems, which may cause the learner to employ metacognition during CR. The use of metacognition during the reasoning process may have improved her reasoning process by allowing her to react to the uncertain features of the clinical problem, and then better integrate or change tactics, refine the articulation of problems, or reduce errors made.[6,9,47,48]

Another explanation for the enhanced interplay among the subjective information acquired, the problems identified, and the objective examination measures identified could relate to the development of a more relative and accurate knowledge base. This enhancement in knowledge could have been produced from soft scaffolds present with the application, which provided sense-making through discipline-specific knowledge supports (ie, embedded expert guidance to help learners use and apply content),[2] as cognitive-based CR may be supported by gains in discipline-specific knowledge.[4,13,15]

Finally, findings that Sara was able to formulate a better relationship between the CR strategy and sequence, used post-intervention, could be attributable to the use of the case-based methodology within the CR-MBIMA. Support for this assertion is found in a study using case-based CBI methodology conducted by Seif et al[20] using a pre-test/post-test design to determine the effects of a sequential, clinically based case, presented through Moodle, a learning management system. From pre- to post-test, improvements from this intervention were found in the cognitive domains of seeking data, comparing information, planning the examination strategy, and hypothesizing reasoning for problems, as well as using experience, or pattern recognition, as a form of CR.[20]

ERRORS IN REASONING

Sara's progress in CR from pre- to post-intervention included a reduction in diagnostic errors; however, her progress did not include a change in her clinical decision to treat the patient, or in the clinical strategies selected, where errors persisted. During Sara's initial interview, errors were made in the diagnostic reasoning process, consistent with novice practitioners tending to have difficulty evaluating hypotheses and making correct clinical decisions once they gather information from the patient.[6,12,13] The errors in the initial session related to not considering disconfirming data that ruled out her initial hypothesis and final hypothesis, and not collecting sufficient data in the collect initial data step of the process, and not integrating data given in all steps to formulating a diagnosis or treatment plan. The commission of error in the initial interview is consistent with 2 types of cognitive sources of error discussed in Section I, Chapter 3, Table 3-3 of this text. First is anchoring, or "the tendency to perceptually lock onto salient features in the diagnostic process, and failing to adjust this initial impression in light of later information."[47] Second is confirmation bias, "the tendency to look for confirming evidence to support a diagnosis rather than look for disconfirming evidence to refute it, despite the latter often being more persuasive and definitive."[47(p777)] In contrast, during her post-interview session, Sara was more organized in her process, using a data-driven method of pattern recognition that was not influenced by biasing errors. This use of clear, unambiguous, decision-making in this session yielded a more accurate diagnosis and could have resulted from the application structure.[3,49,50]

While Sara was able to make more precise and correct decisions related to diagnosis post-intervention, errors persisted from pre- to post-intervention, related to deciding if and how to treat the patient's diagnosis. This commission of error could have related to insufficient experience in making informed decisions[49] toward treatment and treatment interventions, as well as the lack of emphasis on the second part of the HOAC II framework present in the CR-MBIMA related to intervention. Therefore, if enhancing treatment decisions or treatment intervention is a desired impact of the CR-MBIMA, development of this application should focus upon explicitly elaborating treatment strategies to improve CR relative to treatment.

PERCEIVED INFLUENCES ON CLINICAL REASONING

Sara's perceived influences on CR were similar pre- and post-intervention, with a few exceptions. Congruent themes were found pre- and post-intervention for the impact of knowledge and previous experience in supporting the CR process. Interestingly, this supports the development of expert practice in physical therapy that cites the impact of prior professional experience and the need for a patient-centered, well-organized, accessible, comprehensive, relevant, and accurate knowledge base.[5,49,51] This finding is significant because it gives evidence from a novice practitioner for the need for academicians to provide concrete experiences and knowledge supports to allow full development of the cognitive components of CR.[5,49,51]

The implication for DPT educational practice is that students need to be taught how to collect and prioritize subjective and objective information during the development of CR. Researchers[52] suggest that learning to reason involves being contextually immersed in the context of clinical practice and includes values and beliefs of professional socialization and culture. Therefore, based upon this information, it is important for educators to find contextually significant experiences such as case studies (used in the CR-MBIMA), live or videotaped patients, and/or clinical practice experiences that include elements of scope of practice and role definition.

CR-MBIMA Themes

For this case, 3 themes emerged from the post-interview process: the CR-MBIMA structures the process of examination, the CR-MBIMA supports knowledge, and the CR-MBIMA increases the ability to focus upon the problems present within the case to facilitate problem-solving. The emergent themes that the CR-MBIMA can structure the process of examination and support knowledge parallel the works of Friedman et al[53] indicating that CBI via a decisional support system was able to increase physicians' diagnostic performance, hypothesis generation, and CR by providing the information and organization of knowledge needed at point of care.

LIMITATIONS

There are some limitations to this study. First, it is not known if all knowledge acquired by the participant during the investigational test period was solely due to the influence of the CR-MBIMA, as the participant was simultaneously enrolled in DPT coursework. However, this coursework did not strongly emphasize the same content within the CR-MBIMA. Second, it is not known if the effects from the CR-MBIMA on creating higher-order reasoning strategies, better problem identification, more focused subjective and objective data collection, and better organization of the reasoning process will be found in other participants, with early analysis of remaining data trending similarly. Further analysis using a within and across case approach will be used to further confirm or disconfirm these effects. Finally, it is not known if the study participant will continue to demonstrate the ability to use higher-order reasoning strategies or conduct an examination using a sequential procedure like the HOAC II-1, with future cases encountered.

SUGGESTIONS FOR FUTURE RESEARCH

First, subsequent clinical interactions should be observed in these students to determine if the gains in knowledge related to the use of CR strategies and sequencing translate to future clinical performance. Second, a comparison between the cognitive load induced by the think aloud and CR-MBIMA should be conducted to see if the CR-MBIMA does indeed help students manage extraneous cognitive load (ie, load that is not pertinent to the CR process) and induce germane cognitive load that is needed for learning. Third, the mobile application should be implemented using a larger sample size or control group with differing levels of DPT students and residents to determine effects on the sequence and types of CR used. Fourth and finally, the design of the mobile application should be evaluated to see if enhancements can improve the learning process.

CONCLUSION

By using developmental andragogy that focuses on the use of instructional scaffolding with a discipline-specific framework within a CR-MBIMA, it appears that students can acquire improved abilities to perform CR tasks, and progress reasoning more like expert practitioners. This is especially important when considering how effective CR-CBIM mobile technology may be in supporting the reasoning process as students are participating in clinical experiences. As novice students become better equipped to clinically reason through CR-CBIM by using higher-order reasoning strategies, being better able to identify problems, and becoming more sequential in their reasoning process, the gap between novice practitioner and expert CR should narrow. This should allow new graduates to improve the diagnostic process and present with more effective CR-CDM that are in the best interest of their patients/clients, sooner rather than later.

REFERENCES

1. Davidson-Shivers G, Rasmussen K. *Web-Based Learning: Design, Implementation, and Evaluation.* Upper Saddle River, NJ: Merrill Prentice Hall; 2006.
2. Quintana C, Reiser BJ, Davis EA, et al. A scaffolding design framework for software to support science inquiry. *J Learn Sci.* 2004;13(3):337-386.
3. Rothstein JM, Echternach JL, Riddle DL. The hypothesis-oriented algorithm for clinicians II (HOAC II): a guide for patient management. *Phys Ther.* 2003;83(5):455-470.
4. Edwards I, Jones M, Carr J, Braunack-Mayer A, Jensen GM. Clinical reasoning strategies in physical therapy. *Phys Ther.* 2004;84(4):312-330.
5. Terry W, Higgs J. Educational programmes to develop clinical reasoning skills. *Aust J Physiother.* 1993;39(1):47-51.
6. Wainwright SF, Shepard KF, Harman LB, Stephens J. Novice and experienced physical therapist clinicians: a comparison of how reflection is used to inform the clinical decision-making process. *Phys Ther.* 2010;90(1):75-88.

7. Smith M, Higgs J, Ellis E. Factors influencing clinical decision making. In: Higgs J, Jones M, Loftus S, Christensen N, eds. *Clinical Reasoning in the Health Professions*. 3rd ed. Amsterdam, Netherlands: Butterworth-Heinemann Elsevier; 2008:89-100.

8. May S, Greasley A, Reeve S, Withers S. Expert therapists use specific clinical reasoning processes in the assessment and management of patients with shoulder pain: a qualitative study. *Aust J Physiother*. 2008;54(4):261-266.

9. Patel VL, Kaufman DR, Kannampallil TG. Diagnostic reasoning and decision making in the context of health information technology. *Reviews of Human Factors and Ergonomics*. 2013;8(1):149-190.

10. Boshuizen H, Schmidt HG. On the role of biomedical knowledge in clinical reasoning by experts, intermediates and novices. *Cogn Sci*. 1992;16(2):153-184.

11. Embrey DG, Guthrie MR, White OR, Dietz J. Clinical decision making by experienced and inexperienced pediatric physical therapists for children with diplegic cerebral palsy. *Phys Ther*. 1996;76(1):20-33.

12. Gilliland S. Clinical reasoning in first-and third-year physical therapist students. *J Phys Ther Educ*. 2014;28(3):64-77.

13. Doody C, McAteer M. Clinical reasoning of expert and novice physiotherapists in an outpatient orthopaedic setting. *Physiotherapy*. 2002;88(5):258-268.

14. Higgs J. Developing clinical reasoning competencies. *Physiotherapy*. 1992;78(8):575-581.

15. Jensen GM, Shepard KF, Gwyer J, Hack LM. Attribute dimensions that distinguish master and novice physical therapy clinicians in orthopedic settings. *Phys Ther*. 1992;72(10):711-722.

16. Higgs J, Hunt A. Rethinking the beginning practitioner: introducing the "interactional professional." In: Higgs J, Edwards H, eds. *Educating Beginning Practitioners*. Melbourne, Victoria, Australia: Butterworth Heinemann; 1999:10-18.

17. Kenyon LK. The hypothesis-oriented pediatric focused algorithm: a framework for clinical reasoning in pediatric physical therapist practice. *Phys Ther*. 2013;93(3):413-420.

18. Huhn K, McGinnis PQ, Deutsch JE. A comparison of 2 case delivery methods: virtual and live. *J Phys Ther Educ*. 2013;27(3):41-47.

19. Bayliss AJ, Warden SJ. A hybrid model of student-centered instruction improves physical therapist student performance in cardiopulmonary practice patterns by enhancing performance in higher cognitive domains. *J Phys Ther Educ*. 2011;25(3):14.

20. Seif GA, Brown D, Annan-Coultas D. Fostering clinical-reasoning skills in physical therapist students through an interactive learning module designed in the Moodle learning management system. *J Phys Ther Educ*. 2013;27(3):32-40.

21. Thistlethwaite JE, Davies D, Ekeocha S, et al. The effectiveness of case-based learning in health professional education. A BEME systematic review: BEME guide no. 23. *Med Teach*. 2012;34(6):e421-e444.

22. Demetriadis SN, Papadopoulos PM, Stamelos IG, Fischer F. The effect of scaffolding students' context-generating cognitive activity in technology-enhanced case-based learning. *Comput Educ*. 2008;51(2):939-954.

23. Sharma P, Hannafin MJ. Scaffolding in technology-enhanced learning environments. *Interact Learn Environ*. 2007;15(1):27-46.

24. Bruning RH, Schraw GJ, Norby, MM. *Cognitive Psychology and Instruction*. 5th ed. Boston, MA: Pearson; 2011.

25. Cook DA, Erwin PJ, Triola MM. Computerized virtual patients in health professions education: a systematic review and meta-analysis. *Acad Med*. 2010;85(10):1589-1602.

26. Veneri D. The role and effectiveness of computer-assisted learning in physical therapy education: a systematic review. *Physiother Theory Pract*. 2011;27(4):287-298.

27. Ally M. *Mobile Learning: Transforming the Delivery of Education and Training*. Athabasca, Canada: Athabasca University Press; 2009.

28. Hoglund LT. Mobile devices and software applications to promote learning in a musculoskeletal physical therapy class: a case report. *J Phys Ther Educ*. 2015;29(2):54.

29. Mayfield CH, Ohara PT, O'Sullivan PS. Perceptions of a mobile technology on learning strategies in the anatomy laboratory. *Anat Sci Educ*. 2013;6(2):81-89.

30. Noguera JM, Jiménez JJ, Osuna-Pérez MC. Development and evaluation of a 3D mobile application for learning manual therapy in the physiotherapy laboratory. *Comput Educ*. 2013;69:96-108.

31. Kozma RB. Will media influence learning? Reframing the debate. *Educ Technol Res Dev*. 1994;42(2):7-19.

32. Premkumar K. Mobile learning in medicine. In: Kitchenham A, ed. *Models for Interdisciplinary Mobile Learning: Delivering Information to Students*. Hershey, PA: IGI Global; 2011:137-153.

33. Foreman KB, Morton DA, Musolino GM, Albertine KH. Design and utility of a web-based computer-assisted instructional tool for neuroanatomy self-study and review for physical and occupational therapy graduate students. *Anat Rec*. 2005;285(1):26-31.

34. Coulby C, Hennessey S, Davies N, Fuller R. The use of mobile technology for work-based assessment: the student experience. *Br J Educ Technol*. 2011;42(2):251-265.

35. Sharples M, Taylor J, Vavoula G. *Towards a Theory of Mobile Learning*. 2005;1(1):1-9.

36. Schnur JA. *Southern Association of Colleges and Schools, Commission on Colleges* (SACS-COC). Applications files. 2007.

37. Portney LG, Watkins MP. *Foundations of Clinical Research: Applications to Practice*. 3rd ed. Upper Saddle River, NJ: Prentice Hall; 2008.

38. Creswell JW. *Qualitative Inquiry and Research Design: Choosing Among 5 Approaches*. 3rd ed. Thousand Oaks, CA: Sage Publications, Inc; 2012.

39. Creswell JW, Clark VLP. *Designing and Conducting Mixed Methods Research*. 2nd ed. Hoboken, NJ: Wiley Online Library; 2010.

40. DeCuir-Gunby JT, Marshall PL, McCulloch AW. Developing and using a codebook for the analysis of interview data: an example from a professional development research project. *Field Methods*. 2011;23(2):136-155.

41. Polkinghorne DE. Narrative configuration in qualitative analysis. *Int J Qual Stud Educ*. 1995;8(1):5-23.

42. Croskerry P. Achieving quality in clinical decision making: cognitive strategies and detection of bias. *Acad Emerg Med*. 2002;9(11):1184-1204.

43. Patel VL, Arocha JF, Zhang J. Thinking and reasoning in medicine. In: Keith Holyoak, ed. *The Cambridge Handbook of Thinking and Reasoning*. Cambridge, United Kingdom: Cambridge University Press 2005.

44. Patel VL, Arocha JF, Diermeier M, How J, Mottur-Pilson C. Cognitive psychological studies of representation and use of clinical practice guidelines. *Int J Med Inf.* 2001;63(3):147-167.
45. Wessel J, Williams R, Cole B. Physical therapy students' application of a clinical decision-making model. *Internet J Allied Health Sci Pract.* 2006;4(3):8.
46. Case K, Harrison K, Roskell C. Differences in the clinical reasoning process of expert and novice cardiorespiratory physiotherapists. *Physiotherapy.* 2000;86(1):14-21.
47. Croskerry P. The importance of cognitive errors in diagnosis and strategies to minimize them. *Acad Med.* 2003;78(8):775-780.
48. Tan S, Ladyshewsky R, Gardner P. Using blogging to promote clinical reasoning and metacognition in undergraduate physiotherapy fieldwork programs. *Aust J Educ Tech.* 2010;26(3):355-368.
49. Wainwright SF, Shepard KF, Harman LB, Stephens J. Factors that influence the clinical decision making of novice and experienced physical therapists. *Phys Ther.* 2011;91(1):87-101.
50. Croskerry P. Achieving quality in clinical decision making: cognitive strategies and detection of bias. *Acad Emerg Med.* 2002;9(11):1184-1204.
51. Jensen GM, et al. Expert practice in physical therapy. *Phys Ther.* 2000;80(1):28-43.
52. Aljawi R, Higgs J. Learning to reason: a journey of professional socialisation. *Adv Health Sci Educ.* 2008;13(2):133-150.
53. Friedman CP, Elstein AS, Wolf FM, et al. Enhancement of clinicians' diagnostic reasoning by computer-based consultation: a multisite study of 2 systems. *JAMA.* 1999;282(19):1851-1856.

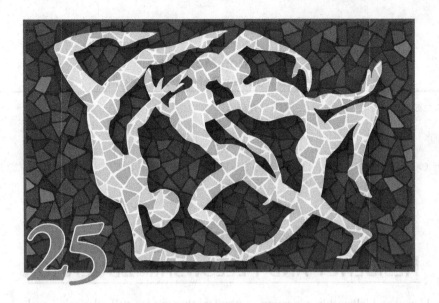

PROMOTING CLINICAL REASONING WITHIN CLINICAL TEACHING IN POST-PROFESSIONAL RESIDENCY AND FELLOWSHIP PROGRAMS

Gregory W. Hartley, PT, DPT, GCS, FNAP and John Seiverd, PT, DPT

OBJECTIVES

- Discuss the evolution of physical therapy residency and fellowship education in the United States and the relationship with clinical reasoning (CR) for expert practice.
- Compare post-professional residency and fellowship education.
- Describe one model outlining clinical skill development progression to enhance CR.
- Explore competency-based assessment of the resident and/or fellow-in-training (FiT).
- Select effective remediation strategies for post-professional residents and FiTs.
- Analyze effective strategies to assess professional behaviors and the affective domain among post-professional residents and FiTs.
- Examine the concept and integration of the hidden curriculum in educating post-professional residents and FiTs.

Musolino GM, Jensen GM, eds. *Clinical Reasoning and Decision-Making in
Physical Therapy: Facilitation, Assessment, and Implementation* (pp 299-319).
© 2020 Taylor & Francis Group.

Reflection Moment:
Points to Ponder Before We Begin

Have you ever considered a residency or FiT? Why or why not?

Why do you think residencies and fellowships are relevant for physical therapists?

How would you expect a resident or FiT to affect society differently than an entry-level doctor of physical therapy (DPT)?

AN OVERVIEW OF PHYSICAL THERAPY
RESIDENCY AND FELLOWSHIP EDUCATION

Post-professional residency and fellowship education in physical therapy are still relatively novel when compared to medicine and some other health professions. Post-professional educational programs (ie, residencies and fellowships) are designed to prepare physical therapists for advanced practice in a defined specialty (residency) or subspecialty (fellowship) area of practice through both didactic and clinical training. Not to be confused with training that occurs in clinical education internships or experiences, these programs are completed post-licensure, are formal in nature (ie, planned by design), and are eligible for accreditation by the American Board of Physical Therapy Residency and Fellowship Education (ABPTRFE), a board of the American Physical Therapy Association (APTA). The overarching goal of post-professional residency and fellowship programs is to produce physical therapists who demonstrate superior and advanced skills and knowledge in all areas of physical therapy including CR, educational techniques, research methodology, professionalism, communication, and administrative practices. An important distinction is that post-professional residents and fellows are not students. Post-professionals are licensed physical therapists who are enrolled in programs designed to elevate their knowledge and skills in a defined area of practice. According to ABPTRFE, a residency is defined as follows:

> *A post-professional planned learning experience in a focused area of practice. Similar to the medical model, a residency program is a structured educational experience (both didactic and clinical) for physical therapists following entry-level education and licensure that is designed to significantly advance the physical therapist's knowledge, skills, and attributes in a specific area of practice (ie, Cardiovascular/Pulmonary, Faculty, Orthopedics, Sports, Pediatrics, etc). It combines opportunities for ongoing mentoring, with a theoretical basis for advanced practice and scientific inquiry based on a Description of Specialty Practice (see definition), Description of Residency Practice (see definition), or valid analysis of practice/comprehensive needs assessment for that specific area of practice. When board certification exists through ABPTS [American Board of Physical Therapy Specialties] for that specialty, the residency training prepares the physical therapist to pass the certification examination following graduation. A residency candidate must be licensed as a physical therapist in the State where the program is located/clinical training will occur prior to entry into the program. Neither "residency" nor "fellowship" is synonymous with the term* internship.[1]

ABPTRFE defines a fellowship program as follows:

> *A post-professional planned learning experience in a focused advanced area of practice. Similar to the medical model, a fellowship is a structured educational experience (both didactic and clinical) for physical therapists which combines opportunities for ongoing mentoring with a theoretical basis for advanced practice and scientific inquiry in a defined area of subspecialization beyond that of a defined specialty area of practice. A fellowship candidate has either completed a residency program in a related specialty area or is a board-certified specialist in the related area of specialty. Fellowship training is not appropriate for new physical therapy graduates.*[2]

Thus, the progression of knowledge, skills, and abilities for the physical therapist could be described objectively in this way: Upon completion of entry-level professional education, the physical therapist has basic information in a vast array of practice areas, encompassing the entire spectrum of the physical therapist's scope of practice. Post-professional residency training then tightens the lens to a single foci of specialty practice (eg, orthopedics, geriatrics, neurology, women's health, oncology, pediatrics, cardiovascular/pulmonary, clinical electrophysiology, sports, and nonclinical faculty), while deepening the level of competence within that specialty. Progression to a fellowship narrows the scope even further (eg, spine, neonatology, movement system, and nonclinical/higher education), all the while increasing the depth of knowledge, skill, and abilities within that area of subspecialization. There should be a general progression of skill acquisition from the novice to the advanced beginner, competent, proficient, and perhaps expert levels of practice as one progresses along the continuum.[3]

Residency programs are planned in the sense that the participants' caseloads, educational projects, and teaching are closely managed—so that if they are in a neurology residency, for example, all their patients have neurological conditions. Participants do not treat other types of patients and have them count toward their required residency hours. Additionally, in what some argue is the hallmark of residency and fellowship education, mentoring occurs in a planned and orchestrated fashion.[4] Therefore, mentors should be highly trained educators who understand andragogy in the context of clinical teaching, and frame mentoring sessions in a planned and structured way that ideally correlates with the didactic content each resident or FiT is learning concurrently. Mentoring faculty should be well versed in the requirements of the post-professional programs. Mentors should be able to teach CR within the population of specialized practice.

Ideally, behavioral milestones for participants should be clear, and residents or FiTs should be educated in ways that foster achievement of established benchmarks, within the planned residency or fellowship curriculum.[4] Skilled faculty manage the curricular progress and processes and facilitate the resident or fellow in achieving curricular goals in a highly clinical context that demands attention to process, structure, and oversight. Post-professional programs have the option of becoming accredited by the ABPTRFE to demonstrate that the curricular characteristics are in place and operating adequately.

ABPTRFE creates and maintains accreditation standards for residency and fellowship post-professional programs.[5] The accreditation process has evolved over the past 20 years, and continues to evolve today. Again, to be clear, post-professional residency and fellowship programs are not the same as clinical education experiences or internships for professional (entry-level) students. To meet accreditation standards, residency and fellowship programs must provide direct oversight of the entire educational process. Even though the resident or fellow is a licensed professional, oversight is provided for the resident's time in the following 3 key areas: patient care, mentoring, and didactic learning. For the resident or fellow in faculty and/or higher education, this may include the correlates of teaching and scholarly works, mentoring, and didactic learning. On average, physical therapy residency and fellowship programs are approximately 1 year in length, though there is variability based upon the chosen focus area of practice and level of training. Specific requirements for accreditation purposes can be found on the ABPTRFE website.[6] During matriculation, residents and FiTs must receive clinical exposure and practice-based learning within the full spectrum of the area of specialty (or subspecialty in the case of fellowships) practice. For nonclinical residencies and fellowships, exposure occurs across all faculty roles, including teaching, scholarship, service, and governance.

An important distinction for post-professional residency and fellowship programs in physical therapy is that they are presently not mandated. Residency education in physical therapy is not required for licensure, nor board certification. Participants in these programs take part voluntarily. Voluntary participation in residency training when board certification is sought lies in stark contrast to medicine.[7] While the individual reasons for enrolling in and completing a post-professional course of study vary widely, there may be tangible advantages of graduating from an accredited post-professional residency program. Namely, graduates are automatically permitted to sit for the relevant ABPTS exam without having to meet additional requirements.[8] Exceptions include residencies in which there is no corresponding ABPTS certification exam. Currently, these include the residency training areas of acute care, wound care, and nonclinical faculty residencies.[6] (Acute and wound care are in developmental stages for exam formulation.) There are likely many other reasons individuals choose to enroll in an accredited post-professional residency or fellowship program, which may include one-to-one mentoring assurance of early career guidance, structured clinical practice, and a formal curriculum tied to their chosen area of specialty practice, forging a path toward rapid skill acquisition and potential expertise.

Even as ABPTRFE accreditation standards set the competency bar for programs, there is wide variability in how these programs are administered. Unlike most health professions, physical therapist residencies and fellowships in physical therapy vary widely in terms of how they are structured and operated. The variability is due in part to the fact that participation in the ABPTRFE programs is voluntary. Therefore, there is no coordinated start date (as in medicine), and the admissions process varies considerably. Additionally, programs may be operated by academic institutions (eg, university or college), a clinical institution (eg, hospital system or a private practice), or a commercial entity (eg, a continuing education provider) or a coordinated effort between entities. Operation of a residency or fellowship program refers to the entity responsible for overall program oversight, admissions, curricular planning, clinical supervision, participant assessment (including written and live patient examinations, or nonclinical teaching and scholarly projects), remediation (where applicable), and faculty training and development.

Adding further to the complexities in physical therapy residencies and fellowships, participants may be in a single clinical site for the entire duration of the program, or they may rotate among a variety of sites, settings, or practices. Programs also vary in other key characteristics such as size (with most admitting 1 to 2 participants per year), didactic teaching methods (remote vs live vs hybrid), and employment relationship with the participant (most pay the participant a salary, while some charge a tuition).[9-11] The profession does not yet have a model of program-level characteristics that predict positive outcomes for the participant (eg, graduation rate, pass rate on the corresponding board examination)—unlike in the profession of medicine, where much research around this question is evident.[12-16] Academicians are just beginning to explore these questions in physical therapy[17] to assist in determining best practice in post-professional education, as well as informing potential participants in selecting a program that is a suitable fit. Most ABPTRFE programs use a centralized application service portal through APTA ABPTRFE and determine fit based upon references, résumés, applicant goals, and often face-to-face and/or telecommunication interviews. Minimal admission requirements include holding a degree in physical therapy as well as current licensure to practice; however, beyond that, admission requirements vary widely depending on program type, operating structure, size, facility mission, vision, and location.

THE ROAD TO SPECIALIZATION

Just as participation in post-professional education in physical therapy is presently voluntary, so is board certification for physical therapists. Board certification for physical therapists is not only voluntary, but it is also nonrestrictive.[18] This means, as an example, that a board-certified pediatric clinical specialist is not restricted from treating geriatric patients. One would argue, however, whether this would be advisable. It is currently up to the individual professional to determine a personal scope of practice.[19] To be eligible to sit for a specific board certification examination, physical therapists must have either completed an accredited residency program in the associated specialty area of practice or must have accrued 2000 hours of clinical practice within the area of specialty practice.[8] Some specialty councils have additional requirements,[20] but all have the hour requirement as described here. Board certification is awarded to those who successfully pass the appropriate board examination, and is valid for up to 10 years. Thus, presently it is possible to become board-certified without completing a residency program. This, too, is very different from other health professions and, arguably, not ideal. Residency education occurs in an environment where CR must be verified by trained faculty, practice at the level of a specialist is witnessed, and competence is explicitly demonstrated. This level of clinical practice is verified before residency graduates can take a written examination that largely tests their cognitive domain knowledge. The profession of physical therapy may begin an evolution toward requiring post-professional residency training to become board-certified. Discussions around this topic are just beginning.[21] (Note: While residency training exists in acute care, wound care, and faculty preparation, presently, board certification is not available in those areas of practice or study.)

What does specialization mean in terms of clinical decision-making (CDM)? If someone pursues specialization via an accredited post-professional residency program, he or she is most likely a new professional, if not a new graduate, or early career professional (2 to 5 years since DPT graduation). Therefore, it is our opinion that he or she should be entering a residency program with, at a minimum, entry-level competence, and ideally exhibit a readiness for residency education through entrustable professional activities or attributes (ie, a short list of integrated activities to be expected of all physical therapy graduates making the transition from physical therapy school to residency), as is done in medicine.[22,23] But upon completion of a residency program, is the graduate an expert in that area of practice? Perhaps some exceptional graduates are expert. Most, however, are farther along the track toward expertise, and likely on a "fast track" via lifelong learning skills gleaned from ABPTRFE training.[24-26]

Ideally, residency programs prepare graduates to sit for, and pass, the corresponding specialty board certification examination. The residency programs would have prepared the graduate by providing in-depth exposure to and clinical mentoring with patients across the diagnostic spectrum within the area of practice. This controlled clinical exposure and guided mentorship serve to cultivate CR through clinical patterns that become easily recognizable to expert clinicians. More experienced skilled clinicians use pattern recognition (ie, forward reasoning) to make large mental leaps, affording them a level of efficiency that is not yet evident in the novice practitioner.[26-28]

THE CONTINUUM OF CLINICAL SKILL DEVELOPMENT

The focus of post-professional education is shifting toward competency-based outcomes of learning.[28] This has created a renewed interest in the Dreyfus model of skill acquisition as a way to frame the development of skill within the area of clinical practice.[3] This model describes stages or phases of development related to the acquisition of new skills. Carraccio et al have eloquently and clearly described the application of the Dreyfus model to the learning of clinical skills.[28] This section is a synopsis of that work, modified to apply to physical therapists. It is important for the reader to understand that the Dreyfus model of skill acquisition as described here is not just describing the traditional image of "clinical skills," but is also strongly grounded in performance, which is the integration of CR, knowledge development, thinking, judgment, CDM, and clinical skills.

The resident physical therapist, who is typically a new graduate physical therapist, would begin the continuum at the novice level. The novice's CDM is rule based, and most reliant on analytic or hypothetico-deductive reasoning. As the learner progresses, knowledge becomes more organized, and patterns begin to be formed. Learners begin to eliminate irrelevant information, choose tests and measures more efficiently, and glean meaningful nuggets of information from patient histories.

The next level, advanced beginner, is characterized by learners who can reflect more on past patient experiences, and distill relevant information based, in part, on those experiences. This ability to recognize patterns for CR with patient presentations allows the learner to begin to make large mental leaps to arrive at a diagnosis. This is forward or nonanalytic reasoning. These learners still use analytic reasoning frequently, but they can integrate nonanalytic reasoning in ways that have not been evident before. While physical therapy professionals all use both forms of reasoning throughout our lives, it is the pattern recognition in the clinical context that allows the resident or FiT to begin to make these mental leaps in CR for CDM. This phase might describe a typical physical therapist resident who is somewhere in the middle of training.

The next phase, competent, is characterized by a learner who may still rely on analytic reasoning, yet the variety of experiences (eg, diagnostic variety, clinical complexity) has expanded, and the learner has reasoning strategies to use based on the clinical presentation.[3,28] For example, in familiar, common, or simple cases, the learner may rely on nonanalytic, forward reasoning via pattern recognition, affording a level of efficiency not seen in novices. However, in more complex, rare, or less familiar cases, the learner will rely more heavily on deductive or analytic reasoning strategies to test working hypotheses. The result is that the learner at this level is capable of functioning quite well regardless of how the patient presents, using CR strategies that are commensurate with the level of familiarity or complexity of the patient presentation. Achieving this level requires adequate exposure to a wide variety of cases, in terms of diagnosis and complexity, across the entire area of specialty practice. This level might describe a resident nearing the end of training or perhaps an FiT at the beginning of his or her study.

The proficient learner is one who is far more reliant on forward reasoning and pattern recognition in CR. These learners can routinely use intuition.[3,28] A hallmark of proficient learners, however, is that they can change plans midstream.[3,28] They are nimble and comfortable with ambiguity, and generally are not fearful of switching gears or approaches. While they may have patterns for many or most clinical diagnoses, they may lack experience with the outcomes of various interventions. These learners will use analytic reasoning and conscious choice when faced with challenging decisions in managing especially difficult cases.[3,28] This level might describe the very exceptional resident at the end of his or her study, a graduating resident who entered a program with some prior clinical experience, or perhaps an FiT near the beginning or middle of his or her study.

The expert learner is one who can use pattern recognition most of the time.[3,28] Further, this learner is characterized by an ability to notice the unexpected.[3,28] The expert is acutely aware of the environment and highly perceptive of even subtle features that do not fit typical patterns.[3,28] Expert learners are comfortable with simple and complex situations and have the experience with outcomes to be able to use forward reasoning and intuition in both diagnostic and therapeutic situations.[3,28] One concern with experts is that they can become complacent, feeling perhaps less challenged.[3,28] This can sometimes lead to performance issues unless they remain challenged in some way. Bereiter and Scardamalia refer to these individuals as "experienced nonexperts."[29] These are clinicians who have moved beyond "proficient" but become stuck or stagnant and unable to perform what most would term an "expert" level; hence, experts remain engaged, stimulated, and challenged. Experts can and do learn from master clinicians. Expert-level professionals might be seen in residents who entered a post-professional program with some experience. It might also describe FiTs at the completion of their training or faculty in a program, without continually challenging their competence in other meaningful ways.

Master clinicians are those who practice in a seemingly effortless way, can see the forest and the trees simultaneously, and notice context, surprise, and culture.[3,28] They are self-motivated, lifelong learners who are committed to their profession.[3,28] They use ongoing self-reflection before, during, and after patient encounters, process both quickly and slowly as the need arises, and have a deep emotional connection and engagement to their work.[3,28] This level might describe the exceptional FiT at the completion of a program or, more likely, and ideally, faculty in the programs.

ASSESSING RESIDENT/FELLOW-IN-TRAINING CLINICAL REASONING

As a requirement of all accredited post-professional residency and fellowship programs, residents and FiTs are assessed in several ways. Currently, there is no single tool used to assess resident and FiT performance. However, the ABPTRFE has begun pilot testing of an assessment tool for core competencies in a residency program. This tool reflects core competencies that are common among all specialty areas. The competencies were developed by an independent work group, and are remarkably similar to those recommended by Furze et al.[30] The tool, once validated, will allow residency faculty to assess the participant in 7 core domains: CR, knowledge for specialty practice, professionalism, communications, education, patient management, and systems-based practice. Each competency domain is described by accompanying behaviors that describe targeted benchmarks. There are 6 levels of competence within each domain. The levels begin at "below entry-level" (Level 0), then progresses to "entry-level" (Level 1), and advances, stepwise, to the "completion" milestone of Level 4. A Level 5 would be used for those residents who excel and exceed expected completion/graduation milestones. It should be noted that this tool was developed to assist residency programs in assessing longitudinal development of clinical skill across the participant's course of study across the competency domains identified. Historically, residency programs have used their own tools for assessing resident performance. These tools vary widely, and most are not validated. However, since nothing specific to physical therapist residency education existed, programs used (or created) tools that met their needs. In the future, it is hoped that a valid, common tool will be available to all programs.

The tool, as described here, focuses on core competencies and milestones within each area of competence. What exactly are milestones? As defined by the Accreditation Council for Graduate Medical Education (ACGME), "A milestone is a significant point in development. For accreditation purposes, the milestones are competency-based developmental outcomes (eg, knowledge, skills, attitudes, performance) that can be demonstrated progressively by residents/fellows from the beginning of their education through graduation to the unsupervised practice of their specialties." Once psychometric properties are established, using the physical therapist residency competency evaluation instrument, developed by ABPTRFE, should work in a similar fashion as the ACGME milestone competencies.

The relevant message here, however, is that the advancing competence of a resident or FiT is assessed periodically throughout his or her matriculation via a measure of clinical performance that is based, at least partly, on the acquisition of advancing levels of CR. This advancing level of CR skill should lead to the creation of heuristics that reduce error in diagnostic and therapeutic reasoning, as well as the development of patterns that facilitate forward reasoning typical among proficient and expert clinicians.[28,31,32] In medicine, the heuristics and pattern recognition used by expert clinicians are commonly referred to as "illness scripts."[33] Perhaps in physical therapy, we are better served to refer to them as "movement scripts."

CR is central to the development of competence and skill among physical therapist residents in all specialty areas of practice. This core area specifically addresses advancing levels of inquiry (ie, evidence-based practice), differential diagnosis, holistic and comprehensive patient-centeredness, interprofessionalism, data analysis and synthesis to guide decision-making, and deep integration of continual self-reflection. Achievement of milestones for CR is therefore integral to the progression of any resident as he or she matriculates through a program of study.

However, the core competencies described, including CR, do not reflect the entire spectrum of knowledge, skills, attitudes, and performance that a resident or FiT should demonstrate prior to completion of a post-professional training program. There is content that is most assuredly specific to each area of specialty practice. Some components within the APTA have begun to define competencies that are essential to their area of practice. For example, the Academy of Geriatric Physical Therapy has published "Essential Competencies in the Care of Older Adults at the Completion of a Physical Therapist Postprofessional Program of Study."[34] Other components of the APTA are certain to develop similar competencies for residency graduates associated with their area of practice in the future. Milestones and benchmarks that are specialty specific (ie, not common among all residents, but unique to a particular area of practice) may be assessed using a variety of measures. However, Objective Structured Clinical Examinations (OSCEs) are frequently used to gauge CR, skill, and performance in very specific, standardized clinical scenarios.

First described by Harden and Gleeson in 1979, OSCEs have become common in both undergraduate (professional level), and graduate (post-professional level) medical education, as well as in many other health professions.[35] OSCEs are a method of assessing a participant's clinical competence, which is objective rather than subjective, and in which the areas tested are carefully planned by the examiners. Generally, standardized patients or high-fidelity manikins are used so that the clinical scenarios are controlled. OSCEs may provide an ideal assessment tool for the performance-related activities that are unique to individual specialty areas of practice. It should be noted, however, that an OSCE is not the same thing as a live patient practical examination. Two live patient practical examinations administered during a participant's course of study are required by ABPTRFE for accreditation purposes.[36] While an OSCE is performed on a mock patient, live patient evaluations are done on actual patients, not actors or simulated patients.

Assessment of the learner should occur using a variety of assessment tools and strategies. Those include a comprehensive competency-based performance measure designed to assess overall learner performance at various points during the curriculum. This can be accomplished using a competency-based assessment tool that evaluates learners in essential or core competency areas of practice and is anchored by milestones along a continuum of clinical and professional development. In addition, learners should receive some OSCEs that are specific to the content area. Learners should also be assessed via live patient practical examinations where performance of the learner is evaluated at a "snapshot" in time, with an expectation that as time passes, reasoning skills improve. Lastly, written examinations should be used to assess knowledge and decision-making at various points in the curriculum. Using a variety of assessments provides faculty with useful insight into the development of knowledge, skill, and performance. It also should easily identify areas for improvement or remediation.

RESIDENT/FELLOW-IN-TRAINING REMEDIATION

When residents or FiTs fail to meet specified programmatic or individualized benchmarks or milestones by the end of their planned experience, it is necessary to consider remediation. Developing an action plan with a specified timeframe for remediation efforts is crucial to mapping out a strategy for allowing the resident or FiT to demonstrate competency in areas that are deficient. When a resident or FiT has deficiencies or shortcomings as they relate to meeting benchmarks or milestones, it should never come as a surprise. Communication should occur frequently between and among mentors, residents/FiTs, training program directors, and administrators (as appropriate) throughout the experience. Expressing concerns or sounding the alarm early on when goals are not being met allows for timely dialogue to plan for a successful outcome.[4]

Deficiencies or shortcomings can be related to clinical competency (which encompasses CDM), professional behaviors/conduct, or a combination. When residents or FiTs are experiencing difficulties, it can be challenging for a clinician preceptor/mentor (especially those with less experience) to identify or put his or her finger on the exact issues or concerns at hand. Using a common, standardized assessment tool, along with other guiding documents (ie, core values, performance elements/expectations, competency assessments), can help preceptors/mentors drill down to the specific attitudes, behaviors, knowledge, skills, or performance/abilities in question. Such a validated assessment tool could prove useful to the processes and systems in place by helping preceptors/mentors quickly and efficiently determine and objectify where problems lie, and the steps that should be taken to begin remediation toward a set of standardized core competencies.[36]

When concerns do arise, having formal policies in place for due process and unsatisfactory progress outlines the exact steps to be taken by either the resident/FiT or the program and faculty. These policies help ensure a fair and equitable process when steps need to be taken toward remediation by delineating roles, responsibilities, and expectations for all parties and stakeholders within the program.

The FATE Model

F: Frame it properly. Be tough on the problem, not the individual. Coming alongside this colleague with respect and unconditional positive regard while trying to effect positive change can be difficult and challenging. However, every effort should be made to be as objective as possible. Avoid the tendency to allow personal feelings and emotions to take over.[37]

A: Accurately define issues. Drill it down by clearly defining the issue(s) at hand. Determine whether it is a matter of clinical competence, professionalism (behavior/conduct), or both. Be sure the exact behaviors or competencies in question are clearly defined and include examples. Use the organization and residency/fellowship program's predetermined assessment tool(s) and policies to assist with progressing toward clinical and professional competencies.

T: Talk straight. Communicate early, directly, openly, and in plain language. Have the difficult and crucial conversation(s) necessary to clearly articulate the undesirable traits and what the expectations and desired outcomes are to effect a change. Use active listening skills and motivational interviewing techniques. Consider using a nonfaculty mentor to facilitate the process.[38]

E: Execute an action plan. While progressing to predetermined benchmarks, set regular meetings with realistic goals and expectations to be accomplished within a reasonable timeframe(s). Adhering to meeting times and following through with the action plan are both vital steps in the remediation process, even when schedules are busy and decisions are difficult.[39] The action plan should be precise and facilitated. Always clearly describe the practice expectation(s), determine a reasonable timeframe, and delineate how they are to be demonstrated (see Appendix A: Action Plan).

Example: Remediating a Clinical Reasoning Deficiency

Problem: Resident failed to recognize mental health/psychiatric comorbidities (depression) or screen for self-harm/suicidal ideation in a patient with obvious signs/symptoms and clear clinical presentation.

Action item: Resident/FiT will identify common mental health/psychiatric symptoms/syndromes/classifications and their effect on treatment and the movement system by 08/01/2019, using independent research, self-study, mental health, online continuing education.

Validation: Mentor feedback, peer review.

It can also prove valuable to have someone from within the organization serve in a nonfaculty mentor role to be available to assist residents or FiTs who are navigating remediation, struggling within the program, or working through personal issues or hardships. The role of a nonfaculty mentor can help to create a neutral and psychologically safe environment. This alternative avenue for residents to communicate outside of their resident role may foster and augment desired change when working through difficult situations. Programs that are part of a sizable organization may have the ability to refer residents or FiTs to an employee assistance program for personal matters that are interfering with the learning experience; guiding counseling referrals to outside resources is also appropriate.

Strategies for Remediation Efforts

When any of the previously mentioned issues or problems occur, it is helpful to have a framework of principles to guide the preceptor/mentor when developing a plan or strategy to remediate resident/FiT competencies or behaviors. Addressing issues early can avoid costly and dangerous medical errors and help influence longstanding desirable behaviors and practices.[40] One novel approach and proposed framework that may help the preceptor/mentor navigate remediation efforts is the FATE Model.

EXTENDED EXPERIENCES

Should a resident or FiT reach the end of the post-professional training experience and still not meet expected/planned benchmarks or milestones, the program must determine if it will allow for a paid or unpaid extension of the ABPTRFE residency or fellowship. An extension, if the resident or FiT is progressing, yet slower than expected, could potentially allow for the resident or FiT to demonstrate competency and successfully complete the program requirements by allowing for additional time and subsequent opportunities (eg, unpaid or paid extension of 2 to 8 weeks in duration with an action plan and specified goals to be met by the end).[6,36] Lack of progression would not warrant an extension.

INFLUENCING PROFESSIONAL BEHAVIORS AND ATTITUDES OF POST-PROFESSIONAL LEARNERS AND MENTORS

As residents and FiTs embark on the road to specialization, all those involved (eg, staff, administrators, clinicians, faculty) within the program should realize the tremendous opportunity they have to profoundly influence the professionalism and character of participants. As most residents and FiTs are likely to be either early career professionals or new graduates, these individuals are impressionable, malleable, and typically eager to be shaped and molded by experienced mentors. This responsibility to model and instill professionalism within the learners should not be taken lightly.[30,41-43] Professionalism, coupled with clinical competency (CR, decision-making, and judgment), is essential to the acquisition of core competencies expected of the post-professional practitioner or clinical specialist.

Professionalism comprises a group of attributes that can be defined as attitudes and behaviors.[44] Each of us has life experiences and comes from differing backgrounds that shape and mold our values, beliefs, world view, attitudes, and behaviors/actions. Depending on the individual, sometimes these personal factors are in line with the values and culture of the profession, organization, or learning environment, and sometimes they are not. This has become increasingly more evident within our culture, where social media has created a mechanism for individuals to live out loud, so to speak, and where others have the ability to observe the way in which we live our personal lives outside of our formal and professional roles. The APTA defines professionalism as follows:

> *Physical therapists consistently demonstrate core values by aspiring to and wisely applying principles of altruism, excellence, caring, ethics, respect, communication, and accountability, and by working together with other professionals to achieve optimal health and wellness in individuals and communities.*[45-47]

Professions possess sets of attributes that set them apart from occupations. Typically, this includes a specialized body of knowledge, unique socialization of student/trainee members, licensure/certification, professional associations, governance by peers, social prestige, vital service to society, a code of ethics, autonomy, equivalence of members, special relationships with clients, belief in service to the public, peer-driven ideas and review processes, self-regulation, a sense of calling to the profession, and autonomy.[44]

To create an environment conducive to learning and encourage positive socialization, post-professional program mentors and faculty should ensure they are making a conscious effort to model the behaviors and attitudes they are attempting to instill in residents and FiTs. The effort should be an intentional, deliberate, and well-thought-out process. Administrators, mentors, and faculty should ideally exhibit an approachable and inviting demeanor that fosters rich mentorship and a willingness to share information, encourages interprofessionalism, and discourages destructive competition.[48]

Encouraging Desirable Behaviors and Attitudes

Successfully and meaningfully influencing the behaviors of others within a program requires being intentional. Intentionally influencing others in a positive way requires knowing your own style, maintaining healthy professional boundaries, promoting a culture of accountability, creating lasting systems, and embracing a core group of shared values.[49-51]

KNOW YOUR PERSONALITY/SOCIAL STYLE

Having self-awareness of one's own style and the knowledge of how different styles effectively interact can help with communication, collaboration, and interpersonal interactions. In the Merrill-Reid model, there are 4 main personal styles: amiable (patient, kind, and fair); analytical (deep, thoughtful, and serious); driver (confident and active); and expressive (social and fun-loving).[48] Realize that regardless of your style, research shows you can be effective when working with others with differing styles as we must with the variety of types and kinds of patients and interprofessional colleagues we encounter daily. By understanding different personality styles and how they best interact, you can effectively collaborate and work with others to accomplish common goals.[41,52]

Model and Encourage Healthy Boundaries

Professional boundaries promote appropriate and effective interactions among residents, FiTs, preceptors, faculty, administrators, and patients. Boundaries serve to establish individual rules, roles, and responsibilities. They also serve to protect trainees, patients, and all those involved by removing unreasonable or unprofessional expectations or demands. Due to diverse cultural backgrounds and varied belief systems within health care settings, it is crucial to define and maintain healthy boundaries among learners, peers, patients, preceptors, and administrators. When boundaries are violated, the learning environment is compromised and negatively impacted. Maintaining healthy boundaries ensures increased psychological safety, an emphasis on learning, and an overall positive experience free from abuse, bullying, undue stress, or coercion.[49,53]

Create a Culture of Accountability

Programs should make every effort to clarify and communicate expectations by providing clear, written expectations and roles for mentors, administrators, and residents/FiTs involved in the program. Part of this process should include developing and communicating a clear set of behaviors and communication methods that are expected, as well as how and when they will be assessed or evaluated. When outlining expectations for residents/FiTs, programs should consider using the Professional Behaviors for the 21st Century: Professional Behaviors Assessment Tool (PBAT), which includes critical professional practice dimensions or elements reflective of post-professional graduates/physical therapists.[54] These dimensions include critical thinking, communication, problem-solving, interpersonal skills, responsibility, professionalism, use of constructive feedback, effective use of time and resources, stress management, and commitment to learning.[55] In the absence of established and validated core competencies, these dimensions can help provide a basis of comparison related to desirable CR skills and behaviors consistent with an autonomous practitioner beyond entry-level.

Establish Lasting Systems

The downfall of many organizations has been placing too much dependence on a single individual or small, elite group of individuals with a specified set of skills or knowledge. When daily operations require the presence of these individuals, the system fails in their absence. By focusing on enduring systems, and not specific individuals with highly specialized training, the system or organization is sustainable.[56]

The devil is in the details, but success is in the systems. —JW Marriott Jr

One such example of this in physical therapy is the guru mentality in patient care. The guru is a clinical specialist physical therapist with a highly specialized skill set that only the guru knows. In his or her absence, no one can treat a patient requiring those highly specialized skills or interventions. Within a successful clinical system, many or all clinicians within a clinical area are cross-trained in the knowledge, skills, and abilities required to effectively care for patients and to mentor others in that specific area of practice. Systems thinking requires selflessly training others who will carry on a tradition and culture of highly specialized care. Within this framework, others step up when the need arises, and the system endures.[50,51,57]

Adopt and Embrace Core Values

It is important that the organization and the program itself have an identity, a set of guiding principles, and a set of core values. Core values serve as a compass or barometer that guides decision-making and positively influences and shapes the systems and processes in place. One such example is the APTA core values of accountability, altruism, compassion/caring, excellence, integrity, professional duty, and social responsibility. The APTA offers a Professionalism in Physical Therapy: Core Values Self-Assessment that speaks to each of these core values with definitions and sample indicators for each element that users can use to self-assess.[58] ABPTRFE embraces the APTA core values and reflects them in its work. However, programs should also consider adopting programmatic core values that speak directly to the team environment and that engage learners and instill creative excitement toward the values, goals, and beliefs held most dear to the program and those involved. Team-specific core values can discourage destructive competition from within and encourage a professional and positive culture of productive team work. One such example, from the James A. Haley Veterans' Hospital physical therapist residency program, was adapted from Coach Anson Dorrance and the University of North Carolina at Chapel Hill women's soccer team (see Appendix B):

1. We don't whine.
2. The truly extraordinary do something every day.
3. We want this year of residency to be rich, valuable, and deep.
4. We work hard.
5. We don't freak out over ridiculous issues, or live in fragile states of emotional catharsis, or create crises where none should exist.
6. We choose to be positive.
7. We treat everyone with respect.
8. We care about each other as colleagues and as human beings.

9. When we don't get our way, we are noble and still support the team and its mission.

10. We work for each other.

11. We are well-led.

12. We want our lives (and not just at work) to be never-ending ascensions, but for that to happen properly, our fundamental attitude about life and our appreciation for it are critical.

Highly effective programs and educators create a safe and nurturing learning environment that promotes a positive culture where healthy boundaries exist. These programs share a set of well-defined core values and are sustainable. In the presence of these core tenets, strong CDM and CR skills can flourish. The residents/FiTs who successfully complete training within these comprehensive programs will be armed with foundational clinical problem-solving and CDM skills that will lead to the provision of exceptional patient care.

THE HIDDEN CURRICULUM

Within post-professional training programs, a didactic curriculum is a necessary and vital piece of the overall learning. In physical therapist residency and fellowship programs, the didactic curriculum is a requirement for accreditation purposes and is intended to supplement or augment the clinical, teaching, or research experiences. The formal, didactic curriculum is well-defined within the program and typically consists of scholarly readings, journal clubs, webinars, learning modules, and exams/quizzes. Didactic curriculums vary somewhat from program to program, with some specialty areas offering curriculum packages or a "canned" curriculum that developing or established programs can purchase. Each APTA academy and specialty area provides guidance, related to the description of specialized, post-professional practices, that speaks to the core knowledge and abilities of a clinical specialist physical therapist within a given specialty. There is also a clinical curriculum designed with planned clinical learning experiences and mentorship opportunities to complement the didactic learning and to advance CR and decision-making skills.

However, there exists a third type of implicit curriculum known as the hidden curriculum. The hidden curriculum, which is more social and often with cultural influences, is often overlooked, less understood, and may be neglected due to the lack of awareness or cognizance on the part of administrators, mentors, and program directors. The hidden curriculum has the greatest potential to make long-lasting and impactful impressions related to behaviors, attitudes, practices, and the subsequent trust and credibility created for the individual and the profession.[41,59] An exit interview process can be an invaluable tool and an enlightening process for programs to self-assess and be aware of strengths and areas for improvement.

Character may almost be called the most effective means of persuasion. —Aristotle

Large or small, every program, clinical area, or group of staff members learners encounter has a certain culture. The cultures and subcultures within ABPTRFE programs can either reinforce or contradict the overarching mission, vision, values, and culture desired by the residency or fellowship program, its parent organization, and even the profession. Experiences and interactions within the culture lead to either positive or negative socialization for the learners, students, residents, and FiTs exposed to the environment and participating in the program. Leaders have a responsibility to themselves, the programs, colleagues, the public, and the profession to model and encourage positive socialization that is in line with all associated programmatic and professional core values. Providing positive socialization and a desirable hidden curriculum begins with intentional leadership and thoughtful mentorship.[48,53]

Begin with the end in mind. —Stephen R. Covey

Intentional Leadership

Great leaders always begin with a vision and a purpose, and an organization or group will eventually take on the personality and character of its leader. Educational and clinical leaders must be intentional and aware of the impact their leadership style will ultimately have on the culture within the organization and, subsequently, the programming throughout. The values, attitudes, behaviors, and culture promoted by leadership will inevitably impact and shape the organization and influence those working within it. This directly influences morale, productivity, and the quality of internal and external services. It also drives and impacts critical components such as performance evaluations, hiring and firing practices, autonomy, sound CDM, and how valued those working within the organization feel. Gordon explains that successful, positive companies with positive employees and positive cultures are created through a set of principles, processes, systems, and habits that are ingrained in the culture,[60] highlighting key tenets within positive organizations:

- A positive environment and culture are everything

- Positive leadership is a requirement

- Trust must permeate the organization[57,60]

Many effective leadership styles and models exist, and there is considerable overlap in the reported best practices. One proven and effective model that has a set of leader behaviors that coincide with desirable practices is servant leadership. Created by Robert Greenleaf, servant leadership has been adopted by the Veterans Administration and consists of a foundational set of 7 pillars: person of character, puts people first, skilled communicator, compassionate collaborator, has foresight, systems thinker, and leads with moral authority. This model also contains 21 core competencies that define the practice of active servant leadership. The success of this model is in a large part due to the nature of how it effectively establishes and encourages employee engagement and creates a psychologically safe work environment. Greenleaf describes servant leaders as being different from other persons of goodwill because they act on what they believe. Servant leadership encourages altruism, courteousness, conscientiousness, and a positive climate—all major tenets of building trust, promoting self-reflection, and developing sound CR skills.[56,61]

The late Stephen Covey stated that the best leaders build trust.[57] He defined trust as confidence born of 2 dimensions: character and competence. Competency can be defined as the ability to do something successfully or efficiently. Character encompasses the mental or moral qualities distinctive to an individual. According to Covey's son, Stephen M. R. Covey, "Trust is equal parts character and competence. You can look at any leadership failure, and it's always a failure of one or the other."[57]

Intentional leaders must be keenly aware of the cultures and subcultures within their teams and organization to promote desired outcomes and have a meaningful influence when positive change is necessary. Often, there is a formal or informal leader established in a group who sets the tone in terms of the acceptable or dominant beliefs, attitudes, and behaviors within the group or work area. Ensuring congruency within all the areas and subcultures within an organization can be challenging. All mentors are leaders and should possess the skills necessary to positively influence others. Using thoughtful mentoring that is planned and well-thought-out can be a catalyst for influencing positive change and the development of strong CR skills.[50,51,62]

The belief that all genuine education comes about through experience does not mean that all experiences are genuinely or equally educative. Experience and education cannot be directly equated to each other. —John Dewey[63]

Thoughtful Mentorship

Traditionally, the mentorship model within residency and fellowship programs is a one-to-one experience with a highly experienced and skilled preceptor. These experiences are regularly scheduled or preplanned and follow a hierarchy of progressively more complex cases requiring the maturation of CR and decision-making skills. Skilled mentors use self-reflection, probing, open-ended questions, case studies/discussion, role-playing, and rubrics to help learners become more efficient problem solvers. These exercises facilitate the transfer of knowledge at a much faster rate than experience alone. Through intentional leadership the mentor facilitates the resident's or FiT's ability to make leaps in CDM and arrive at a diagnosis more efficiently. This includes ruling in or out competing diagnoses and screening for medical referral.

A more progressive and contemporary learning environment that fosters interprofessionalism and teamwork is a collaborative model of clinical education. Collaborative clinical models of learning typically involve a clinic setting with more than one resident or FiT, any number of professional students (ie, DPT students or other disciplines), and one or more mentors. Collaborative models of care can encourage an atmosphere of reliance upon other team members to achieve shared goals. It also can involve providing a unique role or contribution that may be shared with other learners, interdisciplinary staff, and mentors. This form of thoughtful mentorship is beneficial in that it is multidirectional learning and CDM, between and among peers, students (possibly interdisciplinary), residents, FiTs, preceptors/mentors, and administrators.[64] With interactions and communication between more peers and mentors during group mentorship sessions, clinical discussion and problem-solving can be taken to a higher level.

From a programmatic or higher-level view, a well-thought-out and planned mentorship should include multidimensional interactions and multifaceted topics, and should start at the top. A robust post-professional clinical training program should encourage mentorship at all levels. Administrators, program directors, leads, supervisors, managers, staff, and the like should all be seeking out and providing mentorship in a multidirectional approach. Topics such as clinical practice, leadership, professionalism, interprofessionalism, communication, administration, emotional intelligence, and motivational interviewing should be shared and openly discussed. Administrators and higher-level leadership should remain approachable and demonstrate a consistent and predictable mood and behavior. By intentionally modeling desirable behavioral professionalism, administrators create an opportunity to effect positive change through personal influence.

Nobody cares how much you know until they know how much you care. —Theodore Roosevelt

Mentorship should focus on coaching and building teams and one-on-one relationships with the intent of improving employees' ability to maximize their strengths and work cooperatively with others and within other successful systems.[62] This helps clinicians and clinics escape the guru mentality and foster enduring systems with rich learning environments where teaching and learning are valued and shared openly. The ABPTRFE Mentorship Resource Manual, available online, is an exceptional resource and should be required reading for all those faculty, mentors, and administrators involved in the program.[4]

According to Musolino and Mostrom,[65] all physical therapist program curricula should include reflection. If physical therapists are to be more effective as educators, then they are obligated to be reflective as practitioners.[65] Many educators are aware of the need to teach learners to critically think and self-reflect.[65] But, many are too busy telling what they know, and fall short when helping students learn how to learn and think reflectively.[65] Reflection remains a critical component of the scholarship of teaching and learning and assessment.[65] Because of its importance, reflection should also manifest itself within measures of faculty competencies.[65]

There are immeasurable benefits to being part of a post-professional training program. One invaluable aspect related to the spirit of mentorship is the attitude and willingness of staff and faculty to share knowledge and give back. Treating people as whole individuals who are multidimensional beings, and not a thing or an expense to be managed, helps them want to volunteer their best.[50,51] Investing in teams and creating enduring systems and processes can seem like a daunting and overwhelming task, especially for those individuals involved in developing a new program. However, armed with the right focus, tools, and intentions, program directors, administrators, faculty, and mentors can create a solid framework and foundation to develop sophisticated programs dedicated to graduating residents and FiTs who are competent, professional, credible, and highly trusted providers.[66]

REFERENCES

1. American Board of Physical Therapy Residency and Fellowship Education. About clinical residency programs. http://www.abptrfe.org/ResidencyPrograms/About/ClinicalResidencyPrograms/. Accessed March 19, 2018.
2. American Board of Physical Therapy Residency and Fellowship Education. About clinical fellowship programs. http://www.abptrfe.org/FellowshipPrograms/AboutClinicalFellowshipPrograms/. Accessed March 19, 2018.
3. Dreyfus SE, Dreyfus HL. *A Five-Stage Model of the Mental Activities Involved in Directed Skill Acquisition*. Berkeley, CA; 1980.
4. American Board of Physical Therapy Residency and Fellowship Education. ABPTRFE mentoring resource manual 2014. http://www.abptrfe.org/uploadedFiles/ABPTRFEorg/For_Programs/ABPTRFEMentoringResourceManual.pdf. Accessed March 19, 2018.
5. American Board of Physical Therapy Residency and Fellowship Education. What we do. http://www.abptrfe.org/WhatWeDo/. Accessed March 19, 2018.
6. American Board of Physical Therapy Residency and Fellowship Education. http://www.abptrfe.org/home.aspx. Accessed March 19, 2018.
7. Federation of State Medical Boards. State-specific requirements for initial medical licensure. https://www.fsmb.org/licensure/usmle-step-3/state_specific. Accessed March 19, 2018.
8. American Board of Physical Therapy Specialties. Minimum eligibility requirements and general information for all physical therapist specialist certification examinations. http://www.abpts.org/uploadedFiles/ABPTSorg/Specialist_Certification/About_Certification/SpecCertMinimumCriteria.pdf. Accessed March 19, 2018.
9. Hartley G, Harrington K, Roach K. Outcomes of physical therapy clinical residency programs by didactic model and mentor's primary work setting. In: Platform presentation, APTA Combined Sections meeting; 2017; San Antonio, TX.
10. Hartley G, Harrington K, Roach K. Outcomes of physical therapy clinical residency programs by operational structure. In: Poster presentation, APTA Combined Sections meeting; 2017; San Antonio, TX.
11. Hartley G, Harrington K, Roach K. Outcomes of physical therapy clinical residency programs by administrative structure. In: Poster presentation, APTA Combined Sections meeting; 2017; San Antonio, TX.
12. de Virgilio C, Yaghoubian A, Kaji A, et al. Predicting performance on the American Board of Surgery qualifying and certifying examinations: a multi-institutional study. *Arch Surg.* 2010;145:852-856.
13. Falcone JL. Size might matter more than we thought: the importance of residency program size to pass rates on the American Board of Pediatrics certifying examination. *Clin Pediatr.* 2015;54:79-83.
14. Falcone JL, Middleton DB. Pass rates on the American Board of Family Medicine certification exam by residency location and size. *J Am Board Fam Med.* 2013;26:453-459.
15. Mims LD, Mainous AG, Chirina S, Carek PJ. Are specific residency program characteristics associated with the pass rate of graduates on the ABFM certification examination? *Fam Med.* 2014;46:360-368.
16. Sako EY, Petrusa ER, Paukert JL. Factors influencing outcome of the American Board of Surgery certifying examination: an observational study. *J Surg Res.* 2002;105:75-80.
17. Kulig K. Residency education in every town: is it just so simple? *Phys Ther.* 2014;94:151-161.
18. American Physical Therapy Association House of Delegates. *HOD P06-16-10-11: Clinical Specialization in Physical Therapy.* Alexandria, VA; 2016.
19. American Physical Therapy Association. Personal scope of physical therapist practice 2015. http://www.apta.org/ScopeOfPractice/Personal/. Accessed March 19, 2018.
20. American Board of Physical Therapy Specialties. Emergency medical responder certification requirement 2016. http://www.abpts.org/Certification/Sports/EMRRequirement/. Accessed March 19, 2018.
21. American Physical Therapy Association. Best practices. Physical Therapist Clinical Education Task Force report 2017. http://www.apta.org/Educators/TaskForceReport/PTClinicalEducation/. Accessed March 19, 2018.
22. Association of American Medical Colleges. *Core Entrustable Professional Activities for Entering Residency.* Washington, DC: Association of American Medical Colleges; 2014.
23. Chesbro SB, Jensen GM, Boissonnault WG. Entrustable professional activities as a framework for continued professional competence: is now the time? *Phys Ther.* 2018;98(1):3-7.

24. Wainwright SF, Shepard KF, Harman LB, Stephens J. Factors that influence the clinical decision making of novice and experienced physical therapists. *Phys Ther.* 2011;91:87-101.

25. Robertson EK, Tichenor CJ. Post-professional cartography in physical therapy: charting a pathway for residency and fellowship training. *J Orthop Sport Phys Ther.* 2015;45:57-60.

26. Black L, Jensen G, Mostrom E, et al. The first year of practice: an investigation of the professional learning and development of promising novice physical therapists. *Phys Ther.* 2010;90:1758-1773.

27. Durning SJ, Artino AR, Schuwirth L, van der Vleuten C. Clarifying assumptions to enhance our understanding and assessment of clinical reasoning. *Acad Med.* 2013;88:442-448.

28. Carraccio CL, Benson BJ, Nixon LJ, Derstine PL. From the educational bench to the clinical bedside: translating the Dreyfus developmental model to the learning of clinical skills. *Acad Med J Assoc Am Med Coll.* 2008;83:761-767.

29. Bereiter C, Scardamalia M. *Surpassing Ourselves: An Inquiry Into the Nature and Implications of Expertise.* La Salle, IL: Open Court; 1993.

30. Furze J, Tichenor C, Fisher B, Jensen G, Rapport M. Physical therapy residency and fellowship education: reflections on the past, present, and future. *Phys Ther.* 2016;96:949-960.

31. Eva KW. What every teacher needs to know about clinical reasoning. *Med Educ.* 2005;39:98-106.

32. Scott IA. Errors in clinical reasoning: causes and remedial strategies. *BMJ.* 2009;338:b1860.

33. Schmidt HG, Rikers RMJP. How expertise develops in medicine: knowledge encapsulation and illness script formation. *Med Educ.* 2007;41:1133-1139.

34. Hartley G, Jasper A, Brewer K, et al. *Essential Competencies in the Care of Older Adults at the Completion of a Physical Therapist Postprofessional Program of Study.* Madison, WI: Academy of Geriatric Physical Therapy; 2017.

35. Harden RM, Gleeson FA. Assessment of clinical competence using an objective structured clinical examination (OSCE). *Med Educ.* 1979;13:41-54.

36. American Board of Physical Therapy Residency and Fellowship Education. 2018 application resources for clinical residency and fellowship programs: clinical quality standards. http://www.abptrfe.org/uploadedFiles/ABPTRFEorg/For_Programs/Apply/Forms/ABPTRFEClinicalQualityStandards.pdf. Accessed March 19, 2018.

37. Maxfield D, Grenny J, McMillan R, Patterson K, Switzler A. *Silence Kills: The Seven Crucial Conversations for Healthcare.* Provo, UT: VitalSmarts; 2005.

38. Patterson K, Grenny J, McMillan R, Switzler A. *Crucial Conversations: Tools for Talking When Stakes Are High.* New York, NY: McGraw-Hill; 2002.

39. Sparks JW, Landrigan-Ossar M, Vinson A, et al. Individualized remediation during fellowship training. *J Clin Anesth.* 2016;34:452-458.

40. Delisle M, Grymonpre R, Whitley R, Wirtzfeld D. Crucial conversations: an interprofessional learning opportunity for senior healthcare students. *J Interprof Care.* 2016;30:777-786.

41. Coles R. The moral education of medical students. *Acad Med.* 1998;73:55-57.

42. Stern DT, Papadakis M. The developing physician—becoming a professional. *N Engl J Med.* 2006;355:1794-1799.

43. American Physical Therapy Association. *Today's Physical Therapist: A Comprehensive Review of a 21st Century Health Care Profession.* Alexandria, VA: American Physical Therapy Association; 2011.

44. Hammer DP. Professional attitudes and behaviors: the "A's and B's" of professionalism. *Am J Pharm Educ.* 2000;64:455-464.

45. American Physical Therapy Association Board of Directors. *BOD P05-04-02-03: Professionalism in Physical Therapy: Core Values.* Alexandria, VA: American Physical Therapy Association; 2012.

46. Ethics and Judicial Committee. *APTA Guide for Professional Conduct.* Alexandria, VA: American Physical Therapy Association; 2013.

47. American Physical Therapy Association. Professionalism. http://www.apta.org/Professionalism/. Accessed March 19, 2018.

48. Kraut A, Yarris LM, Sargeant J. Feedback: cultivating a positive culture. *J Grad Med Educ.* 2015;7:262-264.

49. Cloud H. *Boundaries for Leaders: Results, Relationships, and Being Ridiculously in Charge.* New York, NY: Harper Business; 2013.

50. Covey S, Merrill R. *The Seven Habits of Highly Effective People: Powerful Lessons in Personal Change.* New York, NY: Simon & Schuster Adult Publishing Group; 1990.

51. Covey S, Merrill R, Merrill R. *First Things First: To Live, to Love, to Learn, to Leave a Legacy.* New York, NY: Simon & Schuster Trade Paperbacks; 1995.

52. Merrill D, Reid R. *Personal Styles & Effective Performance.* Boca Raton, FL: CRC Press; 1981.

53. Weidman JC, Twale DJ, Stein EL. Socialization of graduate and professional students in higher education: a perilous passage? *ASHE-ERIC High Educ Rep.* 2001;28:120.

54. Davis C, Musolino GM, eds. *Patient Practitioner Interaction: An Experiential Manual for Health Care Providers.* 6th ed. Thorofare, NJ: SLACK Incorporated; 2016.

55. May W, Kontney L, Iglarsh Z. Professional behaviors for the 21st century 2010. http://www.marquette.edu/physical-therapy/documents/ProfessionalBehaviors.pdf. Accessed March 19, 2018.

56. Efron L. The three fundamental leadership traits that support enduring organizations. *Forbes.* https://www.forbes.com/sites/louisefron/2015/05/11/the-three-fundamental-leadership-traits-that-support-enduring-organizations/#63064e3c4b7c. Accessed March 19, 2018.

57. Covey S. *The Speed of Trust: The One Thing That Changes Everything.* New York, NY: Simon & Schuster Free Press; 2006.

58. American Physical Therapy Association. Self assess your professional excellence. http://www.apta.org/CoreValuesSelfAssessment/. Accessed March 19, 2018.

59. Hafferty FW. Beyond curriculum reform: confronting medicine's hidden curriculum. *Acad Med.* 1998;73:403-407.

60. Gordon J. *The No Complaining Rule: Positive Ways to Deal With Negativity at Work.* Hoboken, NJ: John Wiley and Sons; 2008.

61. US Department of Veterans Affairs. National Center for Organization Development 2013. https://www.va.gov/NCOD/Servant_ Leadership_In_VA.asp. Accessed March 19, 2018.

62. Gilley A, Gilley JW, McMillan HS. Organizational change: motivation, communication, and leadership effectiveness. *Perform Improv Q.* 2009;21:75-94.

63. Dewey J. *Experience and Education.* New York, NY: Macmillan; 1938.

64. Academy of Acute Care Physical Therapy. Collaborative clinical education in acute care. http://www.acutept.org/?page=CEdge 1114clinicaled. Accessed March 19, 2018.

65. Musolino GM, Mostrom E. Reflection and the scholarship of teaching, learning, and assessment. *J Phys Ther Educ.* 2005;19:52-66.

66. Center for Integrity in Practice. *Preventing fraud, abuse, and waste: A primer for physical therapists.* Alexandria, VA; 2015.

APPENDIX A
SAMPLE ACTION PLAN

Action Plan – Resident A	2019

Foundational, Clinical, Behavioral, & Research Elements: Practice Expectations					
Behavior	**Priority** 1 = low 5 = high	**By When**	**How**	**What**	**Method**
Ability to appropriately synthesize and apply new research information, methods, or instruments to develop evidence-based clinical practice	2	8/1/19	Mentor Indep. Research Self-study Journal Club	Didactic/CEU Mentor time Journal Club	Mentor feedback Peer Review
Ability to explain statistics: e.g. descriptive, inference, testing, statistical power	2	8/1/19	Mentor Indep. Research Self-study Journal Club	Didactic/CEU Mentor time Journal Club	Mentor feedback Peer Review
Ability to apply conflict resolution strategies in a timely manner	3	8/1/19	Mentor Indep. Research Self-study	Mentor Supervised-practice Observation	Mentor feedback Peer review
Ability to apply behavior modification strategies	3	8/1/19	Indep. Research Self-study Neuro-Consort	Didactic time Mentor time	Mentor feedback Peer review
Ability to identify common psychiatric symptoms/ syndromes/ classifications & their effect on tx & the movement system	3	8/1/19	Indep. Research Self-study Mental Health Online/CE	Didactic time Mentor time	Mentor feedback Peer review
Ability to explain neuroplasticity-CNS responses to learning and inquiry; cortical remodeling.	4	8/1/19	Indep. Research Self-study Neuro-Consort	Didactic time Mentor time	Mentor feedback Peer review
Ability to explain motor learning in persons with & without motor, sensory/ perceptual, and/or cognitive pathology	4	8/1/19	Indep. Research Self-study Neuro-Consort	Didactic time Mentor time	Mentor feedback Peer review
Ability to explain theories of motor control	4	8/1/19	Indep. Research Self-study Neuro-Consort	Didactic time Mentor time	Mentor feedback Peer review
Ability to explain neuropathology	4	8/1/19	Indep. Research Self-study Neuro-Consort	Didactic time Mentor time	Mentor feedback Peer review
Ability to explain memory, cognitive processes, & executive functions	4	8/1/19	Indep. Research Self-study Neuro-Consort	Didactic time Mentor time	Mentor feedback Peer review

JAHVH Neurologic PT Residency Program

Action Plan – Resident A | 2019

Ability to explain perceptual disorders	4	8/1/19	Indep. Research Self-study Neuro-Consort	Didactic time Mentor time	Mentor feedback Peer review
Ability to explain hemispheric specialization	4	8/1/19	Indep. Research Self-study Neuro-Consort	Didactic time Mentor time	Mentor feedback Peer review
Documentation skills are at minimum acceptable standards	4	8/1/19	Peer Review Mentor Review	Observation Practice Peer review form	Mentor Feedback/ Peer Review
Educates other PT's, students, & PT residents to enhance knowledge & master skill in neuro PT	4	8/1/19	Mentor Indep. Research Self-study Journal Club	Didactic/CEU Mentor time Journal Club	Mentor feedback Peer Review

Professional Roles, Responsibilities, & Values: Practice Expectations

Behavior	Priority	When	How	What	Method
Ability to apply empathy	5	7/25/19	Supervised-Clinical Practice	Mentor Time Observation	Mentor Feedback/ Observation
Has effective listening & observation techniques	5	7/25/19	Supervised-Clinical Practice	Mentor Time Observation	Mentor Feedback/ Observation
Has effective conflict management techniques	5	7/25/19	Supervised-Clinical Practice	Mentor Time Observation	Mentor Feedback/ Observation
Seeks out ways to be helpful/volunteer, acting as a "team player" in the clinic	5	7/25/19	Supervised-Clinical Practice	Mentor Time Observation	Mentor Feedback/ Observation
Seeks out mentor feedback appropriately & timely	5	7/25/19	Supervised-Clinical Practice	Mentor Time Observation	Mentor Feedback/ Observation
Implements mentor feedback effectively & appropriately in a timely manner	5	7/25/19	Supervised-Clinical Practice	Mentor Time Observation	Mentor Feedback/ Observation
Models professionalism & maturity in decision making & interpersonal interaction	5	7/25/19	Supervised-Clinical Practice	Mentor Time Observation	Mentor Feedback/ Observation
Models respect & compassion for all people	5	7/25/19	Supervised-Clinical Practice	Mentor Time Observation	Mentor Feedback/ Observation

Action Plan – Resident A | 2019

Establishes trustworthy relationships with colleagues, patients, employers & the public	5	7/25/19	Supervised-Clinical Practice	Mentor Time Observation	Mentor Feedback/ Observation
Effectively recognizes & resolves problems in difficult situations	5	7/25/19	Supervised-Clinical Practice	Mentor Time Observation	Mentor Feedback/ Observation
Demonstrates continued pursuit of additional & more advanced knowledge, skills, & abilities	5	7/25/19	Supervised-Clinical Practice	Mentor Time Observation	Mentor Feedback/ Observation
Collaborates with others to solve problems	5	7/25/19	Supervised-Clinical Practice	Mentor Time Observation	Mentor Feedback/ Observation
Appropriate use of personal communication devices (cell phone, tablet, PC) during workday	5	7/25/19	Supervised-Clinical Practice	Mentor Time Observation	Mentor Feedback/ Observation
Prepares appropriately for evaluations & treatment sessions ahead of time	5	7/25/19	Supervised-Clinical Practice	Mentor Time Observation	Mentor Feedback/ Observation
Commitment to sit for the NCS board exam	5	6/30/19	Verbal	ABPTS registration	Verbal/written commitment

Action Plan – Resident A | 2019

It is the plan of the JAHVH Neurologic PT Residency Faculty to ensure you meet the objectives outlined above to improve your understanding and ability to demonstrate accountable, professional behavior and clinical competence. The behaviors outlined above are areas of focus that the faculty believes will offer you the greatest chance of success in possessing and demonstrating appropriate professional behavior and competence in the clinic. The faculty's main concern and desire is your ability to be a successful neurologic clinical specialist PT, coworker, and employee who represents JAHVH, the profession, and yourself positively. Failure to accept or satisfactorily complete this action plan by the specified timeframe may result in probation, unpaid residency extension (for remediation purposes- not to exceed 8 weeks), or early dismissal from the program.

I accept this action plan and intend to work diligently to demonstrate the desirable behaviors and competencies outlined above, by the specified timeframe(s). Furthermore I agree to sit for the NCS board exam at the next available testing date.

Resident Signature: _____   Date: _____

Faculty Mentor: _____   Date: _____

Program Director: _____   Date: _____

JAHVH Neurologic PT Residency Program

APPENDIX B
JAMES A. HALEY VETERANS' HOSPITAL PHYSICAL THERAPY RESIDENCY CORE VALUES

1. Let's begin with this, *we don't whine.* This **tough** individual can handle any situation and never complains about anything in or out of the workplace.

   The true joy in life is to be a force of fortune instead of a feverish, selfish little clod of ailments and grievances complaining that the world will not devote itself to making you happy. —George Bernard Shaw

    TOUGH—from Nordic wheel cross signifying thunder, power, and energy

2. *The truly extraordinary do something every day.* This individual has remarkable **self-discipline,** does what's expected, and every day has a plan to do something to get better or grow.

   Roosevelt, more than any other man living within the range of notoriety, showed the singular primitive quality that belongs to ultimate matter, the quality that medieval theology assigned to God: "he was pure act." —Henry Adams *Theodore Rex*—Desmond Morris

    DISCIPLINED—from "careful" cycle on washing machine

3. *And we want this year of residency to be rich, valuable, and deep.* This is that **focused** individual that is here for the "right reason" to get an education and grow. They lead their life here with the proper balance and an orientation towards intellectual growth, and against the highest public standards and most noble universal ideals, they make good choices to best represent themselves, their team, and the profession.

   College is about books. And by the word books, the proposition means this: College is about the best available tools—books, computers, lab equipment—for broadening your mastery of one or more important subjects that will go on deepening your understanding of the world, yourself, and the people around you.

   This will almost certainly be the last time in your life when other people bear the expense of awarding you 4 years of financially unburdened time. If you use the years primarily for mastering the skills of social life—as though those skills shouldn't already have been acquired by the end of middle school—or if you use these years for testing the degree to which your vulnerable brain and body can bear the strains of the alcoholism with which a number of students depart campus, or the sexual excess that can seem so rewarding (to name only 2 of the lurking maelstroms), then you may ultimately leave this vast table of nutriment as the one more prematurely burnt-out case. —Reynolds Price

    FOCUSED—from camera focus button

4. *We work hard.* This individual embodies the "indefatigable human spirit" and never stops pushing themselves. They are absolutely **relentless** in training and follow through.

   The difference between one person and another, between the weak and the powerful, the great and the insignificant, is energy—invisible determination … This quality will do anything that has to be done in the world, and no talents, no circumstances, no opportunities will make you a great person without it. —Thomas Buxton, philanthropist

   The common denominator of success … [is forming] the habit of doing things that failures don't like to do … Failures are influenced by the desire for pleasing methods … successful [people] are influenced by the desire for pleasing results … We've got to realize right from the start that success is something which is achieved by the minority … and is therefore unnatural and not to be achieved by following your natural likes and dislikes nor by being guided by our natural preferences and prejudices … you won't have to be told how to find your purpose or how to identify it or how to surrender to it. If it's a big purpose, you will be big in its accomplishment. If it's an unselfish purpose, you will be unselfish in accomplishing it. And if it's an honest purpose, you will be honest and honorable in the accomplishment of it. But as long as you live, don't ever forget that while you may succeed beyond your fondest hopes and your greatest expectations, you will never succeed beyond the purpose to which you are willing to surrender. Furthermore, your surrender will not be complete until you have formed the habit of doing the things that failures don't like to do.   —Albert E. N. Gray, *The Common Denominator of Success*

 RELENTLESS—from the symbol for Saturn: god of "relentless natural forces"

5.   *We don't freak out over ridiculous issues or live in fragile states of emotional catharsis or create crises where none should exist.* The best example is the even-keeled stoic that is forever unflappable and **resilient**. The worst example is the "overbred dog," that high maintenance, overly sensitive "flower" that becomes unstable or volatile over nothing significant.

What an extraordinary place of liberties the West really is … exempt from many of the relentless physical and social obligations necessary for a traditional life for survival, they become spoiled and fragile like overbred dogs; neurotic and prone to a host of emotional crises elsewhere.   —Jason Elliot, *An Unexpected Light: Travels in Afghanistan*

 RESILIENT—nautical buoy symbol, which rises and falls with the water, always staying upright

6.   *We choose to be positive.* Nothing can depress or upset this powerful and **positive** life force—no mood swings, not even negative circumstances can affect this "rock."

… everything can be taken from a man but one thing: the last of the human freedoms—to choose one's attitude in any given set of circumstances, to choose one's own way. And there were always choices to make. Every day, every hour, offered the opportunity to make a decision, a decision which determined whether you would or would not submit to those powers which threatened to rob you of your very self, your inner freedom; which determined whether or not you would become the plaything of circumstance … in the final analysis it becomes clear that the sort of person (you are is) the result of an inner decision … therefore, any man can … decide … that (this) last inner freedom cannot be lost.   —Viktor E. Frankl, *Man's Search for Meaning*

 POSITIVE

7.   *We treat everyone with respect.* This is that **classy** individual that goes out of their way to never separate themselves from anyone or make anyone feel beneath them.

Class is the graceful way you treat someone even when they can do nothing for you.   —Doug Smith, Mgr. ('86)

 CLASSY—British hobo symbol for "here live generous people"

8.   *We care about each other as colleagues and as human beings.* This is that nonjudgmental, **caring,** and inclusive friend that never says a negative thing about anyone and embraces everyone because of their humanity, with no elitist separation by academic class, social class, race, religious preference, or sexual orientation.

No man is an island, entire of itself, every man is a piece of the continent, a part of the main … any man's death diminishes me, because I am involved in mankind, and therefore never send to know for whom the bell tolls; it tolls for thee.   —John Donne, *For Whom the Bell Tolls*

 CARING

9.   *When we don't get our own way, we are noble and still support the team and its mission.* This remarkably **noble**, self-sacrificing, generous human being always places the team before themselves.

If there is a meaning in life at all, then there must be a meaning in suffering. Suffering is an ineradicable part of life, even as fate and death. Without suffering and death human life cannot be complete. The way in which a man accepts his fate and all the suffering it entails, the way in which he takes up his cross, gives him ample opportunity—

even under the most difficult circumstances—to add a deeper meaning to his life. It may remain brave, dignified and unselfish. Or in the bitter fight for self-preservation he may forget his human dignity and become no more than an animal. Here lies the chance for a man either to make use of or to forgo the opportunities of attaining the moral values that a difficult situation may afford him. And this decides whether he is worthy of his sufferings or not.
—Viktor E. Frankl, *Man's Search for Meaning*

 NOBLE—Hittite sign for king

10. *We work for each other.* This is the kind of co-worker that works themselves to death covering for all of their teammates in the toughest clinics. Their effort and care (verbal encouragement) make them a pleasure to work with and their **selflessness** in and out of the work environment helps everyone around them.

People don't care how much you know until they know how much you care.   —Note by Rakel Karvelsson (UNC '98)

 SELFLESS—from combination of ancient symbols for "not" and "relating to self"

11. *We are well led.* This is the verbal leader in the clinic that is less concerned about their popularity and more concerned about holding everyone to their highest standards and driving their teammates to their potential. This **galvanizing** person competes (not destructively) all the time and demands that everyone else do as well!

Not long ago, to "believe in yourself" meant taking a principled, and often lonely, stand when it appeared difficult or dangerous to do so. Now it means accepting one's own desires and inclinations, whatever they may be, and taking whatever steps that may be necessary to advance them.   —William Damon, *Greater Expectations*

This is that leader who lives our core values and tries to get those around them to live them as well. They are not shy about calling people out who don't live them and not afraid to protect those not present when others are trashing them. This tribute was paid to Abraham Lincoln by Carl Sandburg. The poet wrote:

Not often in the story of mankind does a man arrive on earth who is both steel and velvet, who is as hard as rock and soft as drifting fog, who holds in his heart and mind the paradox of terrible storm and peace unspeakable and perfect.   —Carl Sandburg about Abraham Lincoln

 GALVANIZING—international symbol for pushbutton or switch

12. *We want our lives (and not just at work) to be never-ending ascensions but for that to happen properly our fundamental attitude about life and our appreciation for it is critical.* This is that humble, gracious high-achiever that is **grateful** for everything that they have been given in life and has a contagious generosity and optimism that lights up a room just by walking into it.

Finally, there is the question of whether we have a duty to feel grateful. Hundreds of generations who came before us lived dire, short lives, in deprivation or hunger, in ignorance or under oppression or during war, and did so partly motivated by the dream that someday there would be men and women who lived long lives in liberty with plenty to eat and without fear of an approaching storm.

Suffering through privation, those who came before us accumulated the knowledge that makes our lives favored; fought the battles that made our lives free; physically built much of what we rely on for our prosperity; and, most important, shaped the ideals of liberty. For all the myriad problems of modern society, we now live in the world our forebears would have wished for us—in many ways, a better place than they dared imagine. For us not to feel grateful is treacherous selfishness.

Failing to feel grateful to those who came before is such a corrosive notion, it must account at some level for part of our bad feelings about the present. The solution—a rebirth of thankfulness—is in our self-interest.   —Gregg Easterbrook, *The Progress Paradox*

 GRATEFUL—Gordian knot indicating a person is "bound" by debt of thanks

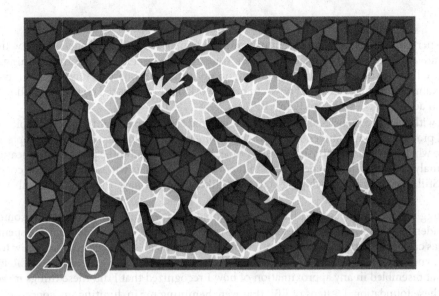

EVOLVING EXPERTISE IN EVIDENCE-BASED PRACTICE WITH CONTEMPORARY CLINICAL REASONING

Eric K. Robertson, PT, DPT and Betsy J. Becker, PT, DPT, PhD

OBJECTIVES

- Compare classic evidence-based practice (EBP) with contemporary evolutions within physical therapy.
- Evaluate clinical reasoning (CR) in relation to expertise and EBP, considering the moral and social aspects of practice.
- Assess a renewed framework for EBP within knowledge networks.
- Examine case considerations expanding the classic view of EBP for a contemporary, media-driven society.

REFLECTIONS FROM A CLINICIAN

To begin this chapter, I (EKR) would like to start with an anecdote that outlines how I arrived at many of the things I will describe in this chapter. I always thought that I understood EBP well, until I realized that I did not. That moment occurred after I was asked by a continuing education provider to help develop a course in advanced EBP. I happily signed up for the task, having held the concepts of EBP in high regard for many years. In fact, when I was in physical therapy school, the term never had a chance to enter our vernacular. However, when I completed a post-professional doctor of physical therapy (DPT) degree several years later, EBP had fully infiltrated academic ranks, and I had been energized and motivated to learn the concepts underlying EBP.

Everyone who has completed a course of study in a health professions educational program since the late 1990s knows about EBP. We know it as having 5 discrete and critical steps, and we know that it is defined by Sackett et al as "the conscientious, explicit and judicious use of current best evidence in making decisions about the care of the individual patient" with integra-

Musolino GM, Jensen GM, eds. *Clinical Reasoning and Decision-Making in Physical Therapy: Facilitation, Assessment, and Implementation* (pp 321-332).

tion of one's clinical expertise, the best available literature, and the patient's values and beliefs.[1] I knew these things too, when I agreed to develop an advanced EBP course. I had even spent time in entry-level DPT programs teaching about EBP, and I was so proud that I had scored several deviations above the norm on my American Board of Physical Therapy Specialties (ABPTS) orthopedic specialist examination! Yet, when I sat down to begin work on the advanced course, I found myself staring at a wall. What exactly formed an advanced course of study in EBP?

I was not altogether without some theories about what my advanced EBP course might contain. I took stock of what I saw and heard from entry-level practitioners and students. I knew that, somehow, I would like to instruct people to be better at critical analysis than they were when they left an entry-level EBP course. I knew I wanted some practical applications, and that perhaps we could expand our analysis to include a deeper dive into the statistical analysis without risking the course transforming into a biostatistics course. Still, the evolving, developing course felt like it did not have the depth and substance I was looking to impart.

I realized I was struggling for the theoretical basis of the course. And, I struggled with that for some time. I read several texts about EBP and evidence-based medicine and evidence-informed practice.[2-5] After a decent time spent working in circles, I finally realized what was causing my frustration: I was attempting to develop an advanced course in how to be a lifelong learner, how to balance patient expectations with research inputs through the lens of one's own expertise, and CR, but I was not thinking of the topic in a way that resembled in any approximation of how I recognized that I did these things myself.

It turns out, it was these foundational 5 steps of EBP that were hemming me in, limiting my conceptualization, and causing the disconnect. Particularly, those 5 steps did not speak to the vast work done related to the development of clinical expertise. They did not tell me about how to be an effective lifelong learner or how to practice so that I could integrate the evidence I was so carefully critiquing. The more layers I peeled back, the more I came to view the courses and texts I had read on the topic as insufficient to take EBP to a more advanced level. As a result, I reimagined the traditional EBP 5-step process and was on my way.

EVIDENCE-BASED PRACTICE: A CURRENT STATE OF AFFAIRS

Before going further, it is valuable to pause and review how EBP has been received and has evolved as part of professional health care practice.

EBP has resulted in an advancement of practice and how students of health professions are taught and acquire knowledge. The development of EBP was due to a need for optimizing quality care for patients in an efficient manner with the onslaught of evidence exceeding one's ability to read everything daily.[1] The process of EBP could guide a clinician to improve quality of care, reduce medical errors, aid in balancing risks and benefits of treatments, challenge views previously based only on beliefs, but now on evidence, and also include patient values into the process.[6] The evidence should be used to inform practice, more effectively CR, but not dictate the final decisions.[7]

However, EBP is not without its critics.[8] It is helpful to examine the strengths and weaknesses of EBP as it was originally framed and continues to be taught and practiced today. While EBP has opened a vector by which evidence can be used in clinics, and based off the latest clinical science, detractors often point out that the process of EBP is time consuming and inefficient.[9] Clinicians may lack access to top quality scientific journals or databases to search. The time it takes to read and filter all the information published is incompatible with life, let alone the demands of a busy clinical practice. Evidence repositories and curated evidence such as clinical practice guidelines (CPGs) and PEDro have attempted to fill a gap and are able to provide clinicians evidence that has already been assessed on its merits or included alongside best practice recommendations.[10] Yet, problems persist, in that CPGs often lack the specificity and guidance that clinical decisions are derived from, and are certainly not available for every type of patient one is to encounter. Although seen as a barrier, one could argue that this gap between evidence and practice is actually the driver for the development of clinical expertise.

A less-discussed but still important limitation of EBP is analyzing its 5 traditional steps and contrasting that with how adults learn. It is through intentional practice, feedback, and mentoring that new skills are acquired and subsequently employed in the clinic. This might explain why, for example, clinicians can sit through a weekend of a 16-hour continuing education course that is richly laden with the best and most current evidence, includes patient cases and examples of application of this evidence, and even includes psychomotor skills practice, but not yield any fruit in terms of change or improvement in their clinical behavior and outcomes.[11-13] This can be due to a number of reasons, but simply, learning a new technique on the weekend does not mean one can apply it effectively in the clinic on Monday. Patient care and technique selection comprise a multifactorial process, which includes much more than psychomotor skills, with a rich plethora of psychosocial factors. Indeed, one course aimed at improving a group of clinicians' beliefs and practice of EBP even found no changes in behavior following the course.[14]

Further still, in the opinion of this author, the concept of expertise, while widely discussed in educational research, is rarely presented or discussed in the context of the science of EBP. While literature discussing expertise references that experts are better able to integrate evidence into their practice, and that they are perhaps more skilled at using a balanced array of patient information, information from evidence sources, and their own experience, it is often a wonder to novices of how exactly these experts attained such skill. An opportunity exists, however, to examine the constructs of EBP alongside those of clinical expertise. In this way, the framework of EBP can expand to include determinants of clinical expertise and evolve in terms of how it is discussed and taught, and so this is the goal of this chapter: to integrate the EBP model with models of clinical expertise. Perhaps we can learn something new together along the way!

Coined in the 1990s, EBP is almost a ubiquitous term in health care today.[1] The APTA has accepted that EBP represents a standard of practice that will lead to the greatest likelihood of positive patient outcomes. To that end, APTA developed a position statement:

> *The physical therapy profession recognizes the use of EBP as central to providing high-quality care and decreasing unwarranted variation in practice. EBP includes the integration of best available research, clinical expertise, and patient values and circumstances related to patient and client management, practice management, and health policy decision-making. Although EBP encompasses more than just applying the best available evidence, many of the concerns and barriers to using EBP revolve around finding and applying research.*[4]

The World Confederation of Physical Therapy also has a policy statement related to EBP and encourages and supports member organizations to "include research methodology and skills to practice as evidence-based practitioners."[15]

THE FIVE STEPS OF EVIDENCE-BASED PRACTICE

Traditionally, EBP is described as having 5 key steps.[16] Each step is dependent upon the others, and full application of the evidence does not occur until each of the steps has been performed on an ongoing basis, couched against the clinician's evaluation of the patient's goals and beliefs, and the clinician's clinical expertise.

Step 1. Developing a clinical question: The entry into EBP begins with the development of a pertinent clinical question. These questions center around patients and are framed in a way that their answer informs the clinician in diagnosis, prognosis, intervention, or another part of patient management. The question should be framed in a way that focuses on foreground more than background material. For example, a question that asks, "What is the preferred intervention for elderly patients with advanced clinical signs of knee osteoarthritis (OA) who exhibit reduced gait speed?" is a more useful question than "How can we treat knee OA?" One common model used when asking the question in this step is the PICO format. In this acronym, P stands for patient, population, or problem; I is intervention exposure or test considered; C means comparison (of intervention, if relevant); and O represents outcome or clinical importance, or the desired effect you are interested in noting. Once a question is formed, we have a framework upon which to begin a literature search.

Step 2. Searching the literature: Having just established a clinically significant question, the clinician then proceeds to his or her favorite database and commences with what he or she hopes will be a tidy literature search. This can take several minutes or several hours depending on the skill of the researcher. Preprocessed evidence collections and databases (eg, PEDro, Cochrane, PTNow.org) or CPGs can assist clinicians in finding pertinent articles or consensus statements related to their topic of interest. Reference librarians are experts in literature searches and are valuable members of the team when it comes to acquiring the evidence. Textbooks are another valuable source of information and should be considered when searching for evidence, as they are not indexed in online databases. Once the search is complete and relevant articles are selected, the clinician moves into the next critical task, which is assessing the validity of the literature.

Step 3. Critiquing the literature: Although only one step out of five, this is the step that is challenging because it includes considering the validity of the study and whether the results will help answer the question established in Step 1. Proper critique of the literature requires a sound understanding of research theory, study design, methods, and statistical analysis, as well as an understanding of the context in which the research study is performed. Judgments can be made as to the internal and external validity of a given trial and thus how generalizable the conclusions are in answering the initially selected question. As no clinical trial is without shortcomings, this step challenges the clinician to carefully scrutinize all aspects of the research in question to reveal further insights. It is recommended to seek primary sources as a preferred piece of literature; ideally, this is a randomized controlled trial.

continued

Step 4. Applying the evidence: At the end of the day, the goal is to learn the answer to the clinical question that impacts patient care, and it happens in this step. If a clinician found evidence that altered his or her CDM about interventions or changed the components of his or her patient education, for example, the next obvious step would be to employ whatever was learned to the patient in question. At this point, it is important to remember that while we may have found literature that we think applies to our patient, it is up to the clinical judgment and expertise of the clinician, as well as the patient's stated goals and inherent values and beliefs, to make the ultimate determination of how much we have learned should be employed.

Step 5. Analyzing the results: This is perhaps an area of EBP that experiences suboptimal engagement.[17-19] It may be because it is so exciting to learn something new, yet often so challenging to accurately measure what we do. However, analyzing the impact of your decisions is a critical step in the process of EBP. It allows clinicians to make judgments that are perhaps more valid in one's own personal practice than any research paper. Analysis of your results in practice could include comparisons of outcomes before and after employing the change in approach, assessment of patient satisfaction, or comparison of outcomes to benchmarked norms, when available.

STRENGTHS AND LIMITATIONS OF EVIDENCE-BASED PRACTICE

EBP has undoubtedly led to much advancement in practice, on both large and small scales. The process of EBP facilitates translation of knowledge into practice, allowing clinicians to focus on the most scientifically supported patient interventions. Providers can leverage the tools of researchers and statisticians to make decisions, expanding their available perspective while inside the clinic. Ideally, this method of improvement in practice will result in more efficient and impactful care, and thus improve the overall state of patient health everywhere. Furthermore, the process of EBP incorporates the provider's experience and the patient's goals and beliefs, resulting in a patient-focused partnership of care.

Unfortunately, the utopian world described above is not always attainable. Critics of EBP point to limitations that make real-world implementation rather challenging.[8] First, a high level of technical skill is required to search and critique the literature. Second, literature searches are not only time consuming but also lead to many articles that clinicians do not have access to, as they are hidden away behind payment gateways. For this reason, despite a clinician's technical adeptness, access to best evidence can be limited without having established strong partnerships and relationships with individuals in universities or large hospital systems. (Note: Being a member of APTA does offer enhanced access to EBP tools and databases for timely and precise evidence for physical therapist practice.)

Last, critics have long pointed out that while the definition of EBP includes clinical expertise as a pillar of evidence, it is seemingly viewed with lowered regard.[20] Perhaps the evidence pyramid is responsible—clinical expertise lies at the very bottom. However, it should be acknowledged that EBP is not synonymous with the evidence pyramid. The evidence pyramid's function is to sort evidence by cause and effect, and does not suggest that clinical expertise is to be deemphasized in comparison. To that end, perhaps the image that should be more popularly promoted is that of the 3-legged stool; the foundation of EBP is held up by the legs of clinical expertise, research evidence, and patient goals and values.

Next, we will share a few limitations to how EBP is described and practiced. Importantly, the 5 steps of EBP, while very logical, do not represent how adult learners general consume, and integrate, information.[21-23] Today, EBP should be taught alongside evolving and developing clinical expertise. It could stand alone as one of the first courses students encounter, but should be reintroduced throughout the curriculum as a dynamic process practiced by all. CR is known to evolve and develop, often looking very different from novice to expert, and the interpretation of EBP is no different. The remainder of this chapter explores this evolution and seeks to delineate it in a way that integrates EBP into what we already know about clinical expertise, CR, and expert patient care.

THE DEVELOPMENT OF CLINICAL REASONING AND CLINICAL EXPERTISE AS IT RELATES TO EVIDENCE-BASED PRACTICE

A prevailing framework describing expert practice is Jensen's theory of expert practice.[24-26] Jensen's work sought to describe differences between experts and novices in clinical practice, consisting of 4 main frameworks that combined to form a philosophy of practice. These frameworks—knowledge, morals and virtues, movement, and CR—come together to form a clinician's philosophy of practice. Pertinent to our discussion is that experts were both quick to innovate and adapt, and they were focused on the patient as a source of evidence. Experts could readily combine the background knowledge they brought to clinic with the novel and unique presentations that patients also bring into the clinic. In addition, the moral compass that experts possess plays an ever-present role in their CDM.

CR by experts is different in many ways than that practiced by novices.[12,25] Pattern recognition, speed, flexibility, and unconscious competence are all characteristics of expert CR. Pattern recognition allows experts to rapidly identify patients and conditions, as well as circumstances that allow CR decisions to occur very quickly.[27] Some expert reasoning is so quick as to appear automatic. Yet experts can have premature closure and make errors in judgment, too. In fact, the upcoming chapter of a resident's reflective self-assessment will provide a clear window into potential errors in CR and CDM, based upon first-hand experiences.

One critical aspect of expert reasoning is that experts also know when not to use a pattern that they might have developed from prior experience. In other words, experts are generally more flexible and can move in and out of pattern recognition, as a form of processing, more adeptly than novices. Likewise, experts are more readily able to adapt new information into circumstances, adapting to new situations, or incorporating new knowledge. In other words, experts possess and use a form of adaptive expertise. Experts are continually learning and refining the very basis of their expertise. In fact, experts have been described as possessing the skills of a master learner![28] It is this very concept of clinician-centered, lifelong learning that has contributed to the emergence of competency-based models of professional development and evaluation.[29] A multitude of constructs converge here, including self-efficacy, self-assessment, and an individual's drive to seek expertise. While an in-depth discourse on these drivers is outside the scope of this chapter (see Section I and Chapter 3), we can find a basis for our advanced EBP concept within them.

EVIDENCE-BASED PRACTICE PROFESSIONALS AS REFLECTIVE, MORAL, AND SOCIAL PRACTITIONERS

The relationship between expertise and EBP extends beyond CR and problem-solving, however. When viewed more broadly, EBP is connected to the larger framework of patient management, and practice in general. The link among all the components of expertise can be realized within the context of a clinician who is also advanced at practicing EBP.

- **EBP as a moral practitioner:** Moral practitioners are able to identify moral and ethical issues, anticipate them, and account for them in practice. Moral practitioners keep the various stakeholders in mind, and the patient, as the primary stakeholder, is a primary determinant of the direction an intervention or treatment takes. The goals and values of the patient factor loom large in CDM. As it relates to EBP, the moral practitioner would never let research findings dominate a discussion with a patient. Instead, the moral practitioner can understand when to apply research findings, and when not to adopt them. The moral practitioner is more likely to incorporate flexibility in his or her thinking and CR, as well as integration of research, in seeking the solution that enables the patient to achieve treatment goals.

- **EBP as a reflective practitioner (RP):** RPs spend time reviewing their decisions and outcomes, and use this review to learn from patients and practice encounters as two of several primary sources of information. EBP includes reflection in the model proposed by Sackett et al,[1] in that the final step of EBP is to analyze one's outcomes. Beyond this, however, RPs can find value in the metacognitive processes that result from reviewing narratives, reflecting and discussing patient cases, and hypothesizing alternate approaches. In other words, RPs can be deeply and positively affected by their critical review of their application of evidence in practice.

- **EBP as a social practitioner:** Social practice involves the link between clinical practice and the context of society and social situations in which that practice occurs. More than simply identifying social aspects of disability, social practitioners partake in both activities and inquiry from a social perspective. Social practitioners inquire through reflective questions that seek to understand how an individual is integrated into his or her social context. Activities consist of practicing in a manner that causes a strengthening of the social context in which both the patient and the practitioner exist. It should be noted that social practice can extend beyond the individual to include the communities and professions in which both patients and/or clinicians exist.

In this section, the concept of expertise in practice was described and placed alongside the concept of EBP. In doing so, we have laid the groundwork to consider EBP not just as a set of steps one completes, but also as a cross-cutting competency that is inextricable from expert practice and CR. Practitioners who exhibit expertise from an EBP perspective must also exhibit expertise as it relates to background knowledge, morals and virtues, CR, and the application of movement as an intervention. EBP is woven in the fabric of the expert practitioners' capabilities, yet experts will not hesitate to even call those principles into question to drive for the best practice for the patients and clients they are serving. Next, we explore how reframing EBP in the context of expertise can provide an enriched framework for teaching and learning about this important aspect of clinical practice.

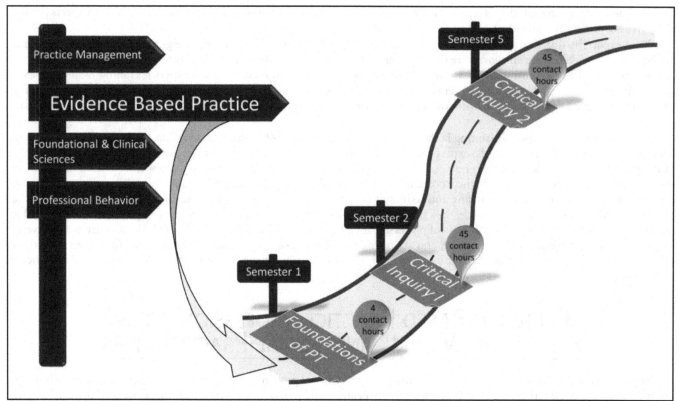

Figure 26-1. One example of incorporating EBP into an entry-level DPT program. The road illustrates the journey of learning and applying EBP early and later during the curriculum. Between the formal EBP instruction milestones, the content is applied in the practice management and clinical science courses. As a result, professional behaviors of a DPT are developed. The road is curved to show the challenges of searching for, interpreting, or contributing to EBP. The road does not end but rather continues on demonstrating the lifelong commitment to creating, evaluating, and applying EBP.

A FRAMEWORK FOR TEACHING AND LEARNING EVIDENCE-BASED PRACTICE

In some health professions education, EBP is presented as a discrete course, which does not allow a student to practice these skills alongside psychomotor and cognitive skill. It teaches EBP as a skill to be learned, with steps the conscientious health care practitioner must take. This course is usually taught early in a curriculum. This is, one might assume, to account for the fact that all subsequent subjects must incorporate the principles of EBP. However, this integration is usually left up to the individual student, or is otherwise left hanging as a directive: "Remember to use your EBP!" Once released out into the real world of practice, clinicians are presented with a multitude of options for continuing competency, but rare among them is advancing one's EBP skills as a topic by itself. Yet, one argues that continuing competency courses themselves are evidence-based, although this low mark is both easily obtained and does little to instill in learners a real improvement in their clinical expertise, or CR directly.

Conversely, one can view EBP as a cross-cutting competency. Instead of a discrete subject, EBP is more a set of foundational principles and a framework that can be applied to all aspects of education and practice. While there is no specific course in expertise per se, the vast collection of experiences clinicians are exposed to all contribute to the attainment of expertise in practice. The argument here is that the very principles of EBP should be considered an essential aspect of the expertise people aim to attain. By increasing the lens of how EBP intersects various aspects of practice, and by dedicating time to reflection, practice, and attainment of these skills and principles, perhaps practice overall can be elevated. This then calls for a review of the essential skills necessary for effective integration of evidence into practice. These include everything from technical research competencies, to technology competencies, to andragogical principles for integrating EBP into entry-level and advanced curricula.

One example of EBP threaded throughout the curriculum is shown in Figure 26-1. EBP is 1 of 4 components of which the curriculum is based and includes content in 3 courses. In addition, EBP is embedded in courses on patient management and CR. The EBP concepts are reinforced throughout the curriculum where students, guided by faculty, ask answerable clinical questions and find evidence to influence patient care decisions.

1. **Technical research competencies:** These encompass more of the traditional skills related to the 5 steps of EBP.

   a. **Search strategies:** In the time-compressed world that is clinical practice, it is essential for clinicians to have the ability to rapidly search and locate key articles and information related to a topic of interest. Too many times clinicians are seen spinning their wheels with databases, using imprecise search terms or ineffective strategies. Resources here include demonstrations of search skills and leveraging medical librarians, as well as the vast array of learning materials related to sites such as PubMed, and appropriate databases for topics under consideration (eg, CINAHL may be more fruitful to pursue for social sciences queries).

   b. **Access to literature:** Although access to literature is often cited as a barrier to EBP, there are ways in which clinicians can maximize their reach. Understanding these strategies can prove critical in the quest for EBP expertise. PubMed Central, Google Scholar, and a host of other online sites offer preprocessed evidence sources. The APTA also has a members-only resource, PTNow.org.

   c. **Statistical competency:** A working knowledge of enough statistical metrics is essential to truly critique a paper or understand the findings of a given analysis (eg, regression, ANOVA). Correctly appraising a study's statistical test for meeting the purpose of the study and research questions is the objective here. Regular employment of minimum clinically important differences, hypothesis testing, measures of association, and effect sizes are all critical to understanding the literature, in relation to a patient case and associated CR/CDM. Health informatics should also be taken into account to improve health care outcomes.

   d. **Critical analysis:** This is similar to the third step of EBP and includes the ability to properly dissect and analyze a given study, groups of studies, and/or health informatics.

   e. **Hierarchy of evidence[20]:** This is seemingly simple, but there is more than meets the eye to understand evidence hierarchies. In terms of associating cause and effect, there is one hierarchy of evidence and another for weighing all sources of information from the patient, literature, and experience. Both need to be appreciated. In addition, meta-analysis, systematic reviews, and CPG review methods should be carefully scrutinized and considered for compliance with national standards before considering the purported patient applications.

2. **Technological competencies:** Technological competencies include understanding how to use social media, as well as digital sources of information, and evaluating online sources of information for veracity and value.

   a. **Social media:** Great opportunities exist within the social media landscape to quickly glean information from journals or colleagues, direct from researchers, and more. Individuals may feel comfortable using social media for personal uses, but academic and professional uses may require additional mentoring to leverage the opportunities here. Most journals have Twitter feeds, and Facebook groups can link people interested in a particular topic. Sources and source data on social media must be carefully scrutinized for fidelity and veracity measures. One should not just jump to face value of the latest tweet, blog statement, or factoid presented and packaged in a fancy marketing manner. Take the time to consider the sources of data, whether methods meet the muster for validity and reliability, and if the sources are trustworthy or driven by ulterior motives.

   b. **Managing workflow and information streams:** One possible drawback to social media is that the valuable information is often delivered alongside copious amounts of noncritical information. Approached in the wrong way, social media can be an enormous opportunity for wasting precious time, just as it is a significant opportunity for saving time when done correctly. Understanding how to curate lists and filter information using native apps or third-party software solutions are a critical aspect to using social media efficiently. Decisions about time investment and what social media platforms to invest in are all part of this competency.

   c. **Evaluating sources and digital literacy:** While it is easier to trust tweets and Facebook posts from official scientific journal sources, the digital environment is rich with sources of misinformation and opportunities to confound rather than enlighten. The burden, therefore, is arguably greater than in traditional scientific environments (eg, the library) in being a skeptical consumer of information and understanding the digital environment enough to know when one is being led astray. Clearly understanding and identifying the original source of information being shared is not always so clear cut, but the ability to do so is just as important as if one were to cite a research paper in a journal. Knowing when something is a retweet, for example, and the date of the retweet relative to the original tweet, is just one example of how social media requires a unique form of digital literacy.

3. **Integration of EBP into CR:** While CR is at the forefront of most professional development pathways, careful attention to how CR is approached, and integration of the principles of EBP during this educational process, can be beneficial. Residency and fellowship training programs are based in mentoring and reflection—in other words, metacognitive processes that enable clinicians to learn from an assigned meaning to their experiences. However, reflection is a skill that can be practiced and improved upon. As students practice reflections and narrative reasoning, close reflection on evidence

should be included. Closely related to this is the concept of deliberative practice. This type of practice is systematic and regular, conducted with purpose, and requiring focused attention to a given objective.[30] Deliberative practice has shown to be beneficial over other forms of less structured practice. Thus, inclusion of EBP principles into deliberative practice related to reflection and the development of CR seems only logical.

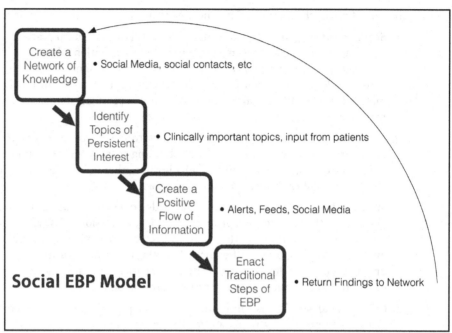

Figure 26-2. A revised, social model of EBP.

4. **Instructional competencies for EBP:** Educators interested in improving the ability for their students to leverage a revised framework for EBP should consider the above points for inclusion in their curricula. Programs from entry-level to residency and fellowship training programs should reflect on which aspects of EBP should be included at a given level, and challenge themselves to continually challenge their students' effectiveness and skill in processing and leveraging information from high-quality sources in their practice. This can result in some instructors investing time in learning more about social media, or the development of new strategies of deliberative practice to best reinforce the principles of EBP in practice.

Viewing EBP as a cross-cutting competency vs a distinct skill or topic can assist both educators and learners in expanding the role that EBP plays in their professional lives. Almost inextricable from the development of clinical expertise, the development of expertise in the principles and practice of EBP are just as critical as any manual therapy technique, psychomotor skill, or communication strategy.

ENVISIONING A NEW FRAMEWORK: A SOCIAL MODEL OF EVIDENCE-BASED PRACTICE

It can be helpful to put all of this conversation together into one picture. To that end, Figure 26-2 outlines a revised model for EBP. This model incorporates and includes the original 5-step process of EBP, while expanding the process of question-gathering to include a network of information.

1. **Develop a network of knowledge.** A knowledge network can be as large or small, as robust and unique as individuals themselves. A network can be highly interconnected, where information sources overlap, leading to triangulation of information to check for accuracy. Networks of knowledge are social in nature, and can consist of colleagues, classic library and journal sources, and less classic information sources such as social media platforms and even radio or television. Since networks of knowledge literature do not exist for physical therapy, we draw from the family medicine literature for an example. Studies show an effective network provided breadth of knowledge, career opportunities, and scholarly activity prospects.[31,32] This supports not only becoming good consumers of the literature, but also contributing to the evidence with their own scholarly work. The more inputs to which you have access, the more likely you are to be able to know, or locate, the information you need. However, one problem with a very large network is managing all the incoming information and filtering out what is unrelated, unnecessary, or inaccurate. The diversity of information or individual characteristics of collaborators within a network can be measured and is explored in more depth in the following chapter. A model of this kind of social network of information informing EBP is diagrammed in Figure 26-3.

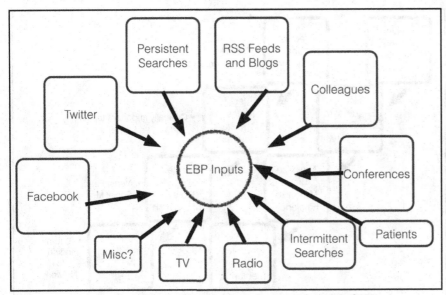

Figure 26-3. A collection of inputs form the basis for a social model of EBP.

2. **Identify persistent questions.** In contrast to typical descriptions of EBP, this model assumes that clinicians operate around certain clinical efficiencies. Geographic, demographic, or other population factors often make it likely that in a given clinical setting, clinicians are aware of the types of patients and conditions they are likely to encounter. Persistent questions can also arise from long-standing interests. For example, a clinician in a given clinic runs a group class on a weekly basis. Instead of formulating a new patient-oriented question and conducting a search each week, the clinician could instead develop a carefully crafted, persistent question related to the effectiveness of class-based or group-based rehabilitation, and input this question into tools that can feed information back to the clinician. Just how this is performed is the next step in our process! It is important to recognize that inputs from patients and lived experiences are as critical here as any other particular source of information.

3. **Create a positive flow of information.** The age of the internet and smartphones has provided us with a multitude of tools to manage the information overflow it has created access to for our judicious utilization. Using tools from Twitter lists, Facebook groups, alerts to RSS feeds (Really Simply Syndication), clinicians can curate their network of knowledge to have key, high-quality information related to their persistent, clinically important questions directed straight to them. Data visualization using infographics is another method to aid in managing the flow of information. A recent study showed higher reader preference and a lower mental effort (eg, cognitive load) when reviewing literature using an infographic summary vs text-only material.[33] There was no difference in the delayed information retention between infographic summaries and text-only material. Future studies could include both formats to better meet the needs of different learning preferences.

4. **Employ the traditional steps of EBP.** While we may feel wondrous in developing rapid, efficient delivery systems of meaningful information at out fingertips, we are not unburdened from the obligation to carefully scrutinize and critically evaluate the information before us. This is where the beauty of the traditional methods of EBP and those classical 5 steps comes to bear.

5. **Return the findings to the network.** As responsible members of any social network, giving is as important as is receiving. To that end, there exists a duty to return that which one learns to the network from which it was gleaned. This could be as simple as a tweet about a topic, or more in-depth writing in a blog post, or even a scholarly product such as an infographic to supplement and summarize literature. Without contributions to the evidence, the profession cannot move forward with the improved patient outcomes for optimizing human movement, the basis of the origins of EBP. So too do our findings return to the network in the embodiment of our treatments, clinical applications, and educational offerings to our colleagues.

Overlaying a Theory of Expertise on a Social Model of Evidence-Based Practice

Missing from the social model of EBP presented in the preceding section is the prior discussion of the theory of expertise. We can envision this as a parallel process that can occur, albeit at a different time scale, as our model of EBP. Figure 26-4 diagrams just one embodiment of the 2 systems of EBP and clinical expertise side by side. Depending on the nuances and focus of a given discussion, we might decide that the contents of the expertise column could shift or change given the sheer breadth of the topic.

The critical aspect, however, is to consider these 2 processes together. Just like the quest for advancing clinical expertise does not have a finishing point, neither should the process and practice of EBP. Two example cases are presented to exemplify the incorporation of this social model of EBP into professional development plans.

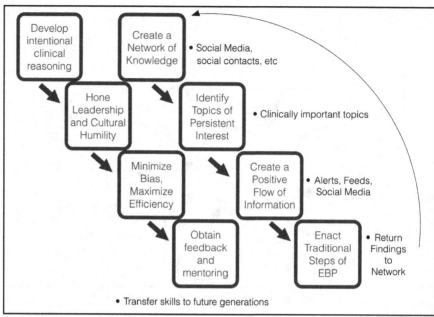

Figure 26-4. Expertise and EBP as parallel processes.

EBP Professional Development Plan: Example Case 1

Background: Jane is an academic faculty member at a physical therapy institution. She has been working for 15 years in academia, and has achieved the rank of professor. Prior to her academic post, she was in practice for 15 years. Jane is ABPTS-certified in geriatrics and has continued clinical practice. She mentors in a residency program and is regarded by her peers as an expert clinician.

Problem: Jane has recognized that her mentees in the clinic are more quickly able to identify newly published research than she is, and that she is somewhat challenged by the new website design from the institution's library. While these self-identified problems do not have a direct impact on patient care, and Jane's outcomes remain strong, she feels that this is an area where she can improve to enhance both her teaching and mentoring, as well as future learning potential.

Solution: Jane seeks out a junior faculty member who has published on EBP and social media, as well as a medical librarian. Jane receives mentoring in social media tools including the use of a Tweet deck to improve the usability of her Twitter account, and subscribes to several geriatric research Facebook and LinkedIn groups. The medical librarian points Jane to several web resources to enhance her database use and spends several sessions mentoring Jane.

Outcome: Jane now is able to challenge her young mentees in who notices new literature on Twitter first. She has included an assignment in her geriatrics management course that requires students to use particular databases at the library and discuss findings on social media. In the process, Jane discovers a new network of professionals and expands her research network.

EBP Professional Development Plan: Example Case 2

Background: Chris is a young professional working in a health system outpatient clinic and sees primarily musculoskeletal patients. Chris has been in practice for 2 years and is an avid user of social media, spending several hours a day on various platforms. Professional development to this point has consisted of going to national conferences and taking continuing education weekend courses in dry needling.

Problem: Chris has received feedback from the clinic leadership that both patient outcomes and satisfaction are lagging behind benchmarked clinic norms. Additionally, Chris is unable to identify a specific cause for this, and expressed frustration that time spent reading the manual therapy journal each month has apparently been wasted.

Solution: Chris meets with a lead clinical mentor for the clinic and gets feedback about patient management based on several observed sessions. A recommendation is made for Chris to complete a clinical residency program to enhance reflection skills and the ability to integrate research into practice. Chris also identifies that the use of social media up to this point has been recreational, and a decision is made to make this time more productive. To that end, Chris reaches out to several peers on social media and finds new groups of clinicians and researchers with whom he can follow and network.

Outcome: Using both the residency program and a vastly enhanced social network, Chris is able to increase his literature consumption dramatically. Mentoring sessions in the clinic have identified deficits in taking a patient history, and this is being addressed. Chris has formed a social network chat session that serves as a virtual journal club to work on critical analysis of key papers each month. Seven months later, well into the residency, clinical outcomes have not improved yet, but patient satisfaction is trending upward, and Chris demonstrates improved fundamentals in practice.

Reflection Moment: Points to Ponder

How has your view of EBP and CR been impacted through your chapter learning?

What surprised you most? What aspects do you find not challenging for your professional development?

Describe the future of how you see digital media continuing to enhance EBP and CR in the health professions for the clinician and our patients' benefit.

REFERENCES

1. Sackett DL, Rosenberg WMC, Gray JAM, Haynes RB, Richardson WS. Evidence based medicine: what it is and what it isn't. *BMJ.* 1996;312(7023):71-72.
2. Woodbury MG, Bscpt, L Msc J, Kuhnke J. Evidence-based practice vs. evidence-informed practice: what's the difference? *Wound Care Can.* 2014;12:18-21.
3. Gwyer J, Hack LM. *Evidence Into Practice: Integrating Judgment, Values, and Research.* Philadelphia, PA: FA Davis Company; 2013.
4. Evidence-based practice & research. http://www.apta.org/EvidenceResearch/. Accessed May 14, 2018.
5. Jewell DV. *Guide to Evidence-Based Physical Therapist Practice.* 4th ed. Burlington, MA: Jones & Bartlett Learning; 2017.
6. Manske RC, Lehecka BJ. Evidence-based medicine/practice in sports physical therapy. *Int J Sports Phys Ther.* 2012;7(5):461-473.
7. Swisher AK. Not resting on our laurels. *Cardiopulm Phys Ther J.* 2011;22(1):4.
8. Scurlock-Evans L, Upton P, Upton D. Evidence-based practice in physiotherapy: a systematic review of barriers, enablers and interventions. *Physiotherapy.* 2014;100(3):208-219.
9. Thomas A, Han L, Osler BP, Turnbull EA, Douglas E. Students' attitudes and perceptions of teaching and assessment of evidence-based practice in an occupational therapy professional master's curriculum: a mixed methods study. *BMC Med Educ.* 2017;17.
10. Bernhardsson S, Johansson K, Nilsen P, Öberg B, Larsson MEH. Determinants of guideline use in primary care physical therapy: a cross-sectional survey of attitudes, knowledge, and behavior. *Phys Ther.* 2014;94(3):343-354.

11. Arnadottir SA, Gudjonsdottir B. Icelandic physical therapists' attitudes toward adoption of new knowledge and evidence-based practice: cross-sectional web-based survey. *Phys Ther.* 2016;96(11):1724-1733.

12. Davies C, Nitz AJ, Mattacola CG, et al. Practice patterns when treating patients with low back pain: a survey of physical therapists. *Physiother Theory Pract.* 2014;30:399-408.

13. Stevenson K, Lewis M, Hay E. Does physiotherapy management of low back pain change as a result of an evidence-based educational programme? *J Eval Clin Pract.* 2006;12(3):365-375.

14. Condon C, McGrane N, Mockler D, Stokes E. Ability of physiotherapists to undertake evidence-based practice steps: a scoping review. *Physiotherapy.* 2016;102(1):10-19.

15. World Confederation for Physical Therapy policy statement on evidence based practice. https://www.wcpt.org/sites/wcpt.org/files/files/PS_Education_Sept2011.pdf. Accessed June 6, 2018.

16. Johnson C. Evidence-based practice in 5 simple steps. *J Manipulative Physiol Ther.* 2008;31(3):169-170.

17. Meerhoff GA, van Dulmen AS, Maas MJM, et al. Development and evaluation of an implementation strategy for collecting data in a national registry and the use of patient-reported outcome measures in physical therapist practices: quality improvement study. *Phys Ther.* 2017;97(8):837-851.

18. McDonnell B, Stillwell S, Hart S, Davis RB. Breaking down barriers to the utilization of standardized tests and outcome measures in acute care physical therapist practice: an observational longitudinal study. *Phys Ther.* 2018;98(6):528-538.

19. Greenberg EM, Greenberg ET, Albaugh J, Storey E, Ganley TJ. Rehabilitation practice patterns following anterior cruciate ligament reconstruction: a survey of physical therapists. *J Orthop Sports Phys Ther.* 2018;48(10):801-811.

20. Murad MH, Asi N, Alsawas M, Alahdab F. New evidence pyramid. *BMJ Evid Based Med.* http://ebm.bmj.com/content/21/4/125. Accessed June 6, 2018.

21. Hayward LM, Black LL, Mostrom E. The first two years of practice: a longitudinal perspective on the learning and professional development of promising novice physical therapists. *Phys Ther.* https://academic.oup.com/ptj/article/93/3/369/2735360?searchresult=1. Accessed May 14, 2018.

22. Cho KK, Marjadi B, Langendyk V, Hu W. Medical student changes in self-regulated learning during the transition to the clinical environment. *BMC Med Educ.* 2017;17(1):59.

23. History of iPhone. Wikipedia. https://en.wikipedia.org/w/index.php?title=History_of_iPhone&oldid=840800323. Accessed June 7, 2019.

24. Jensen GM. Learning: what matters most. *Phys Ther.* 2011;91(11):1674-1689.

25. Jensen GM, Shepard KF, Gwyer J, Hack LM. Attribute dimensions that distinguish master and novice physical therapy clinicians in orthopaedic settings. *Phys Ther.* 1992;72(10):711-722.

26. Jensen GM, Gwyer J, Shepard KF. Expert practice in physical therapy. *Phys Ther.* 2000;80(1):28-43; discussion 44-52.

27. Djulbegovic B, Hozo I, Beckstead J, Tsalatsanis A, Pauker SG. Dual processing model of medical decision-making. *BMC Med Inform Decis Mak.* 2012;12:94.

28. Schumacher DJ, Englander R, Carraccio C. Developing the master learner: applying learning theory to the learner, the teacher, and the learning environment. *Acad Med J Assoc Am Med Coll.* 2013;88(11):1635-1645.

29. Melnyk BM, Gallagher-Ford L, Long LE, Fineout-Overholt E. The establishment of evidence-based practice competencies for practicing registered nurses and advanced practice nurses in real-world clinical settings: proficiencies to improve healthcare quality, reliability, patient outcomes, and costs. *Worldviews Evid Based Nurs.* 2014;11(1):5-15.

30. Duvivier RJ, van Dalen J, Muijtjens AM, et al. The role of deliberate practice in the acquisition of clinical skills. *BMC Med Educ.* 2011;11:101.

31. Sicat BL, O'Kane Kreutzer K, Gary J, et al. A collaboration among health sciences schools to enhance faculty development in teaching. *Am J Pharm Educ.* 2014;78(5).

32. Katerndahl D. Co-evolution of departmental research collaboration and scholarly outcomes. *J Eval Clin Pract.* 18(6):1241-1247.

33. Martin LJ, Turnquist A, Groot B, et al. Exploring the role of infographics for summarizing medical literature. *Health Prof Educ.* 2019;5(1):48-57.

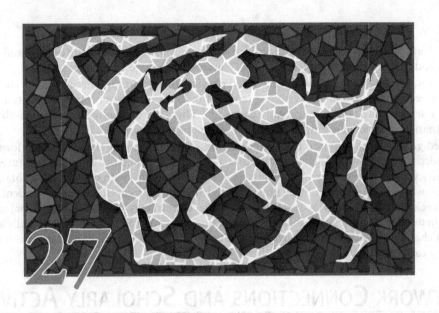

EARLY CAREER FACULTY DEVELOPMENT:
Maximizing Social Capital for Meaningful Clinical Reasoning

Betsy J. Becker, PT, DPT, PhD

OBJECTIVES

- Discuss the concept of agency for the intentional need for early career development of faculty and clinical scholars.
- Examine social network analysis and interconnections concerning scholarship.
- Explore social capital theory, the description of 3 related constructs, and related evidence-based literature.
- Appreciate the relationship of faculty scholarship with clinical reasoning (CR) capacities for teaching and learning.
- Consider preliminary results of a social network analysis with early career physical therapy faculty scholars.

INTRODUCTION

Faculty are responsible for facilitating CR through the scholarship of teaching and learning. Hence, faculty themselves must be capable of CR and related scholarly works. There is evidence in the physical therapy profession of low levels of scholarly activity by program faculty. Scholarly activity is currently measured by a simple count, without accounting for the variety of contributions such as authorship order on publications or grant award amount. Effective network structure and composition have been shown in other professions to aid in improved career advancement, innovation, and collaboration for scholarly activity. Networks can be measured using social network analysis based on the social capital theory. Individual faculty choices about career advancement and decisions about pursuing scholarly activity should be considered by accounting for strategic and intentional actions by faculty. This concept is termed agency. With an accurate understanding of the relationship among agency,

Musolino GM, Jensen GM, eds. *Clinical Reasoning and Decision-Making in Physical Therapy: Facilitation, Assessment, and Implementation* (pp 333-343).

professional networks, and scholarly activity, early career physical therapy faculty could more quickly and appropriately develop success in scholarship and further the development of CR as educators, scholars, and learners.

There are 2899 full-time faculty working in 242 accredited physical therapist programs across the country.[1] Of these, fewer than half (44.8%) have academic doctorates, yet all are required by the Commission on Accreditation in Physical Therapy Education (CAPTE) to demonstrate an active scholarly agenda.[1-3] There are currently 141 full-time physical therapy faculty vacancies, with more than 90 additional openings projected over the next few years.[1]

To sustain continued growth in the physical therapy profession, especially among those who lack formal research training, instruction will be needed for new physical therapist educators regarding social and institutional structures that will affect them during their early faculty years. These faculty will need to establish relationships with colleagues to obtain guidance about setting a scholarly agenda, which is essential for navigating the academy while promoting CR with student learners. Waiting for these connections to develop on their own is an unreliable and ineffective strategy.[4,5] The long-term goal is to provide assistance to early career faculty in developing professional network connections for career advancement, especially as it relates to scholarship. The focus of this chapter provides both the theoretical foundation and pragmatic considerations for research examining social networks of early career faculty within physical therapy.

NETWORK CONNECTIONS AND SCHOLARLY ACTIVITY

The effectiveness of an institution of higher learning is directly related to the quality and vigor of its faculty. Faculty must be capable of facilitating CR and clinical problem-solving (CPS) within the developing physical therapist professional. Therefore, encouraging optimal performance and assisting with the scholarly agenda of new faculty and their career advancement should be a top priority. Scholarship promotes the thinking about learning and teaching within the profession with discovery, integration, application, and teaching from the traditional viewpoint of Boyer's model.[6] However, today, we must also consider the aspects of digital scholarship, as Rumsey described in a scholarly communication at the University of Virginia.[7] Examples of digital scholarship include, but are not limited to, blogs, data visualization, metadata generations, commentaries in virtual spaces, and focused social media groups. Both teachers and learners need to be able to discern these resources for meaning, scholarship, and applications for higher-level learning.

Faculty often describe their early years of establishing new patterns of the teaching, publishing, and service required by the academy as isolating, lonely, and stressful.[5,8] Results from a study of medical faculty showed network connections mattered a great deal in mitigating these issues.[9] There is also evidence that knowledge of the makeup of a faculty network leads to improved performance, innovation, and collaborations.[9-11]

The number of available connections (ie, network size) and how well a faculty member knows about and understands professional connections are as important as the depth and breadth of its member experiences.[12-15] In the practice of family medicine, for example, effective networks provided breadth of knowledge, career opportunities, and scholarly activity prospects.[4,15] Faculty who examined the expertise and demographics of their contacts had a greater likelihood of success in scholarly activity and maintained greater interest in collaboration with faculty from other disciplines.[16,17] One study on the value of research collaborations noted "... No one person is capable of maintaining the deep understanding necessary to conduct truly interdisciplinary research."[18(p272)]

Therefore, it is clearly important to study successful methods to evolve scholarly activity networks. Models for collaboration in research continue to develop, and as another study advocates, for innovation to occur, we must "respond to shifts in the way work is created, completed, and gauged, so that talented clinicians and researchers will be able to flourish in their careers."[19(p462)]

However, to date, the study of how professional relationships are developed and how they contribute to an effective network for scholarly activity has not been applied to the profession of physical therapy, where there is an urgent need to support scholarly activity. Later in the chapter, I will share some preliminary results of my investigation into this novel area of research for the profession.

SCHOLARLY ACTIVITY IN PHYSICAL THERAPY

While it is required that physical therapist faculty have a scholarly agenda,[2] only 21% of physical therapist faculty describe themselves as active in scholarship.[20] A recent study by Hinman and Brown[21] of 2602 physical therapist faculty at 225 accredited physical therapist schools found that scholarly productivity has remained stable over the past 10 years, and yet it was interesting to note that the majority of programs had at least one faculty member who had not yet disseminated a scholarly product. Suggestions included continued focus on teaching and service, as reflected by the greater percentage of time assigned to these areas rather than to scholarship.[21] The reported barriers to maintaining a scholarly agenda among physical therapist faculty are similar to those in other health care research professions, including lack of time and institutional support, few available resources for successful ongoing projects, and, for some, no doctoral training.[21]

Rating	Description
0	no scholarly involvement
1	active, but no products yet
2	less than 5 disseminated products
3	5 to 10 disseminated products
4	more than 10 disseminated products

Figure 27-1. Categories for ranking scholarly productivity by the CAPTE. Hinman MR, Brown T. Changing profile of the physical therapy professoriate—are we meeting CAPTE's expectations? *J Phys Ther Educ.* 2017;31[4]:95-104 and Commission on Accreditation for Physical Therapy Education. Position papers accreditation handbook 2018. http://www.capteonline.org/uploadedFiles/CAPTEorg/About_CAPTE/Resources/Accreditation_Handbook/PositionPapers.pdf.)

MEASURING SCHOLARLY ACTIVITY

Prior studies that explored factors influencing scholarly productivity in physical therapy used simple counts of publications and presentations without describing authorship order, journal impact factor, presentation audience (eg, national or local), and/or peer-review status and/or invited opportunities. Also omitted were grant awards, a very significant contribution of scholarly activity.[21-23] For example, being the first author of a peer-reviewed published paper is universally recognized as a greater contribution than fourth author of seven for a book chapter, but of course, scholarship comprises both. The studies limited the exploration to databases and archival information, rather than primary documents (eg, a faculty curriculum vitae, or CV, would reflect a more complete record of achievement).

CAPTE considers only the quantity of items disseminated, with 5 categories to gauge productivity (Figure 27-1). CAPTE standards expect faculty have "at least one accomplishment for every 2 years of academic service" and "new faculty (<5 years) are not expected to have an established scholarly record yet but should have an appropriate agenda to get there."[24(p12)] Thus, for accreditation purposes, a program could be complying if a faculty member did not have any scholarly output until his or her sixth year in the academy, a very generous time to produce one publication, especially within a doctoring profession. This ranking of scholarly productivity was used to describe the professoriate as a whole in a recent study, but the authors stated that a major limitation was "scholarly productivity is not clearly defined nor weighted by any objective measure of quality such as the type of scholarly product, level of authorship, or impact factor."[21(p103)]

Despite the measurement limitation, prior work can be used to demonstrate the ongoing difficulty with higher academic productivity in physical therapy. Richter et al[25] explored the physical therapist program characteristics associated with the number of publications of physical therapist faculty from 1998 to 2002, and showed that faculty size, whether programs offered a research doctorate, and Carnegie classification were significant. Two studies by Kaufman et al[22,23] that used publications and presentation quantity as outcome measures showed that strong predictors of productivity were highest degree earned, appointment status, and faculty rewards. Kaufman et al[22] also found a gender gap in peer-reviewed publications, with women publishing half as many works as men. Finally, although such studies provide helpful information on the status of scholarly productivity and factors associated with successful presentations and publications, findings might differ if various types of scholarship were weighted.

There are weighted values proposed within other professions, but these have severe limitations that make them unsuitable to implement for physical therapist faculty. For example, a scoring system proposed for lawyers accounts for the length of a publication, and this is not a measurement in physical therapist scoring.[26] A score for athletic trainers does not account for levels of authorship or presentation audience, and leaves out grant awards altogether.[27] A scholarly activity point system was proposed for surgical residents, but gave the same score to all grants regardless of amount awarded or role (this system was developed by 4 persons in-house at one medical center).[28] Some would also argue that a $10,000 to $20,000 funded grant is the same amount of work and process steps as a funded grant of $50,000 to $100,000, yet reporting mechanisms, oversight, and accountability are much greater.

A new scoring system that accounts for the value of variances in scholarly work would be an innovative way to report scholarship in physical therapist training. Boyers' model (see chapter appendix) provides an adequate framework, yet does not address specificity. If rubrics accounted for early work, such as published abstracts or middle authorship, this system would be sensitive enough to show progress by early career faculty. It could also include digital aspects of the scholarship of teaching, learning, and assessment. Gathering all scholarly information—not just presentations and publications from existing databases, but also primary documents including vitaes or personal interviews—would also make this scoring system comprehensive. The system could also improve knowledge for early career faculty of different scholarly items or tracks (eg, educator, researcher, or clinical focus) to better judge where best to expend their limited time and effort for the best outcome. This last point may seem obvious to experienced faculty, but early career faculty may indeed not always know what constitutes valuable scholarly contributions within a particular institution type.

AGENCY

So far, this chapter has covered how faculty network relationships may impact scholarly activity and the state of scholarly activity in physical therapy, including measurement methods. Let us now consider the importance pertaining to individual faculty choices about career advancement and decisions about what scholarly activity to pursue. Agency is defined as taking strategic or intentional actions to achieve meaningful goals, and is shaped by experiences, social capital, and the context in which decisions are made.[29,30] Sociological constructs consider agency as how individuals intentionally plan to influence the trajectory of their careers by creating work situations or opportunities conducive to its development. Agency has also been described as seeking meaningful work, contributing effectively, and being passionate about one's profession.[29]

Agency can be subdivided into agency perspective (ie, self-talk or strategic views in a given situation) and agency behavior (ie, the specific action taken to help one advance).[31] The subdivisions should be familiar to you from earlier chapters related to CR "thinking out loud" and reflective practice perspectives. Similar to the promotion of thinking out loud for CR, self-talk also enhances the faculty members' capacities for meaningful social context to further promote students' CR and CPS abilities. The students are provided a window, so to speak, into the developing faculty scholars' thinking processes, with sharing of self-talk. The exchange of think out loud and sharing of self-talk lends to rich opportunities for CR collaboration for both the student and faculty scholars' development; effectively raising the bar for those who follow.

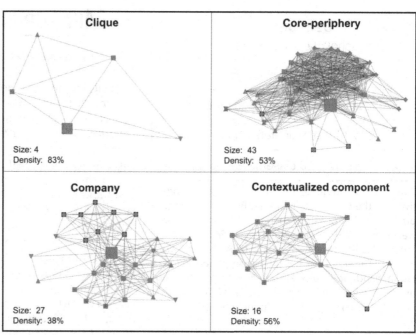

Figure 27-2. Network maps illustrating shape, size, and density structures. The large square is the reference individual whose network is displayed. The shape of the dots indicates where the network member works: square = physical therapist at the institution, triangle = physical therapist at a different institution, circle in a square = non–physical therapist at a different institution, diamond = non–physical therapist at the same institution, hourglass = clinician.

Agency is important in academic career development, where success is typically related to promotion and to tenure awarded for achievement, visibility, and recognition in teaching, scholarly activity, and service.[29,31,32] In this context, it is also important to note that self-motivation is directly related to agency and may depend on the need for achievement, power, and affiliation with a successful group.[33] Those with greater agency are also likely to be concerned with a high standard of excellence, wish to demonstrate a unique accomplishment, and have specific career goals. Terosky and O'Meara,[31] who interviewed and observed hundreds of undergraduate and graduate faculty and faculty development directors, concluded that the sense of personal agency is 1 of 4 aspects related to professional growth, along with learning, professional relationships, and commitment. In a qualitative study about agency and faculty who apply for promotion, results show both social context and relationships with others heavily influenced a sense of agency.[29] Until now, the concept of agency has not been applied in research about the physical therapist profession, but should be considered when studying early career faculty career advancement, and can be measured if desirable. A valid and reliable tool, developed by Campbell and O'Meara,[32] measures agency perspective and agency behavior. There are also valid and reliable methods to measure network relationships that relate to agency, described in the next section.

SOCIAL NETWORK ANALYSIS

Network Structure

Faculty agency and the value of collaborators can be jointly studied within a social context using social network analysis. The methodology uses graph theory to explain how connections form into social structures that influence individuals and the outcomes of the group. Network structure is illustrated using network maps, size, and density measurements. Sample maps are shown in Figure 27-2, where each dot represents a network contact, and lines run among those who know each other. The closer any person appears to another on the map, the more relationships the 2 people have in common.

By studying the maps, it is possible to identify 4 general shapes.[34] The clique shape develops when one's network includes few contacts who provide exclusive support and become partners or even best friends. The second shape is the company, where the network comprises a large group of people who are highly interconnected. It has been compared to a surrogate family, wherein culture and norms form quickly. The other 2 network shapes, core-periphery and contextualized component, form when different contacts are needed for different tasks.[34] For example, an early career faculty member may have long-standing relationships from residency training, and begin to maintain subgroups of contacts related to clinical practice or interprofessional scholarly collaborations.

In addition to maps, the network structure is described by the total number of contacts, or network size. A large network can be beneficial, but can also pose drawbacks. For example, a network with numerous connections can provide information and resources that benefit an early career faculty member who is developing a scholarly agenda. However, maintaining relationships among this high number of connections may require a great deal of energy and effort, manifesting as too many projects that spread one too thin, or communication burdens that limit making new connections.

Density is the third network structure measure and accounts for degrees of interconnection, or the proportion of network contacts who are also connected with each other. When networks are densely interconnected, or closed, ties are redundant and thus theoretically do not contribute new resources or information.[17] In contrast, a less interconnected, or open, network means one has greater control of information and resources because network contacts do not also talk to the others.

Network Composition

In addition to structure measures, networks can be further explored by similarities and differences among persons in the group. Homophily, or determining network contacts based upon similar characteristics, may occur due to preference (physical therapist faculty who prefer other faculty in their department at their university), peer influence (physical therapists encouraging their non–physical therapist contacts to attend a university meeting), or confounding issues (the best time to develop relationships is likely at one's institution, and proximity facilitates collegial connections).[35] Persons tend to form relationships based on similarities, and resources flow more quickly among them. The converse is also true, where dissimilar persons tend to be less likely to share resources.[36]

However, network composition can also be measured by heterogeneity, or how evenly distributed individual characteristics are within the group.[37] For example, one could measure the diversity of contacts by gender, academic rank, or subject expertise. A glossary of information and examples about how to calculate the network structure and composition measures is provided in Table 27-1.[38]

The next section includes a description of the theory behind studying network structure and composition, and a review the literature where these concepts have been applied.

SOCIAL CAPITAL THEORY

The framework used here for social network analysis is the social capital theory, which includes the 3 constructs shown in Figure 27-3. One focuses on access to resources, where network contacts provide information, supplies, or ideas that would not otherwise be available. A second construct emphasizes social cohesion, with strong interconnected ties contributing to robust support and social integration. The third construct highlights brokering across gaps (also called *structural holes*). Brokers facilitate the flow of information, supplies, ideas, or resources across these holes for the benefit of the individual and the group.[39] Social capital can be measured by accounting for the network structure and composition, especially considering those with expert skills or knowledge.[39] In the academy, network members who are published, have grant funding, or are tenured at the rank of professor may be perceived as valuable and much needed mentors for early career faculty members who seek collaborators for scholarly activity.

The value of social capital for the scholarly activity of early career physical therapist faculty is currently unknown. Furthermore, few studies, to date, report effective network structure (eg, shape, size, density) or composition similarities (homophily) or diversity (heterogeneity) for established physical therapist faculty, let alone for those in the early career years. The next section includes examples from other sectors of social network analysis using social capital theory as a framework.

APPLICATION OF SOCIAL CAPITAL THEORY AND NETWORK ANALYSIS

Rodan and Galunic[10] explored the relationship between business manager performance and network structure (size) and composition measure of diversity (heterogeneity). The results showed that networks with contacts who had a variety of knowledge mattered for overall performance, but that network size did not. They also concluded that the ability to exploit position in the network to gain social capital depended on the accuracy of perceptions about network structure and composition. Therefore, if one were not aware of network makeup, being able to access the social capital—the currency of success—was not possible. The Rodan and Galunic[10] study demonstrated that attaining and maintaining contacts and fostering relationships of trust and reciprocity permitted social capital to flow through the network.

Ryan's[40] mixed-methods study showed that not only are network ties significant but having someone in a position of seniority take an interest and give time to aid in the success was also valuable. The networks were a dynamic process that changed depending on tasks and projects. Ryan[40] also reported the value of seemingly fleeting acquaintances because these minor encounters could develop into relationships of high value, given the right circumstances.

	TABLE 27-1
	NETWORK STRUCTURE AND COMPOSITION MEASUREMENT GLOSSARY
Size	Total number of network contacts, excluding the individual whose network is referenced (indicated by the enlarged size).[38] *Calculation:* total contacts minus the network reference *Example:* 21 − 1 = 20 total contacts
Density	Measure of interconnectedness between the individuals who comprise the network. It is the proportion of individuals who are also connected to others.[37] *Calculation:* total ties divided by the total possible number of ties (ranging from 0% to 100%) *Example:* 16 ties / 20 possible ties x 100 = 80% (this is a highly interconnected, closed network)
	Open	Closed Less interconnected	Highly interconnected
Homophily	Measurement of similarity between characteristics of the members in one's network to one's self. It is the tendency for people to build more ties with others who are like themselves. The EI Index is used to measure the number of external ties (E) one has to members in a category different from their own, and the number of internal ties (I), which is the number of members in the same category. The range is from -1 to +1, where a score and EI Index of -1 indicates that one only ties with members in the same category as themselves, which is perfect homophily. A score of +1 means one has ties to members from different categories, which is perfect heterophily.[37] *Calculation:* EI = (E-I)/(E+I) *Example for homophily in work location and profession:* 25 people in one's network = Internal ties: 4 faculty at same institution in PT = 4 total External ties: 8 at different institution in PT + 9 at same institution not PT + 4 clinicians only in academia = 21 total EI index: I = 4, E = 21 ⇨ 21-4/21+4 = .68. This number indicates a high degree of heterophily. When interpreting this number, caution should be taken because this index only considers ties formed without consideration for the population from which the ties have been selected.

continued

TABLE 27-1 (CONTINUED)
NETWORK STRUCTURE AND COMPOSITION MEASUREMENT GLOSSARY

Heterogeneity	Heterogeneity is the measurement of the variety of characteristics each member brings for network diversity. This measure is Agresti's IQV (Index of Qualitative Variation), which gives the amount of diversity among the number of categories. One's network has no diversity or heterogeneity (ie, equal to 0) when one is connected only to those in one group or with one characteristic (eg, all women). One's network has maximum heterogeneity (ie, equal to 1-1/r, where r is the number of different relational types) when one has the same number of connections to those in each group or with each characteristic (eg, an equal number of women and men).[37]
	Calculation: $H/(1-1/r)$
	H formula: $H = 1 - P_1{}^2 - P_2{}^2 - P_3{}^2 \ldots - P_r{}^2$
	Total network members (excluding the early career faculty member, whose network is studied) = 22
	An example includes the following network: P_1: 8 men, P_2: 9 professors and associate professors, P_3: 5 with scholarly activity (r = 3 relation groups)
	Proportion (P) of ties in relation to the total number of members = P_1: 8/22 = .36, P_2: 9/22 = .41, P_3: 5/22 = .23
	$H = 1 - .36^2 - .41^2 - .23^2 = .6494$
	IQV is = .6494 / (1-1/3) = .97. This number indicates diversity.

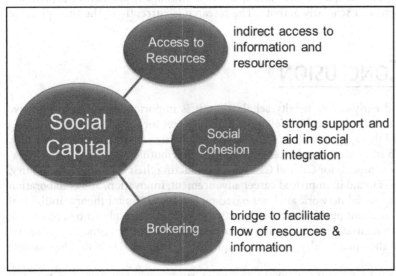

Figure 27-3. Social capital constructs.

A study of medical faculty found high value with connections made at their institution through faculty development programs, which provided access to social capital resources.[9] Network contacts brokered opportunities for increased visibility and allowed mentors who were well connected to make new introductions and thereby expand the faculty network.

Hitchcock et al,[41] describing faculty success and networks, concluded that, "… If one were allowed only one line of inquiry to predict a faculty member's future success in the field, it might well be, 'Tell me about your colleagues.'"[41(p1108)] The findings support the merit of a variety of configurations for relationships among faculty. Although research collaborations were the impetus for the connections, the benefits extended into personal supports. Hitchcock et al[41] reported the value of formal meetings at professional association conferences for new collaborations and a place for idea exchange and project discussions. The value of frequent communication between contacts was also an important characteristic of relationships for medical faculty success.[41]

Faculty development and formal mentorship programs are a reported method to increase collaboration and facilitate introductions for new contacts. In a study of models for medical residents who aspired to clinical academic careers but had insufficient research training, the results showed the importance of having a network with persons already involved in scholarly activity to guide and mentor the new scholar.[42] The authors concluded that when people were surrounded by others who were involved in and encouraged participation in scholarly activity, confidence improved, and it was suggested this could be an answer to the problem of threatened clinical scholarship.[42(p3)] Morzinski and Fisher[43] showed the success of a program for primary care physicians to improve network relationships with peers, mentors, and academic consultants by training in skills that contribute to academic advancement.[42] Morzinski and Fisher[43] also showed that increased network size with new connections external to their institution and links to other influential contacts was significant.

It is unclear whether faculty outside the medical academy, or those within it who emphasize teaching, develop connections in the same way or benefit similarly from relationships with colleagues as do research faculty. While research has pointed out an effective network can improve career success in medicine,[9,42] business,[10,44,45] and social science,[40] perhaps it matters for early career physical therapist faculty too. It is, therefore, this gap in knowledge and understanding that I sought to address by conducting a preliminary study, and the methods and exploratory results are shared here.

PRELIMINARY MIXED-METHODS STUDY

The purpose of the explanatory, mixed-methods study was to investigate agency and the network structure and composition of early career physical therapist faculty as related to scholarly activity.[46] A quantitative study alone would limit the understanding of the depth of faculty experiences. Adding a qualitative phase using a grounded theory approach with in-depth interviews provided information about the processes faculty use for developing a professional network. The 2 inquiries that guided the quantitative phase involved determining effective network structure and composition for predicting success in scholarly productivity over time, and determining if agency scores predict success in scholarly productivity.

Study participants included faculty in their first 5 years working in CAPTE-accredited or candidate for CAPTE accreditation doctor of physical therapy (DPT) programs. Most were women and assistant professors with an average duration as a faculty member of about 2 years.

Preliminary results from the quantitative phase studying early career physical therapist faculty from across the country show that faculty are interested in scholarly activity and have selected a topic. However, few of these faculty, in their first 5 years, have a peer-reviewed publication, the gold standard for scholarship. Agency perspective and agency behavior were high, suggesting individuals are taking strategic and intentional actions to meet their career advancement goals, including scholarship. The professional networks varied in network structure (eg, shape, size, density) and composition (eg, diversity of network contacts). Faculty with more open professional networks appear to have more scholarly work disseminated, when using a weighted scoring system that accounted for quality and quantity of scholarly items. Further analysis using regression models is planned and will include control variables, such as duration as a faculty member, academic rank, and Carnegie classification of their institution, to better predict scholarly activity over time.

The qualitative phase was guided by inquiry to explore the process early career physical therapist faculty use to create a network, and how network connections aid in career advancement. Although the final theory is still under development, initial findings depended on whether the faculty had higher or lower scholarly productivity and the amount of interconnectedness among network collaborators. A joint display to illustrate the quantitative and qualitative findings is planned to explain the findings of agency, network structure and composition, and scholarly activity. The research is currently in the final phase of analysis and planned for dissemination.

CONCLUSION

To advance the profession of physical therapy and early-career faculty scholarship, it is important to consider effective networks for scholarly activity of early-career physical therapist faculty. Networks look different for individuals with varying scholarly productivity. There is evidence in the physical therapy profession of low levels of scholarly activity by program faculty. Faculty must facilitate the skill and practice of CR with students through examples such as contributing to and analyzing literature and applying the best evidence. Faculty serve as role models for CR and CPS when conducting their own scholarly inquiry. Effective networks have been shown in other professions to aid in improved career advancement, innovation, and collaboration for scholarly activity. Networks can be measured using social network analyses based on the social capital theory. Individual faculty choices about career advancement and decisions about pursuing scholarly activity should be considered by accounting for strategic and intentional actions by faculty. With an accurate understanding of the relationship among agency, professional networks, and scholarly activity, early-career physical therapist faculty could more quickly and appropriately develop success in scholarship.

The need for educational research focused on the CR topics of this textbook is critical. Without multi-institutional studies about clinical decision-making in entry-level DPT programs, the profession will be unable to report best practices. Collaborative educational research networks led by physical therapist faculty scholars can aid in more robust study and innovation. Future studies to learn more about networks and faculty career advancement may be guided by the following questions. The network structure and composition can serve as the outcome variable to answer questions such as:

- Does having network contacts with similar interests and characteristics (homophily) predict who becomes collaborators on scholarly activity projects?
- Does being an extrovert or introvert predict who becomes central to a network of an organization?
- How does trust within an organization predict the communication among network contacts within an institution of higher learning?
- Do network structure and composition differ among faculty with primary teaching, administrative, research, or clinical duties?
- Do faculty with an interprofessional network of colleagues achieve more career success with scholarship?
- What are the differences in the mentorship network structure and composition of early-, mid- and later-career faculty?

- Does an effective mentorship network predict career advancement with promotion and tenure?
- Do networks become more effective for faculty after attending formal faculty development programs?
- What are the formal and informal strategies individuals with successful networks use to build and maintain network connections?

The network structure and composition can also serve as the independent variable to answer questions such as the following:

- Do interprofessional relationships predict which faculty have high agency or achieve career advancement such as promotion and tenure?
- Does being central to an organization (ie, network position) predict being selected for prestigious awards, committees, or leadership opportunities?
- Does network structure (ie, size or interconnectedness) predict a group's ability to meet goals for scholarly activity or create a CR project?

Reflection Moment

After reviewing these questions, note your responses and compare them to the future study outcomes disseminated by Becker and her network of research collaborators.

REFERENCES

1. Commission on Accreditation in Physical Therapy Education. Aggregate Program Data 2016-17. Physical Therapist Education Fact Sheets. Vol 20152017.
2. Commission on Accreditation for Physical Therapy Education. Standards and Required Elements for Accreditation of Physical Therapist Education Programs. In: Commission on Accreditation in Physical Therapy Education; 2017.
3. Commission on Accreditation in Physical Therapy Education. Quick facts. http://www.capteonline.org/home.aspx. Accessed March 29, 2017.
4. Sicat BL, O'Kane Kreutzer K, Gary J, et al. A collaboration among health sciences schools to enhance faculty development in teaching. *Am J Pharm Educ.* 2014;78(5):1-5.
5. Stupnisky RH, Weaver-Hightower M, Kartoshkina Y. Exploring and testing the predictors of new faculty success: a mixed methods study. *Stud High Educ.* 2015;40(2):368-390.
6. Boyer EL. Carnegie Foundation for the Advancement of Teaching. *Scholarship Reconsidered: Priorities of the Professoriate.* 1990.
7. Rumsey AS. Scholarly Communication Institute. University of Virginia Library. August 2013. https://libraopen.lib.virginia.edu/downloads/x633f104m. Accessed May 24, 2018
8. Thomas J, Herrin D. Executive master of science in nursing program: incorporating the 14 forces of magnetism. *J Nurs Adm.* 2008;38(2):64-67.
9. Warner ET, Carapinha R, Weber GM, Hill EV, Reede JY. Faculty promotion and attrition: the importance of coauthor network reach at an academic medical center. *J Gen Intern Med.* 2016;31(1):60-67.
10. Rodan S, Galunic C. More than network structure: how knowledge heterogeneity influences managerial performance and innovativeness. *Strateg Manage J.* 2004;25(6):541-562.
11. Law M, Wright S, Mylopoulos M. Exploring community faculty members' engagement in educational scholarship. *Can Fam Physician.* 2016;62(9):e524-e530.
12. Niehaus E, Meara K. Invisible but essential: the role of professional networks in promoting faculty agency in career advancement. *Innov High Educ.* 2015;40(2):159-171.
13. Anderson MH. Social networks and the cognitive motivation to realize network opportunities: a study of managers' information gathering behaviors. *J Organ Behav Manage.* 2008;29(1):51-78.
14. Steffen-Fluhr N, Gruzd A, Collins R, Osatuyi B. *N is for Network: New Tools for Mapping Organizational Change.* National Association of Multicultural Engineering Program Advocates/Women in Engineering Program Advocates Network 4th Joint Conference; April 12-14, 2010; Baltimore, MD.
15. Katerndahl D. Co-evolution of departmental research collaboration and scholarly outcomes. *J Eval Clin Pract.* 2012;18(6):1241-1247.
16. Ponjuan L, Conley VM, Trower C. Career stage differences in pre-tenure track faculty perceptions of professional and personal relationships with colleagues. *J High Educ.* 2011;82(3):319-346.
17. Borgatti SP, Everett MG, Johnson JC. *Analyzing Social Networks.* Thousand Oaks, CA: Sage; 2013.
18. Fiore SM. Interdisciplinarity as teamwork: how the science of teams can inform team science. *Small Group Res.* 2008;39(3):251-277.
19. Pati S, Reum J, Conant E, et al. Tradition meets innovation: transforming academic medical culture at the University of Pennsylvania's Perelman School of Medicine. *Acad Med.* 2013;88(4):461-464.
20. Snyder-Mackler L. Mary McMillan lecture: not eureka. *Phys Ther.* 2015;95(10):1446-1456.

21. Hinman MR, Brown T. Changing profile of the physical therapy professoriate—are we meeting CAPTE's expectations? *J Phys Ther Educ.* 2017;31(4):95-104.
22. Kaufman RR, Chevan J. The gender gap in peer-reviewed publications by physical therapy faculty members: a productivity puzzle. *Phys Ther.* 2011;91(1):122-131.
23. Kaufman RR. Career factors help predict productivity in scholarship among faculty members in physical therapist education programs. *Phys Ther.* 2009;89(3):204-216.
24. Commission on Accreditation for Physical Therapy Education. Position papers accreditation handbook 2018. http://www.capteonline.org/uploadedFiles/CAPTEorg/About_CAPTE/Resources/Accreditation_Handbook/PositionPapers.pdf. Accessed May 12, 2018.
25. Richter RR, Schlomer SL, Krieger MM, Siler WL. Journal publication productivity in academic physical therapy programs in the United States and Puerto Rico from 1998 to 2002. *Phys Ther.* 2008;88(3):376-386.
26. Steinbuch R. On the leiter side: developing a universal assessment tool for measuring scholarly output by law professors and ranking law schools. *Loyola Los Angel Law Rev.* 2011;45(1):87-123.
27. Starkey C, Ingersoll CD. Scholarly productivity of athletic training faculty members. *J Athl Train.* 2001;36(2):156-159.
28. Emerick T, Metro D, Patel R, Sakai T. Scholarly activity points: a new tool to evaluate resident scholarly productivity. *Br J Anaesth.* 2013;111(3):468-476.
29. Gardner SK, Blackston A. Faculty agency in applying for promotion to professor. *J Stud Postsecond Tertiary Educ.* 2017;2:16.
30. O'Meara K. A career with a view: agentic perspectives of women faculty. *J High Educ.* 2015;86(3):331-359.
31. Terosky AL, O'Meara K. The power of strategy and networks in the professional lives of faculty. *Lib Educ.* 2011;97(3):54-59.
32. Campbell C, O'Meara K. Faculty agency: departmental contexts that matter in faculty careers. *Res High Educ.* 2014;55(1):49-74.
33. Dessler G. *Supervision and Leadership in a Changing World.* Upper Saddle River, NJ: Pearson; 2012.
34. Crossley N, Bellotti D, Edwards G, et al. Narratives, typologies and case studies. In: *Social Network Analysis for Ego-Nets.* Thousand Oaks, CA: Sage; 2015:104-125.
35. Isba R, Woolf K, Hanneman R. Social network analysis in medical education. *Med Educ.* 2017;51(1):81-88.
36. Moolenaar NM. A social network perspective on teacher collaboration in schools: theory, methodology, and applications. *Am J Educ.* 2012;119(1):7-39.
37. Crossley N, Bellotti D, Edwards G, et al. Analyzing ego-net data. In: *Social Network Analysis for Ego-Nets.* Thousand Oaks, CA: Sage; 2015:76-104.
38. Borgatti SP, Everett MG, Johnson JC. Data collection. In: *Analyzing Social Networks.* Thousand Oaks, CA: Sage; 2013:44-61.
39. Crossley N, Bellotti D, Edwards G, et al. Social capital and small worlds: a primer. In: *Social Network Analysis for Ego-Nets.* Thousand Oaks, CA: Sage; 2015:23-43.
40. Ryan L. Looking for weak ties: using a mixed methods approach to capture elusive connections. *Sociol Rev.* 2016;64(4):951-969.
41. Hitchcock MA, Bland CJ, Hekelman FP, Blumenthal MG. Professional networks: the influence of colleagues on the academic success of faculty. *Acad Med.* 1995;70(12):1108-1116.
42. Penzner JB, Snow CE, Gordon-Elliott JS, et al. A multi-tiered model for clinical scholarship. *Acad Psychiatry.* 2017;1-3.
43. Morzinski JA, Fisher JC. A nationwide study of the influence of faculty development programs on colleague relationships. *Acad Med.* 2002;77(5):402-406.
44. Seibert SE, Kraimer ML, Liden RC. A social capital theory of career success. *Acad Manage J.* 2001;44(2):219-237.
45. Dobrev SD, Merluzzi J. Stayers versus movers: social capital and early career imprinting among young professionals. *J Organ Behav.* 2018;39(1):67-81.
46. Becker BJ, Sayles H, Woehler M, Rost T, Willett GM. An investigation of professional networks and scholarly productivity of early career physical therapy faculty. *Journal of Physical Therapy Education.* 2019;33:94-102. doi:10.1097/JTE.0000000000000094.

Appendix
Characteristics of Scholarship Chart

IF SCHOLARLY WORK	IT IS TYPICALLY	WITHIN A SCHOLARLY AGENDA, ACCOMPLISHMENT IS TYPICALLY DEMONSTRATED BY	DOCUMENTED, AS APPROPRIATE FOR ACTIVITY, BY
Contributes to development or creation of new knowledge (*Scholarship of Discovery*)	• Primary empirical research • Historical research • Theory development • Methodological studies	• Peer-reviewed publications of research, theory, or philosophical essays • Peer-reviewed professional presentations of research, theory, or philosophical essays • Grant awards in support of research or scholarship	• Bibliographic citation of the accomplishments • Positive external assessment[2] of the body of work
Contributes to the critical analysis and review of knowledge within disciplines or the creative synthesis of insights contained in different disciplines or fields of study (*Scholarship of Integration*)	• Inquiry that advances knowledge across a range of theories, practice areas, techniques, or methodologies • Includes works that interface between physical therapy and a variety of disciplines	• Peer-reviewed publications of research, policy analysis, case studies, integrative reviews of the literature, and others • Copyrights, licenses, patents, or products • Published books • Reports of interdisciplinary programs or service projects • Interdisciplinary grant awards • Peer-reviewed professional presentations • Policy papers designed to influence organizations or governments • Service on editorial board or as peer reviewer	• Bibliographic citation of the accomplishments • Positive external assessment of the body of work • Documentation of role in editorial/ review processes
Applies findings generated through the scholarship of integration or discovery to solve real problems in the professions, industry, government, and the community (*Scholarship of Application/ Practice*)	• Development of clinical knowledge • Application of technical or research skills to address problems	• Activities related to the faculty member's area of expertise (eg, consultation, technical assistance, policy analysis, program evaluation, development of practice patterns) • Peer-reviewed professional presentations related to practice • Consultation reports • Reports compiling and analyzing patient or health services outcomes • Products, patents, license copyrights • Grant awards in support of practice • Reports of meta-analyses related to practice problems • Reports of clinical demonstration projects • Policy papers related to practice	• Formal documentation of a record of the activity and positive formal evaluation by users of the work • Bibliographic citation • Documentation of role in multi-authored products • Positive external assessment of the body of work
Contributes to the development of critically reflective knowledge about teaching and learning (*Scholarship of Teaching/ Learning*)	• Application of knowledge of the discipline or specialty applied in teaching-learning • Development of innovative teaching and evaluation methods • Program development and learning outcome evaluation • Professional role modeling	• Peer-reviewed publications of research related to teaching methodology or learning outcomes, case studies related to teaching-learning, learning theory development, and development or testing of educational models or theories • Successful applications of technology to teaching and learning • Published textbooks or other learning aids • Grant awards in support of teaching and learning • Peer-reviewed professional presentations related to teaching and learning	• Bibliographic citation of the accomplishments • Documentation of scholarly role in creation of multi-authored evaluation reports • Positive external assessment of the body of work
Contributes to the identification, understanding and resolution of significant social, civic, or ethical problems and includes systematic data collection, analysis, interpretation, and impact (*Scholarship of Engagement*)	• Collaborative partnerships involving faculty, community members and organizational representatives (community-based research or interventions)	• Peer-reviewed publications or professional presentations related to development of community-based intervention • Grant awards in support of community-based intervention • Policy papers, presentations, or reports compiling and analyzing community program outcomes that includes analysis and interpretation of data collected and leads to an outcome or plan	• Bibliographic citation of the accomplishments • Positive external assessment of the body of work • Documentation of role in multi-authored products

[2]External assessment = review that occurs outside of the physical therapy unit.

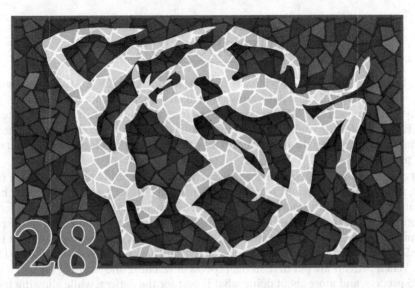

THE DIRECTOR OF CLINICAL EDUCATION LEADING THE WAY:
Facilitating Clinical Reasoning and Clinical Problem-Solving With the Clinical Education Team With Case Exemplars

Gina Maria Musolino, PT, DPT, MSEd, EdD and Alecia Thiele, PT, DPT, MSEd, ATC, LAT, DCE

OBJECTIVES

- Examine the key role of the director of clinical education/academic coordinator of clinical education (DCE/ACCE) in providing resources to assist the clinical instructor (CI)/clinical coordinator of clinical education (CCCE)/site coordinator of clinical education (SCCE) and students for successful clinical reasoning (CR) and clinical problem-solving (CPS).

- Appreciate that CR-CPS and CR-CPS processing takes practice and thoughtful time.

- Understand that one must be effective before one can be efficient.

- Prioritize the CR-CPS process as a foundational element for practice that requires intentional teaching and learning.

- Appraise strategies to take the pressure off the CR-CPS process that can be used to increase effectiveness and proficiency in clinical education (CE).

- Conclude that patients should be included in the CR-CPS process, which builds trust and supports patient-centered care concepts.

- Compare suggestions for CR-CPS remediation.

- Evaluate your approaches to enhance CR-CPS.

Musolino GM, Jensen GM, eds. *Clinical Reasoning and Decision-Making in Physical Therapy: Facilitation, Assessment, and Implementation* (pp 345-362).
© 2020 Taylor & Francis Group.

INTRODUCTION

The director of clinical education/academic coordinator of clinical education (DCE/ACCE) plays an integral role in preparing students for clinical practice. The DCE facilitates teamwork with all clinical education stakeholders to enable success linking academic and clinical physical therapy. DCEs/ACCEs provide resources for clinical instructors (CIs) to assist in the application of CR and CPS within CE. Success for the student moving from didactic education to clinical practice requires the application of CR and CPS skills. This chapter explores the role of the DCE with the CE stakeholders in the facilitation of the foundational elements of professional practice: CR-CPS.

The skill for CR is not only a foundational element for the practice of the doctor of physical therapy (DPT), but is also critical for the ability to *le docre*, meaning "to teach as doctors," our patients and clients. As physical therapy health care educators, we must partner with our patients and clients to address their movement system, optimizing movement for health. The CPS skill is a foundational element of practice for the physical therapist assistant to be a successful member of the physical therapist–physical therapist assistant team for patient/client management. CR is a foundational element of practice for the DPT in patient/client management. CR for the DPT and CPS for the physical therapist assistant are correlates within the CI/DCE purview to facilitate and progress during CE. When patients are put first, in the process of teaching and learning for CE, it is less about being "right or wrong" in the CR-CPS process, and more about doing what is best for the patient, while allowing for possibilities.

CR-CPS is examined from real-case examples of students engaged in clinical experiences who are struggling with CR-CPS and how the DCE serves as a linchpin to bring together all stakeholders, with proactive plans for the students' eventual success in exhibiting appropriate levels of CR-CPS abilities. This chapter addresses the problem-solving in CE used in coordinating and managing academic and clinical education teamwork, with all stakeholders in all practice areas, with the now 5 generations in practice, to facilitate CR-CPS. The chapter authors provide case examples to share their experience in guiding CR in CE, the ever-important red flag item as a foundational element for practice management on the APTA Clinical Performance Instrument (CPI) Assessment.[1,2] CR-CPS clinical readiness and breaking down components of CR-CPS for effective student management and CE instruction are discussed.

Additionally, the APTA CPI[2] criteria for patient management, CR, and CPS, along with sample behaviors, are presented and discussed. The role and need for potential formal remediation are explored. The ever-important APTA CPI performance dimensions are also considered including supervision/guidance, quality, complexity, consistency, and efficiencies of performance.

Self-assessment (SA) is key component to becoming a reflective practitioner (RP) and a lifelong learner (see Section I, Chapter 3). Several chapters within the textbook reiterate the importance of becoming an RP as a developing professional, clinical educator, and seasoned practitioner. The American Physical Therapy Association Clinical Performance Instrument (APTA CPI) calls for the student's SA, along with the CI's assessment, as the licensed professional performing the job for which the student aspires. CIs often have received additional continuing education to best serve as CIs by becoming credentialed through taking the APTA Credentialed Clinical Instructor Program[3] (CCIP), Level 1[4] and Level 2[5] courses. The APTA CCIP (http://www.apta.org/CCIP/), a continuing education professional development course program, is designed to enhance professional development and teaching and learning capacities of CIs. As a component of the Level 1 course, CIs complete a SA of their abilities, considering legal and ethical aspects, effective communication skills, interpersonal relationships, supervisory skills, professional development, assessment and evaluation skills, and capacities for constructive feedback. Through the APTA CCIP Level 1 course, CIs enhance their skills and abilities through professional development and assessment of their performance for credentialing. CIs most frequently complete the course to enhance their CI abilities in (1) communication, (2) feedback and assessment methods, (3) teaching and learning styles, (4) goal-setting and goal-writing, (5) formative and summative feedback, and (6) conflict negotiation/resolution.[6]

To better understand CR-CPS within the CE realm, it is important for one to be aware of common CE terminology and definitions. According to the APTA CCIP, the following terms are defined for clarity[4(pp23-24)]:

- **Director of clinical education/academic coordinator of clinical education (DCE/ACCE):** An individual who manages and coordinates the CE program at the academic institution, including facilitating development of the CE site and clinical educators. This person also coordinates student placements, communicates with the clinical educators about the academic program and student performance, and maintains current information on CE sites.

- **Clinical coordinator of clinical education/site coordinator of clinical education (CCCE/SCCE):** This individual administers, manages, and coordinates CI assignments and learning activities for students during their CE experiences. In addition, this person determines the readiness of others to serve as CIs for students, supervises CIs in the delivery of CE experiences, communicates with academic programs regarding the student performance, and provides essential information about the CE program to the academic physical therapy programs.

- **Clinical instructor (CI):** This individual at the CE site directly instructs and supervises students during the application phase of their CE learning experiences. These individuals carry out learning experiences and assess students' performance in the cognitive, affective, and psychomotor domains of learning as related to entry-level clinical practice and academic clinical performance expectations.

Now that you have a bit of the working terminology for CE in physical therapy, let's, as Covey states, first …

BEGIN WITH THE END IN MIND[7]

Recently, in conversation with a novice DCE, I asked how she facilitated CR-CPS in the classroom. Her response was a timid, *"It's hard, right? I mostly use case studies but haven't really thought about it too much. They either get it or they don't."* Our role as educators is to facilitate the efforts for teaching CR-CPS intentionally to prepare students for clinical education. The responsibility does not lie solely with the clinics, solely with the DCE, or solely with the students, but rather with all faculty, all students in physical therapy, and all clinical educators.

The APTA CPI[1,2] is the highly used performance criteria to assess the performance of the physical therapist and physical therapist assistant in clinical education and readiness for entry into the profession.

Please note that while we are discussing the CR-CPS criteria specifically, the APTA PT/PTA CPI[1,2] must be used in totality, for full-time CEs only, to maintain the psychometric properties, and cannot be used in isolation. Yet for this chapter, we are working, to as Covey[7] states, to "begin with the end in mind" and extract and examine CR-CPS more specifically to work more proactively, for both formative and summative outcomes for CE. By highlighting CR-CPS expectations and shining a light on the outcome expectations, we hope to be able to move the learners along the continuum more readily. If you have a greater understanding of CR-CPS expectations now, you will garner more from your didactic experiences to be capable and better prepared to apply CR-CPS skills for your patients/clients in CE—as they are counting on you, too!

The APTA PT CPI[1] contains 18 performance criteria, and the APTA PTA CPI[2] contains 14 performance criteria that are essential for practice. The **APTA PT CPI** is divided by **professional practice** and **patient management** criteria, with each criterion consisting of sample behaviors for the physical therapist (not an exhaustive list, merely a guide for assessment) and essential skills for the physical therapist assistant. **CR-CPS** are the only **patient management** criteria that are **foundational elements/red flag items** [⚑]. Both [⚑] **CR-CPS** [⚑] are defined on the APTA CPI[1,2] as foundational elements for practice or red flag items. The 4 remaining red flag criteria are contained within the category of **professional practice** and include [⚑] **safety,** [⚑] **professional behavior/clinical behavior,** [⚑] **accountability**, and [⚑] **communication**. Let's examine the foundational elements of practice, as defined by the APTA CPI and essential for the student to progress in the remaining areas. See Table 28-1 for the physical therapist CR criterion and Table 28-2 for the physical therapist assistant CPS criteria.

In terms of the [⚑] red flag or foundational elements of practice, students participating in CE may progress more rapidly in the red flag [⚑] areas than with other performance criteria. Significant concerns related to a performance criterion that is a red flag item warrants immediate attention, more expansive documentation, and a telephone call/text or other notification to the DCE/ACCE, and likely use of the critical incident student performance report in conjunction with the APTA CPI for formal, formative feedback. Possible outcomes from difficulty in performance with a red flag item may include remediation, extension of the experience with a learning contract, and/or dismissal from the CE experience. Alternatively, when a student is given the formative feedback, the student may also progress appropriately once he or she is cognizant of the need to address the criteria more specifically. The intentional facilitator and guidance may be enough to allow the student on CE to then meet expectations. When rating students, CIs are to carefully consider each of the CR-CPS criteria and correlate with the 5 overarching performance dimensions. Both students and CIs complete training, which may be revisited, to properly use the assessment instrument and complete a competency assessment.

TABLE 28-1
APTA PHYSICAL THERAPIST CLINICAL PERFORMANCE INSTRUMENT (PT CPI)

[⊞] CLINICAL REASONING CRITERIA

Clinical reasoning: A systematic process used to assist students and practitioners in inferring or drawing conclusions about patient/client care under various situations and conditions.

APTA CPI Clinical Reasoning for Patient Management

The student applies current knowledge, theory, clinical judgment, and the patient's values and perspective in patient management.

Sample Behaviors (Not Exhaustive)

a. Presents a logical rationale (cogent and concise arguments) for clinical decisions.

b. Makes clinical decisions within the context of ethical practice.

c. Uses information from multiple data sources to make clinical decisions (eg, patient and caregivers, health care professionals, hooked on evidence, databases, and medical records).

d. Seeks disconfirming evidence in the process of making clinical decisions.

e. Recognizes when plan of care and interventions are ineffective, identifies areas needing modification, and implements changes accordingly.

f. Critically evaluates published articles relevant to physical therapy, and applies them to clinical practice.

g. Demonstrates an ability to make clinical decisions in ambiguous situations or where values may be in conflict.

h. Selects interventions based on the best available evidence, clinical expertise, and patient preferences.

i. Assesses patient response to interventions using credible measures.

j. Integrates patient needs and values in making decisions in developing the plan of care.

k. Clinical decisions focus on the whole person rather than the disease.

l. Recognizes limits (learner and profession) of current knowledge, theory, and judgment in patient management.

Adapted from *Physical Therapist Clinical Performance Instrument: Version 2008*, with permission of the American Physical Therapy Association. Copyright © 2008 American Physical Therapy Association.

Reflection Moment (See Tables 28-1 and 28-2)

Consider: What do you see as similar and/or different as you compare the sample behaviors for CR-CPS expected of the physical therapist and the physical therapist assistant? Does anything surprise you? How will you alter your approach to your learning and teaching now that you are more aware of the CR-CPS definitions, expectations, and sample behaviors?

TABLE 28-2

APTA Physical Therapist Assistant Clinical Performance Instrument (PTA CPI)

[🖑] CLINICAL PROBLEM-SOLVING

Clinical problem-solving: Key components: Interview patients/clients, caregivers, family. Communicate understanding of plan of care. Review health care records. Monitor and adjust interventions in the plan of care. Determine when an intervention should not be performed. Demonstrate clinical problem-solving.

Essential Skills

- Presents sound rationale for clinical problem-solving, including review of data collected, and ethical and legal arguments.

- Seeks clarification of plan of care and selected interventions from clinical instructor and/or supervising physical therapist.

- Collects and compares data from multiple sources (eg, chart review, patient, caregivers, team members, and observation) to determine patient's readiness before initiating treatment.

- Demonstrates sound clinical decisions within the plan of care to assess and maximize patient safety and comfort while performing selected interventions.

- Demonstrates sound clinical decisions within the plan of care to assess and maximize intervention outcomes, including patient progression and/or intervention modifications.

- Demonstrates the ability to determine when the clinical instructor and/or supervising physical therapist needs to be notified of changes in patient status, changes or lack of change in intervention outcomes, and completion of intervention expectations (ie, goals have been met).

- Demonstrates the ability to perform appropriately during an emergency situation to include notification of appropriate staff.

Adapted from *Physical Therapy Assistant Clinical Performance Instrument: Version 2008,* with permission of the American Physical Therapy Association. Copyright © 2008 American Physical Therapy Association.

As you have discovered through reading many of the chapters in this CR text, both CPS and CR are inextricably linked to evidence-based practice (EBP), especially for the novice practitioner (see Chapter 26). The patient's values and beliefs must be considered with collaboration in goal-setting with the patient and as part of the clinical decision-making and CPS that occur within the patient/client management. EBP includes the patient's values and beliefs; the current, peer-reviewed research; and the professional's own clinical practice capabilities (expertise). CR-CPS is challenged when any one of the EBP components is missing; for students, this is not usually the evidence. Students come armed with evidence, but applying it and linking to the specific, individual patient case scenario and the patient's values, is the challenge, or sometimes fear, for the novice learner or experienced learner in a novel setting. CR-CPS requires a balance of the 3-pronged stool of EBP—if any leg of the stool is underemphasized, CR-CPS becomes out of balance. Our professional duty is to ensure that all aspects of EBP are not forgotten, and then consider possibilities even beyond EBP (as shared in Chapter 26). When patients are put first in teaching and learning for CE, it is less about being "right or wrong" in the CR-CPS process, and more about doing what is best for the patient, while allowing for possibilities.

Now that you have reviewed the sample behaviors for CR-CPS as foundational elements for practice, and considered the important linkages with EBP, let's consider some examples of CR feedback in CE. Specifically, let's look at some excerpts from the CI and student SA narratives for CR on the APTA CPI. Based on each example presented, consider the learning from this CR text and insert 3 to 4 suggestions for the student and CI to assist in continuing to proactively and intentionally address CR improvement efforts. Consider the APTA CPI CR sample behaviors (provided in Table 28-1) as you develop your planned educational interventions for the students' CR advancement, and all that you have learned in the prior chapters of this textbook. Consider the preferred approach to CR being exhibited and how you might make it more and/or less challenging for the students. Consider the variables of the 5 performance dimensions for practice (eg, supervision/guidance, quality, complexity, consistency, efficiencies of performance) as parameters you may also adjust in your strategies and goals for progression of CR (Table 28-3).

TABLE 28-3

EXAMPLES OF CLINICAL REASONING CRITERION NARRATIVES
APTA PHYSICAL THERAPIST CLINICAL PERFORMANCE INSTRUMENT

CI EXAMPLE A ASSESSMENT	STUDENT EXAMPLE A SELF-ASSESSMENT
The student has demonstrated good SA skills to recognize where limitations are, and she looks for different forms to understand pathology better, using articles, discussion, and past notes. She has demonstrated that she is safe with clinical decision-making, but needs fine-tuning with rationale with decisions initially at the evaluation. Good gathering of objective data at each visit to see progress and justify continuation of skilled services.	*This is something I feel as though I have improved. My CIs have continued to question me about my rationale for my interventions, and I feel as though my ability to answer effectively has improved. Although there is still room for improvement, I feel as though I have continued to improve the size of my "toolbox." One area that I know that I need to improve upon is adjusting sessions on the fly to progress or regress, especially with my higher-functioning patients. I have required cueing from my CI on knowing how to progress exercises when dealing with those higher-functioning patients.*
Suggested Instructional Strategies: 1. 2. 3. 4.	**Suggested Proactive Preparation/Practice:** 1. 2. 3. 4.
CI EXAMPLE B ASSESSMENT	**STUDENT EXAMPLE B SELF-ASSESSMENT**
Student has been encouraged to continually question assess/reassess strategies and interventions and is able to identify without cueing. Initially will ask, "What do you think?" and this CI will reverse the question to continually foster that thirst of CR and critical decision-making. Has made significant strides in being able to correctly provide CR and the "why" we provide that particular intervention.	*I consistently apply current knowledge, theory, clinical judgment, and the patient's values and perspective in my patient management for the well-being of the individual involved. I incorporate a current evidence-based research study into my practice each week. I come into each treatment session with a temporary plan addressing the known limitations, impairments, disabilities, and pathology and adjust accordingly based on the patient's subjective review and response to treatment. I consistently voice my rationale to my CI to ensure proper understanding and gain clinical pearls stemming from her vast clinical experience.*
Suggested Instructional Strategies: 1. 2. 3. 4.	**Suggested Proactive Preparation/Practice:** 1. 2. 3. 4.

As you can see, there are many right answers and/or ways to approach the facilitation of CR. The point is to be certain to keep CR-CPS at the forefront of CE and not let it get lost in the background or not tackled because it is one of the more challenging foundational elements of practice. CR-CPS requires that you bring together multiple skills and abilities and apply and synthesize your learning at higher levels in the affective, cognitive, and psychomotor domains of the learning taxonomies. Metacognition, which was discussed in Chapter 14, may not come naturally. Using concept mapping may assist the learners in seeing the big picture, and/or specific facilitation and guidance through questioning strategies and utilization of frameworks such as the *International Classification of Functioning, Disability and Health* (ICF) and/or Hypothesis-Oriented Algorithm for Clinicians (HOAC II).

The ability to engage in CR and CPS is an active and engaged skill that requires practice—and repeat practice. As many of the examples in the text have elucidated, one must work proactively to improve CR and CPS. Both the DCE and CI offer suggestions, and, as a learner, you should consider how you may also be best guided, and share with your CIs. Students are encouraged to use their own reflective SA, as noted in Chapter 3, to help determine where in your learning the breakdown is occurring. The more you "think out loud," the better your CI and DCE can match teaching strategies to facilitate your specific learning needs, rather than guessing in a vacuum.

Another method of gathering a snapshot of a student's learning in CE is through reflective journals. Guided reflective journals provide another opportunity for the student learner to think out loud in a written narrative, and also provide a window into the student learner's thought processes. Let's examine reflective journal excerpts and consider the role of the DCE in not just culling information from students, but also building upon reflections to promote CR and opportunities for facilitation (Table 28-4).

Reflection Moment (See Table 28-4)

What encouragement would you offer this student, as DCE/ACCE or peer, based upon the reflections? What strategies and/or additional probing questions might you suggest or ask? What ethical principles are revealed? Describe which domain(s) of learning appear to be most challenging for the developing RP learner. Why?

What sample behaviors of CR-CPS do you hear described in the narrative journal? What additional ethical and legal concerns with respect to the physical therapist–physical therapist assistant team were brought to light?

What type of CR approaches do you think the student and/or CI are most dependent upon? What other thoughts come to mind based upon your learning from this CR text? What tools and/or guidance might you provide the learner to specifically ensure movement along the CR learning continuum? Why?

Now that we have worked through mostly positive examples, let's look at some more challenging reports of critical incidents of the students' performance for CR (or lack thereof) with the excerpts provided in Table 28-5. When students are underperforming in CE or not meeting the expectations, CIs are encouraged to activate the **early warning system** (EWS) to formally notify all CE parties (ie, CCCE, CI, student, DCE/ACCE) of the student's critical incident of performance within the APTA CPI criteria. The EWS is especially important for providing formative feedback for the red flag [🏴] foundational elements of practice [🏴] to ensure that all parties are aware and that all efforts can be implemented to assist in addressing the student's learning needs in an effort to help him or her succeed in meeting CE-expected outcomes. The EWS should be perceived as a proactive and positive effort to formatively address areas of needed progression, and an opportunity to progress for the summative assessment outcomes.

When students are put on formal formative notice, they have ample time to progress and generally they do. Many may progress in a timely fashion; some may require additional time, as they will achieve effectiveness without having yet reached needed efficiencies. Others, unfortunately, may not progress, and may even regress. Yet the effort is being made as a gift of formative feedback for notice that intensive and highly intentional efforts are needed for the student to progress. The dimensions of performance are also highlighted in consideration of the student's capabilities. Recall that these include the amount of supervision/guidance being provided, the quality with which the student is performing, the complexity of the scenario, the consistency of the student's performance, and the efficiencies of the student's performance (refer to APTA PT/PTA CPI performance dimensions).

The critical incident report activates the EWS, resulting in a specific and definitive effort to make plans to address the student's deficit areas, working in collaboration with the CE team (ie, CCCE, CI, student, DCE/ACCE) and with resources and support from the academic institution where appropriate. These may include counseling and student services, screening for learning disabilities, disclosure of disabilities, and/or further academic advisement/tutoring.

TABLE 28-4

SAMPLE REFLECTIVE JOURNAL

1. **Share your impressions of a recent patient/client encounter in which you had an "A-ha" moment or experienced surprise in your reflection-in-action or your reflection-on-action.**

   . *I think the most impressionable moment thus far has been an elderly woman stating that she now had reason to keep on living. (I'll also mention that she said this statement while being a little choked up.) The patient had been in a deconditioned state, was not participating in activities that she once had secondary to increased knee pain and difficulty with functional mobility. Through aquatic therapy (which was progressed to more weight-bearing exercise in the gym) she increased her strength, mobility, and confidence in her ability to maintain her independence. She began an exercise class in the community, started using her stationary bike at home, and returned to volunteering at the hospital.*

   . *This patient is a very typical and routine for most therapists, but to me as a student, having her voice this emotion made me realize THAT I CAN MAKE A DIFFERENCE. I have realized this in the past, but with this statement, I think the words finally stuck. And it's not just about what treatment I put a patient through, it's the relationship I form with them, and the motivation, education, and advice I give them on changing their lifestyle. Some patients get better, some patients may get worse, but if I stop to think more about THE PERSON AND HOW I CAN BEST HELP, I may be able to enhance the person's living in some other dimension besides the primary diagnosis.*

2. **Describe how you have used <u>evidence-based practice</u> to best serve your current patients/clients in your progressive case load.**

   . *I've used evidence-based practice for many patients in a couple of different ways. The use of my textbooks for my examinations and use certain special tests with higher sensitivity and specificity. I also have a notebook full of research articles that we have gone over in school (it's divided up by region of the body). I use certain elements of the articles (exercises, treatment methods, and exam techniques) that were found to have a significant improvement on the course of rehabilitation. Also, as a member of the APTA, I get the Physical Therapy Journal monthly. I thumb through the journal and read the articles that are appropriate for my patients and take away little clinical tidbits. Finally, I use online library resources for more information or specific queries that I have about a particular diagnosis (mostly for accessing PubMed).*

3. **With midterm on the horizon, how are you ensuring your continued progression toward achieving your midterm goals?**

   . *I am ensuring my continued progression toward my midterm goals by seeking regular feedback from my CI regarding my clinical and communicative performance and reflecting upon my interactions w/ pts and my CR as it pertains to each person.*

4. **How are you continuing to challenge your own creativity with planning for your patients' care?**

   . *Every night as I plan my interventions for each patient for the next day, I attempt to incorporate a treatment that is new, functional, indicated, and likely tolerated by each patient.*

5. **How has your curiosity been stimulated to continue to learn?**

   . *I have realized that there is so much to learn to become an entry-level physical therapist, not just CR skills, but also treating patients in combination w/ other disciplines, understanding the logistics of health insurance coverages and defensible documentation.*

6. **Describe a specific <u>concrete</u> example of new learning that you have recently experienced with patient care.**

   . *I have recently learned how to verbally cue a patient who is mildly cognitively impaired how to manipulate a weight-activated stance-control prosthetic knee during sit-to-stand transfers.*

7. **Describe 2 ways in which <u>you</u> have exhibited professionalism in the clinic, and describe 2 ways in which you have witnessed <u>your CI</u> exhibit professionalism during CE 2.**

   . *I have professionally, and gently yet firmly, explained to a former patient why she did not qualify for a new POC under Medicare guidelines (this was not fun). I have also remained diplomatic regarding the national elections by abstaining from inappropriate conversation with physical therapists, which may detract from our treatment.*

   . *My CI exhibited professionalism by notifying her boss of an issue w/a physical therapist, who claimed to have performed examination techniques that she did not perform, then allowing one of the physical therapist assistants to treat that patient. My CI also has been very professional by notifying our physical therapists before visits that she is instructing a student, and seeks their permission for me to evaluate those patients beforehand.*

8. **How are you working to improve your ability to self-assess? What barriers do you need to overcome to ensure your success?**

   . *I am working on being honest and open w/myself regarding my clinical and communicative performance, especially when my intuition is screaming that I should rethink a specific line of CR. I then allow myself to reconsider my reasoning w/out being concerned of what my CI or specific patient will think of me if I come to the next visit w/a modified/new direction of treatment in mind. I think I need to continue to work to overcome my own self-consciousness as ...*

TABLE 28-5
CRITICAL INCIDENT REPORTS—CLINICAL REASONING EXAMPLES

EXAMPLE A: CRITERION	DATE/TIME REPORTED
Patient Management: [Pu] Clinical Reasoning [Pu]	08/01/18 06:10 PM—1 week post midterm

Behavior	Antecedent
Student could not present a logical rationale for the patient's exam findings and the connection to the diagnosis he had chosen. Specifically, he (1) could not describe or demonstrate how the patient's joint end feel related to a diagnosis, and (2) could not correct a patient exercise that was painful or explain or demonstrate an understanding of why a change in position reduced the patient's symptoms.	The student has required multiple cues to be able to repeat a sound rationale for exam findings and treatment responses. At the midterm, this was discussed and multiple modes of practice, including patient care, written cases, and CI-student role-play, have been used to improve this skill.

Consequence	CI Comments
Student would not meet the passing criteria for CR if this is not corrected, and would not meet the performance outcome expectations for the CE rotation. The DCE will also be notified.	These instances this week are consistent with difficulties in CR that we discussed at the midterm. The student has improved slowly in this area, especially with written cases, but continues to need cueing to explain a rationale for the findings of most examinations. I am concerned that he will not be able to make significant progress by the end of the clinical rotation.

DCE/ACCE Comments	Date/Time DCE/ACCE Viewed
The CR, critical incidents of student performance also demonstrate additional safety performance errors due to poor clinical judgment. The examples provided demonstrate repeat occurrences of performance in CR that fall below the expectation and compromise patient safety; the CI provided verbal cueing and guidance, coaching, and facilitation. With both live application with patients and simulated practice scenarios, the student was still unable to perform the appropriate CR. Patient management requires demonstration of CR to apply current knowledge, theory, clinical judgment, and the patient's values and perspective in patient management; even with cueing and ample guidance, the student was unable to perform, and on repeat instances, with basic skills and did not respond to patient response to physical therapist interventions. The students' CR performance falls below the expectation and compromises patient safety. Concur with the APTA-credentialed CI's objective report based also upon site visit #2 by DCE with verbal discussion of real-world case. Student exhibited similar challenges in his CR skills and applications. Referral to Student Support Services also completed for student's stress management. Discussed plan with CI to implement use of the CR Tool and provided CR articles to student and CI for review and implementation with cases in the next week with focus on CR. Student may have ample time to address CR deficits in remaining weeks and should be encouraged to continue to work on progress with assistance from CI, faculty, DCE, and working with near-peers.	08/01/18 06:43 PM **Example A:** What are your thoughts regarding the approaches and plan to address CR? Consider from the standpoint of the CE site? CI? Student? DCE? Compare and discuss how Example A differs from **Example B**.

continued

TABLE 28-5 (CONTINUED)
CRITICAL INCIDENT REPORTS—CLINICAL REASONING EXAMPLES

EXAMPLE B: CRITERION	DATE/TIME REPORTED
Patient Management: [꒐] Clinical Reasoning [꒐]	10/03/17 07:31 PM

Behavior	*Antecedent*
Student was unable to differentiate between what was causing a patient with a Baker's cyst who just had a medial meniscectomy to have pinching in the knee and did not know how to modify the exercises that she was going to give the patient based on the above complaint. Student has not provided rationales behind the interventions that she has given patients with different diagnoses up to this point in her clinical internship. Most of her time has been spent on reviewing course material on tests/measures and procedural interventions.	Student knowing how to modify interventions based on patient's response. Instructed student to review over proper progression of therapeutic exercise based on the patient's diagnosis, stage of healing, and level of acuity. Student must develop a basic understanding of different diagnosis and the interventions that needs to be given to treat impairments/limitations first before she can provide proper rationale/clinical judgment behind them.

Consequence	*CI Comments*
Student is at risk for not meeting the passing criteria for CR if this is not corrected.	Student needs guidance and instruction 100% of the time for CR. I am concerned she will not be able to develop the CR skills at the expected level by midterm as she must get the basics of patient safety, tests and measures, and procedural interventions first to develop this skill.

DCE/ACCE Comments
Student has exhibited a repeat pattern of lack of CR skills, which is a red flag item and foundational element for practice. Additionally, the examples provided by the CI of the student's performance also represent a lack of safety, which is also red flag item and foundational element for practice. CR is required for understanding the impact of the POC with patient's physiology and appropriate dosage parameters. Discussed the student performance, which falls below the expectation for year 2, with CCCE and plan to debrief w/CI and student. Additional debriefing sessions planned next week. The CI has provided appropriate verbal cueing, clinical instruction, and facilitation for student, and student requires 100% supervision, which falls below the expectation. The DCE will meet with the student to review learning strategies, references for foundational information, texts and guidance for CR, and referral to Student Support Services. The APTA-credentialed CI has provided objective examples of lack of the fundamental skills of CR. The student's current performance falls below the expectation and compromises patient safety and ability to progress beyond the basic foundational skills. Concur with CI objective report. Patient management requires demonstration of CR to apply current knowledge, basic knowledge, basic skills, theory, clinical judgment, and the patient's values and perspective in patient management. Student should be capable of providing treatment rationales having completed all didactic curriculum. It will be incumbent upon the student to demonstrate daily and weekly progress in the skills of CR. Recommend the student implement the use of the weekly programming planning form to address the goals of CR, patient safety, tests and measures, and procedural interventions, as directed by the CI with feedback regarding the critical incident, a lack of and student performance. The weekly planning form should be immediately implemented by the student, for each identified critical performance criteria, along with student's review of the expected sample behaviors for CR to progress toward expected midterm outcome ratings. EWS activated; all CE parties agreed to plan with safety and CR as top priorities and red flag foundational elements for professionalism and practice management; and all 4 critical incidents to be addressed by Monday with weekly planning goals proactively initiated by student. CI/CCCE/DCE support provided and clinical and academic advisors notified. Discussion of plan of action and instructional suggestions and facilitation completed with student.

continued

Table 28-5 (continued)
Critical Incident Reports—Clinical Reasoning Examples

Final Outcome	Date/Time Final Outcome Filed
CE terminated due to inadequate progression and continued safety risk in CE setting; referred for customized plan for remediation.	10/31/17 10:29 AM Compare and discuss how **Example A** differs from **Example B**. Where do your think the CR problem is occurring?

EXAMPLE C: CRITERION	DATE/TIME REPORTED
Patient Management: [☒] Clinical Reasoning [☒]	03/16/18 04:00 PM

Behavior	Antecedent
On 3/15, student was reviewing a chart and did not understand the definitions of or the difference between the terms "bronchoscopy" and "thoracotomy." Later in the same day, she was reviewing a chart for a patient who was found to have increased troponins during the admitting process. Upon questioning, student indicated she was not familiar with the term "troponin" or its implication.	Student was having difficulty transitioning toward independent management of complex patients because she was not recognizing the implications of items in the medical chart. She was not able to create a picture in her mind of the consequences for the patient, the potential for surgical sites and drains, and the effect on overall patient planning and prognosis

Consequence	CI Comments
The CI was concerned that the student's academic preparation was not adequate for the complex acute care environment. The DCE was contacted for assistance in planning a strategy for the student to successfully complete the rotation.	These difficulties are slowing the process of gaining independence with complex patients. We have initiated use of the weekly planning sheet to break down further goals for each week, and the student has begun to review unknown terminology during breaks and in the evenings.

DCE/ACCE Comments
Discussed onsite visit with student, CI, and CCCE. Student made aware of performance concerns. Debriefing discussion re: student performance, CI, student, and CCCE onsite. Proactive weekly planning form was implemented with fluctuating improvements. Student self-reports using Google to look up medical terminology that she does not know and has not yet secured a medical terminology text or medical dictionary, as of this date. Discussed with student that this recommendation was also made during her prior clinical. CI shared specific examples regarding student's lack of medical terminology and other fundamental knowledge needed for problem-solving and CR. Discussed with CI and student the current critical nature of the exhibited performance level, as being below the expectation for CE. Discussed a plan of action, the week prior that was already initiated to address and provided additional follow-up instructions. Both student and CI willing to continue, CI to complete further report; discussed

continued

TABLE 28-5 (CONTINUED)

CRITICAL INCIDENT REPORTS—CLINICAL REASONING EXAMPLES

with CCCE. CI has implemented an alternating strategy of patient turn-taking to assist student in timely assimilation (CI works with a patient, then student works with a patient); hence pace has decreased. CI reports that often even with patients with diagnoses that the student has seen previously, carry over with CR components is lacking. Student is commended on her professionalism, ability to receive constructive feedback, excellent interpersonal skills, and poise. Student is encouraged to take more initiative in her CR, problem-solving processes with tests and measures and plans of care. Student is highly encouraged to review fundamental knowledge expected from didactics and be more prepared. Student often has challenges recalling information that is expected from both a medical terminology and basic sciences standpoint. The CI was fully open to any additional suggestions to assist the student in her learning processes. Student is experiencing difficulty translating her skills from simple to complex, affecting her overall ability to progress in CE and in progressing her caseload.

CI/CCCE and student agreed to continue the final weeks of CE. It is evident that the performance is below the expectation from midterm and the concerns were addressed with student with her CI and CCCE face to face, at site visit, via telephone consults with CI, student and CCCE. Student has verbally reaffirmed her goal to become a physical therapist during the onsite visit and has no other concerns expressed at this time. Student is aware of her present performance level concerns. Standard referrals were completed for student support services. Discussed with CI the didactic preparation of students in the practice area. Discussed with CI/CCCE student's progressions to date. Discussed with student, onsite, strategies for improvement, increased focus, and the need to use appropriate textbooks, medical dictionary, etc, to support her learning and practice. Discussed challenges with CR.

Final Outcome	*Date/Time Final Outcome Filed*
CE successfully completed.	06/04/18 09:19 AM

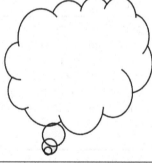

Now considering **Example C**, where do you think the responsibilities could have been improved more proactively? How can the CI hold the student more accountable along the way? What other strategies might you use as a student? CI? Peer? DCE? Consider all the learning from this CR text, what other ideas come to mind in terms of theory, instructional strategies, and innovative methods to facilitate CR?

Reflection Moment

Carefully read through examples A, B, and C in Table 28-5, and consider the roles and responsibilities for all parties. Discuss your impressions, and respond to the follow-up questions.

Consider within each case where the primary area of concern lies, which domain of learning (ie, affective, cognitive, or psychomotor) is most prevalent in need of attention, and how to best address the concern(s). Discuss and compare the approaches and plans in each example, and share any additional ideas and input you might have as a peer, DCE, CI, or academician. Remember the performance dimensions in identifying the student's level of performance with the expectations.

We trust that working through these examples gives you additional insight into the work of the CI and DCE in facilitating CR-CPS for students in physical therapy. The DCE truly appreciates the high-stakes nature of the foundational elements of practice, and will assist the student and CE team in progressing the work by identifying and providing resources that are needed, coaching the CI/CCCE in clinical teaching where needed, and facilitating the student's abilities for CR-CPS by customizing the assistance provided and working with tools (eg, coursework tools, weekly planning forms, CR-CPS articles, CR-Tool,[8] clinical practice guidelines, student program planning flow chart) and guides (eg, CR cycle and descriptions, Figure 3-2, turning descriptions into guiding questions to determine where in the cycle the CR-CPS disruption is occurring).

DCEs take ample time leading discussions with the student and CI to debrief CR-CPS clinical case encounters. Breaking down the patient/client management with the student and CI helps in dissecting where in the learning the CR-CPS interruption is occurring or where faulty reasoning is persisting. The DCE will often observe the student and CI working with the patient together to ascertain if additional opportunities are present to offer advisement and facilitation for CR-CPS or with any performance criteria. Frequently the DCE will also refer the student back to the related course faculty and/or advisors to work one-to-one with faculty or near peers, for brief intervals during CE and/or in a remediation effort.

Table 28-6[8-13] provides examples for posing queries within the CR approaches, building upon the questioning strategies for SA (as discussed in Section I, Chapter 3), to further guide the CI and student learner to discover where to redirect and/or challenge the student who is doing well into a new approach of discovery for CR-CPS. If you are struggling in your clinical decision-making and CPS skills for CR, consider these queries. As a CI, use the sample queries sparingly within the different aspects of CR and/or to facilitate new learning and new approaches. For example, if a student is highly dependent upon the HOAC approach, pose queries that facilitate efforts toward interactive reasoning to move the learner along the CR learning continuum.

TABLE 28-6

QUESTIONING STRATEGIES FOR FACILITATING CLINICAL REASONING TYPES

REASONING TYPE HYPOTHETICO-DEDUCTIVE	QUESTIONING STRATEGIES
Initial data	What information will you use to guide your exam? What do you think is going on with the patient? How will you consider the patient's values and beliefs?
Patient-identified problems	What problems did you identify? Can you identify more than one? What functional limitations/disabilities is your patient experiencing? What are your hypotheses thus far? How will you generate your tests and measures from what you know about the patient thus far? How is any PMH contributing?
Exam	What tests and measures do you want to do to confirm or rule out your hypotheses? What will you do if none of your hypotheses proves out? What will you do if you attain a positive result?
Existing or anticipated patient concerns	Did you identify any existing or anticipated problems that you think may be a problem for your patient? Have you considered the patient's social background? Does the patient have realistic expectations? Why or why not?

continued

TABLE 28-6 (CONTINUED)
QUESTIONING STRATEGIES FOR FACILITATING CLINICAL REASONING TYPES

REASONING TYPE HYPOTHETICO-DEDUCTIVE	QUESTIONING STRATEGIES
Why does this problem exist? Rationale for anticipated problem	Why do you think your patient is experiencing these problems? What is contributing to your patient's problems? How are the impairments linked to the patient's functional limitations and/or disabilities? Do you believe any other problem source is viable?
Refine problem list	Do you want to modify your problem list and/or reprioritize based on what you have now discovered? Does your patient have any problems that require referral to another health care provider and/or community-based resource? What learning needs do you still have? What is your muddiest point? How will you resolve?
Goals	What are your prioritized goals for the patient, and why?
Testing/predictive criteria	How will you know if your hypothesis is correct? How will you determine if physical therapy is effective?
Strategy/tactics	What interventions will you choose to address the problem? What dosage parameter will you elect to address the problem, and why? Will you require additional tests outside the scope of physical therapy practice? If so, why, and how will you achieve? Have you considered home exercise/education programming?
Reassessment	How will you know if your plan is working? When do you anticipate a change? How will you know when your goals have been met? What will you do when goals are met?

FORWARD	QUESTIONING STRATEGIES

Have you seen any patients like this before?
Based on the information, can you speculate as to what might be contributing to the patient's pain?
Based on this information, what things are unlikely to be the cause of pain?
If you see "xyz," what will this mean vs "abc"?
How is this patient's stroke similar or different from the patient we saw yesterday who also had a stroke?
If this patient were now HIV+, how would that change things or not?
If this patient were now 78 instead of 22 years old, how might this change things?

INTERACTIVE	QUESTIONING STRATEGIES

What do you think is the most important to this patient? What is the best way to find out?
What impact did the outcome of the imaging test have on your plan of care, and why?
What will you do if the patient's vitals are altered during the plan of care?
How can you involve the patient in the examination and place of care?
What will be the focus of your intervention?
How did the details of the home situation affect your plan of care for the patient, and why?

CONDITIONAL	QUESTIONING STRATEGIES

Does your hypothesis make sense based on the information gathered through your exam?
Is there anything you might have done differently based on your tests and measures in relation to your hypothesis?
Did you think through your patient's situation thoroughly? Did your hypothesis lead you to the right solution? Did you include the patient in the process? How did the patient respond to you? Your suggestions?

Adapted from Atkinson and Nixon-Cave,[8] Willgens and Sharf,[9] Durning et al,[10] Payton,[11] Duran-Nelson et al,[12] and Musolino and Mostrom.[13]

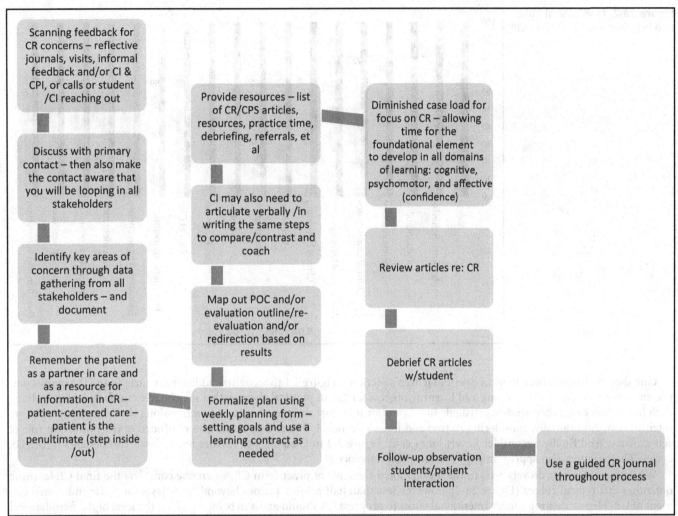

Figure 28-1. Guidelines for process steps: scanning and addressing deficits in clinical education from the DCE perspective (not in lock step order).

Experienced DCEs are inclined to use a stepwise process for problem-solving; the guidelines for the process are provided in Figure 28-1. This remains a flexible framework, as DCEs will continue to scan both the internal and external CE environments to problem-solve, collaborating with the CI, CCCE, and student perspectives to identify solutions, facilitate, and provide tutoring where needed, make necessary referrals, and establish a plan to set up the student for success in foundational elements of practice, especially in terms of CR. While promoting high levels of CR[14] is desired by the profession, the duty belongs to all of us to take responsibility and accountability to ensure that it occurs. We need to continue to teach our learners how to think, as certainly knowledge, technology, research, and innovation will change the future of practice. Yet if we know how to engage in CR and CPS, we can think about our patients and collaborate with them to improve their health. Teaching how to think keeps our learners curious, promoting creative CR and CPS to make connections to design solutions for our patients/clients in an ever-adapting world. Of course, we are subject to errors (see Chapter 3) as human beings, yet practicing CR and CPS allows us to alter our thinking by critical examination through self-awareness.

Figure 28-2. Final clinical education learning outcomes: APTA CPI.

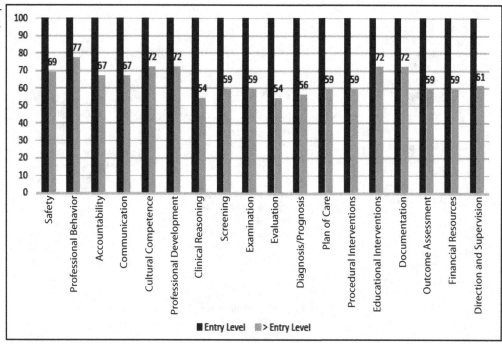

One should also look back to Musolino and Jensen's Section I, Figure 1-1 to recognize additional concepts and the many components contributing in the teaching and learning process for CR in physical therapy that may be relevant for problem-solving each individual case, when students struggle in CE, and/or if we just want to be certain to move along the CR continuum more intentionally. Additionally, considering Artino and Jones's Section I, Figure 2-2, one is also reminded of the important role of self-efficacy. And finally, reconsider Levett-Jones et al' Figure 3-2 in Chapter 3 to further break down components in the CR cycle. (These figures also appear on page 361 for quick reference.)

While most students do very well in the foundational elements of practice in CE, when one considers the final CE learning outcomes of a typical cohort (Figure 28-2), however, less than half achieve ratings beyond entry-level for the foundational element of CR. Hence, making a more intentional effort to progress CR should assist in bringing along the level of the foundational element of practice for all students. The APTA CPI remains both an internally consistent[15] (Cronbach alpha = 0.99) and valid[16] instrument (0.89) for the assessment of students in CE. The APTA CPI should be used specifically in conjunction with the critical incident report of a student's performance, when a student is struggling, most notably with the foundational elements of practice, including CR.

CONCLUSION

Let's **not** fall into the trap of not emphasizing the importance of the need to facilitate higher-level CR with our students and hold them accountable for CR skills while developing in both didactic and clinical education. In a recent mixed-methods study, with focus group interviews,[17] doctor of veterinary medicine graduates believed they had a good levels of reasoning abilities, yet still experienced a deficit in their reasoning capabilities when starting their careers. Overarching themes arising from the data noted that *a lack of responsibility for clinical decisions during the program and the embedded nature of the CR skill within the curriculum could be restricting development.*[17] The purpose of this chapter is to address CR and CPS for a doctoring profession, and to work to intentionally promote CR and CPS to higher performance levels at the entry point to practice. DCEs serve as leaders to facilitate this transition with key stakeholders in clinical education for the doctoring profession.

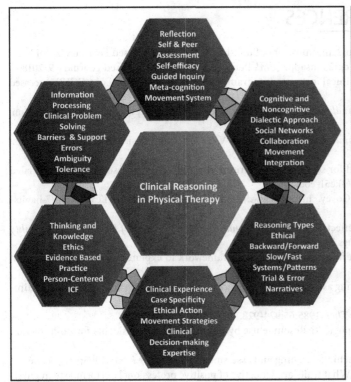

Figure 1-1. CR in physical therapy.

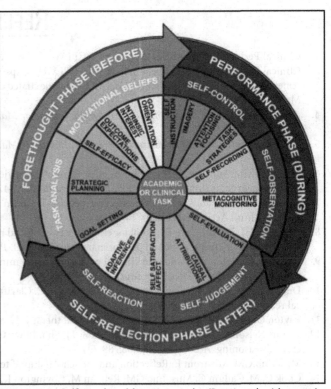

Figure 2-2. Self-regulated learning cycle. (Reprinted with permission from Artino AR Jr, Jones KD. AM last page: self-regulated learning—a dynamic, cyclical perspective. *Acad Med.* 2013;88[7]:1048, as adapted from Zimmerman BJ. Attaining self-regulation: a social cognitive perspective. In: Boekaerts M, Pintrich PR, Zeidner M, eds. *Handbook of Self-Regulation*. San Diego, CA: Academic Press; 2000.)

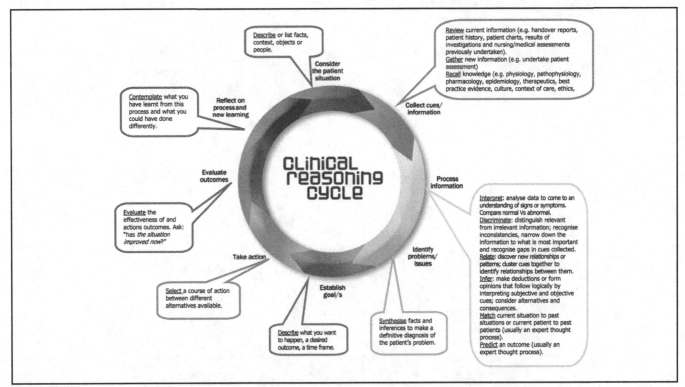

Figure 3-2. Levett-Jones clinical reasoning cycle. (Reprinted with permission from *Nurse Education Today*, 30, Levett-Jones T, Hoffman K, Dempsey J, et al. The "five rights" of clinical reasoning cycle: an educational model to enhance nursing students' ability to identify and manage clinically "at-risk" patients, 515-520, Copyright Elsevier 2010.)

REFERENCES

1. Clinical Performance Instrument. APTA PT-CPI Web. https://cpi2.amsapps.com/. Published June 2006. Accessed February 9, 2018.
2. Clinical Performance Instrument. APTA PTA-CPI Web. https://cpi2.amsapps.com/. Published June 2006. Accessed February 9, 2018.
3. American Physical Therapy Association (APTA). Credentialed clinical instructor program (CCIP). http://www.apta.org/CCIP/. Accessed March 20, 2018.
4. *APTA Credentialed Clinical Instructor Program, Instructor Manual, Level 1.* Alexandria, VA: American Physical Therapy Association; 2009.
5. *APTA Credentialed Clinical Instructor Program, Instructor Manual, Level 2.* Alexandria, VA: American Physical Therapy Association; 2018.
6. Musolino GM, van Duijn J, Noonan, A, et al. Reasons identified for seeking the American Physical Therapy Association Credentialed Clinical Instructor Program in Florida. *J Allied Health,* 2013; 42(3):e51-e60.
7. Covey S. Seven habits of highly effective people. Franklin Covey. https://www.franklincovey.com/Solutions/Leadership/7-habits-signature.html Accessed February 14, 2018.
8. Atkinson HL, Nixon-Cave K. A tool for clinical reasoning and reflection using the *International Classification of Functioning, Disability and Health (ICF)* framework and patient management model. *Phys Ther.* 2011;91:416-430.
9. Willgens AM, Sharf R. Failure in clinical education: using mindfulness as a conceptual framework to explore the lived experiences of 8 physical therapists. *J Phys Ther Educ.* 2015;29(1):70-78.
10. Durning SJ, Antino AR, Schuwirth L, van der Vieuten C. Clarifying assumptions to enhance our understanding and assessment of clinical reasoning. *Acad Med.* 2013;88:442-448.
11. Payton OD. Clinical reasoning process in physical therapy. *Phys Ther.* 1985;65:924-928.
12. Duran-Nelson A, Gladding S, Beattie J, Nixon LJ. Should we Google it? Resource use by internal medicine residents for point-of-care clinical reasoning. *Acad Med.* 2013;88:788-794.
13. Musolino GM, Mostrom E. Reflection and the scholarship of teaching, learning and assessment. *J Phys Ther Educ.* 2005;19(3):52-66.
14. Cook C, McCallum C, Musolino GM, Reiman M, Covington K. What traits are reflective of positive professional performance in physical therapy program graduates? *J Allied Health,* 2018;47(2):96-102.
15. Roach KE, Frost JS, Francis NJ, et al. Validation of the revised physical therapist clinical performance instrument (PT CPI): version 2006. *Phys Ther,* 2012;92(3):416-428.
16. Mori B, Norman KE, Brooks D, Herold J, Beaton DE. Evidence of reliability, validity, and practicality for the Canadian physiotherapy assessment of clinical performance. *Physiother Can.* 2016;68(2):156-169.
17. Vinten CE, Cobb KA, Freeman SL, Mossop LH. An investigation into the clinical reasoning development of veterinary students. *J Vet Med Educ,* 2016;43(4):398-405.

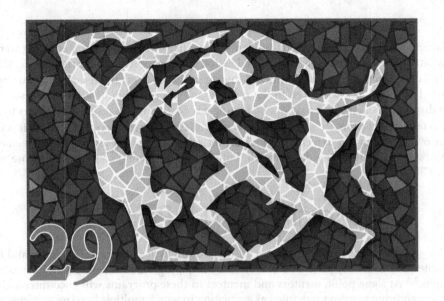

REFLECTION AS A CLINICAL DECISION-MAKING TOOL:
Navigating a Challenging Mentoring Situation— A Case Report Analysis

Theresa Najjar, PT, DPT, NCS, MS

OBJECTIVES

- The learner will reflect about the mentoring he or she provided during a challenging mentoring situation, including any barriers to mentoring that may have contributed to the situation.
- The learner will integrate mentor self-reflection in formal and informal ways as part of further developing intentional mentor skills.
- The learner will display encouragement and support toward other mentors in the process of self-reflection about mentoring when a fellow mentor encounters a challenging mentoring situation.

INTRODUCTION

At some point, a mentor will come across a mentoring situation in which multiple barriers are encountered and a disagreement arises. The purpose of this case report is to demonstrate how reflection can guide a mentor's clinical decision-making (CDM) when encountering a challenging mentoring situation, and develop intentional mentor skills for effective CDM and clinical reasoning (CR).

This chapter discusses a case description of a resident who was a new graduate in her final rotation of a residency program when the mentor identified a challenging mentoring situation. The mentor, who had 4 years of mentoring experience, used

Musolino GM, Jensen GM, eds. *Clinical Reasoning and Decision-Making in Physical Therapy: Facilitation, Assessment, and Implementation* (pp 363-377).

Schön's reflection-in-action and reflection-on-action to identify how her own barriers to mentoring were contributing to the challenging mentoring situation. The mentor then identified actions to overcome those barriers to mentoring.

The mentor actively listened to the resident and worked toward reducing stress the resident felt during mentoring sessions. The mentor also adjusted how feedback was given to the resident and integrated motivational interviewing techniques. Over time, the resident also displayed a change in behaviors indicating a reduction in the resident's barriers to mentoring.

Reflection is a useful tool mentors can use when encountering a challenging mentoring situation. It is important the mentor understands his or her own contribution to a challenging mentoring situation to resolve the disagreement, potential barriers for learning, and set the stage to optimize resident growth. Future research should continue to explore mentor CDM and collaboration for effective CR.

BACKGROUND AND PURPOSE

As of the time of this study, December 2017, the American Board of Physical Therapy Residency and Fellowship Education (ABPTRFE) had accredited 243 residency programs and 50 fellowship programs.[1] Mentoring is a key component of residency and fellowship education.[2,3] At some point, mentors and mentees in these programs will encounter a challenging mentoring situation. A challenging mentoring situation is defined as a situation in which multiple barriers to mentoring (Table 29-1) arise concurrently and possibly result in disagreement between mentor and mentee. While some dissonance can be healthy in mentor relationships, if disagreements are not resolved, they may adversely affect the growth of the resident, lead to conflict with patient/client management, and/or lead to termination of the mentor–mentee relationship.[4-7]

Both mentees and mentors can experience barriers to mentoring. As shown in Table 29-1, barriers fall into 3 main domains: personal, relationship, and program.[4-12] Barriers in the personal domain influence personal and professional development of the individual experiencing the barrier(s) and, as this case report will further explore, likely also impact the other individual in the mentor–mentee relationship. Relationship barriers are related to the mentor–mentee relationship and include topics such as making assumptions about the other person or having prejudices and biases toward that person. Barriers to mentoring can also be attributed to residency or fellowship program structure and include constraints such as time, geographical distance, or even incentives. Like personal barriers, relationship and professional barriers can also impact the complex and rich mentoring partnership.[4-12]

Understanding mentee and mentor barriers to mentoring is an important aspect of mentor growth and development. While the impact of mentoring on a mentee's professional growth and CDM is well-known,[8-10,13-20] research is only beginning to investigate the development and growth of mentors.[11,21-23] Although multiple mentoring frameworks exist,[3,4,6,7,9,12,19,24-35] there is currently no clear guideline or decision tree for mentors to rely on when faced with a challenging mentoring situation. A mentor's ability to handle a challenging mentoring situation can affect the mentor's satisfaction,[36] the mentor–mentee relationship,[3,4,6,7,10-12,19,34,36-38] and the professional growth of both mentor and mentee.[3-8,10,18,21,38] Because a mentor's own barriers to mentoring can impact the complexities of the mentor–mentee relationship,[4,5,8-12,19,24,34,37-39] it is critical for a mentor to reflect and identify his or her own potential barriers when faced with a complex mentoring situation.

Reflection is a key component to learning and developing expertise, serving as a useful tool for gaining new perspectives and insights.[3,16,22,34,40-51] As emphasized in Section I, the literature focus in physical therapy has leaned toward emphasizing the metacognitive (thinking about thinking) aspect of reflection.[16,43,47] In addition to metacognition, reflection encompasses a meta-affective (feeling about feeling) process.[51] A certain amount of self-awareness is required for reflection,[47] emphasizing the foundational skill of self-assessment (SA). Mindfulness, or a nonjudgmental acknowledgment and acceptance of the present moment including one's own thoughts and feelings, may not only be a way of tapping into this self-awareness, but may also influence metacognition and meta-affection.[52,53]

We will now focus on 2 main forms of Schön's reflective practice (RP) for this mentoring analysis. Reflection-in-action is an in-the-moment SA and situational analysis that can often trigger further exploration and experimentation. In contrast, reflection-on-action, or retrospection of a situation, allows it to be reviewed from different angles and potentially leads to a revision of one's CDM.[16,43,47,48,51] The education literature indicates reflection may help a mentor develop intentional mentoring skills.[21,34,38] An intentional mentor is able to assess a mentee with both quantitative and qualitative approaches and continuously strives to build upon the 6 core competencies of mentors in physical therapist residency and fellowship education.[2,3] These 6 core competencies are provided in Figure 29-1 and are defined in detail elsewhere.[2]

The purpose of this case report analysis is to demonstrate how reflection can (1) guide a mentor's CDM when encountering a challenging mentoring situation and (2) develop intentional mentoring skills for effective CDM and CR. While the same holds true and could also be applied for the resident and/or fellow, practicing self-analysis in this regard by the mentor will also promote RP facilitation skills of the mentor for the mentee.

This case report analysis begins with a description of the case, including detailed information about the resident and mentor. The case description is followed by the mentor's clinical impressions regarding the challenging mentoring situation (Mentor Impressions 1 to 3). Mentor impressions are followed by the mentor's examination of herself, including her rationale for and reflection about prior clinical impressions (Mentor, Self-Examinations 1 and 2). The outcomes of the mentor's reflections and

TABLE 29-1		
POSSIBLE BARRIERS TO MENTORING		
MENTEE BARRIERS TO MENTORING		
Personal	*Mentor–Mentee Relationship*	*Program*
• Being disagreement-averse • Lacking confidence • Not being accountable for mentee's role in the journey (passive not self-directed) • Being defensive or sensitive to criticism • Lacking courage to face constructive feedback and make effective changes • Taking things personally (eg, feeling rejected if the mentor cancels) • Having a poor sense of self • Engaging in poor reflection • Having poor self-directed learning • Resenting reflection or journaling • Being a perfectionist • Having poor organization or planning skills • Lacking focus • Assuming entitlement • Not balancing personal time and program commitments	• Making assumptions • Having prejudice or biases based on mentor characteristic or personal relationship • Being jealous • Being competitive • Being manipulative • Being submissive • Having an apathetic attitude • Having a saboteur attitude	• Dealing with time constraints • Having conflicts of interest • Handling a geographical distance between mentor and mentee
MENTOR BARRIERS TO MENTORING		
Personal	*Mentor–Mentee Relationship*	*Program*
• Being disagreement-averse • Engaging in impostership • Not taking accountability for mentor's role in the mentoring journey • Lacking mentoring experience and/or skills (eg, novice mentor) • Having poor reflection • Having a content knowledge gap • Focusing on one mentee-specific problem (overlooking other problems, not self-reflecting on own contributing barriers) • Being uncertain about assessment tools • Having an inability to actively listen • Giving answers or jumping in too soon • Demanding the mentee do it the mentor's way • Trying to solve the mentee's problems • Becoming a permanent leaning post • Suffering burnout and/or stress • Procrastinating	• Making assumptions • Having prejudice or biases based on mentee characteristics or personal relationship • Being jealous • Being competitive • Not understanding mentor role • Not mentoring (eg, teaching or parenting) • Not seeing the mentor–mentee relationship as collegial (eg, teacher-student or boss-employee) • Crossing boundaries • Lacking disclosure with mentee • Facing an ethical dilemma • Having a conflict in the chain of command (eg, mentor signs the paychecks) • Neglecting the mentee • Taking credit for the mentee's work	• Dealing with time constraints • Having conflicts of interest • Dealing with a geographical distance between the mentor and mentee • Having variability between mentors • Having no incentive to mentor

Adapted from Zachary,[4] Zachary and Fischler,[5] McCarthy,[6,7] Cooke et al,[8] Burgess et al,[9] Sambunjak et al,[10] Heeneman and de Grave,[11] and Sng et al.[12]

Figure 29-1. Six core competencies of mentors in physical therapist residency/fellowship education, required for mentors in physical therapist residency and fellowship education. (Adapted from Christensen N, Gerber P, Jensen GM, et al. *American Board of Physical Therapy Residency and Fellowship education mentoring resource manual.* American Board of Physical Therapy Residency and Fellowship Education. http://www.abptrfe.org/uploaded-Files/ABPTRFEorg/For_Programs/ABPTRFEMentoringResourceManual.pdf.)

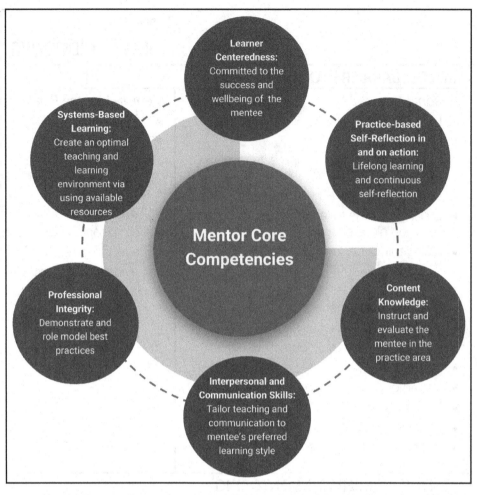

actions are then presented. The report concludes with a discussion and critical analysis of the mentoring case. This case report provides physical therapy residency and fellowship programs and mentors a clear and contemporary example of reflective CDM, facilitating CR during a challenging mentoring situation. It may also serve as a springboard for researchers to create an algorithm or decision tree for mentors who find themselves in a similar situation.

CASE DESCRIPTION

Resident Profile

The resident entered the Kaiser Permanente neurologic physical therapy residency program in August, after having graduated with her doctor of physical therapy degree 3 months prior. The resident's journey through the residency program is described in Figure 29-2. In brief, the resident's 2 acute care rotations took place at the same site, each with a different primary mentor. The resident spent 24 weeks in acute care between August 22 and the following February 10. During that time, she had contact with 3 mentors and received 80 hours of mentoring. Her 2 outpatient rotations consisted of different sites, each with a different primary mentor. She spent 24 weeks in the outpatient setting between February 27 and August 11. During that time, she had contact with 5 mentors and received 93 hours of mentoring. The challenging mentoring situation described in this case was identified by Mentor 1 (M1; the author) during the resident's second outpatient rotation.

Throughout each rotation, the resident was given weekly, written feedback from her mentor about her performance. She also participated in reflective journaling every other week. Upon completion of each rotation, key areas of development during the rotation and recommended areas for growth were identified and discussed with the resident using the program's quantitative and qualitative feedback forms. In addition, barriers to mentoring were observed during each of the rotations. A summary of each rotation's primary mentor's findings is summarized within Figure 29-2.

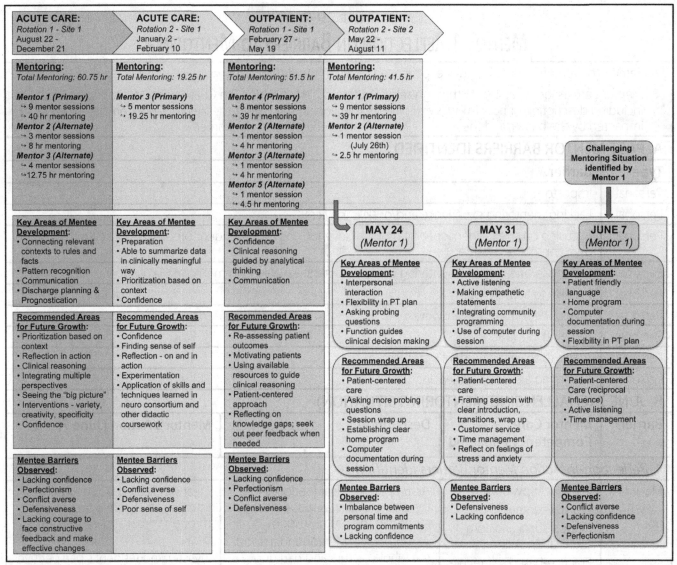

Figure 29-2. Mentor's reflections of resident's progress through the residency program. Reflections of each rotation's primary mentor on the resident's overall key areas of resident development, recommended areas for growth, and overarching barriers to mentoring.

Mentor 1 Profile

At the time the challenging mentoring situation was identified on June 7, M1 had approximately 4 years of experience as a mentor for the Kaiser neurologic physical therapy residency program. While developing as a mentor, she had experienced several barriers to mentoring (Table 29-2, A). She also had self-identified previous experiences with challenging mentoring situations. To develop her mentoring skills, she had sought and received mentoring by her own mentor. In addition, she had reflected on mentoring via reflection-in-action and reflection-on-action through occasional reflective journaling, verbal discussions, participation in mentoring workshops, and completing continuing education courses focused on key concepts of mentoring.

Mentor–Resident Relationship

Prior to mentoring the resident in Outpatient Rotation Part 2 (OR2), M1 had had 36 mentor contact hours with the resident in the acute care setting. During that time, M1 had observed several resident/mentee barriers to mentoring, as well as key areas of resident development and areas for resident growth (see Figure 29-2). During May 24 and May 31 of OR2, M1 broadly identified patient-centered care (PCC), among other areas, as a recommended area for resident growth (see Figure 29-2). After each of those mentor sessions, M1 had given what she believed was clear and constructive verbal and written performance feedback to the resident regarding PCC.

Table 29-2
Mentor 1 Reflection on Barriers to Mentoring

A. Barriers to mentoring intermittently experienced by M1 in the distant past.

B. Mentor barriers identified by M1 through self-reflection during the June 7th Challenging Mentoring Situation, including description of how M1 was exhibiting/experiencing the barrier, the Mentor Core Competencies impacted by the barrier, and the action(s) M1 took after reflecting on the barrier.

A. PAST MENTOR BARRIERS IDENTIFIED

Type	Barrier
Personal	Impostorship
Personal	Lacking mentoring experience and/or skills (novice)
Personal	Focusing on one resident-specific problem (overlooking other resident problems, not self-reflecting on own contributing barriers)
Personal	Lacking in one or more mentoring core competencies/lacking in mentoring skills
Personal	Inability to actively listen
Personal	Giving the resident the answer
Personal	Jumping in too soon
Personal	Trying to solve the resident's problems
Personal	Becoming a permanent leaning post

B. JUNE 7 (CHALLENGING MENTORING SITUATION)

Barrier	Mentor Core Competency Impacted	Description	Mentor's Action (June 7)
1. Reflection-In-Action Mentor Barriers Identified			
Making assumptions	Content knowledge Learner centeredness Interpersonal and communication skills Practice-based self-reflection in and on action	*Assumption 1:* Clear feedback in the area of PCC was made clear by mentor in the past 2 sessions *Assumption 2:* Mentor understood the whole picture and had dug deep enough into the obstacle(s) limiting the resident's growth in PCC *Assumption 3:* Mentor and resident both understood and agreed upon the obstacle(s) limiting the resident's growth in PCC (ie, active listening)	Clearly indicated PCC and active listening as key areas for growth, through verbal and written feedback. Investigated resident's perspective regarding obstacles to providing PCC.
Stress	Content knowledge Learner-centeredness Interpersonal and communication skills Professional integrity Practice-based self-reflection in and on action Systems-based learning	Holding breath Body tense Feeling of anxiety M1 recognized stress likely triggered by presence of disagreement and presence of resident defensiveness	Recognized stress Allowed it to be present Investigated what the mentor needed in that moment with self-kindness Nonidentified (created space) with the stress

continued

	TABLE 29-2 (CONTINUED)		
	MENTOR 1 REFLECTION ON BARRIERS TO MENTORING		
Barrier	**Mentor Core Competency Impacted**	**Description**	**Mentor's Action (June 7)**
Trying to solve resident's problems	Content knowledge Learner-centeredness Interpersonal and communication skills Professional integrity Practice-based self-reflection in and on action	Mentor had provided resident with multiple recommendations to PCC, active listening, caseload, and time management Observed resident defensiveness increasing with increasing recommendations	Identified this as possible contribution to increasing resident defensiveness observed Switched to open-ended questions
Inability to actively listen	Learner-centeredness Interpersonal and communication skills Professional integrity Practice-based self-reflection in and on action	Pre-planning response dialogue Losing focus while resident is talking Not understanding more than just resident's words	Suppressed mentor's internal conversation Refocused on the resident Tried to understand the resident's complete message
2. Reflection-On-Action Mentor Barriers Identified			
Making assumptions	Content knowledge Learner-centeredness Interpersonal and communication skills Practice-based self-reflection in and on action	*Assumption 5:* The mentor had asked for and received a clear commitment from the resident to work on PCC prior to June 7 *Assumption 6:* The resident had the tools she needed to reflect on how her biases, emotions, and actions impact PCC (Principle 1)	Asked resident to begin to set clear goals on written feedback form starting 6/7 to address PCC Principle 1 During mentoring 6/14, asked for resident's clear commitment do deep self-reflection to address PCC principles Provided resident with tools to assist deep reflection within affective domain
Biases based on past resident relationship	Learner-centeredness Interpersonal and communication skills Professional integrity Practice-based self-reflection in and on action	M1 had established biases about the resident due to her experience mentoring the resident in acute care, including identifying several resident barriers to mentoring during that time Biases contributed to M1's stress barrier Biases contributed to M1's active listening barrier	Used mindfulness to bring biases into conscious awareness
Focusing on one resident-specific area	Learner Centeredness Interpersonal and communication skills Practice-based self-reflection in and on action	M1's initial focus on the resident's defensiveness led to increase in stress, ultimately limiting M1's ability to reflect on self-contribution to the disagreement M1's hyper focus on Principle 3 impacted her ability to actively listen to the resident	Increased mindfulness of stress's impact on M1's focus and attention during the session Took a step back Had resident participate in goal-setting

continued

		TABLE 29-2 (CONTINUED)	
		MENTOR 1 REFLECTION ON BARRIERS TO MENTORING	
Barrier	**Mentor Core Competency Impacted**	**Description**	**Mentor's Action (June 7)**
Content knowledge gap	Content knowledge Learner-centeredness Professional integrity Practice-based self-reflection in and on action Systems-based learning	M1 recognized that her knowledge gap in the principles of PCC contributed to a delay in depth and specificity of feedback conveyed to the resident M1 recognized a knowledge gap with motivational interviewing	Reviewed information related to PCC Reviewed and further researched information related to motivational interviewing Encouraged regular reflection-in-action to identify ongoing or new mentor knowledge gaps
Lacking mentoring experience and/or skills	Content knowledge Learner-centeredness Interpersonal and communication skills Professional integrity Practice-based self-reflection in and on action Systems-based learning	Due to the complexity of mentor barriers involved, M1 identified a need for additional guidance during this challenging mentoring situation	Received mentoring from personal mentor Was formally evaluated by personal mentor during a mentoring session with the resident
Variability between mentors and/or sites	Learner-centeredness Interpersonal and communication skills Systems-based learning	Resident recently switched settings and mentors, which contributed to her reports of stress and reduced self-confidence M1 did not realize the impact switching settings and mentors had on this resident and her PCC	Mentor closely read resident's reflective journaling to monitor resident's adjustment to the site Mentor encouraged resident to increase self-care and self-compassion activities during and outside of work to reduce burnout risk

MENTOR IMPRESSION 1

During the 4-hour mentoring session on June 7, M1 noted the resident had made progress toward all prior recommended areas for growth except PCC. M1's previous reflection-on-action, following the May 31 session, allowed her to identify the need for increased specificity of feedback regarding PCC. To provide clear and detailed feedback to the resident, between May 31 and June 7, M1 researched and identified 4 specific PCC principles.[54] These principles are listed in Figure 29-3. On June 7, while observing the resident during patient care, M1 identified PCC Principle 3—reciprocal influence—as a key area for resident growth (see Figure 29-3).

When M1 provided targeted constructive feedback to the resident about this area, she observed the resident exhibiting 4 barriers to mentoring: conflict aversion, lack of confidence, defensiveness, and perfectionism (see Figure 29-2). Several behaviors were observed indicating these barriers were present, as described in Figure 29-4. For example, the resident's barrier of defensiveness was demonstrated by being closed to other's opinions, using blaming language, exhibiting a stiff posture, and shifting away from reflection toward intellectualization (ie, the use of cognitive CR to avoid conflict and feeling through legitimate SA). M1 also observed what she thought to be resident topic avoidance as the resident shifted focus away from M1's feedback on PCC Principle 3 to discuss the resident's personal concerns of stress, caseload size, and time management, as well as how the resident felt these were limiting her growth and development.

M1 identified topic avoidance as a sign of disagreement between the mentor and the resident, as each was identifying a different area she felt was most impacting the resident's growth and development. Due to the presence of barriers to mentoring and a disagreement, M1 further identified the presence of a challenging mentoring situation that, if not resolved, could negatively impact the resident's growth. M1 also realized she had not yet reflected on her own barriers and their potential contribution to this challenging mentoring situation. She recognized that self-reflection was critical to guiding her CDM as an intentional mentor during this challenging mentoring situation.

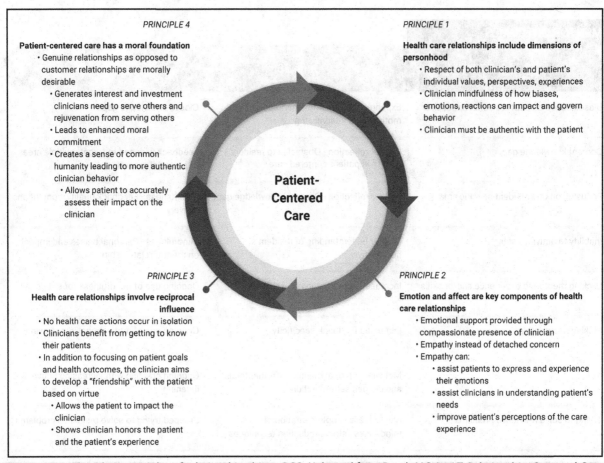

Figure 29-3. The 4 key principles of relationship-driven PCC. (Adapted from Beach MC, Inui T, Relationship-Centered Care Research Network. Relationship-centered care. A constructive reframing. *J Gen Intern Med.* 2006;21[suppl 1]:S3-S8.)

MENTOR SELF-EXAMINATION 1

Reflection-in-Action

As the challenging mentoring situation unfolded, M1 began to use reflection-in-action to guide her CDM (see Table 29-2, B1). She realized she had been functioning under assumptions that were misleading her CDM. First, she assumed she had been specific enough in her original feedback regarding PCC. She now saw more specificity was needed. Second, M1 assumed she had discussed PCC in depth with the resident. By not doing enough initial discovery work in the prior 2 mentor sessions to determine which Principle(s) of PCC (see Figure 29-3) the resident should focus on developing, M1 realized she might not have set the resident up for success. On June 7, following these reflections and the mentor taking on responsibility in the mentor–mentee model, M1 did eventually identify PCC Principle 3 as a key area of focus. However, she then made the third misleading assumption: both she and the resident understood and agreed that Principle 3 was the component of PCC in most need of growth.

It was only when M1 realized she was not actively listening to the resident's differing opinion that a disagreement became apparent. While M1 had zeroed in on PCC Principle 3 as a key area of focus, the resident was instead identifying concerns related to the emotions and reactions the resident believed were governing her behavior and adversely impacting her ability to deliver PCC, which are concerns related to PCC Principle 1.

M1 also realized that identification of a disagreement with the resident evoked feelings of stress, further impeding CDM/CR efforts. This, in turn, was impacting her ability to effectively mentor. After going through a brief mindfulness process to recognize, allow, investigate, and create space from her stressful feelings (see Table 29-2, B1), M1 was able to refocus on the resident. After realizing she was trying to fix things for the resident, M1 was able to switch to more open-ended questions, allowing her to better identify the resident's needs.

MENTOR OUTCOMES		
June 7th	**June 28th**	**August 11th**
Biases based on past resident relationship	Experimentation - Implementation of motivational interviewing	Closed knowledge gaps
Content knowledge gap	Further reflection - Obstacles to resident's growth in patient-centered care	Feedback widened to target multiple areas of potential growth
Focusing on one resident-specific area	Further reflection - Personal knowledge gaps	Mindfulness - Feedback quality, content and delivery
Inability to actively listen	Greater understanding of resident's perspective	Mindfulness - Personal biases and impact on mentor relationship
Lacking mentoring experience and/or skills	Increased active listening	Ongoing use of mindfulness for stress
Making assumptions	Increased feedback specificity	Ongoing use of motivational interviewing
Stress	Met with personal mentor to further focus and deepen self-reflection	Ongoing practice with increasing active listening
Trying to solve resident's problems	Mindfulness - implementation of mindfulness stress reduction techniques	Stopped trying to solve resident's problems

Figure 29-4A. M1's barriers to mentoring, identified on June 7, and the subsequent outcomes on June 28 and August 11.

Mentor Impression 2

M1 began to exercise deeper reflective listening, more fully hearing the resident's perspective. The resident felt stressed and overwhelmed. Perceptions about caseload size, unfamiliarity with the new mentoring site, and struggles with time management were named as the primary contributing factors to the resident's feelings. The resident believed these elements were governing her behavior and negatively affecting her ability to be fully present with the patient, ultimately impacting her ability to provide authentic PCC Principle 1. Once it was determined that these were valid concerns as opposed to the resident lacking accountability for her own journey, M1 realized both PCC Principle 1 and Principle 3 were important areas for the resident's (mentee's) growth. Further, M1 realized that PCC Principle 1 should be targeted first, as the resident's stress was impacting her ability to be mentally and emotionally present and authentic with her patients. Only after the resident was able to be more present and authentic with the patients (PCC Principle 1) could she begin to work on developing relationships with reciprocal influence (PCC Principle 3).

It was also evident that reflection on the part of the mentor and resident produced an opening for learning. It is not uncommon that a learner, even a licensed practicing physical therapist, may fall back into faulty coping patterns or mechanisms when stressed by a challenging situation. When the mentor and resident participated in deep, rich, and honest SA with full disclosures, they landed with full discovery of the impacting factors that needed to be addressed.

M1 also realized the resident had to take a more active role in the mentoring process, especially taking self-initiative with goal-setting for the resident's own lifelong learning and professional development to become a more self-engaged, reflective practitioner. The mentor identified motivational interviewing as a potential tool to assist the resident in making her desired behavior changes around stress and time management. Motivational interviewing is a style of conversation and goal-oriented questioning intending to elicit a behavior change by promoting self-efficacy in a person who may be displaying conflicting beliefs toward a behavior he or she wishes to resolve.[55,56] The resident displayed this ambivalence toward her stress level and time management. For example, she expressed a strong desire to reduce her self-reported stress level of 9 to 10/10, as well as an interest in learning how to reduce her stress. However, when M1 offered ideas on time management and stress reduction and encouraged the resident to ask colleagues for additional suggestions and feedback, the resident hesitated to consider implementing the ideas and to talk with her colleagues, exhibiting barriers to her own professional development.

RESIDENT OUTCOMES		
June 7th	June 28th	August 11th
Accentuating the negative	Body language - Reduced eye contact when conveying differing opinion	Body language - Regular eye contact when conveying differing opinion
Blaming language	Body language - Relaxed posture	Body language - Relaxed posture
Body language - Lack of eye contact when conveying differing opinion	Easily disappointed by unmet goals	Elimination of topic avoidance
Body language - Stiff posture	Fear of failure	Increased active listening during patient care encounters
Closed to other's opinions	Increased openness to other points of view	Increased realistic outlook on unmet goals
Easily disappointed by unmet goals	Increased depth of reflection in and on action	Ongoing increased depth of reflection in and on action
Fear of failure	Reduction in accentuating the negative	Ongoing increased openness to other points of view
Intellectualization	Reduction in blaming language	Ongoing reduction in accentuating the negative
Self-reported stress 9 - 10 / 10	Reduction in intellectualization	Rare use of blaming language
Tears	Reduction in topic avoidance	Rare use of intellectualization
Topic avoidance	Self-directed learning - Participation in weekly goal setting	Reduction in fear of failure
		Self-reported ↑ in mindfulness of biases and emotions during patient care encounters
		Self-reported stress 3 / 10 (July 30th)
		Self-directed learning - Active engagement in the learning process
		Self-directed learning - Actively seeks out feedback from others
		Self-directed learning - Regular participation in weekly and future goal setting

Figure 29-4B. Observed behaviors associated with the mentee's barriers to mentoring (identified by M1 on June 7—see Figure 29-2) and subsequent outcomes over time.

Mentor Self-Examination 2

Reflection-on-Action (see Table 29-2, B2)

Upon completion of the June 7 mentoring session, M1 continued to reflect on the challenging situation. She realized she had made additional assumptions that had impacted her CDM and contributed to the disagreement. Prior to June 7, M1 assumed she had asked for and received a commitment from the resident to work on the area of PCC, but she had not. Further, when the resident identified Principle 1 as an area of concern on June 7, M1 had assumed the resident had the tools she needed to reflect deeply enough on how the resident's biases, emotions, and actions were impacting PCC. As such, M1 had not provided additional resources during mentoring on June 7. The mentor realized these tools would need to be provided to the resident.

In reflecting about her mentor–mentee relationship with the resident, M1 realized that her experience with the resident within the acute care rotation 1 component (see Figure 29-2), particularly regarding previously observed resident barriers to mentoring, had biased the current resident relationship. M1 realized these biases likely contributed to her own previously identified stress and active listening barriers because, based on her previous experiences with the resident, M1 had become quick to attribute any potential disagreement to resident defensiveness. M1 realized her hyperfocus on resident defensiveness not only limited M1's ability to self-reflect on her own contributions to the disagreement but also contributed to an increase in her stress level while mentoring. M1 also had been overly focused on providing feedback regarding PCC Principle 1, impacting her ability to actively listen to the resident.

M1 further reflected on the impact any content knowledge gaps had on her CDM. She recognized that a knowledge gap in PCC Principles contributed to a delay in giving targeted feedback to the resident. M1 also recognized she had a knowledge gap in motivational interviewing and a desire to close that gap so that she could effectively use that tool with her resident.

In addition to knowledge gaps, M1 identified a need for external guidance and mentoring about mentoring due to the complexity of mentor and resident barriers involved. This led M1 to seek out additional guidance from her personal, professional mentor, who helped M1 focus and deepen her self-reflection. Furthermore, M1 recognized a program barrier she had not previously considered: the resident not only had recently switched mentors but also had switched settings. While the resident's reflective journal entries expressed stress over this transition, M1 had not understood the full impact this could have on a resident's PCC. The influence of the environment and types of patient encounters being altered contributed to the experience being much more novel for the resident, even within the same health care system.

Mentor Impression 3

M1 realized that, long before the challenging mentoring situation arose, the resident had given M1 the critical information needed to identify PCC Principle 1 as a primary recommended area for growth via the resident's reflective journaling, interactions during in-person mentor sessions, and responses on written feedback forms. As a mentor, this was a moment of recognition and surprise that M1 had missed the important cues and clues along the way. Due to the mentor's barriers to mentoring, she had missed prior opportunities for more effective active listening. M1 hypothesized the disagreement leading to this challenging mentoring situation might have been avoided if she had identified PCC Principle 1 earlier as an area of focus. M1 shared in the responsibility and accountability for the interprofessional communication, and the need to often read and then reread reflective journals to ascertain full meaning. When in doubt, it is likely best to go ahead and have those needed conversations, which may then shed further light on the potential barriers or reveal changes in missed or confirmed perceptions.

Outcomes

Qualitative analysis of mentor notes and recollections, mentor feedback forms, written resident feedback form responses, and resident reflective journaling from OR2 yielded several mentor and resident outcomes (see Figure 29-4). Reliability and validity of the qualitative and quantitative feedback used in the Kaiser Permanente neurologic residency program have not yet been determined; this is an identified area for further development.

Summary of Short-Term Outcomes (June 7 Through June 28)

In addition to participating in more active listening during mentor sessions, M1 mindfully addressed her stress as it arose during the mentor sessions, allowing her to refocus on the resident with active listening. By increasing the specificity of her qualitative verbal and written feedback, M1 switched from a fixing approach to an open-ended, questioning and facilitation approach. She also began to integrate motivational interviewing techniques related to the resident's goals of reducing stress and improving time management. M1 asked for and received a commitment from the resident to work on PCC, and she provided the resident with tools to assist in deep reflection in the affective learning domain (see Figure 29-4).

As M1 began to address her barriers to mentoring and modify her mentoring approach, the resident's behaviors associated with the resident's barriers to mentoring began to change (see Figure 29-4). In addition, an increase in resident self-directed learning evolved, facilitated by weekly goal-writing in self-identified areas of improvement. The resident also displayed increased openness to other points of view, allowing her not only to be more open to mentor feedback, but also to better understand her patients' perspectives and experiences (ie, PCC Principle 1).

The resident had mixed reports of improvements in stress during this time. For example, during an in-person mentoring session on June 21, she reported a reduction in her overall stress level, but in her reflective journaling on June 25, she reported ongoing high levels of stress and mental exhaustion. Appropriate referrals were completed for additional self-management and assistance with stress management resources and professional assistance support.

Summary of Long-Term Outcomes (June 7 Through August 11)

M1 continued to use reflection to influence her CDM and grow her intentional mentor skills (see Figure 29-4). She also received "mentoring on mentoring" from her personal mentor to facilitate this growth. In addition to reflection, M1 used the tool of mindfulness to help mitigate stress triggered when she observed behaviors indicative of resident defensiveness. M1 closed her knowledge gap related to motivational interviewing. She continued to use motivational interviewing with the resident to promote sustainable goal-setting regarding stress and time management to optimize the resident's ability to be present and authentic with her patients (ie, PCC Principle 1). M1 stopped trying to solve the resident's problems and continued to work on increasing use of active listening during mentor feedback sessions.

The resident also continued to mature (see Figure 29-4). Regarding her stress levels during patient-care encounters, she began to report an increase in mindfulness. The resident also experienced a reduction in self-reported stress, from 9 to 10 out of 10 on July 7 to 3 out of 10 on July 30 (on a scale of 0 being no stress and 10 being the most stress possible). By August 11, the resident had demonstrated a reduction in many of the behaviors associated with her barriers to mentoring. She also showed an increase in self-directed learning and reported an increase in self-confidence. During final program evaluations, the resident achieved progress toward goals related to PCC Principles 1 and 3.

DISCUSSION

Developing advanced practitioners through mentoring involves a 2-way relationship.[3-7] Initially when faced with a challenging mentoring situation, M1 focused on the resident's contribution to the disagreement. With the tool of reflection, M1 was able to identify barriers impacting her ability to be an intentional mentor. By reflecting on and addressing these barriers, she was able to determine her role in the disagreement and adjust her CDM and mentoring of the resident. This, in turn, allowed her to directly address the challenging mentoring situation to positively impact the resident's growth.

By identifying and reflecting on her barriers to mentoring, she also further developed her skills as an intentional mentor, as these barriers each influenced elements of the mentor core competencies. By overcoming her specific barriers to mentoring, M1 was able to better assess her resident quantitatively and qualitatively, while simultaneously continuing her professional development as a mentor. This may have also had an impact on the resident, allowing her to feel as if she could be open to develop and grow in her areas of focus. In short, as the mentor reflected and matured in professional development, the resident also progressed in her own professional development as a mentor.

While reflection has been identified as a key component of learning, developing expertise, new perspectives, and insights,[3,16,22,34,40-51] mentors are not often encouraged to self-reflect on the mentoring they provide or any barriers to mentoring that may exist. M1's self-reflection was in part facilitated by environmental and situational factors. For example, mentor reflection is strongly promoted and encouraged within the Kaiser Permanente neurologic physical therapist residency program. This allowed M1 to feel safe and supported, while undergoing a process that may lead to feelings of judgment and vulnerability.[57] Situationally, M1 had access to her own mentor, who was able to guide M1 to deepen her reflection throughout the challenging mentoring situation (see Table 29-2 and Figure 29-4). While journaling is a useful reflection tool,[43] M1 did not use journaling during this challenging situation. If it had been used, it might have further deepened her reflection experience. As mentor self-reflection becomes more of the norm, residency and fellowship programs that provide a safe and nurturing environment for mentors to reflect will promote more peer-to-peer mentoring.

Because this case report is self-reflective in nature, bias is inevitable. For example, many of the objective findings for M1 were based on her own perceptions of the reflective experience, and therefore carry a personal bias. Other biases may also exist within this case report. For instance, Figure 29-2 summarizes feedback written by multiple mentors including M1. However, because M1 thematically analyzed and summarized the written feedback from other mentors, it is possible her own perspective and bias influenced the interpretation of another mentor's feedback. While the other mentors did review and provide feedback on Figure 29-2, it still contains M1's bias.

Although there are a few other case reports about mentoring in the medical profession, they either focus on qualities of the mentor–mentee relationship[19] or on developing tools to promote resident CR.[16,17] This is the first case report to look at a possible process for a mentor to use when dealing with a challenging mentoring situation for both CDM/CR for the mentor–mentee relationship, and for PCC. In addition to augmenting the RP literature,[3,16,22,34,40-51] it also shows how mentors can use reflection within residencies and fellowships to further develop and deepen intentional mentor skills. Future research on mentoring should continue to explore mentor CDM, possibly creating an algorithm or decision tree for mentoring a resident during challenging mentoring situations.

This case report explored several themes. In addition to reflection, the themes of stress and active listening became key drivers behind the mentor's CDM. Additionally, the tools of motivational interviewing and mindfulness were used repeatedly by the mentor to influence the challenging mentoring situation. As the mentor further developed her intentional mentor skills through the tool of reflection, the resident also grew. Future research in mentoring should further explore the impact these themes and tools have on the mentee, the mentor, and the mentoring relationship. Additional resources for residency and fellowship mentors are also available as a component of the APTA Academy of Physical Therapy Education, Residency and Fellowship Educators Special Interest Group, and the APTA Credentialed Clinical Instructor Level 1 and Level 2 course programs.

REFERENCES

1. American Board of Physical Therapy Residency and Fellowship Education. Accredited residency/fellowship programs through December 31, 2017. http://www.abptrfe.org/uploadedFiles/ABPTRFEorg/ABPTRFEProgramGrowth.pdf. Accessed February 5, 2018.
2. Christensen N, Gerber P, Jensen GM, et al. *American Board of Physical Therapy Residency and Fellowship education mentoring resource manual.* American Board of Physical Therapy Residency and Fellowship Education. http://www.abptrfe.org/uploadedFiles/ABPTRFEorg/For_Programs/ABPTRFEMentoringResourceManual.pdf.
3. Tichenor CJ, Jensen G, Hartley G, Matsui I. *Successful mentorship for residency and fellowship education.* Transcript of course presented at: APTA Learning Center; online: February 27, 2015.
4. Zachary LJ. *The Mentor's Guide: Facilitating Effective Learning Relationships.* 2nd ed. San Francisco, CA: John Wiley & Sons; 2012.
5. Zachary LJ, Fischler LA. *The Mentee's Guide: Making Mentoring Work for You.* San Francisco, CA: John Wiley & Sons; 2009.
6. McCarthy A. *A framework for successful mentoring in physical therapy residencies.* Presented at: Neurologic Physical Therapy Consortium Webinar; 2014.
7. McCarthy A. *Residency mentoring: mentoring in a professional environment.* Presented at: Kaiser Permanente Neurologic Physical Therapy Mentoring Workshop; June 10, 2017; Redwood City, CA.
8. Cooke KJ, Patt DA, Prabhu RS. The road of mentorship. *Am Soc Clin Oncol Educ Book.* 2017;37:788-792.
9. Burgess A, van Diggele C, Mellis C. Mentorship in the health professions: a review. *Clin Teach.* January 2018. doi:10.1111/tct.12756.
10. Sambunjak D, Straus SE, Marusic A. A systematic review of qualitative research on the meaning and characteristics of mentoring in academic medicine. *J Gen Intern Med.* 2010;25(1):72-78.
11. Heeneman S, de Grave W. Tensions in mentoring medical students toward self-directed and reflective learning in a longitudinal portfolio-based mentoring system: an activity theory analysis. *Med Teach.* 2017;39(4):368-376.
12. Sng JH, Pei Y, Toh YP, et al. Mentoring relationships between senior physicians and junior doctors and/or medical students: a thematic review. *Med Teach.* 2017;39(8):866-875.
13. Brooks J. Let's get serious about mentoring. *Br Dent J.* January 2018. doi:10.1038/sj.bdj.2018.39.
14. Geraci SA, Thigpen SC. A review of mentoring in academic medicine. *Am J Med Sci.* 2017;353(2):151-157.
15. Sambunjak D, Straus SE, Marusić A. Mentoring in academic medicine: a systematic review. *JAMA.* 2006;296(9):1103-1115.
16. Atkinson HL, Nixon-Cave K. A tool for clinical reasoning and reflection using the *International Classification of Functioning, Disability and Health (ICF)* framework and patient management model. *Phys Ther.* 2011;91(3):416-430.
17. Baker SE, Painter EE, Morgan BC, et al. Systematic clinical reasoning in physical therapy (SCRIPT): tool for the purposeful practice of clinical reasoning in orthopedic manual physical therapy. *Phys Ther.* 2017;97(1):61-70.
18. Bay EH, Binder C, Lint C, Park S. Mentoring the next generation of neuroscience nurses: a pilot study of mentor engagement within an academic-service partnership. *J Neurosci Nurs.* 2015;47(2):97-103.
19. Rabatin JS, Lipkin M Jr, Rubin AS, Schachter A, Nathan M, Kalet A. A year of mentoring in academic medicine: case report and qualitative analysis of fifteen hours of meetings between a junior and senior faculty member. *J Gen Intern Med.* 2004;19(5 Pt 2):569-573.
20. Lockspeiser TM, Li S-TT, Burke AE, et al. In pursuit of meaningful use of learning goals in residency: a qualitative study of pediatric residents. *Acad Med.* 2016;91(6):839-846.
21. Langdon FJ. Learning to mentor: unravelling routine practice to develop adaptive mentoring expertise. *Teach Dev.* 2017;21(4):528-546.
22. Schatz-Oppenheimer O. Being a mentor: novice teachers' mentors' conceptions of mentoring prior to training. *Prof Dev Educ.* 2017;43(2):274-292.
23. Lopez-Real F, Kwan T. Mentors' perceptions of their own professional development during mentoring. *J Educ for Teach.* 2005;31(1):15-24.
24. Pennanen M, Bristol L, Wilkinson J, Heikkinen HLT. What is "good" mentoring? Understanding mentoring practices of teacher induction through case studies of Finland and Australia. *Pedagogy Cult Soc.* 2016;24(1):27-53.
25. Karallis T, Sandelands E. Making mentoring stick: a case study. *Educ Train.* 2009;51(3):203-209.
26. Jones R, Brown D. The mentoring relationship as a complex adaptive system: finding a model for our experience. *Mentor Tutor.* 2011;19(4):401-418.

27. Nagarur A, O'Neill RM, Lawton D, Greenwald JL. Supporting faculty development in hospital medicine: design and implementation of a personalized structured mentoring program. *J Hosp Med*. October 2017:E1-E4.

28. Akhigbe T, Zolnourian A, Bulters D. Mentoring models in neurosurgical training: review of literature. *J Clin Neurosci*. 2017;45:40-43.

29. Dawson P. Beyond a definition: toward a framework for designing and specifying mentoring models. *Educ Res*. 2014;43(3):137-145.

30. Furze JA, Tichenor CJ, Fisher BE, Jensen GM, Rapport MJ. Physical therapy residency and fellowship education: reflections on the past, present, and future. *Phys Ther*. 2016;96(7):949-960.

31. Klinge CM. A conceptual framework for mentoring in a learning organization. *Adult Learn*. 2015;26(4):160-166.

32. Toh YP, Karthik R, Teo CC, et al. Toward mentoring in palliative social work: a narrative review of mentoring programs in social work. *Am J Hosp Palliat Care*. January 2017:1049909117715216.

33. Schunk DH, Mullen CA. Toward a conceptual model of mentoring research: integration with self-regulated learning. *Educ Psychol Rev*. 2013;25(3):361-389.

34. Mosley Wetzel M, Taylor LA, Vlach SK. Dialogue in the support of learning to teach: a case study of a mentor/mentee pair in a teacher education programme. *Teach Educ*. 2017;28(4):406-420.

35. Neher JO, Gordon KC, Meyer B, Stevens N. A five-step "microskills" model of clinical teaching. *J Am Board Fam Pract*. 1992;5(4):419-424.

36. Overeem K, Driessen EW, Arah OA, Lombarts KMJMH, Wollersheim HC, Grol RPTM. Peer mentoring in doctor performance assessment: strategies, obstacles and benefits. *Med Educ*. 2010;44(2):140-147.

37. Zanchetta MS, Bailey A, Kolisnyk O, et al. Mentors' and mentees' intellectual-partnership through the lens of the Transformative Learning Theory. *Nurse Educ Pract*. 2017;25:111-120.

38. Hudson P. Mentoring as professional development: "growth for both" mentor and mentee. *Prof Dev Educ*. 2013;39(5):771-783.

39. Carmel RG, Paul MW. Mentoring and coaching in academia: reflections on a mentoring/coaching relationship. *Policy Futures Educ*. 2015;13(4):479-491.

40. Black LL, Jensen GM, Mostrom E, et al. The first year of practice: an investigation of the professional learning and development of promising novice physical therapists. *Phys Ther*. 2010;90(12):1758-1773.

41. Edwards I, Jones M, Carr J, Braunack-Mayer A, Jensen GM. Clinical reasoning strategies in physical therapy. *Phys Ther*. 2004;84(4):312-330.

42. Greenfield BH, Bridges PH, Hoy S, et al. Exploring experienced clinical instructors' experiences in physical therapist clinical education: a phenomenological study. *J Phys Ther Educ*. 2012;26(3):40.

43. Greenfield BH, Jensen GM, Delany CM, et al. Power and promise of narrative for advancing physical therapist education and practice. *Phys Ther*. 2015;95(6):924-933.

44. Jensen GM. Learning: what matters most. *Phys Ther*. 2011;91(11):1674-1689.

45. Jensen GM, Gwyer J, Shepard KF. Expert practice in physical therapy. *Phys Ther*. 2000;80(1):28-43.

46. Resnik L, Jensen GM. Using clinical outcomes to explore the theory of expert practice in physical therapy. *Phys Ther*. 2003;83(12):1090-1106.

47. Wainwright SF, Shepard KF, Harman LB, Stephens J. Novice and experienced physical therapist clinicians: a comparison of how reflection is used to inform the clinical decision-making process. *Phys Ther*. 2010;90(1):75-88.

48. Wainwright SF, Shepard KF, Harman LB, Stephens J. Factors that influence the clinical decision making of novice and experienced physical therapists. *Phys Ther*. 2011;91(1):87-101.

49. Wainwright SF, Gwyer J. (How) Can we understand the development of clinical reasoning? *J Phys Ther Educ*. 2017;31(1):4-6.

50. Lowe GM, Prout P, Murcia K. I see, I think I wonder: an evaluation of journaling as a critical reflective practice tool for aiding teachers in challenging or confronting contexts. *Aust J Teach Educ*. 2013;38(6):n6.

51. Wald HS. Professional identity (trans)formation in medical education: reflection, relationship, resilience. *Acad Med*. 2015;90(6):701-706.

52. Jankowski T, Holas P. Metacognitive model of mindfulness. *Conscious Cogn*. 2014;28:64-80.

53. Van der Gucht K, Dejonckheere E, Erbas Y, et al. An experience sampling study examining the potential impact of a mindfulness-based intervention on emotion differentiation. *Emotion*. March 2018. doi:10.1037/emo0000406.

54. Beach MC, Inui T, Relationship-Centered Care Research Network. Relationship-centered care. A constructive reframing. *J Gen Intern Med*. 2006;21(suppl 1):S3-S8.

55. Siengsukon K, Bezner J. *Sleepless in San Antonio: guiding patients to better sleep and wellbeing*. Presented at: American Physical Therapy Association Combined Sections Meeting 2017; February 16, 2017; San Antonio, TX.

56. Benzinger J, Hale JL, Szot L. *Mind over matter: promoting long-term adherence to physical activity post-stroke*. Presented at: APTA Combined Sections Meeting 2017; February 17, 2017; San Antonio, TX.

57. Platzer H, Blake D, Ashford D. Barriers to learning from reflection: a study of the use of groupwork with post-registration nurses. *J Adv Nurs*. 2000;31(5):1001-1008.

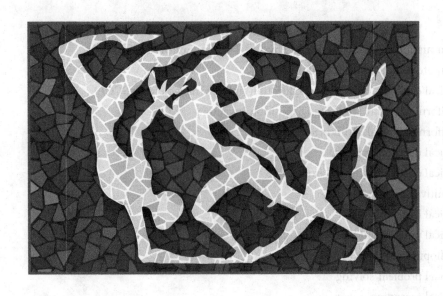

ACRONYMS

For your ease of reference, following are acronyms used throughout the text.

abd	abduction
ABPTRFE	American Board of Physical Therapy Residency and Fellowship Education
ABPTS	American Board of Physical Therapy Specialties
ACCE	academic coordinator of clinical education (interchangeable with DCE)
ACGME	Accreditation Council for Graduate Medical Education
ADDIE	analysis, design, development, implementation, and evaluation
APA	Australian Physiotherapy Association
APTA	American Physical Therapy Association
APTA PT CPI	American Physical Therapy Association Physical Therapist Clinical Performance Instrument
APTA PTA CPI	American Physical Therapy Association Physical Therapist Assistant Clinical Performance Instrument

Musolino GM, Jensen GM, eds. *Clinical Reasoning and Decision-Making in
Physical Therapy: Facilitation, Assessment, and Implementation* (pp 379-381).
© 2020 Taylor & Francis Group.

CAPTE	Commission on Accreditation in Physical Therapy Education
CBIM	computer-based instructional media
CCCE	clinical coordinator of clinical education (interchangeable with SCCE)
CCTDI	California Critical Thinking Disposition Inventory
CCTST	California Critical Thinking Skills Test
CDM	clinical decision-making
CE	clinical education, clinical experience
CFS	cognitive forcing strategies
CI	clinical instructor
CPGs	clinical practice guidelines
CPR	cardiopulmonary resuscitation
CPS	clinical problem-solving
CR	clinical reasoning
CRDM	clinical reasoning and decision-making
CRGR	Clinical Reasoning Grading Rubric
CRLS	clinical reasoning learning session
CR-MBIMA	clinical reasoning mobile-based instructional media application
CRT	Clinical Reasoning and Reflection Tool
CT	critical thinking
DCE	director of clinical education (interchangeable with ACCE)
DPT	doctor of physical therapy
EBP	evidence-based practice
ECHO	Extension for Community Healthcare Outcomes
EPAs	entrustable professional activities
EWS	early warning system
FiRST	Frontiers in Rehabilitation Science and Technology
FiT	fellow-in-training
FSBPT	Federation of State Boards of Physical Therapy
GRE	graduate record examination
HOAC	Hypothesis-Oriented Algorithm for Clinicians
HOD	House of Delegates
HQ-VTC	high-quality video teleconferencing
HSRT	Health Sciences Reasoning Test
HTML	hypertext markup language
ICF	*International Classification of Functioning, Disability and Health*

MAI	Metacognitive Awareness Inventory
MBIMA	mobile-based instructional media application
MDT	Mechanical Diagnosis and Therapy (McKenzie Method)
NPTE	National Physical Therapy Examination
OA	osteoarthritis
OSCE	Objective Structured Clinical Examination
PCC	patient-centered care
PCM	patient/client management
physiotherapist	physical therapist
physiotherapy	physical therapy
POC	plan of care
PT	physical therapist
PTA	physical therapist assistant
ROM	range of motion
RP	reflective practitioner or practice
SA	self-assessment
SCCE	site coordinator of clinical education (interchangeable with CCCE)
SCRIPT	Systematic Clinical Reasoning in Physical Therapy tool
SCT	script concordance test
SIG	special interest group
TASPE	Think Aloud Standardized Patient Examination
TeamSTEPPS	evidenced-based teamwork system addressing quality, safety, and efficiency in health care
TG	telehealth group
TL	transformative learning

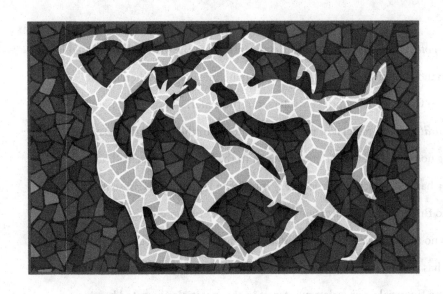

FINANCIAL DISCLOSURES

Dr. Heather Atkinson has no financial or proprietary interest in the materials presented herein.

Dr. Andrew S. Bartlett has no financial or proprietary interest in the materials presented herein.

Dr. Betsy J. Becker has no financial or proprietary interest in the materials presented herein.

Dr. Lisa Black has no financial or proprietary interest in the materials presented herein.

Anita S. Campbell has no financial or proprietary interest in the materials presented herein.

Dr. Nicole Christensen has no financial or proprietary interest in the materials presented herein.

Dr. N. Beth Collier has no financial or proprietary interest in the materials presented herein.

Dr. Chad E. Cook earns honoraria for teaching the content reflected in the book.

Dr. Kyle Covington has no financial or proprietary interest in the materials presented herein.

Dr. Clare Delany has no financial or proprietary interest in the materials presented herein.

Dr. Steven J. Durning has no financial or proprietary interest in the materials presented herein.

Dr. Ian Edwards has no financial or proprietary interest in the materials presented herein.

Dr. Edelle [Edee] Field-Fote has no financial or proprietary interest in the materials presented herein.

Dr. Wing Fu has no financial or proprietary interest in the materials presented herein.

Dr. Jennifer Furze has no financial or proprietary interest in the materials presented herein.

Dr. Margaret M. Gebhardt has no financial or proprietary interest in the materials presented herein.

Dr. Sarah Gilliland has no financial or proprietary interest in the materials presented herein.

Dr. Gregory W. Hartley has no financial or proprietary interest in the materials presented herein.

Dr. Karen Huhn has no financial or proprietary interest in the materials presented herein.

Dr. Gail M. Jensen has no financial or proprietary interest in the materials presented herein.

Dr. A. Daniel Johnson has no financial or proprietary interest in the materials presented herein.

Dr. Daryl Lawson has no financial or proprietary interest in the materials presented herein.

Dr. Alan Chong W. Lee serves as physical therapy telehealth advisor for Bluejay Mobile Health, Inc.

Dr. Gina Maria Musolino has no financial or proprietary interest in the materials presented herein.

Dr. Theresa Najjar has no financial or proprietary interest in the materials presented herein.

Peggy DeCelle Newman has no financial or proprietary interest in the materials presented herein.

Dr. Kim Nixon-Cave has no financial or proprietary interest in the materials presented herein.

Dr. Tricia R. Prokop has no financial or proprietary interest in the materials presented herein.

Dr. Ken Randall has no financial or proprietary interest in the materials presented herein.

Dr. Joseph Rencic has no financial or proprietary interest in the materials presented herein.

Dr. Eric K. Robertson has no financial or proprietary interest in the materials presented herein.

Dr. Trevor Russell has not disclosed any relevant financial relationships.

Dr. John Seiverd has no financial or proprietary interest in the materials presented herein.

Dr. Nancy Smith has no financial or proprietary interest in the materials presented herein.

Dr. Leslie F. Taylor has no financial or proprietary interest in the materials presented herein.

Dr. Alecia Thiele has no financial or proprietary interest in the materials presented herein.

Dr. Yannick Tousignant-Laflamme has no financial or proprietary interest in the materials presented herein.

Dr. Susan Flannery Wainwright has no financial or proprietary interest in the materials presented herein.

Dr. Stephanie A. Weyrauch has no financial or proprietary interest in the materials presented herein.

Brad W. Willis has no financial or proprietary interest in the materials presented herein.

Dr. Steven L. Wolf has no financial or proprietary interest in the materials presented herein.

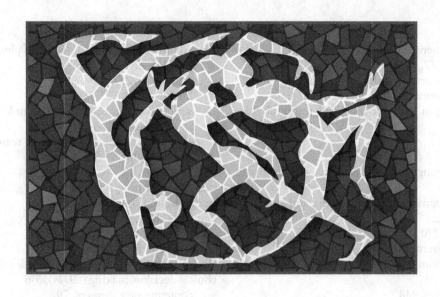

INDEX

Printed in the United States
by Baker & Taylor Publisher Services